Molecular Pathology Library

Series Editor
Philip T. Cagle, MD

For further volumes:
http://www.springer.com/series/7723

Antonia R. Sepulveda • John P. Lynch
Editors

Molecular Pathology of Neoplastic Gastrointestinal Diseases

Springer

Editors
Antonia R. Sepulveda, MD, PhD
Department of Pathology & Cell Biology
Columbia University
New York, NY, USA

John P. Lynch, MD, PhD
Division of Gastroenterology
University of Pennsylvania
Philadelphia, PA, USA

ISSN 1935-987X ISSN 1935-9888 (electronic)
ISBN 978-1-4614-6014-5 ISBN 978-1-4614-6015-2 (eBook)
DOI 10.1007/978-1-4614-6015-2
Springer New York Heidelberg Dordrecht London

Library of Congress Control Number: 2012954430

Printed on acid-free paper

Springer is part of Springer Science+Business Media (www.springer.com)

Preface

Critical molecular mechanisms underlying gastrointestinal (GI) neoplasia have been substantially unraveled in recent years. This has resulted from technological advances such as the genome project data and large-scale "omic" methods, combined with the application of classic molecular and chemical testing approaches and established procedures for pathologic evaluation of tissue and cellular samples. This progress is leading to the development of new approaches for treatments and, in parallel, novel diagnostic workups of gastrointestinal cancers, integrating specific molecular testing in routine pathology practice. Moreover, identification of disease susceptibly genes has enabled the medical community to better manage and prevent diseases that have hereditary traits.

While significant advances have been harnessed, much remains to be learned in the spectrum of neoplastic diseases of the gastrointestinal tract. Critical elements of research that have allowed progress in the various fields of GI neoplastic disease include the availability of animal models, cell culture models, and basic and translational research approaches utilizing prospective or archived specimen material, and such advances are reviewed here.

In this book, we review the molecular aspects that characterize the spectrum of neoplasms that affect the GI tract, providing the reader with up-to-date knowledge at the level of (1) the molecular basis of the individual neoplasms, spanning the carcinomas of esophagus, stomach, small bowel, colon, and rectum; neuroendocrine tumors; and gastrointestinal stromal tumors; (2) molecular testing approaches for diagnosis or for characterization of target genes for selective targeted therapies, with a review of recommended guidelines for clinical application whenever available; (3) molecular testing for hereditary predisposition or disease risk for GI cancers.

The last three chapters in the book are forward-looking, focused on the molecular mechanisms of metastasis, detection of circulating tumor cells and nucleic acids, and the use of tumor markers for gastrointestinal cancers. These are current areas of research interest and future clinical practice and serve to complement the information reviewed for the individual neoplasms.

It is clear that the rapid pace of discovery is unmatched by the definitive validation of many molecular alterations that are identified through ongoing basic and translational research of cancer. Given this scenario we felt it would be impractical to provide coverage of all areas of research in each tumor type, and ultimately, authors for each of the chapters identified what in their opinion are the most relevant topics to cover for each tumor type at the time of writing, realizing that novel findings that may be clinically relevant may become a reality as the book is published. Nevertheless, basic principles of molecular pathogenesis and diagnosis of GI cancers are extensively covered and will remain a foundation for clinical practice as new knowledge emerges.

We expect that this book will be useful to a large spectrum of professionals, from pathologists, laboratorians, clinical gastroenterologists and oncologists, and trainees at various levels such as medical students, residents, fellows, and postdoctoral fellows, as well as investigators interested in the area of gastrointestinal cancer.

New York, NY, USA — Antonia R. Sepulveda, MD, PhD
Philadelphia, PA, USA — John P. Lynch, MD, PhD

Contents

Contributors

Fatima Carneiro, M.D., Ph.D. Department of Pathology and Cancer Genetics Group, Institute of Molecular Pathology and Immunology of the University of Porto, Porto, Portugal

Bruce Giantonio, M.D. Department of Hematology/Oncology, University of Pennsylvania, Philadelphia, PA, USA

Ian S. Hagemann, M.D., Ph.D. Department of Pathology and Immunology, Washington University, St. Louis, MO, USA

Shuko Harada, M.D. Department of Pathology, University of Alabama at Birmingham, Birmingham, AL, USA

Jenia Jenab-Wolcott, M.D., Ph.D. Delaware County Memorial Hospital, Drexel Hill, PA, USA

Loren Joseph, M.D. Department of Pathology, The University of Chicago, Chicago, IL, USA

Jonathan P. Katz, M.D., Ph.D. Division of Gastroenterology, University of Pennsylvania, Philadelphia, PA, USA

John P. Lynch, M.D., Ph.D. Department of Medicine, Division of Gastroenterology, Hospital of the University of Pennsylvania, Philadelphia, PA, USA

Deqin Ma, M.D., Ph.D. Department of Pathology, University of Iowa Hospitals and Clinics, Iowa City, IA, USA

Hiroshi Nakagawa, M.D., Ph.D. Department of Medicine, Gastroenterology Division, University of Pennsylvania School of Medicine, Philadelphia, PA, USA

Carla Oliveira, Ph.D. Cancer Genetics Group, Institute of Molecular Pathology and Immunology of the University of Porto and Medical Faculty of the University of Porto, Porto, Portugal

Joseph R. Pisegna, M.D. Division of Gastroenterology and Hepatology, VA Greater Los Angeles Healthcare System, Los Angeles, CA, USA

Asif Rashid, M.D., Ph.D. Department of Pathology, The University of Texas M. D. Anderson Cancer Center, Houston, TX, USA

Andrew D. Rhim, M.D. Department of Medicine, Gastroenterology Division, University of Pennsylvania School of Medicine, Philadelphia, PA, USA

Frank I. Scott, M.D. Division of Gastroenterology, University of Pennsylvania, Philadelphia, PA, USA

Antonia R. Sepulveda, M.D., Ph.D. Department of Pathology & Cell Biology, Columbia University, New York, NY, USA

Jorge L. Sepulveda, M.D., Ph.D. Department of Pathology & Cell Biology, Columbia University, New York, NY, USA

Raquel Seruca, M.D., Ph.D. Cancer Genetics Group, Institute of Molecular Pathology and Immunology of the University of Porto and Medical Faculty of the University of Porto, Porto, Portugal

Davendra Sohal, M.D., M.P.H. Solid Tumor Oncology, Taussig Cancer Institute, Cleveland Clinic, Cleveland, OH, USA

Weijing Sun, M.D. Department of Medicine, Hematology-Oncology, University of Pittsburgh School of Medicine, UPMC Cancer Pavilion, Pittsburgh, PA, USA

Rohinton S. Tarapore, M.S., Ph.D. Department of Gastroenterology, University of Pennsylvania, Philadelphia, PA, USA

Takeshi Uehara, M.D. Department of Laboratory Medicine, Shinshu University School of Medicine, Matsumoto, Japan

Mamoun Younes, M.D. Department of Pathology, University of Texas Medical School at Houston, Houston, TX, USA

Paul J. Zhang, M.D. Department of Pathology and Lab Medicine, University of Pennsylvania Medical Center, Philadelphia, PA, USA

Part I

Introduction

Mechanisms of Gastrointestinal Carcinogenesis

1

Frank I. Scott and John P. Lynch

Introduction

The burden of neoplastic diseases of the gastrointestinal tract is ever growing. Gastrointestinal malignancies are a leading cause of morbidity worldwide. GLOBOCAN Data from 2008 estimate the overall annual incidence of GI malignancies to be 3.8 million cases per year, with a mortality of 3.2 million persons per year.[1,2] Given these extraordinary numbers of affected patients, a tremendous amount of resources have been expended in a quest to understand, prevent, and treat these diseases over the past 40 years. We now know that malignancies of the gastrointestinal tract are heterogeneous in composition, involving a complex interaction between environmental and host factors. This interaction can result in conversion of normal mucosa to precursor lesions, premalignant lesions, and eventual frank malignancy. Despite differences between malignancies in differing cell types and tissues, there are some common themes shared amongst them.

Cells that have undergone neoplastic transformation lose the ability to respond appropriately to signals regulating cell differentiation, replication, migration, and apoptosis. Neoplasms can develop in any organ of the GI tract and from any tissue in the body and can result in extrinsic compression or invasion, consumption of metabolic resources, and metastatic spread to distant sites in the body. Tumors can therefore significantly impact patient health, regardless of whether they are benign or malignant.

This chapter will aim to demonstrate the underlying molecular mechanisms and genetic basis for gastrointestinal malignancies, focusing on the key principles of oncogenesis and molecular steps involved in initiation, evolution, and progression of gastrointestinal malignancy.

Basic Concepts of Cancer Pathogenesis

Cancer Is a Disease of Gene Mutations

Foremost among the results of the modern molecular revolution is the recognition that many human disease conditions are, fundamentally, caused by mutations in genes. Gastrointestinal cancers are no different. Cancers arise because cells have inherited or acquired mutations in critical genes that regulate cell proliferation, differentiation, and apoptosis. These cells experience disorganized cell division and unregulated growth, which also predisposes the cell to further mutation events. This disordered, unregulated growth leads to the formation of clinically observable tumors. Genetic mutations involved in neoplastic transformation fall into two categories: (1) gain-of-function events, which typically involve oncogene or proto-oncogene activation, and (2) loss-of-function events, typically involving disruption of tumor suppressors.[3] A number of different molecular events can produce gain-of-function (proviral insertion, gene amplification, chromosomal translocations, point mutations, and small deletions) or loss-of-function changes (gene deletions, point mutations, chromosomal rearrangements, and epigenetic gene silencing). One important focus of current research efforts is to utilize novel sequencing and microarray technologies to minutely map and catalogue the many genetic and epigenetic changes that occur in human cancers.

Carcinogenesis Is a Multistep Process

The development of gastrointestinal malignancy usually occurs in a multistep fashion, with malignant neoplastic cells arising from dysplastic tissue (Fig. 1.1). In the colon,

F.I. Scott, M.D.
Division of Gastroenterology, University of Pennsylvania, Philadelphia, PA, USA
e-mail: frankis@mail.med.upenn.edu

J.P. Lynch, M.D., Ph.D. (✉)
Department of Medicine, Division of Gastroenterology, Hospital of the University of Pennsylvania, 4156 Curie Blvd/600 CRB, Philadelphia, PA, USA
e-mail: lynchj@mail.med.upenn.edu

A.R. Sepulveda and J.P. Lynch (eds.), *Molecular Pathology of Neoplastic Gastrointestinal Diseases*, Molecular Pathology Library 7, DOI 10.1007/978-1-4614-6015-2_1,

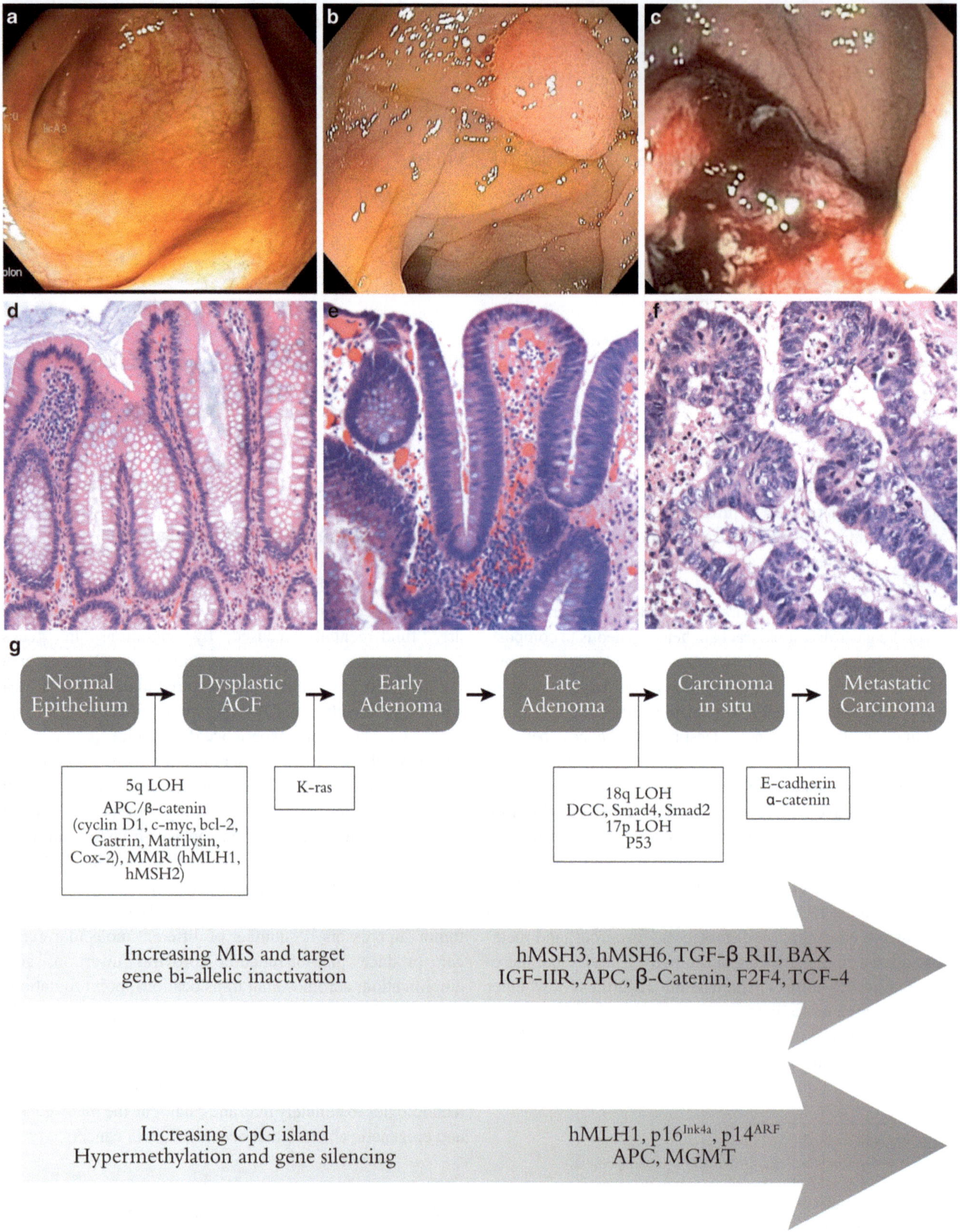

Fig. 1.1 Colon cancer develops in a multistep fashion, progressing from normal mucosa (**a**, **d**) (seen here endoscopically and histologically), with microscopic foci of dysplasia as mutations accumulate. Subsequently, adenomas form (**b**, **e**), with further accumulation of mutations. Neoplastic transformation can then occur with the development of adenocarcinoma (**c**, **f**). An example of the typical progression at the genetic level is also demonstrated (**g**) with examples of mutations that can occur at various points in the progression from normal mucosa to adenoma to carcinoma. *MSI* microsatellite instability. *Pathology images courtesy of Antonia R. Sepulveda, MD, PhD*

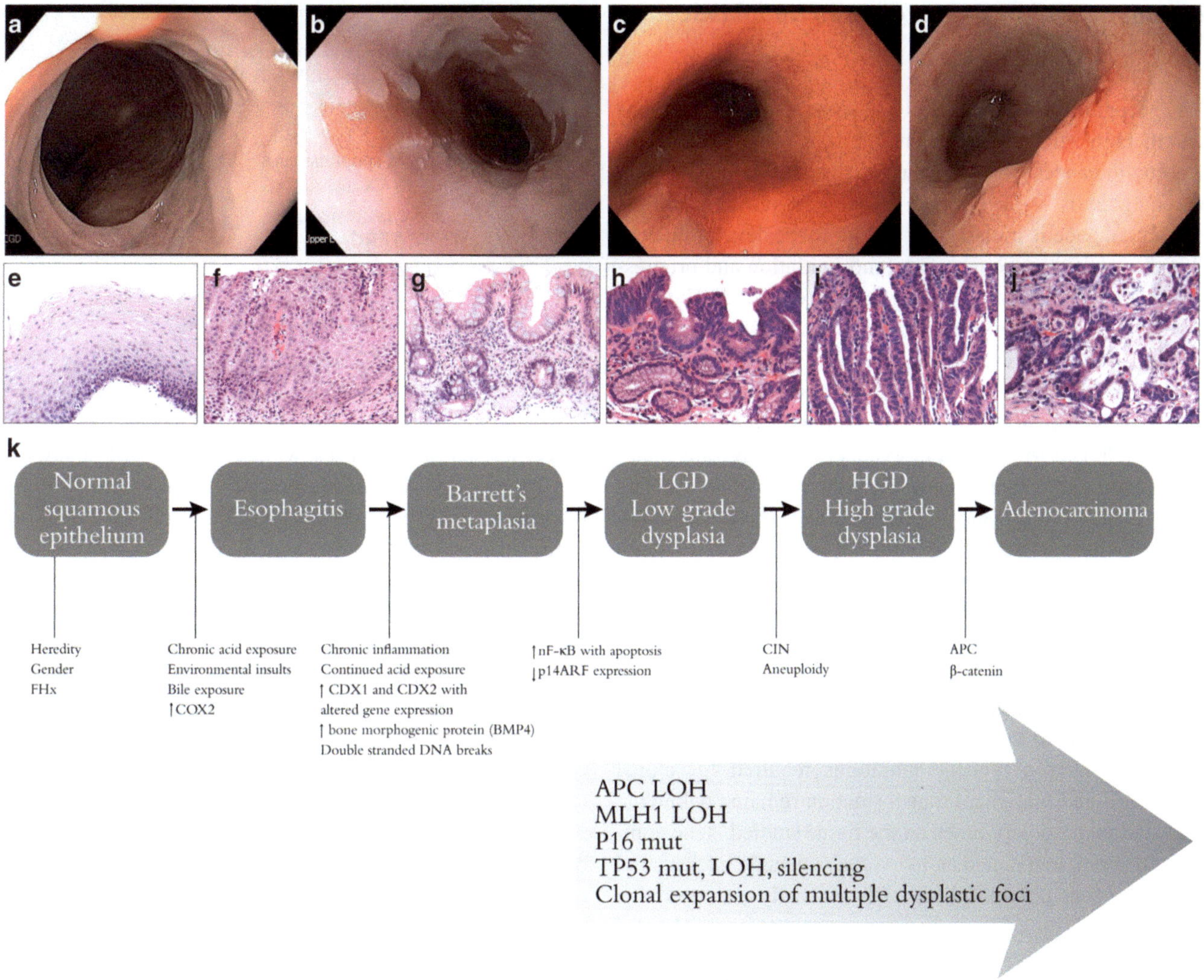

Fig. 1.2 The progression from normal squamous cell mucosa (**a**, **e**) to esophagitis (**f**) to Barrett's esophagus (**b**, **g**), followed by low-grade dysplasia (LGD) (**h**), high-grade dysplasia (HGD) (**c**, **i**), and finally to esophageal adenocarcinoma (**d**, **j**), as seen here endoscopically and histologically, is not as uniform at a genetic level as in colon cancer. Despite this, the process is similar (**k**), with genetic predispositions and environmental insults resulting in chronic inflammation. This inflammation results in Barrett's metaplasia, with subsequent altered gene expression and subsequent development of various mutations and eventual neoplastic transformation. *Endoscopic images courtesy of Dr. Gary W. Falk, M.D., M.Sc. Pathology images courtesy of Antonia R. Sepulveda MD, PhD*

this progression from normal mucosa to dysplastic foci to eventual invasive carcinoma is represented by the adenoma–carcinoma sequence, and has been demonstrated in pathologic, epidemiologic, and animal studies.[4–7] The earliest histologically definable lesions in this sequence are aberrant crypt foci (ACF). ACF are crypts that appear larger and thicker than normal, with increased luminal diameter and an opening that can be slit-like or serrated. They were first identified by methylene blue stain in azoxymethane-treated mice.[8–10] It is estimated that 65–95% of human ACF are hyperplastic, but a significant proportion are dysplastic and are considered to be similar to adenomatous polyps.[11–13] Genetic analysis of these lesions has demonstrated that they share many of the same mutations present in adenomas.[8,13–20]

Similar progressions from normal mucosa to dysplasia to malignancy have been described for esophageal cancer, gastric cancer, and pancreatic cancer. In esophageal adenocarcinoma, malignancy is preceded by a premalignant metaplasia known as Barrett's esophagus. Barrett's is an intestinal-type metaplasia that arises in the setting of chronic gastroesophageal reflux disease.[21] Barrett's metaplasia is not dysplastic, but can progress to dysplasia and adenocarcinoma in a significant number of patients (Fig. 1.2). Similar patterns of progression from established precursor lesions to dysplasia to neoplasia have been documented in the stomach (gastritis > atrophy > intestinal metaplasia > dysplasia > cancer) and in pancreatic cancer (PanIN1a > PanIN1b > PanIN2 > PanIN3) as well.[22,23]

Role of Evolutionary Processes in Neoplastic Transformation

The recognition that cancer is a disease of gene mutations and that biologically there is a recognizable, stepwise pattern leading to cancer led to the current standard model wherein carcinogenesis is a complex process requiring multiple sequential genetic mutations.[24–27] Prior to the development of this theory, it was thought that tumor initiation and progression were distinct biologic and genetic processes.[28] The multistep hypothesis has been supported by growing data that suggest that tumors are clonal, derived from a single progenitor that has acquired the necessary mutations to undergo neoplastic transformation.[24,29] Mutational events are currently believed to be random events, with only rare mutations leading to inappropriate activation of growth promoters or silencing of tumor suppressor pathways. These rare mutations thus impart upon these cells a unique survival advantage over normal adjacent cells.[3,30] These mutations are acquired gradually over a period of time. The survival and competitive advantages of certain mutations permit a clonal expansion. Subsequent acquired mutations may impart a further advantage and another round of clonal expansion, ultimately leading to the formation of a neoplasm.[24,29,31]

The number of genetic mutations required for clonal expansion and malignant transformation remains unknown, and is thought to vary based on the tissue studied, gene combinations employed, and an individual's genetic background including gene polymorphisms. It is currently estimated that for the majority of malignancies the average number of required mutations is between four and seven.[30] This raises an important problem, particularly for epithelial tissues that are constantly turning over. Few cells except stem cells are retained long enough to acquire 3–7 mutations in critical genes, when mutations are believed to be largely random events. This observation then has been used to support the theory that stem cells are involved in carcinogenesis.[32,33] An alternate, unproven hypothesis is that certain mutations can alter population dynamics, with certain non-stem cells acquiring mutations that promote survival or that alter patterns of migration or differentiation.[34,35] This remains an active area of research.

Successfully Transformed Cancer Cells Share a Finite Set of Qualities

While there can be great variety in the processes by which cells acquire cancer-causing mutations, and the genes involved can vary considerably between tissues, it has also been observed that cells that have been successfully transformed typically have obtained a subset of well-defined properties. These properties, while not necessarily unique to malignant cells, are all required for a successfully transformed cell. These six cardinal features were described in a seminal review by Hanahan and Weinberg in 2000.[30] They are (1) self-sufficiency in proliferative signals, (2) ability to ignore anti-proliferative signals, (3) inability to undergo apoptotic cell death or able to evade normal apoptotic cues, (4) telomere maintenance, permitting limitless replication potential, (5) self-directed angiogenesis, improving nutrition and oxygenation to the developing tumor, and, lastly, (6) the capacity to invade tissues locally and metastasize distally (Table 1.1).

Table 1.1 The hallmarks of carcinogenesis

Self-sufficiency in proliferative signals KRAS, cyclin D1, WNT, MYC
Ability to ignore anti-proliferative signals RB, TP53, PTEN, APC
Evasion of apoptotic cues TP53, BAX, bcl-2, FAS
Telomere maintenance TERT, TERC
Self-directed angiogenesis VEGF, PDGF, THBS1
Local invasion and metastatic spread E-cadherin

This is a very flexible model for carcinogenesis, and is better able to describe an individual person's cancer, as any number of gene mutations can yield the same required cancer cell property. Moreover, these properties or hallmark features can be obtained in different orders but still yield a cancer. Several recent studies also indicate that the ability to modulate the immune response should be added to this list as a seventh cancer hallmark feature.[36,37] In addition, this model argues that a beneficial strategy toward cancer therapeutics would be to attack these required features. We will discuss these cardinal features in greater detail later in this chapter.

Biological Factors Contributing to Gastrointestinal Carcinogenesis

Mutations in genes that are crucial for cell proliferation, differentiation, and apoptosis result in disorganized cell division and unregulated growth, which also predispose the cell to further mutation. These mutations can be inherited or sporadic. Exposure to various environmental factors, including chronic inflammatory conditions and carcinogens, can promote these mutations. We will briefly discuss the role of heredity, acquired sporadic mutations, and environmental factors in the pathogenesis of gastrointestinal cancers.

Table 1.2 Signaling pathways involved in familial cancer syndromes of the GI tract

Gene	Associated gastrointestinal malignancy
APC	Familial adenomatous polyposis (FAP)
DNA mismatch repair	Hereditary nonpolyposis colon cancer syndrome (HNPCC)
Base excision repair	MYH adenomatous polyposis (MAP)
ATM	Gastric adenocarcinoma
BRCA2	Pancreatic adenocarcinoma
FA (Fanconi's anemia)	Hepatocellular carcinoma
CDH1/E-cadherin	Gastric adenocarcinoma

Heredity

A familial predisposition for cancer has been recognized for some time. Familial cancer syndromes are recognized for esophageal, gastric, colonic, and pancreatic cancer. Despite the considerable differences between the tissues, familial cancer syndromes share several common features. First, these genetic tendencies are primarily due to inherited (germline) mutations. The mutations confer a significantly increased risk for a particular type of cancer. Moreover, those with a familial cancer syndrome typically develop the cancer at a much younger age than those afflicted with the sporadic type of malignancy. Some germline mutations confer a risk for multiple neoplasms, often in different tissues. In addition, while penetrance for any inherited predisposition can be variable, it is usually the case that in familial cancer syndromes greater than 50% of those carrying the gene mutation will develop a cancer. Lastly, familial cancer syndromes are typically due to inherited mutations in critical tumor suppressor genes.[38]

The inherited colon cancers Hereditary Nonpolyposis Colorectal Cancer (HNPCC), also known as Lynch syndrome, and Familial Adenomatous Polyposis (FAP) illustrate another important principle. HNPCC and FAP kindreds are responsible for approximately 5% of all colon cancers. Research into the causative etiologies of both of these syndromes has illuminated gene pathways involved in the majority of sporadic colon cancers.[4,39,40] This is true for other familial cancer syndromes as well; the study of these disorders has revealed significant insights into the pathogenesis of all malignancies, since many of the genes involved in hereditary cancers are also mutated in sporadic cancers.[41–43] Several common signaling and regulatory pathways are now known to be responsible for the majority of familial cancer syndromes (Table 1.2).

A number of important questions remain unresolved. What are the molecular events that precede the development of malignancy? It is known that biallelic inactivation of tumor suppressor genes is necessary for the genesis of tumors, but the processes causing this are unknown.[44] The reason for this is that the cells retain sufficient function from the remaining normal allele to prevent neoplastic transformation under most circumstances. Molecular studies of the second allele found that they are frequently inactivated by several processes including direct mutation, epigenetic silencing, or gene deletion. A second unanswered question is why neoplastic transformations only occur in a limited set of tissues even though the inherited mutations reside in every cell of the body. One possibility is that these tissues may be uniquely sensitive to or dependent on these genes. The reasons for this selective sensitivity remain unknown. In addition, the penetrance of these mutations can be highly variable in part due to the presence of genetic modifiers. Therefore, there remains much to be learned about the process of carcinogenesis, even when an underlying inherited mutation has been identified.

Sporadic Carcinogenesis

While familial cancer syndromes have been a primary research focus, the majority of all cancers are sporadic. Compared to familial cancers, sporadic malignancies tend to present later in life. This has led to the hypothesis that these tumors are the result of accumulated mutations in the course of a normal life, due to either carcinogen exposures or even errors that occur during DNA replication. It has been estimated that, over decades, these processes can result in the accumulation of several mutations that can collectively result in neoplastic transformation.[24,25] Importantly, although familial and sporadic cancers are mechanistically quite distinct, many of the mutations are common to both processes. Thus, though they may arrive by different means, the path to cancer shares many common elements that will prove useful diagnostically and therapeutically.

One critical difference between familial and sporadic forms of cancer is that the cancer risk is genetically defined for the former but not the latter. Moreover, the sporadic cancer risk can be modified by dietary habits, environmental exposures, and even exercise and fitness levels. Dietary factors, like high salt diets or the Western high-fat diet, have been associated with an increased incidence of gastric cancer and colorectal cancer, respectively.[45–47] Folate supplementation has been associated with a decreased risk of colorectal cancer in a small number of patients.[48,49] Anti-inflammatory medications such as aspirin and other NSAIDs have been associated with a decreased risk of esophageal, gastric, pancreatic, and colorectal cancer in both human[50–54] and animal studies of neoplasia.[55–61] Body habitus, in particular degree of obesity, can increase the risk of cancer of the esophagus, pancreas, and colon.[62,63] One note of caution here is that genetics may not be entirely removed from the risk for sporadic carcinogenesis, as subtle genetic polymorphisms may interact with these dietary and environmental stresses to increase the risk for cancer. Genome-wide association studies are under way to identify these more modest genetic contributions to cancer risk, but much more work needs to be done in this area. In summary, sporadic carcinogenesis is mechanistically distinct from familial forms and the risk for developing a sporadic cancer can be modified by behavior and dietary changes.

Carcinogen Exposure

DNA is typically stable, but can be altered via chemical or physical reactions. Some compounds, such as alkylating agents, can interact and modify DNA directly. These compounds are known as carcinogens. Most agents, however, are procarcinogens, and must first be metabolized to generate active, electrophilic derivatives. These activated compounds can then interact with DNA, modifying individual nucleotides. If not repaired or removed by the cell's DNA repair machinery, these modified nucleotides can then disrupt base pairings during DNA replication. If these chemical modifications are not recognized prior to DNA replication, the mispaired DNA will introduce mutations into the genetic code that will be passed on to subsequent daughter cells. Fortunately, evolution has endowed cells a plethora of mechanisms to protect DNA against potential mutagens[64,65] via repairing mutations that occur[66,67] or initiating apoptosis if necessary in order to prevent transmission of mutant DNA codes to daughter cells.

The gastrointestinal tract is continuously exposed to a number of mutagens via ingestion, and these tissues may therefore be particularly dependent upon these mechanisms for protection. Certain cooking practices can contribute to development of small amounts of carcinogens within food that are then ingested.[68] Food preservation and storage practices may be particularly to blame for inadvertent exposures. Nitrates are preservatives commonly found in processed meats, and historically were included in beer as well. These compounds can function as procarcinogens if converted to N-nitrosamines by gut bacteria. Chronic ingestion of these compounds has been associated with increased rates of gastric and esophageal cancer.[69–72] In contrast, corn, peanuts, and rice storage practices in the developing world frequently lead to contamination by Aspergillus molds. These molds can produce aflatoxin, a procarcinogen that is metabolized by the cytochrome P450 system in the liver. After metabolic conversion, this chemical can form adducts with guanine nucleotides, leading to mutagenesis. Individuals with chronic active HBV infection are especially sensitive to aflatoxin ingestion, as studies have demonstrated that significant amounts of aflatoxin ingestion work in synergy with the virus to increase rates of hepatocellular carcinoma.[73–75] Tobacco smoke is another common environmental exposure that has been linked to gastrointestinal malignancies including head and neck and esophageal squamous cell cancers.[76] Mechanistically, this is due to the 40 different mutagens and carcinogens in tobacco smoke that cause DNA damage. Among these carcinogens are N-nitrosamines, which are thought to directly stimulate colon cancer cell growth, benzo[a]pyrene, which has been associated with esophageal cancer, and polycyclic aromatic hydrocarbons, which are thought to promote *KRAS* mutations in pancreatic cancer.[77] In summary, we are exposed to a number of environmental carcinogens that can play a significant role in introducing DNA mutations and thereby promoting the development of gastrointestinal neoplasia.

Inflammatory Microenvironment

After several decades of observation and study, it was established that chronic inflammatory conditions are associated with cancer in a number of tissues and organ systems. The gastrointestinal organs may be particularly vulnerable for reasons that are not clear at the present time. Every major organ of the GI tract is subject to one or more disease processes that can result in a chronic inflammatory condition. While the etiologies for these processes can vary considerably (chemical, viral, bacterial, genetic) all are known to increase the risk for cancer. These findings have prompted ongoing mechanistic studies into how inflammatory conditions promote carcinogenesis, and have suggested interventions that have begun to reduce the frequency of some GI cancers.

A compelling demonstration of the association between chronic inflammatory conditions and cancer is observed in patients with hereditary pancreatitis. Hereditary pancreatitis is an autosomal dominant condition caused in most kindreds by inherited mutations in the gene encoding cationic trypsinogen (*PRSS1*).[78,79] These mutations augment trypsinogen autoactivation or enhance trypsin stability, leading to episodes of acute pancreatitis.[79] Soon after the recognition of this inherited disorder, it was noted that several family kindreds also experienced high rates of pancreatic cancer.[80] Pancreatic cancers arise only after 20 or more years of recurrent pancreatitis,[81] suggesting that it is the chronic inflammation that causes the cancer, not the *PRSS1* mutation. This pattern thus supports the hypothesis that chronic inflammation can promote carcinogenesis in the pancreas.

Ulcerative colitis (UC) is a chronic, relapsing inflammatory condition of the colon with a strong association with carcinogenesis.[82,83] Initial reports suggested a cumulative cancer risk as high as 60% in UC patients.[84] More recently, this risk has been better defined, and in particular the elements of disease extent, duration, and severity are now recognized to impact the risk for the colon cancer in UC patients.[83] Disease duration is the best-established risk factor, as the annual and cumulative incidences for colon cancer in UC increase from 0.2% and 1.6%, respectively, after 10 years of disease to 1.2% and 18.4%, respectively, after 30 years of UC.[85] Disease extent is also a clinically relevant factor. Pancolitis imparts a 20-fold greater risk for colon cancer than disease limited to the rectum.[85,86] Together, these correlations support the conclusion that the chronic inflammatory process can promote carcinogenesis.

Lastly, epidemiological studies examining aspirin and nonsteroidal anti-inflammatory use and cancer incidence have generally confirmed that frequent users of aspirin or other NSAIDS have reduced rates of esophageal, gastric, and colon cancers.[50,53,54,87] Meta-analyses have further concluded that regular aspirin or NSAID use may be chemoprotective for gastric and esophageal cancers[50] or in patients with familial adenomatous polyposis (FAP), an inherited predisposition to colon cancer.[88,89] In summary, there is substantial epidemiologic, biologic, and pharmacologic evidence implicating the inflammatory environment as a causative factor for many human gastrointestinal cancers.

Molecular Mechanisms Promoting Neoplastic Transformation

As was discussed previously, there are a great variety of mutations cancer cells can accumulate. This has challenged our ability to understand the process mechanistically and develop effective therapeutic modalities. However, Hanahan and Weinberg in 2000 suggested an alternative model, recognizing six hallmark features that all cancers need to acquire to become a "successful" cancer.[30] These are (1) self-sufficiency in proliferative signals, (2) ability to ignore anti-proliferative signals, (3) inability to undergo apoptotic cell death or able to evade normal apoptotic cues, (4) telomere maintenance, permitting limitless replication potential, (5) self-directed angiogenesis, improving nutrition and oxygenation to the developing tumor, and, lastly, (6) the capacity to invade tissues locally and metastasis distally. We will explore several of these topics in greater depth next.

Self-Sufficiency in Growth Signals

The concept that genetic mutations could result in gained functionality and unrestrained cell proliferation was first appreciated via the study of DNA viruses and retroviruses that were known to be associated with tumors in humans and animals. In these initial studies, viral genes were identified that could induce neoplastic transformation. These genes were called oncogenes.[90] Subsequent research demonstrated similar sequences in the human genome. These human genes are now known as 'proto-oncogenes', and further research has demonstrated that proto-oncogenes and their regulators are frequently mutated in human malignancies, resulting in their constitutive activation.[91] Since the initial discovery of the human oncogene *HRAS*,[92] more than 80 human proto-oncogenes have been identified, and new candidates are constantly being evaluated.

Proto-oncogenes fall into four broad categories: peptide growth factors, receptor and non-receptor tyrosine kinases, signal transduction proteins associated with cell membranes, and nuclear transcription factors.[93] All have been found to play significant roles in cell cycle regulation, proliferation, and differentiation. Several proto-oncogenes can be activated simultaneously in gastrointestinal cancers, and continued functionality is mandatory for tumor growth. Disruption of these stimulatory signals not only results in inhibition of tumor growth but can also trigger induction of apoptosis and cell death.[94] This has led to the suggestion that cancers are "oncogene dependent", and therapeutic strategies to take advantage of this dependency are being explored.

Several types of mutations involving proto-oncogenes can lead to the development of neoplasia.[3,93] Gene rearrangements, point mutations, and insertion/deletion events can permanently alter the conformation of the gene product, resulting in chronically active proteins. These same mechanisms can interfere with or inactivate proto-oncogene regulatory domains. Mutations can also increase oncogene mRNA production. All of these mutations, therefore, result in either loss of proto-oncogene regulator function or inappropriate proto-oncogene expression. The result is uncontrolled cell division, proliferation, and delayed differentiation.

While several proto-oncogenes are typically activated simultaneously in transformed cells, the combination of genes is highly variable between tissues and even within the same cancer. Critical growth-signaling pathways often will contain several proto-oncogenes in epistatic succession. Phenotypically, these mutations would all produce the same effect. One example is the epithelial growth factor signaling cascade. EGF, the receptor *EGFR*, *KRAS*, *JUN* (*c-jun*), and *MYC* (*c-myc*) are all linked in this signaling pathway. *KRAS* mutations are present in up to 90% of pancreatic cancers and 50% of colorectal cancers, but are much less common in cancers of the esophagus. Therefore, while 90% of esophageal squamous cell carcinomas do not have KRAS mutations, these tumors still exhibit increased EGFR activity due to EGFR gene amplification. In summary, one essential feature of neoplastic cells is gain-of-function mutations of proto-oncogenes, with subsequent self-sufficiency in proliferation.

Immunity to Growth-Inhibitory Signals

While proto-oncogenes function to promote cell division, tumor suppressor genes normally function to tightly control this process. The discovery of genes responsible for tightly regulating proliferation emerged from studying the pediatric disease retinoblastoma. Retinoblastoma is a rare pediatric malignancy of the retina, with both familial and sporadic forms. The sporadic form was noted to be considerably rarer than its familial counterpart. In 1971, Alfred Knudson theorized that there was a genetic link between these two forms of this rare disease based on an epidemiologic review of 48 cases.[95,96] He postulated that this disease was caused by two mutations in the same gene. This hypothesis would come to be known as "the two-hit hypothesis." In the familial form of retinoblastoma, one of these mutations was inherited in the germline, and the second mutation was acquired. In the sporadic form, both copies had to undergo mutation via somatic processes and hence the much lower incidence of this form of the disease. In 1973, David Comings elaborated on Knudson's hypothesis, theorizing that the product involved may play a role in tumor suppression and that the mutation involved led to inactivation of this gene.[97] It would be another 13 years before this theory was definitively confirmed, when the retinoblastoma gene *RB* was cloned in 1986.[98] Since this discovery, over 20 tumor suppressor genes have been identified.

Mutations involving tumor suppressor genes are strictly loss-of-function events. As with retinoblastoma, all tumor suppressors require biallelic inactivation for neoplastic progression. In familial disorders involving tumor suppressor mutations, the first allele has been rendered nonfunctional in the germline. The second allele is typically inactivated via either epigenetic gene silencing or allelic loss, known as loss of heterozygosity (LOH). Promoter hypermethylation has been shown to play an important role in silencing multiple tumor suppressor genes. This, along with other types of epigenetic modification, will be discussed later in this chapter. LOH is a result of nonreciprocal translocation or missegregation during cell division, resulting in loss of the second functional allele in a daughter cell. Several tumor suppressor genes have been discovered by identifying regions of chromosomes susceptible to LOH and looking within them for candidate tumor suppressor genes.[99–106]

Tumor suppressor genes can serve as intracellular signaling proteins, transcription factors, adhesion proteins, cell surface receptors, or apoptotic signaling proteins. RB is a crucial regulator of the cell cycle, and is responsible for regulation of the transition from the G1 to the S phase. RB inhibits the exit from G1 by binding several transcription factors in the E2F family, silencing the expression of genes normally regulated by these factors.[107,108] These E2F target genes are necessary for nucleotide synthesis and DNA replication, which occur during the normal S phase.[109–112] RB is tightly regulated via phosphorylation by cyclin-dependent kinases (CDKs), lowering its binding affinity for these transcription factors.[109,112] RB inactivation allows for unbridled progression through the cell cycle and unrestricted cell division.[113,114] Modulation of RB function is therefore an important step in many neoplastic processes.

RB itself is not mutated in gastrointestinal malignancies. Many GI cancers exhibit alternative methods of altering RB's normal function, however.[115–117] Human malignancies have demonstrated several mechanisms of RB inhibition, including cyclin-dependent kinase (CDK) upregulation or stabilization, as well as inhibition of CDK inhibitors (CDKIs), p21, p27, and p16, via mutation or silencing.[38,114] Attempting to reconstitute the function of these CDKIs in tumors is an active area of research, as they represent possible novel therapeutic targets.

Another tumor suppressor frequently affected in malignancy is p53. Dysfunction of this gene product is thought to be present in as many as 50% of human malignancies.[118] P53 was initially felt to promote immortalization, as it was found to induce neoplastic transformation in primary rat embryonic fibroblasts.[119,120] This was disputed when it was discovered that *TP53* mutation was responsible for Li–Fraumeni Syndrome,[121] as well as multiple other malignancies, including colorectal cancer.[122] It was also discovered that some *TP53* mutations had a dominant-negative phenotype; this p53 was capable of binding and inhibiting its wild-type counterpart.[123,124]

After significant further research, it was discovered that p53 is a transcription factor that is activated by direct DNA damage, aberrant growth signals, and metabolic stressors.[125] When DNA is damaged, the DNA Damage Response (DDR) system is activated. This system, in turn, activates the protein kinases ataxia telangiectasia mutated (ATM) and Chk2, which phosphorylate and stabilize p53. P53 accumulates in the nucleus, and participates in transcription regulation via DNA binding. Several other factors can stimulate p53 function. Aberrant growth signals can induce p53 function. These signals stimulate the expression of the tumor suppressor p14 ARF, a protein that can bind the p53 inhibitor Mdm2, blocking its interaction with p53.[126,127] Oxidative and metabolic stressors can also induce p53 via kinases involved in Mdm2 regulation.[128] Several of these kinases also function as post-transcriptional modifiers, adding or removing moieties from the p53 molecule to alter its confirmation and improve its stability.

P53 has many downstream effects, including cell cycle regulation, induction of apoptosis, and inhibition of neovascularization.[25,122,129] P53 can inhibit progression through the cell cycle via induction of the CDKI p21$^{WAFI/CIPI}$.[130] p21$^{WAFI/CIPI}$ is a potent inhibitor of CDK, which is involved in the Rb pathway. P53 also plays a role in the induction of apoptosis via increased expression of cell surface markers such as Fas, PIDD, and Killer/DR5. P53 also results in the expression of proteins such as BAX, NOXA, and p53AIP1, which disrupt

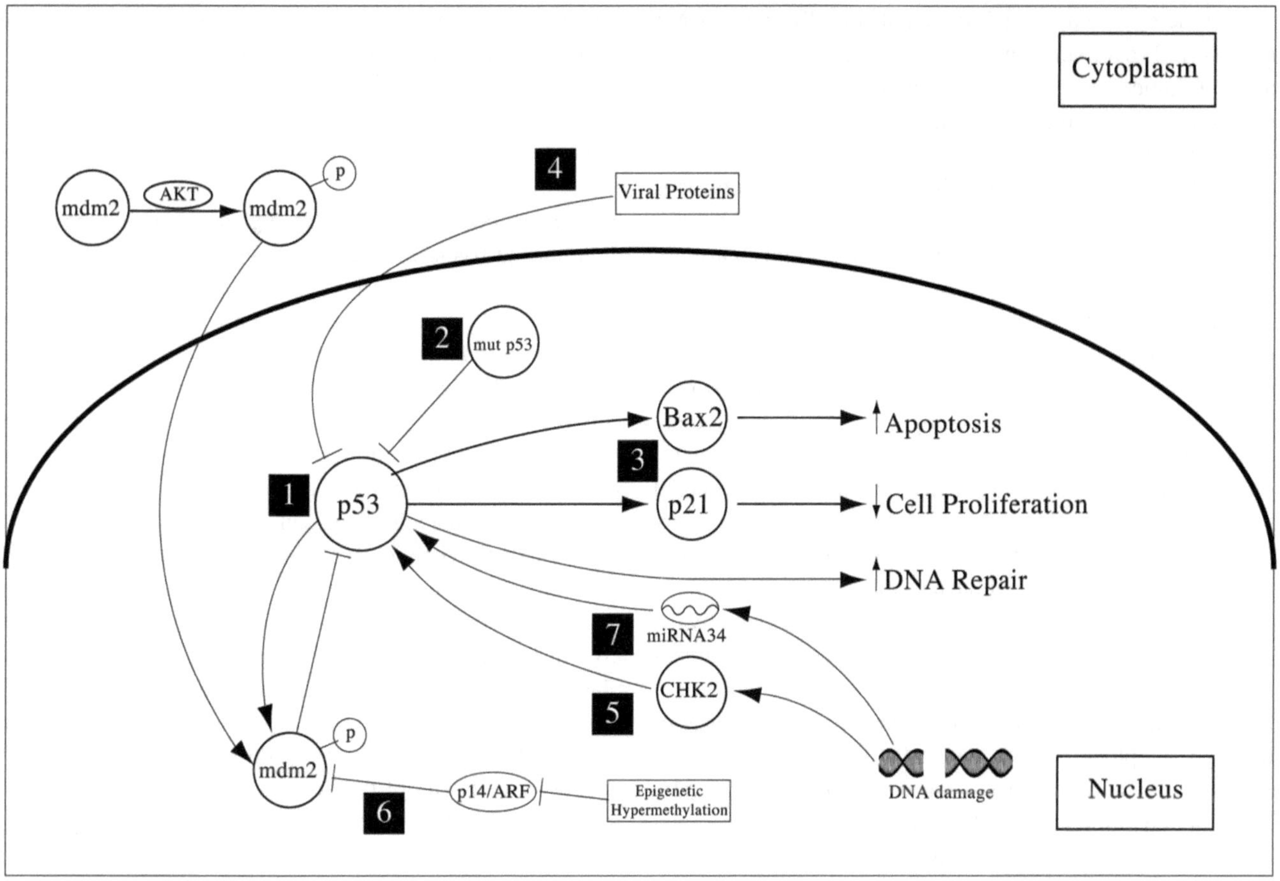

Fig. 1.3 Mechanisms of p53 regulation in malignancy. There are a multitude of ways that neoplastic cells can inhibit p53 function. Direct mutations can occur in p53 itself (1). When one copy of p53 develops a mutation, this mutant p53 can bind to and inhibit wild-type p53 (2). Downstream targets of pr53 such as Bax2 and p21 can be affected by mutation as well (3). Several viruses have proteins that can inhibit p53 function directly (4). Regulators of p53 such as CHK2 and MDM2 can undergo mutation, disrupting their upregulatory or inhibitory effects on p53 (5 and 6). Lastly, miRNA regulators of p53 mRNA have been discovered as well, such as miRNA34 (7)

mitochondrial function, hastening cell death.[25, 122, 129] Lastly, p53 can induce the synthesis of thrombospondin 1 and maspin, key proteins involved in the inhibition of neovascularization.[131,132] Given its broad range of effects critical to tumor suppression, a number of compounds are actively being tested in an attempt to restore wild-type functionality to mutant p53's.[133]

P53 function is normally regulated by the protein Mdm2. This protein binds to p53, and can also ubiquitinate it, demarcating it for proteosomal degradation. Mdm2 is upregulated by p53, resulting in negative feedback inhibition.[122,129] ATM and Chk2 can also phosphorylate Mdm2, inhibiting its effect on p53.[134,135] P53 is also under posttranscriptional regulation via the antisense RNA Wrap53. Wrap53 binds to p53 mRNA, stabilizing it in the setting of DNA damage. Wrap53 knockdown models demonstrate significantly reduced levels of p53 target synthesis, suggesting that Wrap53 plays a key role in augmenting p53 levels.[136]

TP53 function can be altered via a number of different mechanisms in malignancy (Fig. 1.3). Direct nonsense mutations can result in no viable gene product. Missense mutations can result in a nonfunctional protein that can bind functional p53, inactivating it. Mutations in the regulatory pathway of mdm2 have also been observed. Finally, mutations in the downstream effectors of p53 result in decreased function as well. In summary, p53 function is crucial to a cell's ability to progress appropriately through the cell cycle or induce apoptosis if necessary. Given its broad range of functionality, it is not surprising that p53 or one of its mediators is inactivated in most gastrointestinal malignancies.

Limitless Replication Potential

Normal human cells can only undergo a set number of cell divisions before permanently withdrawing from the cell cycle. This limit is known as the 'Hayflick Limit' and it represents a powerful inhibitor of neoplastic transformation.[137,138] This function is lost in malignant cells, which can divide without limit and are said to be "immortalized." The regulation of replication potential is mediated via structures at the end of each chromosome known as telomeres.

Telomeres are comprised of a number of TTAGGG DNA repeats, a 3′ overhang, and several associated binding proteins. Telomeres serve multiple purposes, one of which is maintenance of chromosomal integrity and facilitation of DNA replication.[139,140] The structure of telomeres prevents the DDR system from recognizing the end of chromosomes as double strand breaks, and also provides a 5′ template for priming DNA polymerase, allowing for accurate chromosomal replication.

Telomere length is dynamic and functions as a tumor suppressor. Telomeres are maintained at the ends of each chromosome via two enzymes: telomerase reverse transcriptase (TERT) and telomerase RNA component (TERC). Telomere synthesis correlates with TERT activity. In adult humans, only activated lymphocytes and hematopoietic and epithelial stem cells demonstrate significant levels of TERT activity.[141–143] Without the function of these enzymes, telomeres are continually degraded with each cell division. Eventually, double-stranded DNA is exposed which is recognized by the cell as a double strand break. The DDR system recognizes this and activates p53. As this double strand break is not reparable, normal cells will then either enter senescence or undergo apoptosis.[144] The particular senescence pathway varies significantly amongst tissues, and may involve p16, AKT, or activation of NK cells.[145]

Alternatively, cells can continue to undergo continued slow proliferation after the telomeres have been eroded. This results in the development of massive genome instability and cell death, a process known as "telomere crisis." Studies of dysplastic tissues such as colonic adenomas have demonstrated loss of telomeres, minimal TERT function, and significant genome instability.[146] Rarely, cells can emerge from this slow proliferative phase without further restrictions in proliferative capability. This results in immortalization, and has been demonstrated in murine, yeast, and human cell lines.[147–153] Human cancer cells are universally immortalized and demonstrate the ability to maintain some degree of telomere integrity.[154–158] The majority of these immortalized cells have regained some degree of TERT function. While TERT reactivation is the predominant mechanism seen in cancer, approximately 10–15% of malignancies are thought to employ an alternative means of telomere biosynthesis known as alternative lengthening of telomeres (ALT).[159–161] This mechanism involves homologous recombination-based exchange of telomeres over several cell division cycles to reconstitute the telomere. Cells undergoing ALT are characterized by highly heterogeneous chromosome length, the presence of extrachromosomal telomeric DNA, and PML nuclear bodies. The exact mechanisms of recombination are incompletely understood. Activation of the ALT pathway may be associated with a poor prognosis.[162] In summary, telomerase length functions as a critical safeguard against immortalization and neoplastic transformation. Malignancies can circumvent this mechanism via reactivation of TERC or via the ALT pathway, allowing for unlimited replication.

Sustained Angiogenesis

Neoplastic cells exhibit much higher metabolic demands than normal tissues. Increased oxygen and nutrient requirements often outpace what is already available at the site of tumorigenesis. It has been shown that without increasing the supply of blood flow to new tumors, growth is markedly constrained.[163] The process of new vascular formation, or angiogenesis, is tightly controlled in normal human adult tissue, and is both focal and limited in duration. Pathologic angiogenesis, on the other hand, is markedly disorganized, can result in active bleeding, and can occur indefinitely.

A number of chemical messengers have been implicated in the regulation of neovascularization. Several pro-angiogenic factors have been discovered, including vascular endothelial growth factor (VEGF), fibroblast growth factor (FGF), and platelet-derived growth factor (PDGF). Similarly, there are a number of anti-angiogenic factors as well, including thrombospondin 1, angiostatin, and endostatin. Discovering how neoplastic cells co-opt the normal angiogenic machinery to increase their blood supply has been an area of ongoing research, with potential therapeutic implications.

There are several mechanisms by which tumors can modulate angiogenesis to their benefit. Thrombospondin 1 (THBS1) is a potent inhibitor of neovascularization, and is produced by fibroblasts found in stromal tissue.[164] THBS1 appears to be downregulated in a number of human malignancies. Some tumors have even demonstrated the ability to secrete small molecules that inhibit THBS1 function, allowing further growth.[165] There also appears to be an interaction between THBS1 and a number of known oncogenes such as RAS. Murine models have demonstrated that activation of THBS1 is necessary for tumor regression, even when primary oncogenes have been inactivated.[166]

Vascular endothelial growth factor (VEGF) is another potent mediator of angiogenesis, inducing neovascularization by binding to the tyrosine kinase receptor (VEGFR) and activating a number of signaling pathways. VEGF is found to be overexpressed in a number of human tumors.[167] Given this commonality amongst several cancers, VEGF has become a target for pharmacotherapy. Bevacizumab is a humanized monoclonal IgG1 mAb against VEGF that has been shown to inhibit formation of new blood vessels and cause regression of microvasculature.[168] This compound has been shown, in combination with other chemotherapeutic regimens such as 5-FU/Leucovorin or FOLFOX, to improve median survival and mortality.[169–171] Vatalanib is a small molecule aimed at the VEGFR tyrosine kinase that is being evaluated, but appears to be less effective compared to bevacizumab when combined with FOLFOX.[172] Sunitinib is an inhibitor of multiple tyrosine kinases, including PDGFR, VEGFR, KIT (c-Kit), and RET, and is also undergoing evaluation as a potential chemotherapeutic.[173] In summary, angiogenesis is a pivotal and necessary requirement for tumor growth, and various neoplastic processes have found a number of ways to enhance neovascularization. This area represents an exciting opportunity for pharmacologic intervention, with several compounds being developed and studied.

The Inflammatory Microenvironment

It has been argued by some that inflammation, or immune modulation, constitutes a seventh cancer hallmark.[36] It is understandable why this has been proposed; however, the necessity of this as a true hallmark remains controversial. The underlying neoplastic effects of inflammation are still being delineated. These mechanisms likely involve several distinct contributions including (1) promotion of a mutagenic environment, (2) enhancement of classic cancer hallmarks, and (3) alterations of immune cancer surveillance. A chronic inflammatory microenvironment is very mutagenic due to activated inflammatory cells that generate reactive oxygen and nitrogen species (ROS and RNS). These nucleophiles are highly reactive and can chemically react with and damage DNA, RNA, lipids, and proteins. DNA damage not repaired can lead to mutagenesis and neoplastic transformation.[174, 175] This is made more likely due to the fact that other inflammatory mediators like cytokines and eicosanoids make tumor suppressor and DNA repair mechanisms less effective by promoting cell proliferation and inhibiting apoptosis.

Eicosanoids are oxygenated lipid derivatives produced in arachidonic acid metabolism.[176–178] Eicosanoids are released by many cell types with activation of the inflammatory response. Examples of eicosanoids include prostaglandins, thromboxanes, and leukotrienes. Eicosanoid biosynthesis itself produces ROS and contributes to DNA mutagenesis. In addition, these factors provoke many cancer hallmarks in cells including promoting proliferation, inhibiting apoptosis,[179–182] and inducing angiogenesis.[183] Eicosanoids also induce chemokine and cytokine synthesis and secretion, further increasing the degree of inflammation present.[184–186] Lastly, there is evidence suggesting that eicosanoids can also suppress immune cancer surveillance mechanisms, making neoplastic transformation more likely.[187–190] Because of these prolific pro-neoplastic effects, many tumors exhibit increased eicosanoid synthesis.

Cytokines and chemokines also likely play a pivotal role in promoting carcinogenesis. As with the eicosanoids, these factors can promote the acquisition of several cancer hallmarks (Fig. 1.4).[191–195] These small molecules work in autocrine and paracrine manners to (1) induce cell proliferation, (2) inhibit apoptosis, (3) promote cell migration and cancer cell metastasis, and (4) induce angiogenesis. Neoplastic cells also secrete chemokines and cytokines capable of inhibiting immune surveillance for malignancy. Moreover, lymphocyte infiltration promoted by these factors aids in the degradation of stromal elements and likely enhances cancer cell migration and metastatic spread.[191,194–196]

In conclusion, the recognition of hallmark features of cancers has dramatically altered how we view cancer pathogenesis. No longer is it a complicated set of various gene mutations. Rationally, we can now appreciate the key events. They are those mutations that endow the cancer cells with qualities that allow them to successfully form a tumor. This new perspective guides our therapeutic approach as well. Novel therapies are being successfully applied directed more at these hallmark features rather than specific gene mutations.

Genetic Instability and Gastrointestinal Carcinogenesis

Point mutations, altered methylation, and gene rearrangements are all common events observed in human malignancy. All of these mechanisms have been observed in cells that have undergone neoplastic transformation.[29,197,198] In colorectal cancer, genetic instability has been observed in aberrant crypt foci and several familial colon cancer syndromes.[14,20,25,44,199] Despite these observations, in vitro studies and several computational models have demonstrated neoplastic transformation without the aid of genetic instability.[43,200–202] As mentioned above, it is evident that genetic instability is playing a contributory role in the promotion of neoplastic progression, even if it is not mandatory in the initial stages of transformation.

There are several forms of genetic instability. They include chromosomal instability (CIN), microsatellite instability (MSI), epigenetic modification, and inactivation of normal DNA repair mechanisms such as DNA mismatch repair (MMR), nucleotide excision repair (NER), and base excision repair (BER). Four of these mechanisms play a common role in the pathogenesis of gastrointestinal malignancy: MSI, CIN, epigenetic modification, and BER inactivation.[146,203–205]

Microsatellite Instability

The contribution of microsatellite instability (MSI or MIN) to malignancy is the best understood of the genetic mechanisms involved in gastrointestinal malignancy.[44,72,206,207] Although DNA replication occurs with great fidelity, on rare occasions base mismatches and short insertion–deletion mispairings can occur. Short segments of DNA with repeated

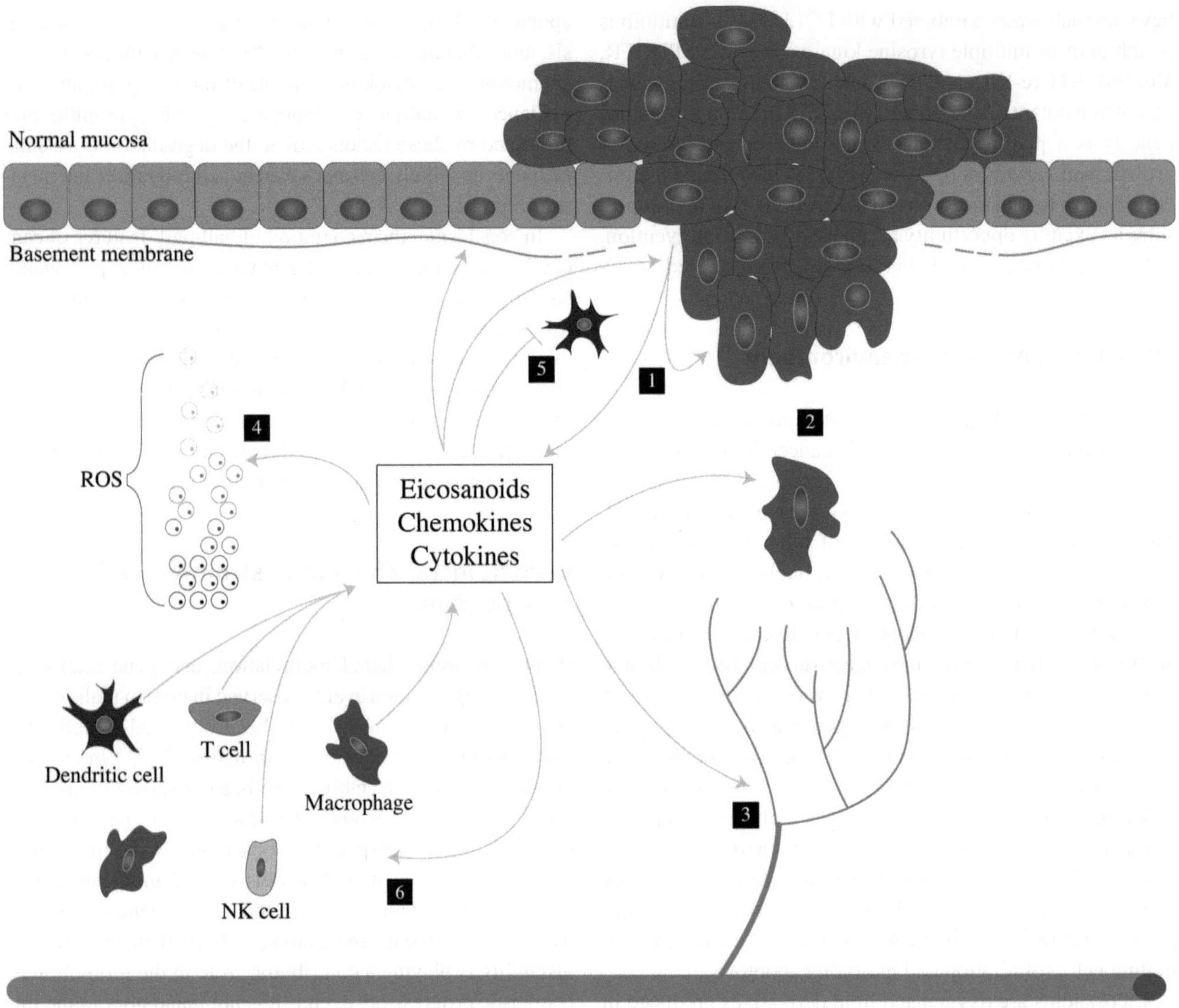

Fig. 1.4 The inflammatory microenvironment. The inflammatory microenvironment can have several pro-neoplastic effects, many mediated by the release of chemical messengers such as eicosanoids, chemokines, and cytokines. These molecules can induce proliferation and inhibit apoptosis in the tumor itself (1), induce tumor cell invasion and metastatic spread (2), promote neovascularization via angiogenesis (3), increase production of ROS, resulting in DNA damage and mutagenesis (4), inhibit tumor surveillance by immune cells (5), and finally promote further inflammation via cytokine and eicosanoid release, as well as increased tissue infiltration by inflammatory cells (6)

bases known as microsatellites are particularly prone to this type of error.[44,197,203,206] Most microsatellites are located in noncoding regions of DNA.[208–211] When a mismatch occurs, it results in the formation of an insertion–deletion loop (IDL) which can be recognized by the Mismatch Repair (MMR) multimer.[212] The MMR multimer is a complex consisting of MutS (MSH2, MSH3, MSH5) and MutL (MLH1, MLH3, PMS1, PMS2) subunits that recognize these errors and then signals for repair. Genes that contain these repetitive sequences in their coding regions are highly susceptible to mutation when the MMR system has been inactivated. Colorectal, gastric, and pancreatic cancers can possess mutations in the MMR system. These MSI-related malignancies tend to remain diploid. They also typically tend to be more resistant to DNA-damaging chemotherapeutics, though they have better overall survival rates.[198,206]

MSI mutations usually lead to inactivation of their target genes via frameshift mutations. APC, β(beta)-catenin, TGF-β(beta)II, and Insulin-like growth factor II have all been shown to be affected by MSI.[208–210,213–216] While p53 is not typically affected by MSI, its downstream targets can be.[211,217] The KRAS pathway is also affected by MSI via mutations in the downstream target BRAF, although the mechanism for this mutation remains unclear as this gene does not contain a classic repeat.[218] In summary, loss of MMR function promotes the accumulation of frameshift mutations in microsatellites. These nucleotide repeats are present in multiple genes, and these mutations result in inactivation of tumor suppressors, promotion of tumor growth, and accelerated malignant transformation.

HNPCC accounts for approximately 5% of all colorectal cancers. MSI was first demonstrated to be an important component of HNPCC in 1983. These patients frequently have germline mutations in *MLH1* or *MSH2*. Various mutations in these two genes account for 60% of HNPCC kindreds.[219,220] Mutations in other MMR subunits have also been documented, though less frequently.[221–227] Mutations in *PMS2* and *MSH6* are seen in "non-classic" HNPCC families, exhibiting later onset of colorectal cancer and an increased frequency of extra-intestinal malignancies such as endometrial cancer.[228] Approximately one-third of HNPCC patients do not possess an identifiable germline mutation, suggesting that there may be an unrecognized component or gene product involved in MMR. As with other familial cancer syndromes, silencing of the remaining allele is required to fully inactivate the MMR multimer. Allelic loss and epigenetic silencing of the remaining allele are a common mechanism observed in gastrointestinal cancers.[229]

Microsatellite instability can also occur in sporadic cancers, and is thought to account for 10–15% of sporadic colorectal cancer. Similar to HNPCC, sporadic MSI colorectal cancer tends to occur more proximally, have a greater mucinous component, be poorly differentiated, lack aneuploidy, and have a better overall survival.[230–233] Patients with sporadic MSI colon cancers tend to be older than their familial counterparts, and decreased *MLH1* expression has been documented with increasing age.[234] At the genetic level, sporadic MSI is quite different from familial microsatellite instability, and is thought to primarily involve epigenetic silencing of both alleles of the *hMLH1* gene without a direct genetic mutation.[229,235–237]

The presence of MSI also appears to have prognostic value, as it may be a marker for cancers poorly responsive to specific chemotherapy agents. Initial data suggested that patients with MSI colorectal cancer might be more responsive to chemotherapy,[238] though subsequent studies have demonstrated minimal benefit and possible increased mortality with standard chemotherapeutic regimens involving 5-FU in this population[239–248] (further discussed in Chap. 2). This is thought to be secondary to decreased tumor effect coupled with the known immunosuppressive effects of these regimens. There may be a role for less toxic therapies in these patients, given the minimal benefit of typical regimens.[212]

In summary, while MIN is seen in both familial cancer syndromes and sporadic malignancies, the genetic mechanisms underlying each can be quite different. Regardless of the mechanism, however, data suggest that these patients are less likely to derive benefit from standard 5-FU chemotherapeutic regimens, and may require more tailored therapy involving other agents.

Chromosomal Instability

CIN is a defining characteristic of many human malignancies, including several in the gastrointestinal tract. In CIN, large portions of entire chromosomes are lost during division. This loss of genetic material at the chromosomal level is known as aneuploidy. CIN has been documented in most dysplastic lesions and increases as dysplasia advances. The timing of CIN in the progression of transformation remains controversial, however. Several studies of sporadic adenomas and familial adenomatous polyposis syndrome (FAP) utilizing single nucleotide polymorphisms (SNPs) have demonstrated high frequencies of allelic disruptions via CIN.[249–251] The mechanisms behind CIN remain incompletely understood and have been difficult to study, with each neoplasm demonstrating a unique karyotype. The effects of chromosomal instability have been well documented, however; CIN can result in gene amplification of proto-oncogenes as well as loss of tumor suppressors via LOH, thereby promoting tumor growth and transformation.[252–254]

There are multiple possible etiologies for CIN. Proposed mechanisms include the dysfunction of the DNA damage repair (DDR) complex, altered cell cycle or telomere regulation, and chromosomal segregation errors.[198,255,256] Inactivation of any of the mechanisms involved in DDR can result in increased tolerance to severe DNA damage and mutation, increasing the risk of mutagenesis. Examples of such genes associated with human malignancy include *ATM*, *BRCA1* and *BRCA2*, and *TP53*.[44,198] Chromosome missegregation also plays a significant role in CIN. Cell cycle and mitotic checkpoints represent a major cell cycle control mechanism, ensuring fidelity of chromosomal segregation and delaying anaphase until all chromatids are appropriately aligned at the metaphase plate. Dysfunction of the genes involved in this process, such as *CHFR*, can directly lead to aneuploidy. *CHFR* expression has been found absent in up to 30% of human colon, esophageal, and gastric cancers, due to epigenetic silencing.[257–259] Several genes involved in mitotic spindle sensing have also been associated with CIN and malignancy, including the mitotic arrest-deficient (MAD) and the budding uninhibited by benzimidazole (BUB) families. Mutations in genes in both of these families have been documented in several human malignancies, including colon cancer.[255,260,261] Mutations in APC, also involved in this process, are commonly seen in colorectal cancer.[262,263] There have also been documented mutations in the proteins present in the kinetochore and centromere in colorectal cancer.[264,265]

Telomere maintenance can also play a role in chromosomal instability. Inactivation of tumor suppressors typically activated with telomere erosion can allow the cell cycle to proceed erroneously, with continued attempts at double strand break (DSB) repair. The results of this inappropriate repair can be disastrous, with formation of dicentric chromosomes, breakage–fusion–breakage cycles, recurrent DSBs, and an incredible amount of genomic instability. This model has been demonstrated in vitro and in vivo, and has been documented both in adenomatous polyps and in pancreatic precursors (PanIN-1A lesions),[266,267] as well as *terc*-deficient murine models.[268] In summary, it appears that telomere stability and telomerase dysfunction play a critical role in the chromosomal instability seen in malignancy.

Base Excision Repair

DNA nucleotide bases are rarely altered via interaction with ROS or via methylation, acetylation, or deamination, particularly in the setting of cellular stressors. Altering individual bases in DNA can result in modified binding affinities, disrupting the normal non-covalent interactions that occur between base pairs. This subsequently can result in mispairing and transition or transversion mutations during DNA replication.[203] These types of changes in the DNA sequence can result in both missense and nonsense mutations. Nonsense mutations cause premature protein truncations and are therefore usually inactivating. Missense mutations, in contrast, can inactivate a tumor suppressor like APC, or cause an activating mutation as is observed in KRAS.[43,203,269] The Base Excision Repair (BER) pathway recognizes these base modifications and activates repair mechanisms. It is important to note that while CIN and MSI are thought to be mutually exclusive,[197] BER defects have been appreciated in both CIN+ and MSI+ colorectal cancers, as well as tumors that are both MIN and CIN stable.[203,270,271]

Two mutations in the BER pathway have been associated with malignancies of the gastrointestinal tract. These genes are *MYH* and *MED1(MBD4)*.[41–43,203,272–274] *MYH*, along with two other enzymes, detects and repairs oxidative damage to guanine bases. Germline mutations in *MYH* result in the FAP-like syndrome MYH Adenomatous Polyposis (MAP).[41–43] MAP-associated colon cancer requires that two mutant *MYH* alleles be inherited, rather than one. When an individual inherits two copies of the mutant allele, oxidative damage to guanine bases slowly accumulates over many years, resulting in mutations in a specific set of proteins, including APC and KRAS.[41–43,269] Other tumor suppressors frequently inactivated in colorectal cancer, such as p53, SMAD4, and TGF-β(beta)IIR, are not typically mutated in MAP-associated colon cancers. It remains unclear if *MYH* heterozygotes are at increased risk for CRC, or if sporadic MYH mutations play a role in CRC. *MYH*'s role in other malignancies of the GI tract, particularly gastric cancer, is being assessed as well.[274] Another BER gene frequently involved in malignancy is *MED1(MBD4)*. This gene encodes for a glycosylase involved in the repair of deaminations of methylcytosines, preventing the transition C→T. This enzyme is frequently mutated in MIN+ tumors.[272,275]

While not part of the classical BER pathway, methylguanine methyl transferase (MGMT) is another gene involved in DNA repair thought to be associated with gastrointestinal malignancy.[270,271,276] MGMT repairs alkyl adducts of guanine and thymine.[276] This enzyme is not technically a member of the BER pathway, but is vital in protecting cells from the cytotoxic effects of methylating chemotherapeutic agents and a number of carcinogens.[276] *MGMT* is silenced in a number of gastrointestinal malignancies, including colon, gastric, and esophageal cancer via promoter hypermethylation.[276,277] In *MGMT*-inactive tumors, Ki-RAS and p53 mutations are frequent, and such mutations activate and inactivate these genes, respectively.[278–280] In summary, damage to the genes encoding the enzymes involved in BER can result in significant genetic instability, as well as missense and nonsense mutations, with a typical pattern of mutation and subsequent malignancy.

Epigenetic Modification

Epigenetic modification refers to the modification of DNA and genes in an inheritable fashion without changing the actual base pair sequence. This process was first appreciated in 1983, when Feinberg and Vogelstein demonstrated a significant degree of hypomethylation in neoplastic tissues compared to normal human tissue.[281,282] This was then confirmed via liquid chromatography of various neoplastic tissues, and demonstrated in colonic adenomas and cancer as well.[281,283–285] Since this early work, the underlying mechanisms of epigenetic modification in neoplastic transformation and progression have been further elucidated.

Epigenetic mechanisms include DNA methylation, gene imprinting, and histone acetylation. These mechanisms allow the transfer of information via cell division without altering the actual nucleotide sequence and are utilized by cells to silence gene expression.[286,287] DNA methylation involves the regulated methylation of cytosine bases of concentrated CpG dinucleotides found in regions known as CpG islands. It is estimated that nearly 50% of genes possess CpG islands within their promoters. The degree of methylation present in these islands is strongly regulated. Fully methylated regions are rare, and are only found in genes regulated by imprinting and in inactivated X chromosomes in females.[288] Imprinting is the selective methylation of one allele of a gene, resulting in expression of only the paternal or maternal copy of a gene.[289,290]

DNA methylation of CpG islands functions to control whether chromatin is in an open, transcriptionally active conformation, or closed state, more tightly bound with histones and transcriptionally silent. This process is regulated by a class of enzymes known as DNA methyltransferases.[288,291] CpG methylation allows methyl-CpG Domain proteins (MBDs) to bind DNA. MBDs then recruit other enzymes to form a multi-protein complex. These enzymes modify histones, allowing for the formation of compact nucleosomes, modifying the conformation of DNA. This compact form of DNA is transcriptionally silent.[292] The resultant methylation status is passed through cell division and maintained in daughter cells.

There is growing evidence that dysfunctional methylation of CpG islands and loss of imprinting (LOI) are both involved in the pathogenesis of a number of GI malignancies.[236,292–297] Dysfunctional methylation can result in hypomethylation or hypermethylation, and can modify the property of chromosomes and even individual bases.[282] Hypomethylation has been implicated in the activation of numerous proto-oncogenes in colon, gastric, and pancreatic cancers.[296,298–307] Both hypomethylation and hypermethylation have been shown to promote chromosomal instability and CIN.[257,258,308–312]

Hypermethylation of CpG islands in gene promoters has been shown to result in silencing of tumor suppressors, as well as DNA repair genes. One example of this is the sporadic inactivation of *MLH1*. The silencing of tumor suppressors via hypermethylation is thought to be the predominant contribution of epigenetic mechanisms to neoplastic transformation.[281,313] CpG methylation may also contribute to tumor progression via promotion of base mutations. After methylation, cytosine can stably undergo deamination, resulting in missense and nonsense mutations. It is estimated that 50% of inactivating point mutations in *p53* occur as a result of such transition mutations.[314] Methylated CpG dinucleotides are also more easily mutated by UV light and benzo[a]pyrene diol epoxide in tobacco smoke.[315,316]

Aberrant hypermethylation of CpG islands occurs gradually. Much of the CpG island methylation that has been observed is associated with advancing age.[317–319] While it is unclear whether age-related hypermethylation contributes significantly towards transformation, it has been demonstrated that this can result in silencing of tumor suppressor genes. *APC*, *SFRP*, *CDH1* (*E-cadherin*), and *CDKN2A* (p16) have all been shown to be silenced by hypermethylation in colon, gastric, and pancreatic cancer.[20,293,320] Hypermethylation can also inhibit p14/ARF, affecting the p53 pathway,[321–323] and has been implicated in silencing of several other tumor suppressors.[270,271,317,318] CpG hypermethylation has been shown to play a role in neovascularization and cancer cell metastasis as well.[277 320,324–329]

Some malignancies have multiple genes silenced via hypermethylation simultaneously. This has been coined the CpG island methylator phenotype (CIMP).[270,271,317,318,330–332] BRAF and KRAS appear to be frequently affected by activating mutations in CIMP+ tumors.[333] It has also been suggested that there may be several classes of CIMP cancers, with different groups of genes silenced in each. In the colon, CIMP positivity is strongly associated with the formation of proximal serrated adenomas, as well as hyperplastic polyps.[270,271] This suggests that hyperplastic polyps may not be entirely benign and that some may have malignant potential. A lack of definitive diagnostic criteria has made studying this disorder difficult thus far.[237] It remains an area of active research.

In summary, epigenetic modification of DNA allows for the transfer of information to daughter cells without requiring modification of the DNA sequence. Both hypomethylation and hypermethylation appear to play a key role in many of the genetic mechanisms discussed already.

New Insights and Paradigms

Cancer Cells, Stem Cells, and Cancer Stem Cells

The role of stem cells and stem cell biology in gastrointestinal carcinogenesis has been a very active area of research, and controversial. There are several possible roles for stem cells in cancer pathogenesis. First, cancer may be a disease of stem cells. Stem cells are long-lived and thus are around long enough to acquire the multiple mutations that are needed for transformation. Other cell types have shorter life spans and are typically sloughed off.[334–336] Moreover, adult stem cells can undergo a limitless number of cell divisions since they retain telomerase expression. Thus they have already acquired a potent cancer hallmark.

Stem cells may also be more susceptible to transformation than other cell types. This has been suggested by experiments in transgenic mice. Parallel investigation by two separate groups demonstrated in the colon that induction of an oncogenic mutation in stem cells frequently yielded gross tumors. Induction of the same mutation in transit amplifying or differentiated cells produced only microadenomas that did not progress.[337, 338] Based on these observations, the authors concluded that intestinal stem cells are uniquely vulnerable to neoplastic transformation. Whether this principle is true in other gastrointestinal tissues remains to be determined. Lastly, many markers for tissue stem cells are also detected in subsets of cancer cells. This suggests that cancer cells may have originated from the stem cell compartment and retained expression of these markers. *PROM-1*, *DCAML-1*, *LGR5*, and *MSI-1* are examples of this. All have been proposed to mark tissue stem cells, and all have been shown to be expressed in a subpopulation of colon and gastric cancers.[334,339]

This finding of tissue stem cell markers in a subset of cancer cells led in part to the hypothesis that not all cells within the tumor are equivalent. It is speculated that cancers, like normal tissues, contain stem cells that divide and give rise to cells that populate the tumor.[334,339,340] A corollary of this is that most cells in the tumor cannot divide and produce an unlimited number of daughter cells. Cancer stem cells have been reportedly identified in gastric, colon, pancreatic, and hepatocellular cancers.[339,340] A number of investigators have reported putative cancer stem cell markers, based on xenograft studies in immune-deficient mice. The basic methodology has been to identify a subpopulation of cells based on cell surface markers and flow cytometry that can form a tumor with very few cells upon injection into a mouse. Certain subpopulations may require several thousand cells to form a tumor, others as few as 10.[334,339] Those subpopulations requiring the fewest cells are thought to be enriched with cancer stem cells. However, questions remain as to whether these methods are appropriately rigorous enough, and whether these subpopulations are in fact an artifact of the techniques used.[341] This will remain an important area for future investigations.

MicroRNAs and Gastrointestinal Cancers

Given the discovery of a multitude of tumor suppressors and oncogenes, as well as the growing role of epigenetic regulation of these genes and pathways, it is quite clear that the development of neoplastic transformation is an extremely complicated and incompletely understood process. The recent discovery of microRNA adds yet another layer of complexity to this picture. MicroRNAs were first discovered by Lee et al in 1993 while studying the gene lin-4, a gene involved in *Caenorhabditis elegans* development.[342,343] This gene appeared to encode a very small RNA molecule that was complementary to the promoter region of the gene lin-14. When present, lin-4 repressed synthesis of lin-14, as well as lin-28, resulting in abnormal development.[344,345] Based on its sequence and size, Lee et al hypothesized that this small piece of RNA was incapable of encoding a protein. This small RNA molecule would be the first in a new class of noncoding RNAs, known as microRNAs. Since their initial discovery, advancements in technology have resulted in the discovery of hundreds of members of this new class of mRNA regulator.

MicroRNAs (miRNAs) are a diverse class of small, noncoding RNA molecules, involved in the regulation of cell differentiation, development, apoptosis, and proliferation.[346] miRNA precursors are initially 60–110 bps in length, with a hairpin-loop structure, known as pri-miRNA.[347–349] This hairpin-loop structure is cleaved in the nucleus by an RNase III enzyme known as Drosha to form the pre-miRNA molecule (Fig. 1.5). The pre-miRNA is transported into the cytoplasm where it is cleaved by the enzyme Dicer.[350] This results in the formation of a final miRNA product, typically only about 20 bp in length and double stranded. One of these strands is then incorporated into a complex containing Dicer and several other proteins known as the microRNA ribonucleoprotein complex (miRNP).[351,352] Once the miRNP complex has formed, it is capable of binding multiple mRNA molecules and silencing them. MicroRNAs have been found to play a role in many pivotal processes in cell and tissue differentiation, function, and maintenance, including hematopoiesis, proliferation, apoptosis, angiogenesis, and stem cell differentiation.[353–362]

Given their broad range of effects, it is not surprising that miRNAs have been implicated in a number of human malignancies. The first malignancy found to have altered levels of miRNA was B-cell chronic lymphocytic leukemia (CLL). In 2002, Calin et al demonstrated that in approximately 60% of patients with B-cell CLL, there was a significant downregulation of the miRNA molecules miR-15a and miR-16–1 secondary to a small deletion in chromosome 13q14.[363] These microRNAs have since been implicated in the regulation of Bcl-2, a known inhibitor of apoptosis.[359] At normal levels, they function as tumor suppressors, inhibiting levels of Bcl-2. When downregulated, Bcl-2 mRNA levels increase, resulting in decreased apoptosis. Alteration of miRNA may also have a pro-oncogenic effect. The gene *BIC*, which encodes the microRNA miR-155, has been demonstrated to promote lymphoma formation in several animal models.[364,365] miR-17–92 has also shown similar effects, via its effects on E2F1, in transgenic *c-Myc* mouse models of carcinogenesis.[366]

The development of high-throughput miRNA detection techniques has allowed for the measurement of many microRNAs at once, with neoplastic tissue uniformly yielding altered patterns of microRNA expression. Each neoplastic tissue evaluated has been shown to demonstrate a unique profile compared to its normal counterpart.[367] These patterns have also been shown to be distinct amongst different malignancies and within the same malignancy at different stages of transformation.[367–369] A number of studies have demonstrated differing profiles of miRNA expression in GI malignancies. One study of colon cancer cells demonstrated 21 miRNAs that appear to be upregulated, and one that was downregulated.[367] Another study looking at 156 known miRNAs in colon cancer identified 13 specific miRNAs that frequently demonstrated altered expression, and one that was significantly upregulated in late stages of disease.[370] Similar studies have noted specific patterns of miRNA regulation in Barrett's esophagus and esophageal adenocarcinoma,[371–374] with differences in patterns of expression at each stage of progression.[375] One significant problem that remains, however, is that the function of these miRNAs, and their specific roles in their respective malignancies, is unknown. This remains an area of active research.

A number of specific microRNAs have been implicated in malignancies of the gastrointestinal tract, and active research into their function is ongoing. Upregulation of the microRNA mIR-21 has been shown to be associated with metastatic spread of colon cancer via suppression of the cell cycle regulator Pdcd4.[376] mIR-21 has also been shown to be upregulated in both Barrett's esophagus and esophageal adenocarcinoma.[377,378] miR-194 is another microRNA observed to be upregulated in cancer. miR-194 is elevated in Barrett's Esophagus, esophageal adenocarcinoma, and metastatic pancreatic cancer, though its function is unclear.[375,379, 380] In contrast, miR-143 and miR-145 have both been shown to be downregulated in colon adenomas,

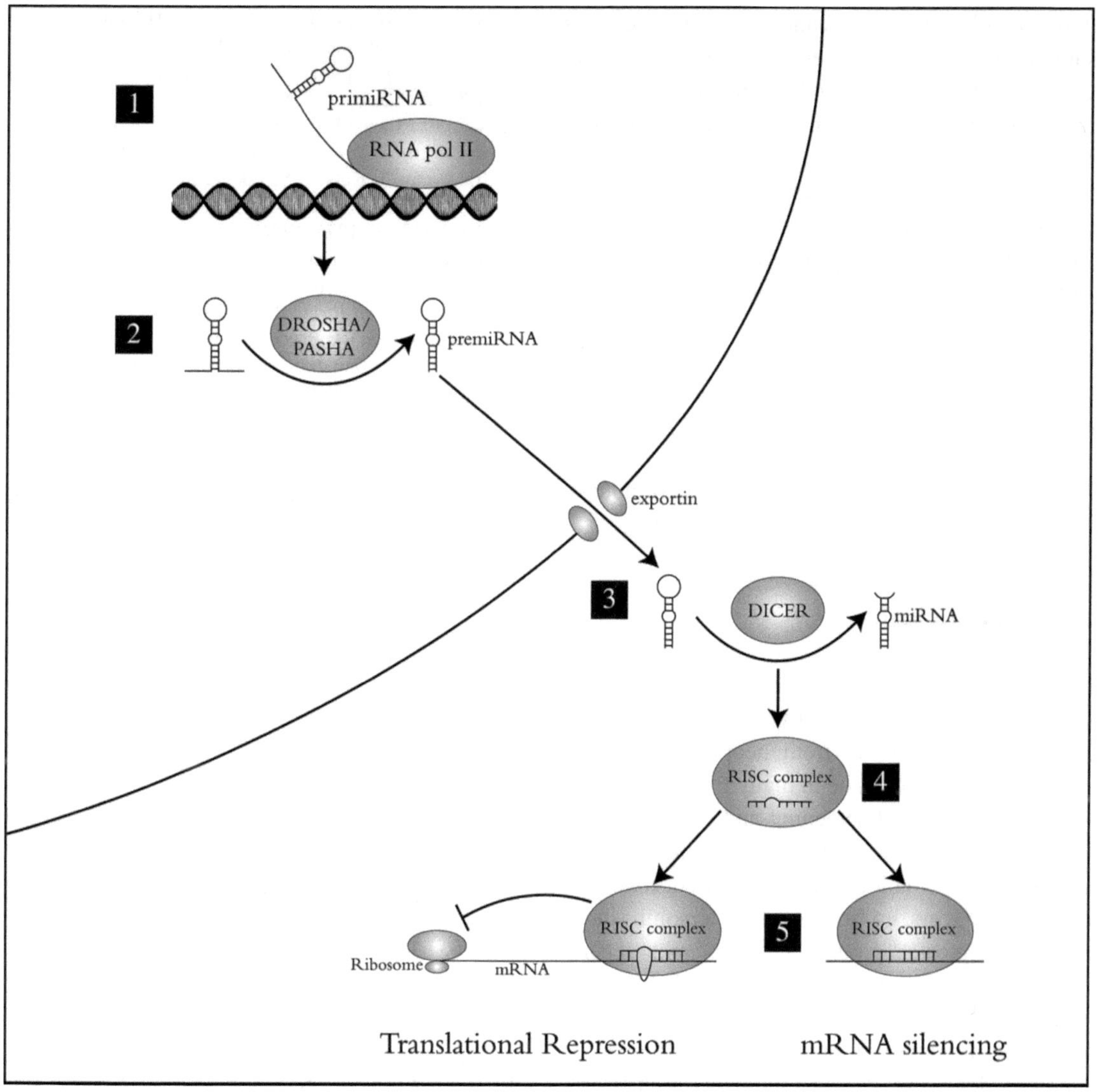

Fig. 1.5 The synthesis of microRNA is a multistep process. The synthesis of microRNA occurs in multiple steps and at multiple sites within the cell. The first step occurs in the nucleus, as RNA polymerase II synthesizes the first precursor, pri-miRNA (1). This hairpin-loop structure is cleaved via Drosha, to form pre-miRNA (2). Pre-miRNA leaves the nucleus and the hairpin loop is cleaved by Dicer in the cytoplasm (3). A single strand of the remaining miRNA molecule is included in the formation of the RISC complex along with several other proteins (4). This multimer can then bind mRNA (5). If the miRNA has mismatches, a loop forms, resulting in translational repression. If the miRNA and mRNA are complementary, the mRNA molecule is degraded

colon cancer, and esophageal adenocarcinoma.[375,381–383] It is anticipated that these miRNAs act to prevent neoplastic transformation, but the mechanism for their effect is presently unknown.

Many of the same mechanisms involved in the dysregulation of tumor suppressors and oncogenes are thought to play a role in miRNA dysregulation as well. Epigenetic modification has been shown to play a role, with a recent study demonstrating epigenetic silencing of a proposed tumor suppressor mIR-137 in 100% of colorectal cancer cell lines, and in 82% of adenomas and resected carcinomas.[384] This silencing was not present in normal mucosa. Disruptions in the process of miRNP formation can also result in modified miRNA expression. Alterations in levels of the enzymes Dicer and Drosha have been reported in several human malignancies, including NSCLC and gastric cancer.[385–387] In intestinal-type gastric cancer, both Dicer and Drosha have been shown to be significantly upregulated in neoplastic tissue compared to non-neoplastic tissue, although interestingly Drosha-negative cancer cells were associated with the worst prognosis.[387] Finally, mutations and chromosomal rearrangements may result in loss and/or amplification of critical cancer-associated miRNAs, respectively. Genome-wide associations have demonstrated that a majority of miRNA genes are found in regions particularly prone to mutation or alteration in cancer.[388] These regions are known as cancer-associated genomic regions (CAGRs).[346] miRNA loci have been shown to have a high frequency of mutation in human cancers.[389] This theory is further supported by evidence demonstrating significant concordance with DNA copy number and miRNA over-expression and under-expression in breast cancer.[390] However, it is not yet known whether this is a predominant mechanism in gastrointestinal cancers as well.

In summary, microRNAs are small RNA molecules involved in regulating the stability and translation of mRNA via complementary binding. miRNAs are involved in multiple aspects of cellular regulation including apoptosis, cell cycle regulation, and terminal differentiation. Patterns of miRNA expression appear to be unique to each malignancy at each stage of progression to metastatic disease. The processes regulating the expression of each of these molecules, as well as the mechanisms underlying their dysregulation with gastrointestinal carcinogenesis, remain an active area of research.

Summary and Conclusions

The National Cancer Act of 1971 is perceived as the start of our modern 'war' on cancer morbidity and mortality. Forty years later, too many still die from neoplastic diseases. However, progress has been made in many fronts, including cancer prevention (improved screening and early interventions), identification of increased-risk populations, and cancer therapeutics (stage IV colon cancer median survival with treatment is nearly 2 years, up from less than 6 months in the 1970s). Perhaps the greatest progress has been made regarding our understanding of cancer pathogenesis. The mechanisms discussed at length in this chapter are the fruit of 40 years of labor into the question of why we develop cancer. There is ample evidence to expect that future research efforts, building on these discoveries, will yield more sensitive screening and preventative strategies, as well as more effective therapeutics.

Acknowledgements The authors would like to acknowledge the assistance of Stephanie Icken, who contributed to the design of the figures used in this chapter.

References

1. Ferlay J, Shin HR, Bray F, Forman D, Mathers C, Parkin DM. Estimates of worldwide burden of cancer in 2008: GLOBOCAN 2008. *Int J Cancer*. 2010;127:2893–2917.
2. Ferlay J, S.H.R, Bray F, Forman D, Mathers C, and Parkin DM. GLOBOCAN 2008, Cancer incidence and mortality worldwide. *IARC CancerBase No. 10* 2010; (Available from: http://globocan.iarc.fr. Accessed Access, 2010).
3. Ponder BA. Cancer genetics. *Nature*. 2001;411(6835):336–341.
4. Lynch JP, Hoops TC. The genetic pathogenesis of colorectal cancer. *Hematol Oncol Clin North Am*. 2002;16(4):775–810.
5. Winawer SJ, Zauber AG, Ho MN, et al. Prevention of colorectal cancer by colonoscopic polypectomy. The National Polyp Study Workgroup. *N Engl J Med*. 1993;329(27):1977–1981.
6. Winawer SJ, Zauber AG, O'Brien MJ, et al. The National Polyp Study. Design, methods, and characteristics of patients with newly diagnosed polyps. The National Polyp Study Workgroup. *Cancer*. 1992;70(5 Suppl):1236–1245.
7. Kim EC, Lance P. Colorectal polyps and their relationship to cancer. *Gastroenterol Clin North Am*. 1997;26(1):1–17.
8. Takayama T, Katsuki S, Takahashi Y, et al. Aberrant crypt foci of the colon as precursors of adenoma and cancer. *N Engl J Med*. 1998;339(18):1277–1284.
9. Roncucci L, Pedroni M, Vaccina F, Benatti P, Marzona L, De Pol A. Aberrant crypt foci in colorectal carcinogenesis. Cell and crypt dynamics. *Cell Prolif*. 2000;33(1):1–18.
10. Tudek B, Bird RP, Bruce WR. Foci of aberrant crypts in the colons of mice and rats exposed to carcinogens associated with foods. *Cancer Res*. 1989;49(5):1236–1240.
11. Siu IM, Pretlow TG, Amini SB, Pretlow TP. Identification of dysplasia in human colonic aberrant crypt foci. *Am J Pathol*. 1997;150(5):1805–1813.
12. Siu IM, Robinson DR, Schwartz S, et al. The identification of monoclonality in human aberrant crypt foci. *Cancer Res*. 1999; 59(1):63–66.
13. Nucci MR, Robinson CR, Longo P, Campbell P, Hamilton SR. Phenotypic and genotypic characteristics of aberrant crypt foci in human colorectal mucosa. *Hum Pathol*. 1997;28(12):1396–1407.
14. Heinen CD, Shivapurkar N, Tang Z, Groden J, Alabaster O. Microsatellite instability in aberrant crypt foci from human colons. *Cancer Res*. 1996;56(23):5339–5341.
15. Pedroni M, Sala E, Scarselli A, et al. Microsatellite instability and mismatch-repair protein expression in hereditary and sporadic colorectal carcinogenesis. *Cancer Res*. 2001;61(3):896–899.
16. Shivapurkar N, Huang L, Ruggeri B, et al. K-ras and p53 mutations in aberrant crypt foci and colonic tumors from colon cancer patients. *Cancer Lett*. 1997;115(1):39–46.
17. Shpitz B, Bomstein Y, Shalev M, et al. Oncoprotein coexpression in human aberrant crypt foci and minute polypoid lesions of the large bowel. *Anticancer Res*. 1999;19(4B):3361–3366.
18. Takayama T, Ohi M, Hayashi T, et al. Analysis of K-ras, APC, and beta-catenin in aberrant crypt foci in sporadic adenoma, cancer, and familial adenomatous polyposis. *Gastroenterology*. 2001;121(3):599–611.
19. Smith AJ, Stern HS, Penner M, et al. Somatic APC and K-ras codon 12 mutations in aberrant crypt foci from human colons. *Cancer Res*. 1994;54(21):5527–5530.
20. Suzuki H, Watkins DN, Jair KW, et al. Epigenetic inactivation of SFRP genes allows constitutive WNT signaling in colorectal cancer. *Nat Genet*. 2004;36(4):417–422.
21. Stairs DB, Kong J, Lynch JP. Cdx genes, inflammation, and the pathogenesis of intestinal metaplasias. In: Kaestner K, ed. *Molecular Biology of Digestive Organs*. Vol 96: Elsevier; 2010:231–270.
22. Hruban RH, Adsay NV, Albores-Saavedra J, et al. Pancreatic intraepithelial neoplasia: a new nomenclature and classification system for pancreatic duct lesions. *Am J Surg Pathol*. 2001;25(5):579–586.
23. Hruban RH, Takaori K, Klimstra DS, et al. An illustrated consensus on the classification of pancreatic intraepithelial neoplasia and intraductal papillary mucinous neoplasms. *Am J Surg Pathol*. 2004;28(8):977–987.
24. Nowell PC. The clonal evolution of tumor cell populations. *Science*. 1976;194(4260):23–28.
25. Vogelstein B, Kinzler KW. Cancer genes and the pathways they control. *Nat Med*. 2004;10(8):789–799.
26. Yuasa Y. Control of gut differentiation and intestinal-type gastric carcinogenesis. *Nat Rev Cancer*. 2003;3(8):592–600.
27. Fearon ER, Vogelstein B. A genetic model for colorectal tumorigenesis. *Cell*. 1990;61(5):759–767.
28. Blair DG, Oskarsson M, Wood TG, McClements WL, Fischinger PJ, Vande Woude GG. Activation of the transforming potential of

a normal cell sequence: a molecular model for oncogenesis. *Science*. 1981;212(4497):941–943.

29. Cahill DP, Kinzler KW, Vogelstein B, Lengauer C. Genetic instability and Darwinian selection in tumours. *Trends Cell Biol.* 1999;9(12):M57–M60.
30. Hanahan D, Weinberg RA. The hallmarks of cancer. *Cell.* 2000;100(1):57–70.
31. Muto T, Bussey HJ, Morson BC. The evolution of cancer of the colon and rectum. *Cancer*. 1975;36(6):2251–2270.
32. Reya T, Morrison SJ, Clarke MF, Weissman IL. Stem cells, cancer, and cancer stem cells. *Nature*. 2001;414(6859):105–111.
33. Taipale J, Beachy PA. The Hedgehog and Wnt signalling pathways in cancer. *Nature*. 2001;411(6835):349–354.
34. Shih IM, Wang TL, Traverso G, et al. Top-down morphogenesis of colorectal tumors. *Proc Natl Acad Sci USA*. 2001;98(5):2640–2645.
35. Wright NA, Poulsom R. Top down or bottom up? Competing management structures in the morphogenesis of colorectal neoplasms. *Gut*. 2002;51(3):306–308.
36. Colotta F, Allavena P, Sica A, Garlanda C, Mantovani A. Cancer-related inflammation, the seventh hallmark of cancer: links to genetic instability. *Carcinogenesis*. 2009;30(7):1073–1081.
37. Mantovani A. Cancer: inflaming metastasis. *Nature*. 2009; 457(7225):36–37.
38. Sherr CJ. Principles of tumor suppression. *Cell*. 2004;116(2): 235–246.
39. Chung DC. The genetic basis of colorectal cancer: insights into critical pathways of tumorigenesis. *Gastroenterology*. 2000;119(3): 854–865.
40. Kinzler KW, Vogelstein B. Lessons from hereditary colorectal cancer. *Cell*. 1996;87(2):159–170.
41. Jones S, Emmerson P, Maynard J, et al. Biallelic germline mutations in MYH predispose to multiple colorectal adenoma and somatic G:C–>T:A mutations. *Hum Mol Genet*. 2002;11(23):2961–2967.
42. Sampson JR, Dolwani S, Jones S, et al. Autosomal recessive colorectal adenomatous polyposis due to inherited mutations of MYH. *Lancet*. 2003;362(9377):39–41.
43. Sieber OM, Lipton L, Crabtree M, et al. Multiple colorectal adenomas, classic adenomatous polyposis, and germ-line mutations in MYH. *N Engl J Med*. 2003;348(9):791–799.
44. Nagy R, Sweet K, Eng C. Highly penetrant hereditary cancer syndromes. *Oncogene*. 2004;23(38):6445–6470.
45. Slattery ML, Boucher KM, Caan BJ, Potter JD, Ma KN. Eating patterns and risk of colon cancer. *Am J Epidemiol*. 1998;148(1): 4–16.
46. Reddy BS, Sharma C, Mathews L, Engle A. Fecal mutagens from subjects consuming a mixed-western diet. *Mutat Res*. 1984;135(1): 11–19.
47. Correa P, Piazuelo MB, Camargo MC. The future of gastric cancer prevention. *Gastric Cancer*. 2004;7(1):9–16.
48. Lashner BA, Heidenreich PA, Su GL, Kane SV, Hanauer SB. Effect of folate supplementation on the incidence of dysplasia and cancer in chronic ulcerative colitis. A case–control study. *Gastroenterology*. 1989;97(2):255–259.
49. Giovannucci E, Stampfer MJ, Colditz GA, et al. Folate, methionine, and alcohol intake and risk of colorectal adenoma. *J Natl Cancer Inst*. 1993;85(11):875–884.
50. Gonzalez-Perez A, Garcia Rodriguez LA, Lopez-Ridaura R. Effects of non-steroidal anti-inflammatory drugs on cancer sites other than the colon and rectum: a meta-analysis. *BMC Cancer*. 2003;3:28.
51. Anderson KE, Johnson TW, Lazovich D, Folsom AR. Association between nonsteroidal anti-inflammatory drug use and the incidence of pancreatic cancer. *J Natl Cancer Inst*. 2002;94(15):1168–1171.
52. Coogan PF, Rosenberg L, Palmer JR, et al. Nonsteroidal anti-inflammatory drugs and risk of digestive cancers at sites other than the large bowel. *Cancer Epidemiol Biomarkers Prev*. 2000; 9(1):119–123.
53. Akre K, Ekstrom AM, Signorello LB, Hansson LE, Nyren O. Aspirin and risk for gastric cancer: a population-based case–control study in Sweden. *Br J Cancer*. 2001;84(7):965–968.
54. Langman MJ, Cheng KK, Gilman EA, Lancashire RJ. Effect of anti-inflammatory drugs on overall risk of common cancer: case–control study in general practice research database. *BMJ*. 2000;320(7250):1642–1646.
55. Chen X, Li N, Wang S, et al. Aberrant arachidonic acid metabolism in esophageal adenocarcinogenesis, and the effects of sulindac, nordihydroguaiaretic acid, and alpha-difluoromethylornithine on tumorigenesis in a rat surgical model. *Carcinogenesis*. 2002;23(12):2095–2102.
56. Buttar NS, Wang KK, Leontovich O, et al. Chemoprevention of esophageal adenocarcinoma by COX-2 inhibitors in an animal model of Barrett's esophagus. *Gastroenterology*. 2002;122(4): 1101–1112.
57. Carlton PS, Gopalakrishnan R, Gupta A, et al. Piroxicam is an ineffective inhibitor of N-nitrosomethylbenzylamine-induced tumorigenesis in the rat esophagus. *Cancer Res*. 2002;62(15):4376–4382.
58. Hahm KB, Song YJ, Oh TY, et al. Chemoprevention of Helicobacter pylori-associated gastric carcinogenesis in a mouse model: is it possible? *J Biochem Mol Biol*. 2003;36(1):82–94.
59. Furukawa F, Nishikawa A, Lee IS, et al. A cyclooxygenase-2 inhibitor, nimesulide, inhibits postinitiation phase of N-nitrosobis(2-oxopropyl)amine-induced pancreatic carcinogenesis in hamsters. *Int J Cancer*. 2003;104(3):269–273.
60. Schuller HM, Zhang L, Weddle DL, Castonguay A, Walker K, Miller MS. The cyclooxygenase inhibitor ibuprofen and the FLAP inhibitor MK886 inhibit pancreatic carcinogenesis induced in hamsters by transplacental exposure to ethanol and the tobacco carcinogen NNK. *J Cancer Res Clin Oncol*. 2002;128(10):525–532.
61. Wenger FA, Kilian M, Bisevac M, et al. Effects of Celebrex and Zyflo on liver metastasis and lipidperoxidation in pancreatic cancer in Syrian hamsters. *Clin Exp Metastasis*. 2002;19(8):681–687.
62. Calle EE, Rodriguez C, Walker-Thurmond K, Thun MJ. Overweight, obesity, and mortality from cancer in a prospectively studied cohort of U.S. adults. *N Engl J Med*. 2003;348(17):1625–1638.
63. Harriss DJ, Atkinson G, George K, et al. Lifestyle factors and colorectal cancer risk (1): systematic review and meta-analysis of associations with body mass index. *Colorectal Dis*. 2009;11(6):547–563.
64. Lawley PD. From fluorescence spectra to mutational spectra, a historical overview of DNA-reactive compounds. *IARC Sci Publ*. 1994;125:3–22.
65. Gonzalez FJ, Gelboin HV. Role of human cytochromes P450 in the metabolic activation of chemical carcinogens and toxins. *Drug Metab Rev*. 1994;26(1–2):165–183.
66. Friedberg EC. DNA damage and repair. *Nature*. 2003;421(6921): 436–440.
67. Heinen CD, Schmutte C, Fishel R. DNA repair and tumorigenesis: lessons from hereditary cancer syndromes. *Cancer Biol Ther*. 2002;1(5):477–485.
68. Sugimura T. *Food and cancer Toxicology*. 2002;181–182:17–21.
69. Bartsch H, Ohshima H, Shuker DE, Pignatelli B, Calmels S. Exposure of humans to endogenous N-nitroso compounds: implications in cancer etiology. *Mutat Res*. 1990;238(3):255–267.
70. Kamiyama S, Ohshima H, Shimada A, et al. Urinary excretion of N-nitrosamino acids and nitrate by inhabitants in high- and low-risk areas for stomach cancer in northern Japan. *IARC Sci Publ*. 1987;84:497–502.
71. Lu SH, Ohshima H, Fu HM, et al. Urinary excretion of N-nitrosamino acids and nitrate by inhabitants of high- and low-risk areas for esophageal cancer in Northern China: endogenous formation of nitrosoproline and its inhibition by vitamin C. *Cancer Res*. 1986;46(3):1485–1491.
72. Zatonski W, Ohshima H, Przewozniak K, et al. Urinary excretion of N-nitrosamino acids and nitrate by inhabitants of high- and

low-risk areas for stomach cancer in Poland. *Int J Cancer.* 1989;44(5):823–827.
73. Groopman JD, Cain LG, Kensler TW. Aflatoxin exposure in human populations: measurements and relationship to cancer. *Crit Rev Toxicol.* 1988;19(2):113–145.
74. Wogan GN. Aflatoxins as risk factors for hepatocellular carcinoma in humans. *Cancer Res.* 1992;52(7 Suppl):2114s-2118s.
75. Scholl P, Musser SM, Kensler TW, Groopman JD. Molecular biomarkers for aflatoxins and their application to human liver cancer. *Pharmacogenetics.* 1995;Spec No 5:S171–176.
76. Enzinger PC, Mayer RJ. Esophageal cancer. *N Engl J Med.* 2003;349(23):2241–2252.
77. Seitz HK, Cho CH. Contribution of alcohol and tobacco use in gastrointestinal cancer development. *Methods Mol Biol.* 2009;472:217–241.
78. Whitcomb DC, Gorry MC, Preston RA, et al. Hereditary pancreatitis is caused by a mutation in the cationic trypsinogen gene. *Nat Genet.* 1996;14(2):141–145.
79. Teich N, Rosendahl J, Toth M, Mossner J, Sahin-Toth M. Mutations of human cationic trypsinogen (PRSS1) and chronic pancreatitis. *Hum Mutat.* 2006;27(8):721–730.
80. Whitcomb DC, Pogue-Geile K. Pancreatitis as a risk for pancreatic cancer. *Gastroenterol Clin North Am.* 2002;31(2):663–678.
81. Howes N, Lerch MM, Greenhalf W, et al. Clinical and genetic characteristics of hereditary pancreatitis in Europe. *Clin Gastroenterol Hepatol.* 2004;2(3):252–261.
82. Bargen JA. Chronic ulcerative colitis associated with malignant disease. *Arch Surg.* 1928;17:561–576.
83. Loftus EV Jr. Epidemiology and risk factors for colorectal dysplasia and cancer in ulcerative colitis. *Gastroenterol Clin North Am.* 2006;35(3):517–531.
84. Devroede GJ, Taylor WF, Sauer WG, Jackman RJ, Stickler GB. Cancer risk and life expectancy of children with ulcerative colitis. *N Engl J Med.* 1971;285(1):17–21.
85. Eaden JA, Abrams KR, Mayberry JF. The risk of colorectal cancer in ulcerative colitis: a meta-analysis. *Gut.* 2001;48(4):526–535.
86. Ekbom A, Helmick C, Zack M, Adami HO. Ulcerative colitis and colorectal cancer. A population-based study. *N Engl J Med.* 1990;323(18):1228–1233.
87. Kune GA, Kune S, Watson LF. Colorectal cancer risk, chronic illnesses, operations, and medications: case control results from the Melbourne Colorectal Cancer Study. *Cancer Res.* 1988;48(15):4399–4404.
88. Giardiello FM, Yang VW, Hylind LM, et al. Primary chemoprevention of familial adenomatous polyposis with sulindac. *N Engl J Med.* 2002;346(14):1054–1059.
89. Phillips RK, Wallace MH, Lynch PM, et al. A randomised, double blind, placebo controlled study of celecoxib, a selective cyclooxygenase 2 inhibitor, on duodenal polyposis in familial adenomatous polyposis. *Gut.* 2002;50(6):857–860.
90. Czernilofsky AP, Levinson AD, Varmus HE, Bishop JM, Tischer E, Goodman HM. Nucleotide sequence of an avian sarcoma virus oncogene (src) and proposed amino acid sequence for gene product. *Nature.* 1980;287(5779):198–203.
91. Suarez HG. Activated oncogenes in human tumors. *Anticancer Res.* 1989;9(5):1331–1343.
92. Parada LF, Tabin CJ, Shih C, Weinberg RA. Human EJ bladder carcinoma oncogene is homologue of Harvey sarcoma virus ras gene. *Nature.* 1982;297(5866):474–478.
93. Cantley LC, Auger KR, Carpenter C, et al. Oncogenes and signal transduction. *Cell.* 1991;64(2):281–302.
94. Felsher DW. Cancer revoked: oncogenes as therapeutic targets. *Nat Rev Cancer.* 2003;3(5):375–380.
95. Knudson AG Jr. Mutation and cancer: statistical study of retinoblastoma. *Proc Natl Acad Sci USA.* 1971;68(4):820–823.
96. Knudson AG. Cancer genetics. *Am J Med Genet.* 2002;111(1):96–102.
97. Comings DE. A general theory of carcinogenesis. *Proc Natl Acad Sci USA.* 1973;70(12):3324–3328.
98. Friend SH, Bernards R, Rogelj S, et al. A human DNA segment with properties of the gene that predisposes to retinoblastoma and osteosarcoma. *Nature.* 1986;323(6089):643–646.
99. Hahn SA, Schutte M, Hoque AT, et al. DPC4, a candidate tumor suppressor gene at human chromosome 18q21.1. *Science.* 1996;271(5247):350–353.
100. Thiagalingam S, Lengauer C, Leach FS, et al. Evaluation of candidate tumour suppressor genes on chromosome 18 in colorectal cancers. *Nat Genet.* 1996;13(3):343–346.
101. Borresen AL. Oncogenesis in ovarian cancer. *Acta Obstet Gynecol Scand Suppl.* 1992;155:25–30.
102. Kinzler KW, Nilbert MC, Su LK, et al. Identification of FAP locus genes from chromosome 5q21. *Science.* 1991;253(5020):661–665.
103. Huiping C, Sigurgeirsdottir JR, Jonasson JG, et al. Chromosome alterations and E-cadherin gene mutations in human lobular breast cancer. *Br J Cancer.* 1999;81(7):1103–1110.
104. Suzuki H, Komiya A, Emi M, et al. Three distinct commonly deleted regions of chromosome arm 16q in human primary and metastatic prostate cancers. *Genes Chromosomes Cancer.* 1996; 17(4):225–233.
105. Wu MS, Chang MC, Huang SP, et al. Correlation of histologic subtypes and replication error phenotype with comparative genomic hybridization in gastric cancer. *Genes Chromosomes Cancer.* 2001;30(1):80–86.
106. Sakakura C, Mori T, Sakabe T, et al. Gains, losses, and amplifications of genomic materials in primary gastric cancers analyzed by comparative genomic hybridization. *Genes Chromosomes Cancer.* 1999;24(4):299–305.
107. Weintraub SJ, Prater CA, Dean DC. Retinoblastoma protein switches the E2F site from positive to negative element. *Nature.* 1992;358(6383):259–261.
108. Helin K, Harlow E, Fattaey A. Inhibition of E2F-1 transactivation by direct binding of the retinoblastoma protein. *Mol Cell Biol.* 1993;13(10):6501–6508.
109. Harbour JW, Luo RX, Dei Santi A, Postigo AA, Dean DC. Cdk phosphorylation triggers sequential intramolecular interactions that progressively block Rb functions as cells move through G1. *Cell.* 1999;98(6):859–869.
110. Yan Z, DeGregori J, Shohet R, et al. Cdc6 is regulated by E2F and is essential for DNA replication in mammalian cells. *Proc Natl Acad Sci USA.* 1998;95(7):3603–3608.
111. Leone G, DeGregori J, Yan Z, et al. E2F3 activity is regulated during the cell cycle and is required for the induction of S phase. *Genes Dev.* 1998;12(14):2120–2130.
112. Lundberg AS, Weinberg RA. Functional inactivation of the retinoblastoma protein requires sequential modification by at least two distinct cyclin-cdk complexes. *Mol Cell Biol.* 1998;18(2):753–761.
113. Nevins JR. The Rb/E2F pathway and cancer. *Hum Mol Genet.* 2001;10(7):699–703.
114. Classon M, Harlow E. The retinoblastoma tumour suppressor in development and cancer. *Nat Rev Cancer.* 2002;2(12):910–917.
115. Lukas J, Bartkova J, Bartek J. Convergence of mitogenic signalling cascades from diverse classes of receptors at the cyclin D-cyclin-dependent kinase-pRb-controlled G1 checkpoint. *Mol Cell Biol.* 1996;16(12):6917–6925.
116. Ayhan S, Isisag A, Saruc M, Nese N, Demir MA, Kucukmetin NT. The role of pRB, p16 and cyclin D1 in colonic carcinogenesis. *Hepatogastroenterology.* 2010;57(98):251–256.
117. Feakins RM, Nickols CD, Bidd H, Walton SJ. Abnormal expression of pRb, p16, and cyclin D1 in gastric adenocarcinoma and its lymph node metastases: relationship with pathological features and survival. *Hum Pathol.* 2003;34(12):1276–1282.
118. Soussi T, Wiman KG. Shaping genetic alterations in human cancer: the p53 mutation paradigm. *Cancer Cell.* 2007;12(4):303–312.

119. Parada LF, Land H, Weinberg RA, Wolf D, Rotter V. Cooperation between gene encoding p53 tumour antigen and ras in cellular transformation. *Nature*. 1984;312(5995):649–651.
120. Eliyahu D, Raz A, Gruss P, Givol D, Oren M. Participation of p53 cellular tumour antigen in transformation of normal embryonic cells. *Nature*. 1984;312(5995):646–649.
121. Malkin D, Li FP, Strong LC, et al. Germ line p53 mutations in a familial syndrome of breast cancer, sarcomas, and other neoplasms. *Science*. 1990;250(4985):1233–1238.
122. Vogelstein B, Lane D, Levine AJ. Surfing the p53 network. *Nature*. 2000;408(6810):307–310.
123. Eliyahu D, Goldfinger N, Pinhasi-Kimhi O, et al. Meth A fibrosarcoma cells express two transforming mutant p53 species. *Oncogene*. 1988;3(3):313–321.
124. Hinds P, Finlay C, Levine AJ. Mutation is required to activate the p53 gene for cooperation with the ras oncogene and transformation. *J Virol*. 1989;63(2):739–746.
125. Finlay CA, Hinds PW, Levine AJ. The p53 proto-oncogene can act as a suppressor of transformation. *Cell*. 1989;57(7):1083–1093.
126. Eischen CM, Weber JD, Roussel MF, Sherr CJ, Cleveland JL. Disruption of the ARF-Mdm2-p53 tumor suppressor pathway in Myc-induced lymphomagenesis. *Genes Dev*. 1999;13(20):2658–2669.
127. Zhang Y, Xiong Y, Yarbrough WG. ARF promotes MDM2 degradation and stabilizes p53: ARF-INK4a locus deletion impairs both the Rb and p53 tumor suppression pathways. *Cell*. 1998;92(6): 725–734.
128. Vousden KH, Ryan KM. p53 and metabolism. *Nat Rev Cancer*. 2009;9(10):691–700.
129. Oren M. Decision making by p53: life, death and cancer. *Cell Death Differ*. 2003;10(4):431–442.
130. el-Deiry WS, Tokino T, Velculescu VE, et al. WAF1, a potential mediator of p53 tumor suppression. *Cell*. 1993;75(4):817–825.
131. Dameron KM, Volpert OV, Tainsky MA, Bouck N. The p53 tumor suppressor gene inhibits angiogenesis by stimulating the production of thrombospondin. *Cold Spring Harb Symp Quant Biol*. 1994;59:483–489.
132. Gansauge S, Gansauge F, Gause H, Poch B, Schoenberg MH, Beger HG. The induction of apoptosis in proliferating human fibroblasts by oxygen radicals is associated with a p53- and p21WAF1CIP1 induction. *FEBS Lett*. 1997;404(1):6–10.
133. Farnebo M, Bykov VJ, Wiman KG. The p53 tumor suppressor: a master regulator of diverse cellular processes and therapeutic target in cancer. *Biochem Biophys Res Commun*. 2010;396(1): 85–89.
134. Maya R, Balass M, Kim ST, et al. ATM-dependent phosphorylation of Mdm2 on serine 395: role in p53 activation by DNA damage. *Genes Dev*. 2001;15(9):1067–1077.
135. Hirao A, Kong YY, Matsuoka S, et al. DNA damage-induced activation of p53 by the checkpoint kinase Chk2. *Science*. 2000;287(5459):1824–1827.
136. Mahmoudi S, Henriksson S, Corcoran M, Mendez-Vidal C, Wiman KG, Farnebo M. Wrap53, a natural p53 antisense transcript required for p53 induction upon DNA damage. *Mol Cell*. 2009;33(4):462–471.
137. Wright WE, Shay JW. The two-stage mechanism controlling cellular senescence and immortalization. *Exp Gerontol*. 1992;27(4): 383–389.
138. Maser RS, DePinho RA. Connecting chromosomes, crisis, and cancer. *Science*. 2002;297(5581):565–569.
139. Sharpless NE, DePinho RA. Telomeres, stem cells, senescence, and cancer. *J Clin Invest*. 2004;113(2):160–168.
140. Chan SR, Blackburn EH. Telomeres and telomerase. *Philos Trans R Soc Lond B Biol Sci*. 2004;359(1441):109–121.
141. Weng NP, Levine BL, June CH, Hodes RJ. Regulated expression of telomerase activity in human T lymphocyte development and activation. *J Exp Med*. 1996;183(6):2471–2479.
142. Wright WE, Piatyszek MA, Rainey WE, Byrd W, Shay JW. Telomerase activity in human germline and embryonic tissues and cells. *Dev Genet*. 1996;18(2):173–179.
143. Broccoli D, Young JW, de Lange T. Telomerase activity in normal and malignant hematopoietic cells. *Proc Natl Acad Sci USA*. 1995;92(20):9082–9086.
144. Krizhanovsky V, Xue W, Zender L, Yon M, Hernando E, Lowe SW. Implications of cellular senescence in tissue damage response, tumor suppression, and stem cell biology. *Cold Spring Harb Symp Quant Biol*. 2008;73:513–522.
145. Krizhanovsky V, Yon M, Dickins RA, et al. Senescence of activated stellate cells limits liver fibrosis. *Cell*. 2008;134(4):657–667.
146. van Heek NT, Meeker AK, Kern SE, et al. Telomere shortening is nearly universal in pancreatic intraepithelial neoplasia. *Am J Pathol*. 2002;161(5):1541–1547.
147. Hastie ND, Dempster M, Dunlop MG, Thompson AM, Green DK, Allshire RC. Telomere reduction in human colorectal carcinoma and with ageing. *Nature*. 1990;346(6287):866–868.
148. Harley CB, Futcher AB, Greider CW. Telomeres shorten during ageing of human fibroblasts. *Nature*. 1990;345(6274):458–460.
149. Harley CB, Vaziri H, Counter CM, Allsopp RC. The telomere hypothesis of cellular aging. *Exp Gerontol*. 1992;27(4):375–382.
150. Counter CM, Avilion AA, LeFeuvre CE, et al. Telomere shortening associated with chromosome instability is arrested in immortal cells which express telomerase activity. *EMBO J*. 1992;11(5):1921–1929.
151. Rudolph KL, Chang S, Lee HW, et al. Longevity, stress response, and cancer in aging telomerase-deficient mice. *Cell*. 1999;96(5): 701–712.
152. Rudolph KL, Millard M, Bosenberg MW, DePinho RA. Telomere dysfunction and evolution of intestinal carcinoma in mice and humans. *Nat Genet*. 2001;28(2):155–159.
153. Chin L, Artandi SE, Shen Q, et al. p53 deficiency rescues the adverse effects of telomere loss and cooperates with telomere dysfunction to accelerate carcinogenesis. *Cell*. 1999;97(4):527–538.
154. Plentz RR, Wiemann SU, Flemming P, et al. Telomere shortening of epithelial cells characterises the adenoma-carcinoma transition of human colorectal cancer. *Gut*. 2003;52(9):1304–1307.
155. Blasco MA, Rizen M, Greider CW, Hanahan D. Differential regulation of telomerase activity and telomerase RNA during multistage tumorigenesis. *Nat Genet*. 1996;12(2):200–204.
156. Yoshida R, Kiyozuka Y, Ichiyoshi H, et al. Change in telomerase activity during human colorectal carcinogenesis. *Anticancer Res*. 1999;19(3B):2167–2172.
157. Nowak J, Januszkiewicz D, Lewandowski K, et al. Activity and expression of human telomerase in normal and malignant cells in gastric and colon cancer patients. *Eur J Gastroenterol Hepatol*. 2003;15(1):75–80.
158. Yang SM, Fang DC, Luo YH, Lu R, Battle PD, Liu WW. Alterations of telomerase activity and terminal restriction fragment in gastric cancer and its premalignant lesions. *J Gastroenterol Hepatol*. 2001;16(8):876–882.
159. Henson JD, Neumann AA, Yeager TR, Reddel RR. Alternative lengthening of telomeres in mammalian cells. *Oncogene*. 2002;21(4):598–610.
160. Bryan TM, Englezou A, Dalla-Pozza L, Dunham MA, Reddel RR. Evidence for an alternative mechanism for maintaining telomere length in human tumors and tumor-derived cell lines. *Nat Med*. 1997;3(11):1271–1274.
161. Opitz OG, Suliman Y, Hahn WC, Harada H, Blum HE, Rustgi AK. Cyclin D1 overexpression and p53 inactivation immortalize primary oral keratinocytes by a telomerase-independent mechanism. *J Clin Invest*. 2001;108(5):725–732.
162. Cesare AJ, Reddel RR. Alternative lengthening of telomeres: models, mechanisms and implications. *Nat Rev Genet*. 2010;11(5): 319–330.
163. Folkman J. Tumor angiogenesis: therapeutic implications. *N Engl J Med*. 1971;285(21):1182–1186.

164. Volpert OV, Lawler J, Bouck NP. A human fibrosarcoma inhibits systemic angiogenesis and the growth of experimental metastases via thrombospondin-1. *Proc Natl Acad Sci USA*. 1998;95(11):6343–6348.
165. Kang WC, Han SH, Ahn TH, Shin EK. Images in cardiology. Unusual dominant course of left circumflex coronary artery with absent right coronary artery. *Heart*. 2006;92(5):657.
166. Giuriato S, Ryeom S, Fan AC, et al. Sustained regression of tumors upon MYC inactivation requires p53 or thrombospondin-1 to reverse the angiogenic switch. *Proc Natl Acad Sci USA*. 2006;103(44):16266–16271.
167. Ferrara N, Gerber HP, LeCouter J. The biology of VEGF and its receptors. *Nat Med*. 2003;9(6):669–676.
168. Fujita Y, Abe R, Shimizu H. Clinical approaches toward tumor angiogenesis: past, present and future. *Curr Pharm Des*. 2008;14(36):3820–3834.
169. Kabbinavar F, Hurwitz HI, Fehrenbacher L, et al. Phase II, randomized trial comparing bevacizumab plus fluorouracil (FU)/leucovorin (LV) with FU/LV alone in patients with metastatic colorectal cancer. *J Clin Oncol*. 2003;21(1):60–65.
170. Giantonio BJ, Catalano PJ, Meropol NJ, et al. Bevacizumab in combination with oxaliplatin, fluorouracil, and leucovorin (FOLFOX4) for previously treated metastatic colorectal cancer: results from the Eastern Cooperative Oncology Group Study E3200. *J Clin Oncol*. 2007;25(12):1539–1544.
171. Hurwitz H, Fehrenbacher L, Novotny W, et al. Bevacizumab plus irinotecan, fluorouracil, and leucovorin for metastatic colorectal cancer. *N Engl J Med*. 2004;350(23):2335–2342.
172. Los M, Roodhart JM, Voest EE. Target practice: lessons from phase III trials with bevacizumab and vatalanib in the treatment of advanced colorectal cancer. *Oncologist*. 2007;12(4):443–450.
173. Winder T, Lenz HJ. Vascular endothelial growth factor and epidermal growth factor signaling pathways as therapeutic targets for colorectal cancer. *Gastroenterology*. 2010;138(6):2163–2176.
174. Ohshima H, Tatemichi M, Sawa T. Chemical basis of inflammation-induced carcinogenesis. *Arch Biochem Biophys*. 2003;417(1):3–11.
175. Marks F, Furstenberger G. Cancer chemoprevention through interruption of multistage carcinogenesis. The lessons learnt by comparing mouse skin carcinogenesis and human large bowel cancer. *Eur J Cancer*. 2000;36(3):314–329.
176. Thun MJ, Henley SJ, Patrono C. Nonsteroidal anti-inflammatory drugs as anticancer agents: mechanistic, pharmacologic, and clinical issues. *J Natl Cancer Inst*. 2002;94(4):252–266.
177. Krishnan K, Brenner DE. Prostaglandin inhibitors and the chemoprevention of noncolonic malignancy. *Gastroenterol Clin North Am*. 2001;30(4):981–1000.
178. Crofford LJ. Prostaglandin biology. *Gastroenterol Clin North Am*. 2001;30(4):863–876.
179. Goodlad RA, Lee CY, Levin S, Wright NA. Effects of the prostaglandin analogue misoprostol on cell proliferation in the canine small intestine. *Exp Physiol*. 1991;76(4):561–566.
180. Goodlad RA, Madgwick AJ, Moffatt MR, Levin S, Allen JL, Wright NA. The effects of the prostaglandin analogue, misoprostol, on cell proliferation and cell migration in the canine stomach. *Digestion*. 1990;46(Suppl 2):182–187.
181. Rudnick DA, Perlmutter DH, Muglia LJ. Prostaglandins are required for CREB activation and cellular proliferation during liver regeneration. *Proc Natl Acad Sci USA*. 2001;98(15):8885–8890.
182. Dormond O, Foletti A, Paroz C, Ruegg C. NSAIDs inhibit alpha V beta 3 integrin-mediated and Cdc42/Rac-dependent endothelial-cell spreading, migration and angiogenesis. *Nat Med*. 2001;7(9):1041–1047.
183. Fosslien E. Review: molecular pathology of cyclooxygenase-2 in cancer-induced angiogenesis. *Ann Clin Lab Sci*. 2001;31(4):325–348.
184. Hilkens CM, Snijders A, Snijdewint FG, Wierenga EA, Kapsenberg ML. Modulation of T-cell cytokine secretion by accessory cell-derived products. *Eur Respir J Suppl*. 1996;22:90s-94s.
185. Marcinkiewicz J. Regulation of cytokine production by eicosanoids and nitric oxide. *Arch Immunol Ther Exp (Warsz)*. 1997;45(2–3):163–167.
186. Shao J, Lee SB, Guo H, Evers BM, Sheng H. Prostaglandin E2 stimulates the growth of colon cancer cells via induction of amphiregulin. *Cancer Res*. 2003;63(17):5218–5223.
187. Roper RL, Phipps RP. Prostaglandin E2 regulation of the immune response. *Adv Prostaglandin Thromboxane Leukot Res*. 1994;22:101–111.
188. Kucharzik T, Lugering N, Winde G, Domschke W, Stoll R. Colon carcinoma cell lines stimulate monocytes and lamina propria mononuclear cells to produce IL-10. *Clin Exp Immunol*. 1997;110(2):296–302.
189. Kambayashi T, Alexander HR, Fong M, Strassmann G. Potential involvement of IL-10 in suppressing tumor-associated macrophages. Colon-26-derived prostaglandin E2 inhibits TNF-alpha release via a mechanism involving IL-10. *J Immunol*. 1995;154(7):3383–3390.
190. Wang Z, Chen Y, Zheng R, et al. In vitro effects of prostaglandin E2 or indomethacin on the proliferation of lymphokine-activated killer cells and their cytotoxicity against bladder tumor cells in patients with bladder cancer. *Prostaglandins*. 1997;54(5):769–779.
191. Mocellin S, Wang E, Marincola FM. Cytokines and immune response in the tumor microenvironment. *J Immunother*. 2001;24(5):392–407.
192. Saito S, Kitayama J, Jin ZX, et al. Beta-chemokine, macrophage inflammatory protein-1beta (MIP-1beta), is highly expressed in diffuse type human gastric cancers. *J Exp Clin Cancer Res*. 2003;22(3):453–459.
193. Salcedo R, Oppenheim JJ. Role of chemokines in angiogenesis: CXCL12/SDF-1 and CXCR4 interaction, a key regulator of endothelial cell responses. *Microcirculation*. 2003;10(3–4):359–370.
194. White ES, Strieter RM, Arenberg DA. Chemokines as therapeutic targets in non-small cell lung cancer. *Curr Med Chem Anticancer Agents*. 2002;2(3):403–417.
195. Balkwill F. Tumor necrosis factor or tumor promoting factor? *Cytokine Growth Factor Rev*. 2002;13(2):135–141.
196. Farrow B, Evers BM. Inflammation and the development of pancreatic cancer. *Surg Oncol*. 2002;10(4):153–169.
197. Lengauer C, Kinzler KW, Vogelstein B. Genetic instabilities in human cancers. *Nature*. 1998;396(6712):643–649.
198. Lengauer C, Kinzler KW, Vogelstein B. Genetic instability in colorectal cancers. *Nature*. 1997;386(6625):623–627.
199. Augenlicht LH, Richards C, Corner G, Pretlow TP. Evidence for genomic instability in human colonic aberrant crypt foci. *Oncogene*. 1996;12(8):1767–1772.
200. Hahn WC, Counter CM, Lundberg AS, Beijersbergen RL, Brooks MW, Weinberg RA. Creation of human tumour cells with defined genetic elements. *Nature*. 1999;400(6743):464–468.
201. Zimonjic D, Brooks MW, Popescu N, Weinberg RA, Hahn WC. Derivation of human tumor cells in vitro without widespread genomic instability. *Cancer Res*. 2001;61(24):8838–8844.
202. Sieber O, Heinimann K, Tomlinson I. Genomic stability and tumorigenesis. *Semin Cancer Biol*. 2005;15(1):61–66.
203. Jiricny J, Marra G. DNA repair defects in colon cancer. *Curr Opin Genet Dev*. 2003;13(1):61–69.
204. Breivik J, Gaudernack G. Genomic instability, DNA methylation, and natural selection in colorectal carcinogenesis. *Semin Cancer Biol*. 1999;9(4):245–254.
205. Sancar A, Lindsey-Boltz LA, Unsal-Kacmaz K, Linn S. Molecular mechanisms of mammalian DNA repair and the DNA damage checkpoints. *Annu Rev Biochem*. 2004;73:39–85.

206. Peltomaki P. Deficient DNA, mismatch repair: a common etiologic factor for colon cancer. *Hum Mol Genet*. 2001;10(7):735–740.
207. Kolodner RD, Marsischky GT. Eukaryotic DNA mismatch repair. *Curr Opin Genet Dev*. 1999;9(1):89–96.
208. Huang J, Papadopoulos N, McKinley AJ, et al. APC mutations in colorectal tumors with mismatch repair deficiency. *Proc Natl Acad Sci USA*. 1996;93(17):9049–9054.
209. Miyaki M, Iijima T, Kimura J, et al. Frequent mutation of beta-catenin and APC genes in primary colorectal tumors from patients with hereditary nonpolyposis colorectal cancer. *Cancer Res*. 1999;59(18):4506–4509.
210. Parsons R, Myeroff LL, Liu B, et al. Microsatellite instability and mutations of the transforming growth factor beta type II receptor gene in colorectal cancer. *Cancer Res*. 1995;55(23):5548–5550.
211. Rampino N, Yamamoto H, Ionov Y, et al. Somatic frameshift mutations in the BAX gene in colon cancers of the microsatellite mutator phenotype. *Science*. 1997;275(5302):967–969.
212. Boland CR, Goel A. Microsatellite instability in colorectal cancer. *Gastroenterology*. 2010;138(6):2073–2087.
213. Samowitz WS, Holden JA, Curtin K, et al. Inverse relationship between microsatellite instability and K-ras and p53 gene alterations in colon cancer. *Am J Pathol*. 2001;158(4):1517–1524.
214. Losi L, Ponz de Leon M, Jiricny J, et al. K-ras and p53 mutations in hereditary non-polyposis colorectal cancers. *Int J Cancer*. 1997;74(1):94–96.
215. Souza RF, Appel R, Yin J, et al. Microsatellite instability in the insulin-like growth factor II receptor gene in gastrointestinal tumours. *Nat Genet*. 1996;14(3):255–257.
216. Grady WM, Rajput A, Myeroff L, et al. Mutation of the type II transforming growth factor-beta receptor is coincident with the transformation of human colon adenomas to malignant carcinomas. *Cancer Res*. 1998;58(14):3101–3104.
217. Yagi OK, Akiyama Y, Nomizu T, Iwama T, Endo M, Yuasa Y. Proapoptotic gene BAX is frequently mutated in hereditary nonpolyposis colorectal cancers but not in adenomas. *Gastroenterology*. 1998;114(2):268–274.
218. Wang L, Cunningham JM, Winters JL, et al. BRAF mutations in colon cancer are not likely attributable to defective DNA mismatch repair. *Cancer Res*. 2003;63(17):5209–5212.
219. Liu B, Parsons R, Papadopoulos N, et al. Analysis of mismatch repair genes in hereditary non-polyposis colorectal cancer patients. *Nat Med*. 1996;2(2):169–174.
220. Peltomaki P, Vasen HF. Mutations predisposing to hereditary nonpolyposis colorectal cancer: database and results of a collaborative study. The International Collaborative Group on Hereditary Nonpolyposis Colorectal Cancer. *Gastroenterology*. 1997;113(4):1146–1158.
221. Beauchamp RD, Sheng HM, Shao JY, Thompson EA, Ko TC. Intestinal cell cycle regulations. Interactions of cyclin D1, Cdk4, and p21Cip1. *Ann Surg*. 1996;223(5):620–627.
222. Kolodner RD, Tytell JD, Schmeits JL, et al. Germ-line msh6 mutations in colorectal cancer families. *Cancer Res*. 1999;59(20):5068–5074.
223. Wu Y, Berends MJ, Sijmons RH, et al. A role for MLH3 in hereditary nonpolyposis colorectal cancer. *Nat Genet*. 2001;29(2):137–138.
224. Akiyama Y, Sato H, Yamada T, et al. Germ-line mutation of the hMSH6/GTBP gene in an atypical hereditary nonpolyposis colorectal cancer kindred. *Cancer Res*. 1997;57(18):3920–3923.
225. Miyaki M, Konishi M, Tanaka K, et al. Germline mutation of MSH6 as the cause of hereditary nonpolyposis colorectal cancer. *Nat Genet*. 1997;17(3):271–272.
226. Huang J, Kuismanen SA, Liu T, et al. MSH6 and MSH3 are rarely involved in genetic predisposition to nonpolypotic colon cancer. *Cancer Res*. 2001;61(4):1619–1623.
227. Liu T, Yan H, Kuismanen S, et al. The role of hPMS1 and hPMS2 in predisposing to colorectal cancer. *Cancer Res*. 2001;61(21):7798–7802.
228. Wijnen J, de Leeuw W, Vasen H, et al. Familial endometrial cancer in female carriers of MSH6 germline mutations. *Nat Genet*. 1999;23(2):142–144.
229. Kane MF, Loda M, Gaida GM, et al. Methylation of the hMLH1 promoter correlates with lack of expression of hMLH1 in sporadic colon tumors and mismatch repair-defective human tumor cell lines. *Cancer Res*. 1997;57(5):808–811.
230. Ionov Y, Peinado MA, Malkhosyan S, Shibata D, Perucho M. Ubiquitous somatic mutations in simple repeated sequences reveal a new mechanism for colonic carcinogenesis. *Nature*. 1993;363(6429):558–561.
231. Lothe RA, Peltomaki P, Meling GI, et al. Genomic instability in colorectal cancer: relationship to clinicopathological variables and family history. *Cancer Res*. 1993;53(24):5849–5852.
232. Thibodeau SN, Bren G, Schaid D. Microsatellite instability in cancer of the proximal colon. *Science*. 1993;260(5109):816–819.
233. Sinicrope FA, Rego RL, Halling KC, et al. Prognostic impact of microsatellite instability and DNA ploidy in human colon carcinoma patients. *Gastroenterology*. 2006;131(3):729–737.
234. Kakar S, Burgart LJ, Thibodeau SN, et al. Frequency of loss of hMLH1 expression in colorectal carcinoma increases with advancing age. *Cancer*. 2003;97(6):1421–1427.
235. Herman JG, Umar A, Polyak K, et al. Incidence and functional consequences of hMLH1 promoter hypermethylation in colorectal carcinoma. *Proc Natl Acad Sci USA*. 1998;95(12):6870–6875.
236. Veigl ML, Kasturi L, Olechnowicz J, et al. Biallelic inactivation of hMLH1 by epigenetic gene silencing, a novel mechanism causing human MSI cancers. *Proc Natl Acad Sci USA*. 1998;95(15):8698–8702.
237. Grady WM, Carethers JM. Genomic and epigenetic instability in colorectal cancer pathogenesis. *Gastroenterology*. 2008;135(4):1079–1099.
238. Elsaleh H, Joseph D, Grieu F, Zeps N, Spry N, Iacopetta B. Association of tumour site and sex with survival benefit from adjuvant chemotherapy in colorectal cancer. *Lancet*. 2000;355(9217):1745–1750.
239. de Vos tot Nederveen Cappel WH, Meulenbeld HJ, Kleibeuker JH, et al. Survival after adjuvant 5-FU treatment for stage III colon cancer in hereditary nonpolyposis colorectal cancer. *Int J Cancer*. 2004;109(3):468–471.
240. Jover R, Zapater P, Castells A, et al. Mismatch repair status in the prediction of benefit from adjuvant fluorouracil chemotherapy in colorectal cancer. *Gut*. 2006;55(6):848–855.
241. Popat S, Hubner R, Houlston RS. Systematic review of microsatellite instability and colorectal cancer prognosis. *J Clin Oncol*. 2005;23(3):609–618.
242. Kim GP, Colangelo LH, Wieand HS, et al. Prognostic and predictive roles of high-degree microsatellite instability in colon cancer: a National Cancer Institute-National Surgical Adjuvant Breast and Bowel Project Collaborative Study. *J Clin Oncol*. 2007;25(7):767–772.
243. Storojeva I, Boulay JL, Heinimann K, et al. Prognostic and predictive relevance of microsatellite instability in colorectal cancer. *Oncol Rep*. 2005;14(1):241–249.
244. Lanza G, Gafa R, Santini A, Maestri I, Guerzoni L, Cavazzini L. Immunohistochemical test for MLH1 and MSH2 expression predicts clinical outcome in stage II and III colorectal cancer patients. *J Clin Oncol*. 2006;24(15):2359–2367.
245. Des Guetz G, Schischmanoff O, Nicolas P, Perret GY, Morere JF, Uzzan B. Does microsatellite instability predict the efficacy of adjuvant chemotherapy in colorectal cancer? A systematic review with meta-analysis. *Eur J Cancer*. 2009;45(10):1890–1896.

246. Bertagnolli MM, Niedzwiecki D, Compton CC, et al. Microsatellite instability predicts improved response to adjuvant therapy with irinotecan, fluorouracil, and leucovorin in stage III colon cancer: Cancer and Leukemia Group B Protocol 89803. *J Clin Oncol*. 2009;27(11):1814–1821.
247. Ribic CM, Sargent DJ, Moore MJ, et al. Tumor microsatellite-instability status as a predictor of benefit from fluorouracil-based adjuvant chemotherapy for colon cancer. *N Engl J Med*. 2003;349(3):247–257.
248. Benatti P, Gafa R, Barana D, et al. Microsatellite instability and colorectal cancer prognosis. *Clin Cancer Res*. 2005;11(23):8332–8340.
249. Shih IM, Zhou W, Goodman SN, Lengauer C, Kinzler KW, Vogelstein B. Evidence that genetic instability occurs at an early stage of colorectal tumorigenesis. *Cancer Res*. 2001;61(3):818–822.
250. Cardoso J, Molenaar L, de Menezes RX, et al. Chromosomal instability in MYH- and APC-mutant adenomatous polyps. *Cancer Res*. 2006;66(5):2514–2519.
251. Pino MS, Chung DC. The chromosomal instability pathway in colon cancer. *Gastroenterology*. 2010;138(6):2059–2072.
252. Sunpaweravong P, Sunpaweravong S, Puttawibul P, et al. Epidermal growth factor receptor and cyclin D1 are independently amplified and overexpressed in esophageal squamous cell carcinoma. *J Cancer Res Clin Oncol*. 2005;131(2):111–119.
253. Hollstein MC, Smits AM, Galiana C, et al. Amplification of epidermal growth factor receptor gene but no evidence of ras mutations in primary human esophageal cancers. *Cancer Res*. 1988;48(18):5119–5123.
254. Ormandy CJ, Musgrove EA, Hui R, Daly RJ, Sutherland RL. Cyclin D1, EMS1 and 11q13 amplification in breast cancer. *Breast Cancer Res Treat*. 2003;78(3):323–335.
255. Cahill DP, Lengauer C, Yu J, et al. Mutations of mitotic checkpoint genes in human cancers. *Nature*. 1998;392(6673):300–303.
256. Bharadwaj R, Yu H. The spindle checkpoint, aneuploidy, and cancer. *Oncogene*. 2004;23(11):2016–2027.
257. Honda T, Tamura G, Waki T, Kawata S, Nishizuka S, Motoyama T. Promoter hypermethylation of the Chfr gene in neoplastic and non-neoplastic gastric epithelia. *Br J Cancer*. 2004;90(10):2013–2016.
258. Shibata Y, Haruki N, Kuwabara Y, et al. Chfr expression is down-regulated by CpG island hypermethylation in esophageal cancer. *Carcinogenesis*. 2002;23(10):1695–1699.
259. Corn PG, Summers MK, Fogt F, et al. Frequent hypermethylation of the 5' CpG island of the mitotic stress checkpoint gene Chfr in colorectal and non-small cell lung cancer. *Carcinogenesis*. 2003;24(1):47–51.
260. Li Y, Benezra R. Identification of a human mitotic checkpoint gene: hsMAD2. *Science*. 1996;274(5285):246–248.
261. Jin DY, Spencer F, Jeang KT. Human T cell leukemia virus type 1 oncoprotein Tax targets the human mitotic checkpoint protein MAD1. *Cell*. 1998;93(1):81–91.
262. Fodde R, Kuipers J, Rosenberg C, et al. Mutations in the APC tumour suppressor gene cause chromosomal instability. *Nat Cell Biol*. 2001;3(4):433–438.
263. Kaplan KB, Burds AA, Swedlow JR, Bekir SS, Sorger PK, Nathke IS. A role for the Adenomatous Polyposis Coli protein in chromosome segregation. *Nat Cell Biol*. 2001;3(4):429–432.
264. Wang Z, Cummins JM, Shen D, et al. Three classes of genes mutated in colorectal cancers with chromosomal instability. *Cancer Res*. 2004;64(9):2998–3001.
265. Ewart-Toland A, Briassouli P, de Koning JP, et al. Identification of Stk6/STK15 as a candidate low-penetrance tumor-susceptibility gene in mouse and human. *Nat Genet*. 2003;34(4):403–412.
266. Hermsen M, Postma C, Baak J, et al. Colorectal adenoma to carcinoma progression follows multiple pathways of chromosomal instability. *Gastroenterology*. 2002;123(4):1109–1119.
267. Engelhardt M, Drullinsky P, Guillem J, Moore MA. Telomerase and telomere length in the development and progression of premalignant lesions to colorectal cancer. *Clin Cancer Res*. 1997;3(11): 1931–1941.
268. Artandi SE, Chang S, Lee SL, et al. Telomere dysfunction promotes non-reciprocal translocations and epithelial cancers in mice. *Nature*. 2000;406(6796):641–645.
269. Lipton L, Halford SE, Johnson V, et al. Carcinogenesis in MYH-associated polyposis follows a distinct genetic pathway. *Cancer Res*. 2003;63(22):7595–7599.
270. Jass JR. Hyperplastic polyps and colorectal cancer: is there a link? *Clin Gastroenterol Hepatol*. 2004;2(1):1–8.
271. Jass JR, Whitehall VL, Young J, Leggett BA. Emerging concepts in colorectal neoplasia. *Gastroenterology*. 2002;123(3): 862–876.
272. Riccio A, Aaltonen LA, Godwin AK, et al. The DNA repair gene MBD4 (MED1) is mutated in human carcinomas with microsatellite instability. *Nat Genet*. 1999;23(3):266–268.
273. Petronzelli F, Riccio A, Markham GD, et al. Biphasic kinetics of the human DNA repair protein MED1 (MBD4), a mismatch-specific DNA N-glycosylase. *J Biol Chem*. 2000;275(42): 32422–32429.
274. Kambara T, Whitehall VL, Spring KJ, et al. Role of inherited defects of MYH in the development of sporadic colorectal cancer. *Genes Chromosomes Cancer*. 2004;40(1):1–9.
275. Bader S, Walker M, Hendrich B, et al. Somatic frameshift mutations in the MBD4 gene of sporadic colon cancers with mismatch repair deficiency. *Oncogene*. 1999;18(56):8044–8047.
276. Gerson SL. MGMT: its role in cancer aetiology and cancer therapeutics. *Nat Rev Cancer*. 2004;4(4):296–307.
277. Lind GE, Thorstensen L, Lovig T, et al. A CpG island hypermethylation profile of primary colorectal carcinomas and colon cancer cell lines. *Mol Cancer*. 2004;3(1):28.
278. Esteller M, Toyota M, Sanchez-Cespedes M, et al. Inactivation of the DNA repair gene O6-methylguanine-DNA methyltransferase by promoter hypermethylation is associated with G to A mutations in K-ras in colorectal tumorigenesis. *Cancer Res*. 2000;60(9): 2368–2371.
279. Nakamura M, Watanabe T, Yonekawa Y, Kleihues P, Ohgaki H. Promoter methylation of the DNA repair gene MGMT in astrocytomas is frequently associated with G:C -> A:T mutations of the TP53 tumor suppressor gene. *Carcinogenesis*. 2001;22(10): 1715–1719.
280. Park TJ, Han SU, Cho YK, Paik WK, Kim YB, Lim IK. Methylation of O(6)-methylguanine-DNA methyltransferase gene is associated significantly with K-ras mutation, lymph node invasion, tumor staging, and disease free survival in patients with gastric carcinoma. *Cancer*. 2001;92(11):2760–2768.
281. Feinberg AP, Tycko B. The history of cancer epigenetics. *Nat Rev Cancer*. 2004;4(2):143–153.
282. Feinberg AP, Vogelstein B. Hypomethylation distinguishes genes of some human cancers from their normal counterparts. *Nature*. 1983;301(5895):89–92.
283. Gama-Sosa MA, Slagel VA, Trewyn RW, et al. The 5-methylcytosine content of DNA from human tumors. *Nucleic Acids Res*. 1983;11(19):6883–6894.
284. Goelz SE, Vogelstein B, Hamilton SR, Feinberg AP. Hypomethylation of DNA from benign and malignant human colon neoplasms. *Science*. 1985;228(4696):187–190.
285. Feinberg AP, Gehrke CW, Kuo KC, Ehrlich M. Reduced genomic 5-methylcytosine content in human colonic neoplasia. *Cancer Res*. 1988;48(5):1159–1161.
286. Walsh CP, Chaillet JR, Bestor TH. Transcription of IAP endogenous retroviruses is constrained by cytosine methylation. *Nat Genet*. 1998;20(2):116–117.

287. Yoder JA, Walsh CP, Bestor TH. Cytosine methylation and the ecology of intragenomic parasites. *Trends Genet.* 1997;13(8): 335–340.
288. Baylin SB, Herman JG. DNA hypermethylation in tumorigenesis: epigenetics joins genetics. *Trends Genet.* 2000;16(4):168–174.
289. Li E. Chromatin modification and epigenetic reprogramming in mammalian development. *Nat Rev Genet.* 2002;3(9):662–673.
290. Reik W, Dean W, Walter J. Epigenetic reprogramming in mammalian development. *Science.* 2001;293(5532):1089–1093.
291. Tycko B. Epigenetic gene silencing in cancer. *J Clin Invest.* 2000;105(4):401–407.
292. Lund AH, van Lohuizen M. Epigenetics and cancer. *Genes Dev.* 2004;18(19):2315–2335.
293. Strathdee G. Epigenetic versus genetic alterations in the inactivation of E-cadherin. *Semin Cancer Biol.* 2002;12(5):373–379.
294. Nie Y, Liao J, Zhao X, et al. Detection of multiple gene hypermethylation in the development of esophageal squamous cell carcinoma. *Carcinogenesis.* 2002;23(10):1713–1720.
295. Cruz-Correa M, Cui H, Giardiello FM, et al. Loss of imprinting of insulin growth factor II gene: a potential heritable biomarker for colon neoplasia predisposition. *Gastroenterology.* 2004;126(4): 964–970.
296. Cui H, Onyango P, Brandenburg S, Wu Y, Hsieh CL, Feinberg AP. Loss of imprinting in colorectal cancer linked to hypomethylation of H19 and IGF2. *Cancer Res.* 2002;62(22):6442–6446.
297. Cunningham JM, Christensen ER, Tester DJ, et al. Hypermethylation of the hMLH1 promoter in colon cancer with microsatellite instability. *Cancer Res.* 1998;58(15):3455–3460.
298. Cravo M, Pinto R, Fidalgo P, et al. Global DNA hypomethylation occurs in the early stages of intestinal type gastric carcinoma. *Gut.* 1996;39(3):434–438.
299. Akiyama Y, Maesawa C, Ogasawara S, Terashima M, Masuda T. Cell-type-specific repression of the maspin gene is disrupted frequently by demethylation at the promoter region in gastric intestinal metaplasia and cancer cells. *Am J Pathol.* 2003;163(5): 1911–1919.
300. Oshimo Y, Nakayama H, Ito R, et al. Promoter methylation of cyclin D2 gene in gastric carcinoma. *Int J Oncol.* 2003;23(6): 1663–1670.
301. Yanagawa N, Tamura G, Honda T, Endoh M, Nishizuka S, Motoyama T. Demethylation of the synuclein gamma gene CpG island in primary gastric cancers and gastric cancer cell lines. *Clin Cancer Res.* 2004;10(7):2447–2451.
302. Nishigaki M, Aoyagi K, Danjoh I, et al. Discovery of aberrant expression of R-RAS by cancer-linked DNA hypomethylation in gastric cancer using microarrays. *Cancer Res.* 2005;65(6): 2115–2124.
303. Feinberg AP, Vogelstein B. Hypomethylation of ras oncogenes in primary human cancers. *Biochem Biophys Res Commun.* 1983; 111(1):47–54.
304. Nakamura N, Takenaga K. Hypomethylation of the metastasis-associated S100A4 gene correlates with gene activation in human colon adenocarcinoma cell lines. *Clin Exp Metastasis.* 1998; 16(5):471–479.
305. Miki Y, Nishisho I, Horii A, et al. Disruption of the APC gene by a retrotransposal insertion of L1 sequence in a colon cancer. *Cancer Res.* 1992;52(3):643–645.
306. Suter CM, Martin DI, Ward RL. Hypomethylation of L1 retrotransposons in colorectal cancer and adjacent normal tissue. *Int J Colorectal Dis.* 2004;19(2):95–101.
307. Karpinski P, Sasiadek MM, Blin N. Aberrant epigenetic patterns in the etiology of gastrointestinal cancers. *J Appl Genet.* 2008;49(1): 1–10.
308. Xu GL, Bestor TH, Bourc'his D, et al. Chromosome instability and immunodeficiency syndrome caused by mutations in a DNA methyltransferase gene. *Nature.* 1999;402(6758):187–191.
309. Okano M, Bell DW, Haber DA, Li E. DNA methyltransferases Dnmt3a and Dnmt3b are essential for de novo methylation and mammalian development. *Cell.* 1999;99(3):247–257.
310. Qu GZ, Grundy PE, Narayan A, Ehrlich M. Frequent hypomethylation in Wilms tumors of pericentromeric DNA in chromosomes 1 and 16. *Cancer Genet Cytogenet.* 1999;109(1):34–39.
311. Cohen D, Musch A. Apical surface formation in MDCK cells: regulation by the serine/threonine kinase EMK1. *Methods.* 2003;30(3):269–276.
312. Toyota M, Sasaki Y, Satoh A, et al. Epigenetic inactivation of CHFR in human tumors. *Proc Natl Acad Sci USA.* 2003;100(13): 7818–7823.
313. Jones PA, Baylin SB. The fundamental role of epigenetic events in cancer. *Nat Rev Genet.* 2002;3(6):415–428.
314. Rideout WM 3rd, Coetzee GA, Olumi AF, Jones PA. 5-Methylcytosine as an endogenous mutagen in the human LDL receptor and p53 genes. *Science.* 1990;249(4974):1288–1290.
315. Pfeifer GP. p53 mutational spectra and the role of methylated CpG sequences. *Mutat Res.* 2000;450(1–2):155–166.
316. Pfeifer GP, Tang M, Denissenko MF. Mutation hotspots and DNA methylation. *Curr Top Microbiol Immunol.* 2000;249:1–19.
317. Kondo Y, Issa JP. Epigenetic changes in colorectal cancer. *Cancer Metastasis Rev.* 2004;23(1–2):29–39.
318. Toyota M, Ahuja N, Ohe-Toyota M, Herman JG, Baylin SB, Issa JP. CpG island methylator phenotype in colorectal cancer. *Proc Natl Acad Sci USA.* 1999;96(15):8681–8686.
319. Issa JP, Ottaviano YL, Celano P, Hamilton SR, Davidson NE, Baylin SB. Methylation of the oestrogen receptor CpG island links ageing and neoplasia in human colon. *Nat Genet.* 1994;7(4):536–540.
320. Ueki T, Toyota M, Sohn T, et al. Hypermethylation of multiple genes in pancreatic adenocarcinoma. *Cancer Res.* 2000;60(7):1835–1839.
321. Esteller M, Cordon-Cardo C, Corn PG, et al. p14ARF silencing by promoter hypermethylation mediates abnormal intracellular localization of MDM2. *Cancer Res.* 2001;61(7):2816–2821.
322. Esteller M, Corn PG, Baylin SB, Herman JG. A gene hypermethylation profile of human cancer. *Cancer Res.* 2001;61(8):3225–3229.
323. Esteller M, Tortola S, Toyota M, et al. Hypermethylation-associated inactivation of p14(ARF) is independent of p16(INK4a) methylation and p53 mutational status. *Cancer Res.* 2000;60(1): 129–133.
324. Kuroki T, Trapasso F, Yendamuri S, et al. Allele loss and promoter hypermethylation of VHL, RAR-beta, RASSF1A, and FHIT tumor suppressor genes on chromosome 3p in esophageal squamous cell carcinoma. *Cancer Res.* 2003;63(13):3724–3728.
325. Kang GH, Shim YH, Jung HY, Kim WH, Ro JY, Rhyu MG. CpG island methylation in premalignant stages of gastric carcinoma. *Cancer Res.* 2001;61(7):2847–2851.
326. Xu XL, Yu J, Zhang HY, et al. Methylation profile of the promoter CpG islands of 31 genes that may contribute to colorectal carcinogenesis. *World J Gastroenterol.* 2004;10(23):3441–3454.
327. Tamura G, Sato K, Akiyama S, et al. Molecular characterization of undifferentiated-type gastric carcinoma. *Lab Invest.* 2001;81(4): 593–598.
328. Klein C, Pillot T, Chambaz J, Drouet B. Determination of plasma membrane fluidity with a fluorescent analogue of sphingomyelin by FRAP measurement using a standard confocal microscope. *Brain Res Brain Res Protoc.* 2003;11(1):46–51.
329. Ahuja N, Mohan AL, Li Q, et al. Association between CpG island methylation and microsatellite instability in colorectal cancer. *Cancer Res.* 1997;57(16):3370–3374.
330. Rashid A, Shen L, Morris JS, Issa JP, Hamilton SR. CpG island methylation in colorectal adenomas. *Am J Pathol.* 2001;159(3): 1129–1135.

331. Toyota M, Ohe-Toyota M, Ahuja N, Issa JP. Distinct genetic profiles in colorectal tumors with or without the CpG island methylator phenotype. *Proc Natl Acad Sci USA*. 2000;97(2): 710–715.
332. Iino H, Jass JR, Simms LA, et al. DNA microsatellite instability in hyperplastic polyps, serrated adenomas, and mixed polyps: a mild mutator pathway for colorectal cancer? *J Clin Pathol*. 1999;52(1):5–9.
333. Weisenberger DJ, Siegmund KD, Campan M, et al. CpG island methylator phenotype underlies sporadic microsatellite instability and is tightly associated with BRAF mutation in colorectal cancer. *Nat Genet*. 2006;38(7):787–793.
334. Zou GM. Cancer initiating cells or cancer stem cells in the gastrointestinal tract and liver. *J Cell Physiol*. 2008;217(3):598–604.
335. van der Flier LG, Clevers H. Stem cells, self-renewal, and differentiation in the intestinal epithelium. *Annu Rev Physiol*. 2009;71:241–260.
336. Hiyama E, Hiyama K. Telomere and telomerase in stem cells. *Br J Cancer*. 2007;96(7):1020–1024.
337. Barker N, Ridgway RA, van Es JH, et al. Crypt stem cells as the cells-of-origin of intestinal cancer. *Nature*. 2009;457(7229): 608–611.
338. Zhu L, Gibson P, Currle DS, et al. Prominin 1 marks intestinal stem cells that are susceptible to neoplastic transformation. *Nature*. 2009;457(7229):603–607.
339. Todaro M, Francipane MG, Medema JP, Stassi G. Colon cancer stem cells: promise of targeted therapy. *Gastroenterology*. 2010;138(6):2151–2162.
340. Takaishi S, Okumura T, Wang TC. Gastric cancer stem cells. *J Clin Oncol*. 2008;26(17):2876–2882.
341. Quintana E, Shackleton M, Sabel MS, Fullen DR, Johnson TM, Morrison SJ. Efficient tumour formation by single human melanoma cells. *Nature*. 2008;456(7222):593–598.
342. Lee R, Feinbaum R, Ambros V. A short history of a short RNA. *Cell*. 2004;116(2 Suppl):S89-S92. 81 p following S96.
343. Lee RC, Feinbaum RL, Ambros V. The C. elegans heterochronic gene lin-4 encodes small RNAs with antisense complementarity to lin-14. *Cell*. 1993;75(5):843–854.
344. Olsen PH, Ambros V. The lin-4 regulatory RNA controls developmental timing in Caenorhabditis elegans by blocking LIN-14 protein synthesis after the initiation of translation. *Dev Biol*. 1999;216(2):671–680.
345. Bagga S, Bracht J, Hunter S, et al. Regulation by let-7 and lin-4 miRNAs results in target mRNA degradation. *Cell*. 2005;122(4): 553–563.
346. Calin GA, Croce CM. MicroRNA signatures in human cancers. *Nat Rev Cancer*. 2006;6(11):857–866.
347. Ambros V. The functions of animal microRNAs. *Nature*. 2004;431(7006):350–355.
348. Bartel DP. MicroRNAs: genomics, biogenesis, mechanism, and function. *Cell*. 2004;116(2):281–297.
349. Pasquinelli AE, Hunter S, Bracht J. MicroRNAs: a developing story. *Curr Opin Genet Dev*. 2005;15(2):200–205.
350. Gregory RI, Chendrimada TP, Shiekhattar R. MicroRNA biogenesis: isolation and characterization of the microprocessor complex. *Methods Mol Biol*. 2006;342:33–47.
351. Rana TM. Illuminating the silence: understanding the structure and function of small RNAs. *Nat Rev Mol Cell Biol*. 2007;8(1): 23–36.
352. Ji X. The mechanism of RNase III action: how dicer dices. *Curr Top Microbiol Immunol*. 2008;320:99–116.
353. Brennecke J, Hipfner DR, Stark A, Russell RB, Cohen SM. bantam encodes a developmentally regulated microRNA that controls cell proliferation and regulates the proapoptotic gene hid in Drosophila. *Cell*. 2003;113(1):25–36.
354. Chen CZ, Li L, Lodish HF, Bartel DP. MicroRNAs modulate hematopoietic lineage differentiation. *Science*. 2004;303(5654): 83–86.
355. Fazi F, Rosa A, Fatica A, et al. A minicircuitry comprised of microRNA-223 and transcription factors NFI-A and C/EBPalpha regulates human granulopoiesis. *Cell*. 2005;123(5):819–831.
356. Chen JF, Mandel EM, Thomson JM, et al. The role of microRNA-1 and microRNA-133 in skeletal muscle proliferation and differentiation. *Nat Genet*. 2006;38(2):228–233.
357. Krichevsky AM, Sonntag KC, Isacson O, Kosik KS. Specific microRNAs modulate embryonic stem cell-derived neurogenesis. *Stem Cells*. 2006;24(4):857–864.
358. Esau C, Kang X, Peralta E, et al. MicroRNA-143 regulates adipocyte differentiation. *J Biol Chem*. 2004;279(50):52361–52365.
359. Cimmino A, Calin GA, Fabbri M, et al. miR-15 and miR-16 induce apoptosis by targeting BCL2. *Proc Natl Acad Sci USA*. 2005;102(39):13944–13949.
360. Chan JA, Krichevsky AM, Kosik KS. MicroRNA-21 is an antiapoptotic factor in human glioblastoma cells. *Cancer Res*. 2005;65(14):6029–6033.
361. He L, Thomson JM, Hemann MT, et al. A microRNA polycistron as a potential human oncogene. *Nature*. 2005;435(7043): 828–833.
362. Dews M, Homayouni A, Yu D, et al. Augmentation of tumor angiogenesis by a Myc-activated microRNA cluster. *Nat Genet*. 2006;38(9):1060–1065.
363. Calin GA, Dumitru CD, Shimizu M, et al. Frequent deletions and down-regulation of micro- RNA genes miR15 and miR16 at 13q14 in chronic lymphocytic leukemia. *Proc Natl Acad Sci USA*. 2002;99(24):15524–15529.
364. Tam W, Hughes SH, Hayward WS, Besmer P. Avian bic, a gene isolated from a common retroviral site in avian leukosis virus-induced lymphomas that encodes a noncoding RNA, cooperates with c-myc in lymphomagenesis and erythroleukemogenesis. *J Virol*. 2002;76(9):4275–4286.
365. Costinean S, Zanesi N, Pekarsky Y, et al. Pre-B cell proliferation and lymphoblastic leukemia/high-grade lymphoma in E(mu)-miR155 transgenic mice. *Proc Natl Acad Sci USA*. 2006;103(18): 7024–7029.
366. O'Donnell KA, Wentzel EA, Zeller KI, Dang CV, Mendell JT. C-Myc-regulated microRNAs modulate E2F1 expression. *Nature*. 2005;435(7043):839–843.
367. Volinia S, Calin GA, Liu CG, et al. A microRNA expression signature of human solid tumors defines cancer gene targets. *Proc Natl Acad Sci USA*. 2006;103(7):2257–2261.
368. Lu J, Getz G, Miska EA, et al. MicroRNA expression profiles classify human cancers. *Nature*. 2005;435(7043):834–838.
369. Garzon R, Pichiorri F, Palumbo T, et al. MicroRNA fingerprints during human megakaryocytopoiesis. *Proc Natl Acad Sci USA*. 2006;103(13):5078–5083.
370. Bandres E, Cubedo E, Agirre X, et al. Identification by Real-time PCR of 13 mature microRNAs differentially expressed in colorectal cancer and non-tumoral tissues. *Mol Cancer*. 2006;5:29.
371. Feber A, Xi L, Luketich JD, et al. MicroRNA expression profiles of esophageal cancer. *J Thorac Cardiovasc Surg*. 2008;135(2):255–260. discussion 260.
372. Kan T, Sato F, Ito T, et al. The miR-106b-25 polycistron, activated by genomic amplification, functions as an oncogene by suppressing p21 and Bim. *Gastroenterology*. 2009;136(5):1689–1700.
373. Maru DM, Singh RR, Hannah C, et al. MicroRNA-196a is a potential marker of progression during Barrett's metaplasia-dysplasia-invasive adenocarcinoma sequence in esophagus. *Am J Pathol*. 2009;174(5):1940–1948.
374. Mathe EA, Nguyen GH, Bowman ED, et al. MicroRNA expression in squamous cell carcinoma and adenocarcinoma of the

esophagus: associations with survival. *Clin Cancer Res.* 2009;15(19):6192–6200.

375. Watson DI, Wijnhoven BP, Michael MZ, Mayne GC, Hussey DJ. Hp24 microRNA expression profiles in barrett's oesophagus. *ANZ J Surg.* 2007;77(Suppl 1):45.
376. Asangani IA, Rasheed SA, Nikolova DA, et al. MicroRNA-21 (miR-21) post-transcriptionally downregulates tumor suppressor Pdcd4 and stimulates invasion, intravasation and metastasis in colorectal cancer. *Oncogene.* 2008;27(15):2128–2136.
377. Krichevsky AM, Gabriely G. miR-21: a small multi-faceted RNA. *J Cell Mol Med.* 2009;13(1):39–53.
378. Smith CM, Watson DI, Michael MZ, Hussey DJ. MicroRNAs, development of Barrett's esophagus, and progression to esophageal adenocarcinoma. *World J Gastroenterol.* 2010;16(5):531–537.
379. Hino K, Tsuchiya K, Fukao T, et al. Inducible expression of microRNA-194 is regulated by HNF-1alpha during intestinal epithelial cell differentiation. *RNA.* 2008;14(7):1433–1442.
380. Mees ST, Mardin WA, Wendel C, et al. EP300–a miRNA-regulated metastasis suppressor gene in ductal adenocarcinomas of the pancreas. *Int J Cancer.* 2010;126(1):114–124.
381. Michael MZ, O'Connor SM, van Holst Pellekaan NG, Young GP, James RJ. Reduced accumulation of specific microRNAs in colorectal neoplasia. *Mol Cancer Res.* 2003;1(12):882–891.
382. Akao Y, Nakagawa Y, Naoe T. MicroRNAs 143 and 145 are possible common onco-microRNAs in human cancers. *Oncol Rep.* 2006;16(4):845–850.
383. Akao Y, Nakagawa Y, Naoe T. MicroRNA-143 and −145 in colon cancer. *DNA Cell Biol.* 2007;26(5):311–320.
384. Balaguer F, Link A, Lozano JJ, et al. Epigenetic silencing of miR-137 is an early event in colorectal carcinogenesis. *Cancer Res.* 2010;70(16):6609–6618.
385. Thomson JM, Newman M, Parker JS, Morin-Kensicki EM, Wright T, Hammond SM. Extensive post-transcriptional regulation of microRNAs and its implications for cancer. *Genes Dev.* 2006;20(16):2202–2207.
386. Karube Y, Tanaka H, Osada H, et al. Reduced expression of Dicer associated with poor prognosis in lung cancer patients. *Cancer Sci.* 2005;96(2):111–115.
387. Tchernitsa O, Kasajima A, Schafer R, et al. Systematic evaluation of the miRNA-ome and its downstream effects on mRNA expression identifies gastric cancer progression. *J Pathol.* 2010;222: 310–319.
388. Calin GA, Sevignani C, Dumitru CD, et al. Human microRNA genes are frequently located at fragile sites and genomic regions involved in cancers. *Proc Natl Acad Sci USA.* 2004;101(9): 2999–3004.
389. Zhang L, Huang J, Yang N, et al. microRNAs exhibit high frequency genomic alterations in human cancer. *Proc Natl Acad Sci USA.* 2006;103(24):9136–9141.
390. Iorio MV, Ferracin M, Liu CG, et al. MicroRNA gene expression deregulation in human breast cancer. *Cancer Res.* 2005;65(16): 7065–7070.

Part II

Epithelial Neoplastic Disease

2 Targeted Therapies and Molecular Diagnostics of Gastrointestinal Cancers

Davendra Sohal, Antonia R. Sepulveda, and Weijing Sun

Introduction

Clinical applications of genomic medicine and molecular diagnostics based on testing of tumor tissues are becoming a reality in clinical practice, with significant impact on personalized therapies for cancer patients. Advances in targeted therapies for cancers of the gastrointestinal tract have recently emerged and are rapidly moving targets. In this chapter, we review the targeted therapies that are currently standard of practice in colorectal and gastric cancers, requiring specific molecular testing for selection of candidate patients for therapy.

Gastric and Gastroesophageal Cancers

EGFR Pathways

The epidermal growth factor receptor (EGFR) family of transmembrane receptor tyrosine kinases includes four members: HER1 (also known as the EGFR and ErbB-1), HER2 (p185, HER2/neu, ErbB-2), HER3 (ErbB-3), and HER4 (ErbB-4). The molecular structures of EGFRs comprise an extracellular ligand-binding domain, a short transmembrane domain, and an intracellular domain with tyrosine kinase (TK) activity, except HER3. The binding of different ligands, including epidermal growth factor (EGF) and TGF-alpha to the extracellular domain, initiates a signal transduction cascade that elicits cell cycle progression, cell proliferation, anti-apoptotic signals, and survival, adhesion, migration, and differentiation.[1] Ligand binding to the EGFR extracellular domain induces EGFR homodimerization as well as heterodimerization with other types of HER proteins. HER2 does not bind to any known ligand, but it is the preferred heterodimerization partner for other members of the HER family. Ligand binding to EGFR followed by dimerization results in phosphorylation of the intracellular tyrosine kinase which triggers a series of intracellular signals including the activation of mitogen-activated kinase (MAPK): (KRAS/NRAS/RAF/MEK/ERK) or the phosphatidylinositol-3 kinase (PI3K) (PI3K/PTEN/AKT/mTOR) pathways (reviewed in[2]; Fig. 2.1).

Targeting HER2 Receptors

The human epidermal growth factor receptor 2 (Her2 or ErbB-2) was first described in gastric cancer in 1986.[3] HER2 has no known ligand (orphan receptor), and preferentially heterodimerizes with HER3, which lacks intrinsic tyrosine kinase activity. The HER2 and the HER2/HER3 heterodimers are likely to be the most effective complex for activating downstream pathways.[4,5]

Overexpression and amplification of HER2 have been described in 6–35% of gastric and gastroesophageal junction (GEJ) adenocarcinomas.[6-9] Up to about a third of all GEJ adenocarcinomas and a quarter of non-GEJ gastric cancers have HER2 overexpression.

Importantly, as in breast cancer, HER2 overexpression has been linked to prognosis in gastric cancer. An early Japanese study showed 5-year survival rates of 11% and 50% for HER2-positive vs. HER2-negative gastric cancer, respectively.[10] Another study showed that HER2 was an independent prognostic marker in resected gastric cancer, and overall survival was significantly associated with HER2

D. Sohal, M.D., M.P.H.
Solid Tumor Oncology, Taussig Cancer Institute, Cleveland Clinic, 9500 Euclid Avenue, R35 Cleveland, OH 44195, USA
e-mail: sohald@ccf.org

A.R. Sepulveda, M.D., Ph.D.
Department of Pathology & Cell Biology, Columbia University, 630 W 168th Street, VC-14 RM 212, New York, NY 10032, USA
e-mail: as4400@columbia.edu

W. Sun, M.D. (✉)
Department of Medicine, Hematology-Oncology, University of Pittsburgh School of Medicine, UPMC Cancer Pavilion, 5150 Centre Avenue, Fifth Floor, Pittsburgh, PA 15232, USA
e-mail: sunw@upmc.edu

A.R. Sepulveda and J.P. Lynch (eds.), *Molecular Pathology of Neoplastic Gastrointestinal Diseases*, Molecular Pathology Library 7,
DOI 10.1007/978-1-4614-6015-2_2,

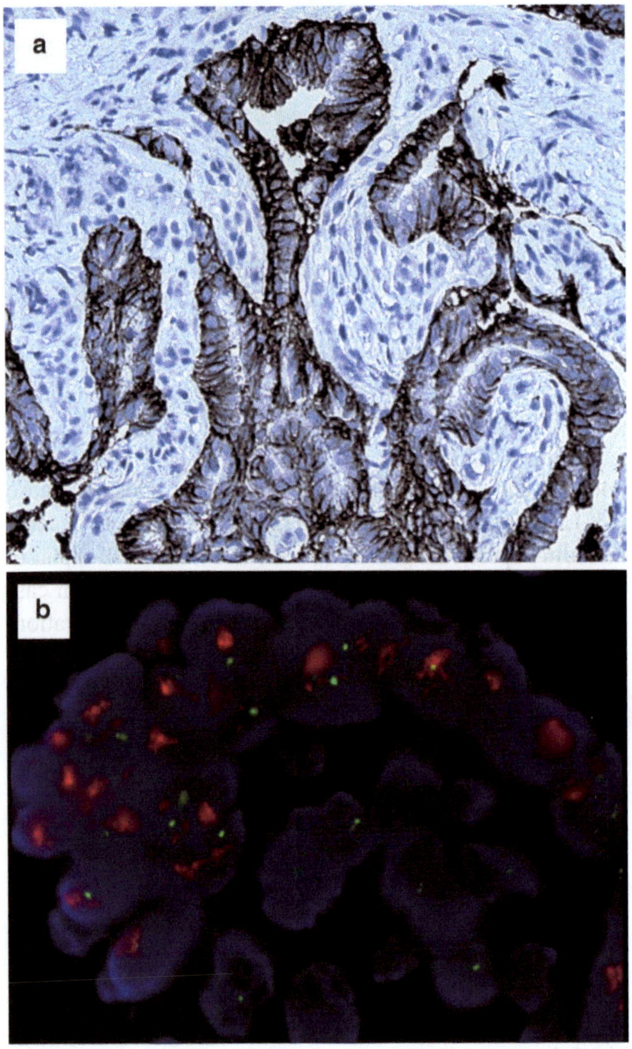

Fig. 2.1 Immunohistochemistry and FISH for HER2 in gastric adenocarcinoma. (**a**) Immunohistochemistry for HER2 shows a positive (3+) moderately differentiated adenocarcinoma. (**b**) FISH analysis reveals positive HER2 amplification by FISH (*red dots*). Courtesy of Dr. Paul Zhang MD, University of Pennsylvania

expression levels.[8] HER2/neu-positivity rates have been reported to be more frequent in intestinal type gastric cancer (21.5%) than in diffuse gastric cancer (2%) or mixed types (5%).[6] Overall, HER2/neu amplification in gastric carcinoma is associated with poor outcome[6,11] and has been shown to be an independent prognostic factor.[12]

Trastuzumab is a monoclonal antibody that specifically targets HER2 protein by directly binding the extracellular domain of the receptor. Trastuzumab enhances survival rates in both primary and metastatic HER2-positive breast cancer patients. The efficacy of trastuzumab in breast cancer has led to investigation of its antitumor activity in patients with other HER2-positive cancers, including gastric and GEJ adenocarcinomas. In preclinical studies, treatment with trastuzumab inhibited growth of gastric cancer cell lines.[6] Based on the preclinical data in gastric cancer and clinical evidence in breast cancer, early phase trials of trastuzumab in metastatic gastric cancer wherein tumors overexpressed HER2 were conducted and the antibody therapy was shown to confer improved clinical outcomes. Thereafter, a large randomized phase 3 clinical trial (the ToGA trial) was concluded, definitively establishing the utility of targeting HER2 in advanced gastric cancer.[13] In this study, metastatic gastric or gastroesophageal adenocarcinoma cases where the tumor overexpressed HER2 were randomized to receive standard chemotherapy (a fluoropyrimidine [5-fluorouracil or capecitabine] and platinum combination) with or without trastuzumab.[13] Overall survival was improved in the trastuzumab arm, with little added toxicity. Median overall survival was 13.8 months in those assigned to trastuzumab plus chemotherapy compared with 11.1 months in those assigned to chemotherapy alone (HR 0.74, $p=0.0046$). Therefore, testing HER2 and adding trastuzumab to the chemotherapy regimen for HER2-positive tumors have become the standard of care for advanced gastric adenocarcinoma. In this trial, a HER2 scoring system modified from the protocol in breast cancer was used: a score of immunohistochemistry (IHC) 3+ and/or fluorescent in situ hybridization (FISH) positive (HER2:CEP17 ratio ≥2) was defined as HER2 positive. The study reported an overall HER2-positivity rate of 22.1% evaluated from 3,665 patients.[13] An example of HER2-positive tumor by IHC and FISH is shown in Fig. 2.1.

Criteria for interpretation of HER2 modified for gastric and GEJ adenocarcinoma have been recently reviewed.[14–19] Studies have shown good correlation of HER2 expression in primary vs. metastatic carcinoma lesions.[20] Notably, HER2 overexpression is already observed in early gastric cancers.[21] Heterogeneity of HER2 expression occurs frequently in gastric and GEJ adenocarcinoma; however, testing is often done in biopsies when no resection specimen is available.[16] The College of American Pathologists (CAP) reviewed current guidelines for interpretation of HER2 expression.[13,14,19,22] Importantly, criteria for interpreting HER2 IHC on gastric and GEJ carcinomas differ significantly from the criteria used in breast cancer. First, gastric carcinoma interpretation criteria use 10% tumor cell staining as a cutoff to distinguish negative from 1+. In gastric carcinoma, the distinction between 1+, 2+, and 3+ depends on the intensity of staining presuming that more than 10% of tumor cells show HER2 expression (Table 2.1). Second, gastric cancers only show expression along the basolateral or lateral cell membranes, while apical membranes are negative. Therefore, the criteria for 2+ and 3+ staining in gastric cancer require only lateral

Table 2.1 Criteria for scoring and reporting HER2 expression in gastric and esophageal adenocarcinomas by immunohistochemistry

Staining pattern Resection specimen	Biopsy specimen	HER2 expression Interpretation
No reactivity or membranous reactivity in <10% of tumor cells	No reactivity in any tumor cell	Negative
Faint or barely detected membranous reactivity in ≥10% tumor cells Cells are reactive only in part of their membrane	Tumor cell cluster of ≥5 cells with faint or barely detected membranous reactivity irrespective of percentage of tumor cells stained	Negative
Weak to moderate complete, basolateral, or lateral membranous reactivity in ≥10% tumor cells	Tumor cell cluster of ≥5 cells with weak to moderate complete, basolateral, or lateral membranous reactivity irrespective of percentage of tumor cells stained	Equivocal
Strong complete, basolateral, or lateral membranous reactivity in 10% or more of tumor cells	Tumor cell cluster of ≥5 cells with strong complete, basolateral, or lateral membranous reactivity irrespective of percentage of tumor cells stained	Positive

FISH testing for *HER2* gene amplification should be performed when the IHC is equivocal (2+). Modified from the College of American Pathologists (CAP) web site[78] and based on studies reported by[13,22]

or basolateral staining, in contrast to breast cancer criteria which require complete, circumferential staining. Third, the criteria for HER2 overexpression differ when interpreting biopsy and resection specimens due to heterogeneity of HER2 expression in gastric and gastroesophageal junction carcinomas (Table 2.1).

Colon Cancer

Molecular Testing of Colorectal Cancers for Targeted and Conventional Therapy

Molecular testing of colorectal cancer (CRC) tissues has important implications for treatment selection in these patients. We will discuss recently introduced therapy approaches that use information from molecular testing of CRC tumor tissues for selection of individualized therapy, representing the principles of personalized tumor diagnostics and targeted therapy. One application of tissue molecular testing discussed here considers the DNA mismatch repair status of CRC and takes into consideration the mutational status of the EGFR signaling pathway to select targeted therapy.

DNA Mismatch Repair Defects and Microsatellite Instability

Approximately 15% of all CRCs show underlying defects in DNA mismatch repair (dMMR) and the tumor tissues show microsatellite instability (MSI), discussed in detail in Chaps. 1, 7, and 8. In 3–5% of MSI-positive CRC patients harbor germline mutations related to the Lynch syndrome and the remaining 12% or so are sporadic-type CRC cases.[23] Microsatellites are short tandem repeats of nucleotides that occur throughout the genome. In cells with deficient mismatch repair, errors in DNA replication accumulate and are detectable in these regions, identified as microsatellite instability (MSI).[24–26] Therefore, MSI, particularly when a tumor is identified to have a high level of MSI (MSI-H), acts as a marker of deficient MMR.[24] MSI-positive status correlated with the tumors being in the proximal colon and with improved survival.[26] This was soon followed by the identification of the genes responsible for hereditary nonpolyposis colorectal cancer (HNPCC) *MSH2*[27,28] and *MLH1*.[29,30] Subsequently, MSI has been shown to play a role in sporadic colorectal cancers also.[31] In humans, at least six different genes (*MSH2*, *MLH1*, *PMS1*, *hPMS2*, *MSH6*, and *MLH3*) encode the mismatch repair system.[32] In hereditary defects, recessive mutation of one allele followed by somatic inactivation of the other is the mechanism of gene silencing.[33] In sporadic CRC cases, the most prevalent mechanism of MMR gene inactivation is biallelic inactivation by methylation and transcriptional silencing of the *MLH1* promoter region.[34–39] Assessment of MSI status can be done by immunohistochemistry to evaluate expression of DNA mismatch repair proteins or by PCR-based DNA testing for MSI to assess instability at microsatellite sequences.[24,40] Combining testing for *BRAF* V600E activating mutation and CpG island methylation status of the promoter region of *MLH1* gene helps determine whether a MSI-positive tumor with loss of *MLH1* expression is likely to be an inherited Lynch syndrome/HNPCC tumor (*BRAF* mutation-negative and *MLH1* promoter methylation-negative) or sporadic-type CRC (*BRAF* mutation-positive in up to 70% of cases and *MLH1* promoter methylation-positive) (reviewed in Chap. 7).

An interesting aspect of MSI is its distinct relationship to colorectal cancer behavior. It was shown in a large series that MSI occurs in 17% of colon cancer cases in young (less than 50 years) individuals and this MSI was associated with a lower likelihood of tumor metastasis to regional lymph nodes as well as distant organs, leading to an overall survival advantage, independent of stage of disease.[41] Another study reported that MSI-H tumors were more likely than MSI-low level tumors to be in younger individuals, right-sided, poorly differentiated with mucin production, and with an overall better prognosis.[42] In addition to being a prognostic marker, MSI has a predictive role also.[43] While earlier studies did not bear this out,[44] improved outcomes were seen with chemotherapy for advanced stage III colorectal cancers that were MSI-H.[45] However, another study showed that patients with stage II tumors characterized by deficient DNA mismatch repair and therefore an MSI-positive status receiving fluorouracil (5-FU) had no improvement in disease-free survival, and in fact, treatment was associated with reduced overall survival.[46] Larger trials are needed to determine with certainty the utility of these markers for treatment selection in routine patient care.[47] However, regimens with 5-FU alone should be avoided in patients with stage II CRC who may be candidates for chemotherapy.

Targeting EGFR Signaling Pathways in CRC

Aberrant activation of EGRF signaling pathways is frequent in CRC, and is primarily associated with activating mutations of genes in these pathways (MAPK and PI3K). Tyrosine kinase inhibitors targeting the intracellular domain of the EGFR, namely erlotinib and gefitinib, have not been shown to have meaningful clinical efficacy in this disease, given that activating mutations in the *EGFR* gene are not a feature of CRC.[48,49] Based on data in the literature, the following are the proportions of cases harboring various mutations in EGFR pathway genes[50]: MAPKinase pathway: *KRAS* (40–45%), *NRAS* (2.5%), *BRAF* (5–10%); PI3Kinase pathway: *PIK3CA* (15%), *PTEN* (10–20%), *AKT* (5%); and combined mutations: *KRAS/NRAS* and *PI3K* (10%). An interesting finding is that in CRC as in other tumors, *RAS* and *RAF* mutations are mutually exclusive.[51,52] Therefore, together, *BRAF* and *KRAS* are mutated in about half of all CRC cases.

KRAS mutations are found in about 40–45% of all colorectal cancers and occur mostly at exon 2 [codon 12 (70–80%) or 13 (20–30%)], while there are rare mutations in codons 61 and 146.[53] *BRAF* mutations occur most commonly at exon 15 with thymine to adenine transversion at nucleotide position 1796, which leads to the substitution of valine for glutamate (a substitution mutation termed V600E), and are found in about 5–10% of all colorectal cancers[50]. Importantly *BRAF* V600E mutation occurs in 4–12% of DNA mismatch repair proficient tumors (microsatellite stable) and in 40–74% of MSI-H sporadic CRC (MLH1-deficient), but is not found in MLH1-deficient MSI-H CRC in HNPCC/Lynch syndrome-associated CRC.[51,54,55]

Mutations in the PI3K axis are seen in about 20% of all colorectal cancer cases.[50,51] Interestingly, mutations across the two EGFR signaling axes are not mutually exclusive, and about 5% of tumors harbor mutations in genes from both arms of the pathway.[51]

The role of EGFR pathway gene mutations in the clinical management of colorectal cancer has been extensively studied. In terms of prognosis, *KRAS* mutations do not confer a poor prognosis by themselves, probably because they appear very early in cancer development.[56–58] However, *BRAF* mutations confer a significantly poorer prognosis, as compared to wild-type *BRAF* tumors. It is still early to say if PI3K axis mutations play a prognostic role in CRC.[56,57]

More importantly, the EGFR pathway has become an important therapeutic target. Cetuximab and panitumumab are anti-EGFR antibodies that target the extracellular domain of the receptor. They have been shown to improve progression-free, and in some cases, overall survival in metastatic colorectal cancer.[59] A landmark paper by Karapetis et al published in 2008 showed that in patients with wild-type *KRAS* tumors, treatment with cetuximab as compared with supportive care alone significantly improved overall survival (median, 9.5 vs. 4.8 months). In contrast, among patients with mutated *KRAS* tumors, there was no significant difference between those who were treated with cetuximab and those who were not. This study concluded that patients with a colorectal tumor bearing mutated *KRAS* did not benefit from cetuximab, whereas patients with wild-type *KRAS* CRC did benefit from cetuximab therapy.[60] *KRAS* mutations render these agents ineffective, because activated KRAS is downstream of EGFR and constitutive activation of the former leads to independence from the latter[51,60] (Fig. 2.2). Therefore, given evidence from phase II and III clinical trials using monoclonal antibodies as monotherapy or in combination with chemotherapy for metastatic CRC (Stage IV: any T, any N, M1) that tumors with *KRAS* mutation in codons 12, 13, or 61 did not benefit from treatment with cetuximab or panitumumab,[61] patients with metastatic CRC who are candidates for anti-EGFR antibody therapy should have their tumor tested for *KRAS* mutations in a CLIA-accredited laboratory.[61] There is up to 40% response rate to anti-EGFR therapy in wild-type CRC while the remainder 60% wild-type tumors will not respond, presumably due to other gene/protein alterations in the EGFR or other signaling pathways.[61]

For CRC with an activated mutant *KRAS*, a number of drugs that may inhibit downstream signaling molecules (such as inhibitors of mTOR, RAF, and MEK) are under evaluation[62] (Fig. 2.2). The predictive role of *BRAF* mutational studies in CRC is still unclear. While *BRAF* activating mutations should act similar to *KRAS* in terms of predicting

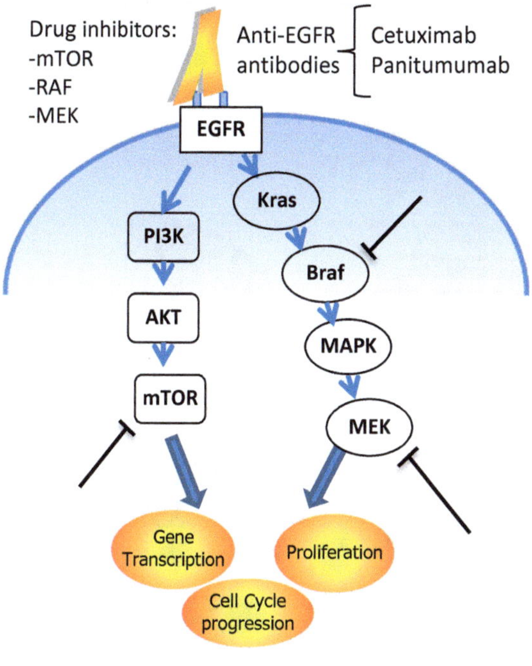

Fig. 2.2 EGFR signaling pathways: mutation targets and targeted therapies

response to EGFR antibody therapy, the markedly poor prognosis that a *BRAF* mutation confers, along with the relatively low proportion of cases with *BRAF* mutations in clinical trials, makes it difficult to assess this role clearly.[57] Although *BRAF* inhibitors have been tested in early studies, larger trials are needed to determine if colorectal cancer will respond to these agents in a manner similar to what is now seen in melanoma.[63] It has been demonstrated recently that colon cancer cells, in contrast to melanoma cells, are unresponsive to the BRAF inhibitor vemurafenib by employing rapid feedback activation of EGFR, which neutralizes the benefit of vemurafenib.[64] Therefore, a dual strategy of targeting BRAF and EGFR may be needed to effect clinical responses in BRAF-mutant CRC.

Preclinical data have shown that a *PIK3CA* or *PTEN* mutation (which leads to constitutive activation of the PI3K pathway) causes resistance of cancer cells to cetuximab.[65] Indirect evidence stems from preclinical work showing that *PIK3CA* mutation uncouples cell proliferation signaling from the KRAS pathway, leading to failure of inhibitors targeting the MAPK axis.[66] Initially, small studies showed conflicting roles of *PIK3CA* mutation in response to EGFR antibodies,[67,68], but a recent large study has demonstrated that *PIK3CA* mutation is associated with poor response to cetuximab.[51] Preclinical models indicate that in these tumors, inhibition of the PI3K axis may be required to achieve cancer control. Blocking the PI3K pathway in cancer cells with activating *PI3KCA* mutations has been shown to inhibit cell growth and induce apoptosis.[69,70] A study by de Roock et al found that *BRAF*, *NRAS*, and *PIK3CA* exon 20 mutations are significantly associated with a low response rate to cetuximab targeted therapy, in that objective response rates could be improved by stratifying patients by additional genotyping of *BRAF*, *NRAS*, and *PIK3CA* exon 20 mutations in a *KRAS* wild-type population.[51,71]

In addition, when mutations in both EGFR pathway axes exist, dual inhibition with MEK and AKT/PI3K inhibitors is required to control cell growth.[70,72] Thus, work is ongoing on various inhibitors of these signal transduction molecules to see if collective inhibition of some or all constitutively activated genes will achieve clinical benefit.

Molecular Testing for CRC Targeted Therapies

EGFR mutational testing is not indicated for CRC since activating *EGFR* mutations in CRC are rare and do not confer sensitivity to tyrosine kinase inhibitors or to cetuximab therapy.[73] Further, EGFR IHC is not warranted for selection or exclusion of patients for cetuximab therapy, as it was observed that cetuximab shows activity in CRC patients with tumors that do not express the epidermal growth factor receptor by IHC.[74] Currently, the standard of practice for selection of CRC patients with metastatic disease who are candidates for targeted therapies with anti-EGFR antibodies is primarily based on mutational status of *KRAS*.[61] The mutational status of *BRAF*, *NRAS*, *PI3KCA*, and other genes downstream of EGFR may affect response to anti-EGFR targeted therapy.[71] Therefore, testing for mutations in these genes may be indicated in candidate patients, particularly in the setting of clinical trials, at the present time.

Interestingly, in contrast to other activating mutations in *KRAS*, use of cetuximab among patients with chemotherapy-refractory colorectal cancer with the *KRAS* G13D mutation may be associated with longer overall and progression-free survival,[52] although this remains a matter of debate.

Regarding the choice of tissue for DNA mutational analysis, since *KRAS* mutations occur early in colorectal carcinogenesis, most clinical trials tested the primary tumor site and published studies showed good correlation between *KRAS* mutation status in primary vs. metastatic colon cancer lesions with high average concordance of 93% (76–100%).[75,76] Therefore testing tumor tissue from the primary site or from metastatic lesions is appropriate. Pathologists should select a block of formalin-fixed, paraffin-embedded (FFPE) tissue with the highest % of viable tumor and largest tumor area

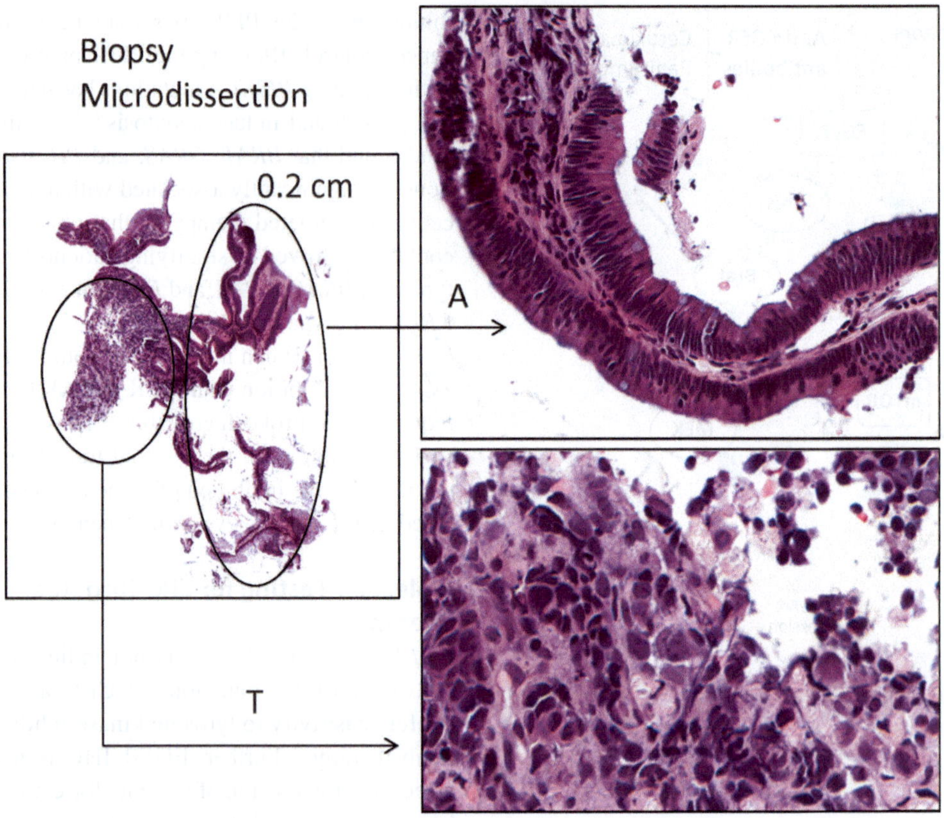

Fig. 2.3 Tissue microdissection from a small CRC biopsy sample (0.2 cm). Two tissue areas, *T* tumor, *A* adenoma, were separately marked to enrich the tumor area for DNA extraction. Microdissection was then performed using unstained slides matching the H&E stained guide slide, shown in the figure

possible. Individual laboratories may have different requirements depending on the assay used. The technical approaches for mutational testing vary widely among laboratories and follow requirements for validation and interpretation, particularly for laboratory developed tests. Such methods include Sanger sequencing, allele-specific PCR, melt curve analysis, pyrosequencing, fluorescent bead detection assay, MassARRAY MALDI-TOF mass spectrometry, and newer next-generation deep sequencing approaches.

Adequate DNA amount can be obtained by pooling macro- or micro-dissected tissue from multiple tissue levels (Fig. 2.3). Importantly, a biopsy may be preferable to the resection specimen if the resection was done after neoadjuvant therapy (Fig. 2.4), and minimal numbers of residual tumor cells persist, making the tissue inadequate for molecular testing.

In summary, *KRAS* mutational analysis of CRC tumor tissues is recommended as the standard of care in patients who are candidates for targeted anti-EGFR antibody therapy. Additional mutational testing of other EGFR pathway genes may be helpful to better select patients for targeted therapies with improved outcomes, as suggested by published studies, but a general consensus about which genes should be tested is not yet established. In large practice centers, the trend is to test all colorectal adenocarcinomas for *KRAS* codon 12–13 mutations, for *BRAF* V600E mutations, and for microsatellite instability, thus allowing for selection of patients for conventional therapy as well as targeted therapy.[77]

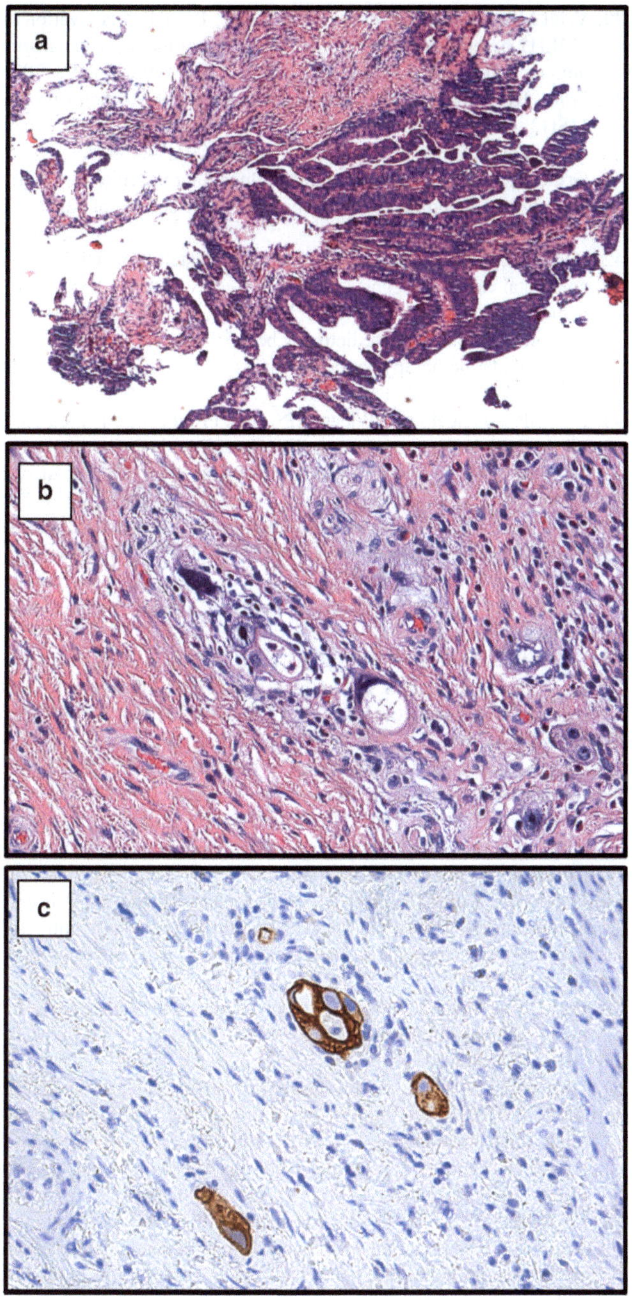

Fig. 2.4 Selection of CRC tissue specimen for DNA extraction and mutational analysis. A pretreatment small biopsy (**a**) with representative CRC was used for DNA testing in a patient with rectal cancer who received neoadjuvant therapy. *Panels* (**b**) and (**c**) represent rare residual tumor cells in the resection specimen. The limited number of tumor cells embedded in the background of fibrous tissue and muscularis rendered the resection specimen inadequate for molecular testing due to insufficient tumor cellularity

References

1. Lurje G, Lenz HJ. EGFR signaling and drug discovery. *Oncology*. 2009;77:400–10.
2. Arkenau HT. Gastric cancer in the era of molecularly targeted agents: current drug development strategies. *J Cancer Res Clin Oncol*. 2009;135:855–66.
3. Sakai K, Mori S, Kawamoto T, et al. Expression of epidermal growth factor receptors on normal human gastric epithelia and gastric carcinomas. *J Natl Cancer Inst*. 1986;77:1047–52.
4. Srinivasan R, Leverton KE, Sheldon H, Hurst HC, Sarraf C, Gullick WJ. Intracellular expression of the truncated extracellular domain of c-erbB-3/HER3. *Cell Signal*. 2001;13:321–30.
5. Hirata A, Hosoi F, Miyagawa M, et al. HER2 overexpression increases sensitivity to gefitinib, an epidermal growth factor receptor tyrosine kinase inhibitor, through inhibition of HER2/HER3 heterodimer formation in lung cancer cells. *Cancer Res*. 2005;65:4253–60.
6. Tanner M, Hollmen M, Junttila TT, et al. Amplification of HER-2 in gastric carcinoma: association with Topoisomerase IIalpha gene amplification, intestinal type, poor prognosis and sensitivity to trastuzumab. *Ann Oncol*. 2005;16:273–8.
7. Gravalos C, Jimeno A. HER2 in gastric cancer: a new prognostic factor and a novel therapeutic target. *Ann Oncol*. 2008;19:1523–9.
8. Allgayer H, Babic R, Gruetzner KU, Tarabichi A, Schildberg FW, Heiss MM. c-erbB-2 is of independent prognostic relevance in gastric cancer and is associated with the expression of tumor-associated protease systems. *J Clin Oncol*. 2000;18:2201–9.
9. Yano T, Doi T, Ohtsu A, et al. Comparison of HER2 gene amplification assessed by fluorescence in situ hybridization and HER2 protein expression assessed by immunohistochemistry in gastric cancer. *Oncol Rep*. 2006;15:65–71.
10. Yonemura Y, Ninomiya I, Ohoyama S, et al. Expression of c-erbB-2 oncoprotein in gastric carcinoma. Immunoreactivity for c-erbB-2 protein is an independent indicator of poor short-term prognosis in patients with gastric carcinoma. *Cancer*. 1991;67:2914–8.
11. Ananiev J, Gulubova M, Manolova I, Tchernev G. Prognostic significance of HER2/neu expression in gastric cancer. *Wien Klin Wochenschr*. 2011;123:450–4.
12. Park DI, Yun JW, Park JH, et al. HER-2/neu amplification is an independent prognostic factor in gastric cancer. *Dig Dis Sci*. 2006;51:1371–9.
13. Bang YJ, Van Cutsem E, Feyereislova A, et al. Trastuzumab in combination with chemotherapy versus chemotherapy alone for treatment of HER2-positive advanced gastric or gastro-oesophageal junction cancer (ToGA): a phase 3, open-label, randomised controlled trial. *Lancet*. 2010;376:687–97.
14. Ruschoff J, Hanna W, Bilous M, et al. HER2 testing in gastric cancer: a practical approach. *Mod Pathol*. 2012;25(5):637–50.
15. Mrklic I, Bendic A, Kunac N, et al. Her-2/neu assessment for gastric carcinoma: validation of scoring system. *Hepatogastroenterology*. 2012;59:300–3.
16. Kim MA, Lee HJ, Yang HK, Bang YJ, Kim WH. Heterogeneous amplification of ERBB2 in primary lesions is responsible for the discordant ERBB2 status of primary and metastatic lesions in gastric carcinoma. *Histopathology*. 2011;59:822–31.

17. Giuffre G, Ieni A, Barresi V, Caruso RA, Tuccari G. HER2 status in unusual histological variants of gastric adenocarcinomas. *J Clin Pathol*. 2012;65:237–41.
18. Park YS, Hwang HS, Park HJ, et al. Comprehensive analysis of HER2 expression and gene amplification in gastric cancers using immunohistochemistry and in situ hybridization: which scoring system should we use? *Hum Pathol*. 2012;43:413–22.
19. Hofmann M, Stoss O, Shi D, et al. Assessment of a HER2 scoring system for gastric cancer: results from a validation study. *Histopathology*. 2008;52:797–805.
20. Bozzetti C, Negri FV, Lagrasta CA, et al. Comparison of HER2 status in primary and paired metastatic sites of gastric carcinoma. *Br J Cancer*. 2011;104:1372–6.
21. Moelans CB, Milne AN, Morsink FH, Offerhaus GJ, van Diest PJ. Low frequency of HER2 amplification and overexpression in early onset gastric cancer. *Cell Oncol (Dordr)*. 2011;34:89–95.
22. Ruschoff J, Dietel M, Baretton G, et al. HER2 diagnostics in gastric cancer-guideline validation and development of standardized immunohistochemical testing. *Virchows Arch*. 2010;457: 299–307.
23. de la Chapelle A, Hampel H. Clinical relevance of microsatellite instability in colorectal cancer. *J Clin Oncol*. 2010;28:3380–7.
24. Sepulveda A. Microsatellite: Medscape, 2009.
25. Ionov Y, Peinado MA, Malkhosyan S, Shibata D, Perucho M. Ubiquitous somatic mutations in simple repeated sequences reveal a new mechanism for colonic carcinogenesis. *Nature*. 1993;363: 558–61.
26. Thibodeau SN, Bren G, Schaid D. Microsatellite instability in cancer of the proximal colon. *Science*. 1993;260:816–9.
27. Leach FS, Nicolaides NC, Papadopoulos N, et al. Mutations of a mutS homolog in hereditary nonpolyposis colorectal cancer. *Cell*. 1993;75:1215–25.
28. Fishel R, Lescoe MK, Rao MR, et al. The human mutator gene homolog MSH2 and its association with hereditary nonpolyposis colon cancer. *Cell*. 1993;75:1027–38.
29. Bronner CE, Baker SM, Morrison PT, et al. Mutation in the DNA mismatch repair gene homologue hMLH1 is associated with hereditary non-polyposis colon cancer. *Nature*. 1994;368:258–61.
30. Papadopoulos N, Nicolaides NC, Wei YF, et al. Mutation of a mutL homolog in hereditary colon cancer. *Science*. 1994;263:1625–9.
31. Liu B, Farrington SM, Petersen GM, et al. Genetic instability occurs in the majority of young patients with colorectal cancer. *Nat Med*. 1995;1:348–52.
32. Miyaki M, Konishi M, Tanaka K, et al. Germline mutation of MSH6 as the cause of hereditary nonpolyposis colorectal cancer. *Nat Genet*. 1997;17:271–2.
33. Moslein G, Tester DJ, Lindor NM, et al. Microsatellite instability and mutation analysis of hMSH2 and hMLH1 in patients with sporadic, familial and hereditary colorectal cancer. *Hum Mol Genet*. 1996;5:1245–52.
34. Benachenhou N, Guiral S, Gorska-Flipot I, Michalski R, Labuda D, Sinnett D. Allelic losses and DNA methylation at DNA mismatch repair loci in sporadic colorectal cancer. *Carcinogenesis*. 1998;19:1925–9.
35. Cunningham JM, Christensen ER, Tester DJ, et al. Hypermethylation of the hMLH1 promoter in colon cancer with microsatellite instability. *Cancer Res*. 1998;58:3455–60.
36. Kane MF, Loda M, Gaida GM, et al. Methylation of the hMLH1 promoter correlates with lack of expression of hMLH1 in sporadic colon tumors and mismatch repair-defective human tumor cell lines. *Cancer Res*. 1997;57:808–11.
37. Miyakura Y, Sugano K, Konishi F, et al. Extensive methylation of hMLH1 promoter region predominates in proximal colon cancer with microsatellite instability. *Gastroenterology*. 2001;121:1300–9.
38. Toyota M, Ahuja N, Ohe-Toyota M, Herman JG, Baylin SB, Issa JP. CpG island methylator phenotype in colorectal cancer. *Proc Natl Acad Sci USA*. 1999;96:8681–6.
39. Veigl ML, Kasturi L, Olechnowicz J, et al. Biallelic inactivation of hMLH1 by epigenetic gene silencing, a novel mechanism causing human MSI cancers. *Proc Natl Acad Sci USA*. 1998;95:8698–702.
40. Stone JG, Robertson D, Houlston RS. Immunohistochemistry for MSH2 and MHL1: a method for identifying mismatch repair deficient colorectal cancer. *J Clin Pathol*. 2001;54:484–7.
41. Gryfe R, Kim H, Hsieh ET, et al. Tumor microsatellite instability and clinical outcome in young patients with colorectal cancer. *N Engl J Med*. 2000;342:69–77.
42. Benatti P, Gafa R, Barana D, et al. Microsatellite instability and colorectal cancer prognosis. *Clin Cancer Res*. 2005;11:8332–40.
43. Ribic CM, Sargent DJ, Moore MJ, et al. Tumor microsatellite-instability status as a predictor of benefit from fluorouracil-based adjuvant chemotherapy for colon cancer. *N Engl J Med*. 2003;349: 247–57.
44. Kim GP, Colangelo LH, Wieand HS, et al. Prognostic and predictive roles of high-degree microsatellite instability in colon cancer: a National Cancer Institute-National Surgical Adjuvant Breast and Bowel Project Collaborative Study. *J Clin Oncol*. 2007;25:767–72.
45. Bertagnolli MM, Niedzwiecki D, Compton CC, et al. Microsatellite instability predicts improved response to adjuvant therapy with irinotecan, fluorouracil, and leucovorin in stage III colon cancer: Cancer and Leukemia Group B Protocol 89803. *J Clin Oncol*. 2009;27:1814–21.
46. Sargent DJ, Marsoni S, Monges G, et al. Defective mismatch repair as a predictive marker for lack of efficacy of fluorouracil-based adjuvant therapy in colon cancer. *J Clin Oncol*. 2010;28:3219–26.
47. Kerr DJ, Midgley R. Defective mismatch repair in colon cancer: a prognostic or predictive biomarker? *J Clin Oncol*. 2010;28:3210–2.
48. Kozuch P, Malamud S, Wasserman C, Homel P, Mirzoyev T, Grossbard M. Phase II trial of erlotinib and capecitabine for patients with previously untreated metastatic colorectal cancer. *Clin Colorectal Cancer*. 2009;8:38–42.
49. Fisher GA, Kuo T, Ramsey M, et al. A phase II study of gefitinib, 5-fluorouracil, leucovorin, and oxaliplatin in previously untreated patients with metastatic colorectal cancer. *Clin Cancer Res*. 2008;14:7074–9.
50. Bardelli A, Siena S. Molecular mechanisms of resistance to cetuximab and panitumumab in colorectal cancer. *J Clin Oncol*. 2010;28:1254–61.
51. De Roock W, Claes B, Bernasconi D, et al. Effects of KRAS, BRAF, NRAS, and PIK3CA mutations on the efficacy of cetuximab plus chemotherapy in chemotherapy-refractory metastatic colorectal cancer: a retrospective consortium analysis. *Lancet Oncol*. 2010;11:753–62.
52. De Roock W, Jonker DJ, Di Nicolantonio F, et al. Association of KRAS p.G13D mutation with outcome in patients with chemotherapy-refractory metastatic colorectal cancer treated with cetuximab. *JAMA*. 2010;304:1812–20.
53. Bos JL, Fearon ER, Hamilton SR, et al. Prevalence of ras gene mutations in human colorectal cancers. *Nature*. 1987;327:293–7.
54. Deng G, Bell I, Crawley S, et al. BRAF mutation is frequently present in sporadic colorectal cancer with methylated hMLH1, but not in hereditary nonpolyposis colorectal cancer. *Clin Cancer Res*. 2004;10:191–5.
55. Palomaki GE, McClain MR, Melillo S, Hampel HL, Thibodeau SN. EGAPP supplementary evidence review: DNA testing strategies aimed at reducing morbidity and mortality from Lynch syndrome. *Genet Med*. 2009;11:42–65.
56. Roth AD, Tejpar S, Delorenzi M, et al. Prognostic role of KRAS and BRAF in stage II and III resected colon cancer: results of the translational study on the PETACC-3, EORTC 40993, SAKK 60–00 trial. *J Clin Oncol*. 2010;28:466–74.
57. Hutchins G, Southward K, Handley K, et al. Value of mismatch repair, KRAS, and BRAF mutations in predicting recurrence and benefits from chemotherapy in colorectal cancer. *J Clin Oncol*. 2011;29:1261–70.

58. Rizzo S, Bronte G, Fanale D, et al. Prognostic vs predictive molecular biomarkers in colorectal cancer: is KRAS and BRAF wild type status required for anti-EGFR therapy? *Cancer Treat Rev.* 2010;36(Suppl 3):S56–61.
59. Grothey A. EGFR antibodies in colorectal cancer: where do they belong? *J Clin Oncol.* 2010;28:4668–70.
60. Karapetis CS, Khambata-Ford S, Jonker DJ, et al. K-ras mutations and benefit from cetuximab in advanced colorectal cancer. *N Engl J Med.* 2008;359:1757–65.
61. Allegra CJ, Jessup JM, Somerfield MR, et al. American Society of Clinical Oncology provisional clinical opinion: testing for KRAS gene mutations in patients with metastatic colorectal carcinoma to predict response to anti-epidermal growth factor receptor monoclonal antibody therapy. *J Clin Oncol.* 2009;27:2091–6.
62. Prenen H, Tejpar S, Van Cutsem E. New strategies for treatment of KRAS mutant metastatic colorectal cancer. *Clin Cancer Res.* 2010;16:2921–6.
63. Flaherty KT, Puzanov I, Kim KB, et al. Inhibition of mutated, activated BRAF in metastatic melanoma. *N Engl J Med.* 2010;363:809–19.
64. Prahallad A, Sun C, Huang S, et al. Unresponsiveness of colon cancer to BRAF(V600E) inhibition through feedback activation of EGFR. *Nature.* 2012;483:100–3.
65. Jhawer M, Goel S, Wilson AJ, et al. PIK3CA mutation/PTEN expression status predicts response of colon cancer cells to the epidermal growth factor receptor inhibitor cetuximab. *Cancer Res.* 2008;68:1953–61.
66. Halilovic E, She QB, Ye Q, et al. PIK3CA mutation uncouples tumor growth and cyclin D1 regulation from MEK/ERK and mutant KRAS signaling. *Cancer Res.* 2010;70:6804–14.
67. Prenen H, De Schutter J, Jacobs B, et al. PIK3CA mutations are not a major determinant of resistance to the epidermal growth factor receptor inhibitor cetuximab in metastatic colorectal cancer. *Clin Cancer Res.* 2009;15:3184–8.
68. Sartore-Bianchi A, Martini M, Molinari F, et al. PIK3CA mutations in colorectal cancer are associated with clinical resistance to EGFR-targeted monoclonal antibodies. *Cancer Res.* 2009;69:1851–7.
69. Brachmann SM, Hofmann I, Schnell C, et al. Specific apoptosis induction by the dual PI3K/mTor inhibitor NVP-BEZ235 in HER2 amplified and PIK3CA mutant breast cancer cells. *Proc Natl Acad Sci USA.* 2009;106:22299–304.
70. Serra V, Markman B, Scaltriti M, et al. NVP-BEZ235, a dual PI3K/mTOR inhibitor, prevents PI3K signaling and inhibits the growth of cancer cells with activating PI3K mutations. *Cancer Res.* 2008;68:8022–30.
71. De Roock W, De Vriendt V, Normanno N, Ciardiello F, Tejpar S. KRAS, BRAF, PIK3CA, and PTEN mutations: implications for targeted therapies in metastatic colorectal cancer. *Lancet Oncol.* 2011;12:594–603.
72. She QB, Halilovic E, Ye Q, et al. 4E-BP1 is a key effector of the oncogenic activation of the AKT and ERK signaling pathways that integrates their function in tumors. *Cancer Cell.* 2010;18:39–51.
73. Ogino S, Meyerhardt JA, Cantor M, et al. Molecular alterations in tumors and response to combination chemotherapy with gefitinib for advanced colorectal cancer. *Clin Cancer Res.* 2005;11:6650–6.
74. Chung KY, Shia J, Kemeny NE, et al. Cetuximab shows activity in colorectal cancer patients with tumors that do not express the epidermal growth factor receptor by immunohistochemistry. *J Clin Oncol.* 2005;23:1803–10.
75. Cejas P, Lopez-Gomez M, Aguayo C, et al. Analysis of the concordance in the EGFR pathway status between primary tumors and related metastases of colorectal cancer patients: Implications for cancer therapy. *Curr Cancer Drug Targets.* 2012;12(2):124–31.
76. Baas JM, Krens LL, Guchelaar HJ, Morreau H, Gelderblom H. Concordance of predictive markers for EGFR inhibitors in primary tumors and metastases in colorectal cancer: a review. *Oncologist.* 2011;16:1239–49.
77. Funkhouser WK Jr, Lubin IM, Monzon FA, et al. Relevance, pathogenesis, and testing algorithm for mismatch repair-defective colorectal carcinomas: a report of the association for molecular pathology. *J Mol Diagn.* 2012;14:91–103.
78. CAP. Frequently Asked Questions About ER/PgR Testing Guidelines, 2012.

Molecular Pathology of Barrett's Metaplasia and Esophageal Adenocarcinoma

3

Mamoun Younes

Introduction

Barrett's metaplasia (BM), also called Barrett's esophagus, is a condition in which the normal squamous lining of the esophagus is replaced by specialized columnar epithelium containing goblet cells as a result of chronic gastroesophageal reflux disease (GERD).[1] BM is associated with an increased risk for esophageal adenocarcinoma (EAC). The incidence of EAC has been rising in the United States and Western Europe since the 1970s.[2,3] Most EAC is discovered at a late stage and is associated with poor prognosis although survival has generally been improving over time.[2,4] Patients with BM are enrolled in surveillance programs where esophageal endoscopy and biopsy are performed at certain intervals largely determined by the degree of dysplasia in the biopsy tissue.[1] Understanding the molecular changes that occur during the progression from normal squamous epithelium to BM and eventually to EAC is essential for developing effective prevention and treatment strategies.

There are two major processes during the progression from normal esophagus to EAC: metaplasia and neoplasia, illustrated in Fig. 1.2 (Chap. 1). The molecular mechanisms underlying these two changes are numerous, some unique to each step but some contribute to both. Obviously, we cannot cover every reported molecular change in this chapter. As a result, we will focus mostly on changes that were generally reported at least two or three times in the literature, realizing that some molecular changes that we do not have a chance to cover in this chapter may prove very important in future studies.

M. Younes, M.D. (✉)
Department of Pathology, University of Texas Medical School at Houston, 6413 Fannin, MSB 2.270, Houston, TX 77030, USA
e-mail: mamoun.younes@uth.tmc.edu

The Role of Acid and Bile

Both acid and bile play a role in the metaplastic as well as the neoplastic processes. Acid reflux may activate the NADPH oxidase NOX5-S and increase the production of reactive oxygen species, which in turn increases p16 promoter methylation, downregulates p16 expression, and increases cell proliferation.[5] Acidic pH has been also shown to induce topoisomerase-II (TOP2)-mediated DNA damage and p53 protein upregulation in cultured human cell lines[6] and increases the expression of COX-2 in the squamous epithelium.[7]

While acid suppression therapy reduces heartburn, inflammation, and proliferative activity in BM, it appears to have no effect on oxidative DNA damage, apoptosis, the expression of COX-2, c-myc, p53, O6-methylguanine methyl transferase (MGMT), or on aberrant DNA methylation.[8–10] Bile acids, especially Deoxycholic acid (DCA), cause reactive oxygen species (ROS)-mediated chromosome damage and mutation induction in the human p53 gene, both at neutral and acidic pH although this was considerably increased at acidic pH.[11] Since bile acids can induce DNA damage at neutral pH, acid suppression therapy may not eliminate DNA damage or the carcinogenic potential of the refluxate.[8,11,12] Bile acids also activate NF-kappaB in BM.[13] In BM epithelial cells, DCA-induces genotoxicity while simultaneously inducing activation of the NF-kappaB pathway therefore enabling cells with DNA damage to resist apoptosis.[14]

CDX

The caudal-related homeobox genes CDX1 and CDX2 play an important role in intestinal epithelial differentiation.[15] CDX1 mRNA and CDX2 mRNA are expressed in gastric intestinal metaplasia[16] and ectopic expression of either CDX1 or CDX2 in the gastric epithelium of transgenic mice induces intestinal metaplasia.[17–19]

A.R. Sepulveda and J.P. Lynch (eds.), *Molecular Pathology of Neoplastic Gastrointestinal Diseases*, Molecular Pathology Library 7,
DOI 10.1007/978-1-4614-6015-2_3, © Springer Science+Business Media New York 2013

Acidic pH induces transcription of the CDX2 gene in mouse esophageal keratinocytes.[20] In a rat model, cholic acid and deoxycholic acid activate CDX2 promoter via NF-kappaB and stimulate production of CDX2 protein in esophageal keratinocytes and production of intestinal-type mucin.[21] In cultured human EAC cell line, deoxycholate and acid increase NF-kappaB activity which leads to expression of CDX2, which in turn mediates intestinal metaplasia and expression of Guanylyl cyclase C (GC-C), an intestine-specific tumor suppressor.[22]

In human biopsy tissue, CDX2 mRNA can be detected in both esophagitis and BM epithelium, but CDX2 protein is detected only in BM (not in esophagitis).[16,23] CDX1 mRNA is expressed only in BM epithelium.[16,24] The specific expression of CDX1 mRNA in only BM, and not in squamous or gastric epithelium, is thought to be due to the methylation status of the CDX1 promoter. Conjugated bile salts and TNF-alpha and IL-1beta, mediated by NF-kappaB signaling, can increase CDX1 mRNA expression in vitro, but only when the CDX1 promoter was unmethylated or partially methylated.[24]

Factors secreted from fibroblasts have been recently proposed to induce columnar phenotype in adjacent squamous epithelium. Human fibroblasts exposed to acidified medium show significant upregulation of Heparin-binding EGF-like growth factor (HB-EGF). Biopsy specimens from patients with reflux esophagitis show a strong expression of HB-EGF in fibroblasts underlying the damaged epithelium. Furthermore, in vitro stimulation of HET1A human squamous epithelial cells with HB-EGF increases CDX2 expression in a dose-dependent manner, and also upregulates cytokeratin 7 and villin.[25]

Because in several studies of esophageal biopsies CDX2 expression has been detected in columnar cells that do not show "intestinal metaplasia," as well as those with "intestinal metaplasia," it has been proposed that CDX2 may serve as a marker of BM when "intestinal metaplasia" is not present in the biopsy. In one study, CDX2 protein expression was detected in 23 of 67 (34%) samples with only cardiac-type mucosa and this was associated with increased likelihood of finding intestinal metaplasia in another biopsy set of columnar-lined esophagus from the same patients. Fifty-two percent of biopsies with only cardiac mucosa positive for CDX2 showed intestinal metaplasia in a second set of biopsies. Based on these findings, the authors suggested that CDX2 expression in cardiac-type mucosa might be able to predict the presence of undetected intestinal metaplasia in columnar-lined esophagus, and thus may be a putative marker for the presence of intestinal metaplasia in the absence of goblet cells.[26] Unfortunately, this approach may lead to a significant number of patients labeled as having BM based on CDX2 immunostaining when they do not have BM. In the Kerkhof study, a full 48% of patients with cardiac only mucosa and positive CDX2 did not show intestinal metaplasia in a second set of biopsies. It may be prudent, at least for the time being, to take a conservative approach on this issue because we need prospective follow-up studies from more than one center to show what happens to patients with cadia only epithelium and positive CDX2 on long follow up, taking into consideration the effect of reflux treatment on progression of these CDX2 positive cells to intestinal metaplasia. If one feels excited about immunostaining biopsies with cardia only epithelium for CDX2, it is probably better to report the results as positive (or negative) for CDX2, and comment that positive CDX2 immunostaining was found to be associated with an increased probability of finding intestinal metaplasia on another set of biopsies, therefore clinical correlation and follow up is suggested, without giving the patient a diagnosis of BM.

COX-2

Expression of the proinflammatory enzyme Cyclooxynage-2 (COX-2) in the esophagus increases with exposure to acid[7] and Gastrin.[27] COX-2 mRNA is elevated in esophageal squamous mucosa with reflux compared to no reflux,[28] and expression in patients with BM was found to increase with time,[27] probably due to prolonged and repeated exposure to gastroesophageal reflux. Ferguson and colleagues reported that polymorphic variants in COX-2, especially the COX-2 8473 C allele, were associated with a significantly increased risk of esophageal adenocarcinoma.[29]

There are contradicting reports regarding the level of COX-2 expression in BM, dysplasia, and EAC, and the effect of acid suppressive therapy and other treatments on COX-2 expression. While COX-2 mRNA levels were said to be elevated in BM and to increase with progression to EAC,[30] studies utilizing immunohistochemistry (IHC) showed different results.[31,32] Similarly, antireflux surgery and acid suppression therapy were associated with reduced COX-2 expression in BM in some studies,[28] while others reported no effect of acid suppression therapy on COX-2.[9,10] These differing results may be due to differences of COX-2 detection and assay methods used and lack of standardization.

Cyclin D1

Cyclin D1 was found to be expressed in BM, and its expression decreased in patients on proton pump inhibitors (PPI), H2-blockers, and antacids. The greatest decrease in Cyclin D1 levels was associated with PPI followed by H2-blockers and least effective were antacids.[33] Cyclin D1 adenine 870 polymorphism is associated with increased Cyclin D1 expression, cancer onset at an early age, and aggressive tumors.[34]

EGFR

CDX2 induction by deoxycholic acid occurs through ligand-dependent transactivation of the epidermal growth factor receptor (EGFR).[35] DCA, at neutral and acidic pH or acid alone can upregulate EGFR mRNA in vitro which in the case of neutral pH DCA was NF-kappaB dependent.[36]

EGFR gene amplification was detected initially in 30.8% of EAC and in 20% of BM[37] but a later study found EGFR amplification in only 8% of EAC.[38]

Using semiquantitative IHC, EGFR was reported to be overexpressed in 35% of BM with high-grade dysplasia (HGD) and 80% of EAC when compared to BM. EGFR overexpression was accompanied by aneuploidy of chromosome 7 in addition to amplification of the EGFR locus.[36]

EGFR signaling is in part mediated by the Raf/MEK/ERK (MAPK) kinase pathway, which may be activated as an early event in the development of Barrett's adenocarcinoma. *RAS* or *BRAF* mutations were detected in about 32% of all Barrett's adenocarcinomas and in a proportion of high-grade dysplasia lesions.[39]

Her-2/erbB-2/neu

c-erbB2 was found to be amplified, both by IHC and by FISH, in a significant number of EAC and in dysplastic BM.[37,38,40,41] Significant heterogeneity in immunostaining and amplification (FISH) was found in EAC and dysplastic foci ranging from completely negative to strongly positive/amplified.[42] Walch and colleagues found that polysomy 17 without *Her-2/neu* gene amplification in roughly half the cases of EAC and BM with HGD and that was associated with a normal or moderately elevated mRNA expression and no or weak immunostaining. There was no locus-specific *Her-2/neu* amplification in cases of BM with low-grade dysplasia (LGD), but polysomy 17 was present in a few of these, suggesting that chromosome 17 polysomy without *Her-2/neu* gene amplification precedes *Her-2/neu* gene amplification in HGD and EAC.[41]

HER-2/neu oncogene amplification, determined by FISH, correlates with shortened patient survival and independently predicts poor outcome in patients with EAC.[43] Results of the ToGA clinical trial, which included gastric and gastroesophageal junction adenocarcinoma showed a significant survival benefit for patients treated with a combination of Trastuzumab and standard chemotherapy in patients with positive *Her2/neu*.[44] Currently, oncology practice is employing assessment of *HER-2/neu* expression by immunohistochemistry with reflex testing for gene amplification by FISH in advanced esophageal adenocarcinomas to select patients for targeted therapy. Interestingly, Hu et al reported that no *HER2* amplification or overexpression was identified in BM or low-grade dysplasia.[45]

Microsatellite and Chromosomal Instability

Genetic defects in the DNA mismatch repair are not believed to play an important role in EAC,[46] although roughly 15–20% of EAC have been reported to have microsatellite instability at 1 or more chromosomal loci[47,48] and low-level microsatellite alterations can be seen in the majority of EAC.[49] Chromosomal instability represent the most frequent associated changes underlying neoplastic development and progression in Barrett's associated neoplasia. Gene losses are most common but gene amplifications may also occur.[50] Hyperploidy of chromosomes 4 and 8 was found in at least 70% of nondysplastic BM and up to 100% of EAC, suggesting that genetic instability arises before dysplasia in BM.[51]

Genome wide analyses of the Barrett's esophagus-dysplasia sequence have shown a significant trend toward increasing loss of chromosomes with higher progression stage in the Barrett's, dysplasia and adenocarcinoma stepwise sequence. In low-grade dysplasia, loss of 3p14.2 (68.4%) and 16q23.1 (47.4%) was limited to narrow regions within the *FHIT* (3p14.2) and *WWOX* (16q23.1) genes, whereas loss of 9p21 (68.4%) occurred in larger regions. A significant increase in the loss of other chromosomal regions was seen in HGD and EAC. Loss of 17p (47.6%) is one of the most frequent events in EAC.[50]

Cytokines

Polymorphisms of *IL23R* gene was found to be a risk variant for the development of BM,[52] and a genetic profile predisposing to a strong pro-inflammatory host response, mediated by IL-12p70 and partially dependent on IL-10, was also found to be associated with BM.[53] This risk further increases when this genotype coincides with a hiatal hernia, suggesting that exposure to gastroesophageal reflux in the presence of a pro-inflammatory genetic background is important for the development of BE.[53] Physiological levels of DCA can activate NF-kappaB and induce NF-kappaB target gene expression, particularly IkappaB and IL-8.[13]

IL-1 receptor antagonist and IL-10 and IL-1 gene polymorphism are more commonly found in patients with BM or EAC than those with esophagitis,[54] and IL-6 expression and secretion are increased in BM tissue.[55] IL-8 mRNA expression is increased in patients with reflux, and the highest levels are seen in dysplastic BM and EAC.[56] IL-1beta, IL-8, and interferon gamma (IFN-gamma) are increased in reflux esophagitis, with a modest increase in anti-inflammatory IL-10; both IL-10 and IL-4 are increased in BM.[57,58] Nissen fundoplication, an anti-reflux surgery, significantly decreases IL-8 expression compared with preoperative levels.[56]

DNA Methylation

Promoter hypermethylation is a common mechanism of gene inactivation. In BM, and during malignant progression, several genes involved in protection from oxidative DNA damage, tumor suppression, Wnt pathway, apoptosis, and cytokine signaling have been reported to be regulated by epigenetic mechanisms involving CpG island methylation.

Hypermethylation of *ESR1* (estrogen receptor-alpha) is seen at high frequency in inflammatory reflux esophagitis and at all subsequent stages, whereas *APC* and *CDKN2A* (p16) hypermethylation is found in Barrett's metaplasia, dysplasia, and EAC.[59] APC gene promoter hypermethylation can be seen in up to 90% of patients with EAC and 40% of patients with BM but not in matching normal esophageal tissues. Moreover, hypermethylated *APC* DNA was detected in the plasma of 25% of EAC patients and were associated with reduced patient survival.[60] *APC* promoter methylation in BM is associated with inactivation of the *APC* gene and increase the risk of malignant progression.[61, 62] Downregulation of the Wnt inhibitory factor-1 (*WIF-1*) correlated with promoter hypermethylation. EAC tissue samples showed higher levels of *WIF-1* methylation compared to normal epithelium, and BM samples from patients with EAC show more *WIF-1* hypermethylation than samples from patients without EAC.[63]

Glutathione peroxidase-3 (GPx3) is a secretory protein with potent extracellular antioxidant activity. Consistently reduced levels of GPx3 mRNA is seen in 91% of EAC. *GPx3* promoter hypermethylation was detected in 62% of Barrett's metaplasia, 82% of dysplasia, and 88% of EAC, and hypermethylation of both alleles of *GPx3* is found most frequently in EAC.[64]

P16, *RUNX3*, and *HPP1* displayed increasing methylation frequencies in BM, and the increase in methylation occurred early at the interface between BM and LGD. Hypermethylation of *p16*, *RUNX3*, and *HPP1* is independently associated with an increased risk of progression to HGD or EAC.[65]

Reprimo, a candidate tumor-suppressor gene, regulates p53-mediated cell cycle arrest at G2 phase. In BM, HGD, and EAC, the level and frequency of *Reprimo* methylation were significantly higher than in normal esophagus. *Reprimo* methylation was not detected in samples from normal squamous esophageal mucosa, but was present in 36% of BM, 64% of HGD, and 63% of EAC, suggesting that this epigenetic alteration is an early event in the neoplastic process in BM.[66]

Downregulation of Smad4 in BM occurs due to several different mechanisms, including methylation, deletion, and protein modification.[67] Methylation of the suppressors of cytokine signaling (*SOCS*) *SOCS-3* and *SOCS-1* was not seen in reflux esophagitis. However, *SOCS-3* methylation occurred in 13% of BM without dysplasia and hypermethylated *SOCS-3* promoter was found in 74% of EAC, 69% of HGD, and 22% of LGD.[68] Hypermethylation of the proapoptotic death-associated protein kinase *DAPK* promoter was detected in 20% of normal esophageal mucosa, 50% of BM, 53% of BM with dysplasia, and 60% of EAC, and resulted in a marked decrease in DAPK protein expression, which in turn was associated with increased depth of tumor invasion and advanced tumor stages. The severity of reflux esophagitis correlated significantly with the hypermethylation rate of the *DAPK* promoter.[69] Hypermethylation of the DNA repair protein O6-methylguanine methyl transferase (*MGMT*) was detected in 78.9% of EAC, 100% of BM with dysplasia, 88.9% of BM without dysplasia, and 21.4% of normal esophageal mucosa, and correlated significantly with downregulation of *MGMT* transcripts and protein expression.[70]

MYC

Using in situ hybridization with biotinylated probes, and a small sample of patients with BM, Abdelatif and coworkers found enhanced *c-myc* expression in all grades of dysplasia and carcinoma.[71] A larger study in which *c-myc* was quantitated by PCR and Southern blot analysis showed *c-myc* gene to be amplified in only 4.6% of EAC.[38] Others have reported that the chromosome containing *c-myc* (8q24) was amplified in 37% of EAC.[50] c-myc protein expression was also determined by immunohistochemical analysis and assessed using the Immunoreactive Scoring System (IRS). Overexpression of *c-myc* was found in 9.6% of normal esophageal tissue, 37.2% of BM without dysplasia, 45.5% of BM with dysplasia, and 73% of EAC.[72]

RAS and *RAF*

EGFR signaling is in part mediated by the Raf/MEK/ERK (MAPK) kinase pathway, which may be activated as an early event in the development of EAC by RAS or BRAF activation. Abdelatif and coworkers found *H-ras* to be consistently expressed in HGD and EAC but not in low-grade dysplasia,[71] and, in another study, high levels of H-ras mRNA were found in 40% EAC and one Barrett's specimen.[73] *KRAS* amplification was found in just 10% of EAC.[38] Point mutations in *K-ras*/codon 12 were found rarely in BM without dysplasia (0.4%) and in roughly 4% of BM with dysplasia and 35% of EAC; *K-ras*/codon 13 mutation (GGCgly → GACasp) was not observed.[74]

Sommerer et al reported *KRAS2* mutations in 21% of EAC and 11% of HGD, but not in LGD or normal gastric or esophageal mucosa, while *BRAF* activating mutations were rare.[39]

CDKN2 (p16)

The *CDKN2* gene, located on chromosome 9p21, that encodes the p16 inhibitor of cyclinD/Cdk4 complexes is a target of allelic loss and inactivation in a variety of human cancers and cell lines. 9p21 allelic losses and *CDKN2* mutations develop as early lesions in diploid cells before aneuploidy and cancer during neoplastic progression in BM.[75] Evidence from cell culture experiments suggests that NADPH oxidase NOX5-S, which mediates acid-induced H_2O_2 production and oxidative DNA damage, is involved in acid-induced hypermethylation of p16 gene promoter and downregulation of p16 mRNA.[5] A study of biopsies from 304 patients with BM revealed a mutation spectrum consistent with that caused by oxidative damage and chronic inflammation.[76]

Loss of heterozygosity (LOH) of 9p21, which contains the p16INK4a tumor suppressor gene locus, is one of the most frequent genetic abnormalities in human neoplasia, including esophageal EAC. Only a minority of EAC with 9p21 LOH has a somatic mutation in the remaining p16 allele, and none have been found to have homozygous deletions. Promoter hypermethylation with LOH was found to be a common mechanism for inactivation of p16 in the pathogenesis of EAC.[77,78] P16 promoter hypermethylation was detected in 3% of BM without dysplasia, 60% of BM indefinite for dysplasia, 56% LGD, and 75% of HGD.[79] However, others found p16 promoter hypermethylation in 66% of BM without dysplasia, 47% of IND/LGD, and 81% of HGD and any *p16* abnormality (9pLOH, p16 mutation, and hypermethylation) in 88% of BM without dysplasia, 87% of IND/LGD, and 86% of HGD. These findings led to the conclusion that BM contains genetic and/or epigenetic *p16* lesions and has the ability to undergo clonal expansion, creating a field in which other abnormalities can arise that can lead to EAC.[80] Maley and colleagues further expanded on this and proposed that *p16* loss of heterozygosity, promoter methylation, and sequence mutations have strong, independent, advantageous effects on BM early in progression. Second lesions in *p16* and *p53* are associated with later selective sweeps. They hypothesize that virtually all of the other lesion expansions, including microsatellite shifts, could be explained as hitchhikers on *p16* lesion clonal expansions.[81] However, by studying clonality at the crypt level, Leedham and colleagues dispute this hypothesis. They showed that BM heterogeneity arises from multiple independent clones.[82]

TP53

Specimens of BM from separate sites were found to have identical *p53* mutations suggesting a clonal origin, however, cancers arising in mutant epithelium may not have similar mutations to those found in the BM.[83] Both 17p allelic deletions and p53 protein overexpression are frequently involved in carcinogenesis in BM,[84] and *p53* gene mutations and p53 protein immunostaining were shown to be present in a majority of Barrett's adenocarcinomas.[85]

Overexpression of p53 was found in 5% of BM negative for dysplasia, 15% of indefinite for dysplasia (IND)/LGD, 45% of HGD, and 53% EAC by flow cytometry.[86] Similarly, studies utilizing immunohistochemistry (IHC) on formalin fixed and paraffin embedded biopsy tissue found p53 protein accumulation (positive staining) in 0% of BM negative for dysplasia, 9% of IND/LGD, 55% of HGD, and 87% of EAC.[87] In a retrospective analysis of 24 patients with follow-up biopsies, two patients who showed low-grade dysplasia and who were positive for p53 on biopsy showed high-grade dysplasia in follow-up biopsies which led the authors to hypothesize that positive immunostaining for p53 may be an objective marker of neoplastic progression in BM.[87] Later, it was shown that p53 protein accumulation as detected by immunohistochemistry is more specific and has better predictive value for subsequent development of HGD/EAC than histologic diagnosis of LGD.[88,89] Allelic losses at 17p and *p53* mutations were also shown to precede the development of high-grade dysplasia, aneuploidy, and EAC.[90,91]

Although *p53* mutations in exons 5–8 were detected in 53% of EAC and p53 accumulation was observed in a similar percentage (57%) of these, *p53* gene mutation and p53 protein accumulation had a significant discordance.[92] In another study, all samples containing *p53* mutations displayed p53 protein accumulation; however, in the majority of cases, p53 protein accumulation was not associated with mutations. Gene expression analysis found no differences in p53 and mdm-2 transcription levels between the cases with and without p53 protein accumulation.[93] Based on these and similar reports, it appears that *p53* gene mutations are not the primary cause of protein accumulation and positive immunostaining for p53.

There is a highly significant association between nitrotyrosine (NTS), a stable reaction product of nitric oxide (NO) reflecting chronic NO-induced cellular protein damage, and endogenous p53 mutations at CpG dinucleotides. This suggests that an active inflammatory process, most likely a consequence of GERD, underlies molecular progression to EAC.[94] It has been previously postulated that in BM gastroesophageal reflux causes oxidative DNA damage which leads to cell cycle arrest at the G0G1 or G2M phases of the cell cycle to enable repair of damaged DNA. In some cases this would be followed sequentially by p53 gene mutation and protein accumulation, DNA aneuploidy, HGD, and EAC.[95] Failure of acid suppression therapy (AST) to alter malignant progression in BM may be due, at least in part, to defects in DNA repair and cell cycle control resulting from p53 gene mutation, present before the initiation of AST. Therefore, although AST may be effective in preventing further DNA damage, it is unlikely to alter progression in genetically unstable cells.[8]

DNA Ploidy Abnormalities

Patients with dysplasia or adenocarcinoma had evidence of genomic instability (aneuploidy) or abnormalities of mucosal proliferation by flow cytometry, even when the dysplasia was focal or difficult to recognize histologically.[96] The percentage of biopsies with an aneuploid DNA content, and the mean S and G2M fraction threshold values, increased with the histologic grade of dysplasia. Aneuploidy or G2M fraction greater than 6% was the best discriminating criteria between those two distinct groups of patients. All patients with high-grade dysplasia or cancer had aneuploid cell populations or increased G2M fraction, none of the patients whose biopsies were negative for dysplasia had evidence of genomic instability or increased G2M fraction, however, flow cytometric abnormalities were found in 40% of patients with biopsies IND or LGD.[97] Nine of 13 patients who showed aneuploid or increased G2/tetraploid populations in their initial flow-cytometric analysis developed HGD or EAC during follow-up but none of the 49 patients without these abnormalities progressed.[98] A similar predictive value could be obtained from flow cytometry performed on formalin-fixed and paraffin-embedded biopsies of BM.[99,100] In situ hybridization on BM cells with and without dysplasia and EAC showed that genetic instability arises well before dysplasia in BM, with chromosome 4 and 8 hyperploidy representing the earliest and most common alterations.[51]

Multiple Molecular Abnormalities

In addition to the many studies reporting on the significance of single molecular abnormalities in the development of BM or dysplasia and EAC in BM, there are a few studies that examined the clinical significance of two or more combined molecular changes.

In one study, the sizes of clones with p53 loss of heterozygosity or ploidy abnormalities was found to predict progression to EAC better than the mere presence of such clones, and the combination of clonal expansion and genetic instability was a better predictor of cancer outcome than either alone.[101] In another study, ten-year cumulative incidence of EAC in patients with BM who had no baseline abnormality was 12%, but was as high as 79% in patients with baseline 17p LOH, DNA content abnormalities, and 9p LOH.[102] The panel of abnormalities that includes 17p LOH, DNA content tetraploidy and aneuploidy, and 9p LOH was found to be the best predictor of progression to EAC.[102]

Hypermethylation of both *p16* and *APC* was a strong predictor of subsequent progression to HGD or EAC.[103] Others have proposed that promoter methylation levels of a panel of eight genes (*p16*, *HPP1*, *RUNX3*, *CDH13*, *TAC1*, *NELL1*, *AKAP12*, and *SST*) could be of value in predicting neoplastic progression in BM.[104]

MicroRNAs

Several microRNAS (miRNAs) were found to be downregulated or upregulated during different stages of malignant progression in BM; some of these were found to be particularly involved in progression from low-grade dysplasia to cancer, and some were shown to act as oncogenes by mainly suppressing the activity of known tumor suppressor genes.[105]

Concluding Remarks

Several molecular changes are present at the same time at any point during progression from normal squamous epithelium, reflux esophagitis, BM without dysplasia, and BM with dysplasia and EAC. The clinical significance of most of the molecular changes reported in the literature is still unknown because most studies are retrospective and look at snapshots of different stages of the disease with no follow up. Because of this, the exact sequence of the many molecular changes during malignant progression in BM remains unknown or speculative at this point.

Unfortunately, and perhaps for the lack of better alternative, the vast majority of studies look at molecular changes in BM in relation to the degree of dysplasia, which is a moving target with high inter and intra-observer variability. This is responsible, at least in part, for some of the differences in molecular changes reported by different investigators. Of equal importance is that the vast majority of studies do not take the of antireflux treatment on molecular changes or disease progression into account. For example, several studies (some mentioned above) showed that exposure of the esophageal epithelium, whether squamous or BM, to acid, bile, or both induces molecular changes in the epithelial cells, and it is therefore likely that the extent of these changes varies between individuals with GERD as the treatment and its effectiveness varies.

References

1. Wang KK, Sampliner RE. Updated guidelines 2008 for the diagnosis. Surveillance and therapy of Barrett's Esophagus. *Am J Gastroenterol*. 2008;103(3):788–797.
2. Younes M, Miller CC. Incidence and survival trends of esophageal carcinoma in the United States: racial and gender differences by histological type. *Scand J Gastroenterol*. 2002;37(12): 1359–1365.
3. Brown LM, Devesa SS, Chow WH. Incidence of adenocarcinoma of the esophagus among white Americans by sex, stage, and age. *J Natl Cancer Inst*. 2008;100(16):1184–1187.
4. Cen P, Banki F, Cheng L, Khalil K, Du XL, Fallon M, et al. Changes in age, stage distribution, and survival of patients with esophageal adenocarcinoma over three decades in the United States. *Ann Surg Oncol*. 2012;19:1685–1691.
5. Hong J, Resnick M, Behar J, Wang LJ, Wands J, DeLellis RA, et al. Acid-induced p16 hypermethylation contributes to development of esophageal adenocarcinoma via activation of NADPH oxidase NOX5-S. *Am J Physiol Gastrointest Liver Physiol*. 2010;299(3):G697–706.
6. Xiao H, Li T-KK, Yang J-MM, Liu LF. Acidic pH induces topoisomerase II-mediated DNA damage. *Proc Natl Acad Sci USA*. 2003;100(9):5205–5210.
7. Hamoui N, Peters JH, Schneider S, Uchida K, Yang D, Vallb ohmer D, et al. Increased acid exposure in patients with gastroesophageal reflux disease influences cyclooxygenase-2 gene expression in the squamous epithelium of the lower esophagus. *Arch Surg*. 2004;139(7):712-6. discussion 716–7.
8. Carlson N, Lechago J, Richter J, Sampliner RE, Peterson L, Santella RM, et al. Acid suppression therapy may not alter malignant progression in Barrett's metaplasia showing p53 protein accumulation. *Am J Gastroenterol*. 2002;97(6):1340–1345.
9. Lao-Sirieix P, Roy A, Worrall C, Vowler SL, Gardiner S, Fitzgerald RC. Effect of acid suppression on molecular predictors for esophageal cancer. *Cancer Epidemiol Biomarkers Prev*. 2006;15(2): 288–293.
10. Abu-Sneineh A, Tam W, Schoeman M, Fraser R, Ruszkiewicz AR, Smith E, et al. The effects of high-dose esomeprazole on gastric and oesophageal acid exposure and molecular markers in Barrett's oesophagus. *Aliment Pharmacol Ther*. 2010;32(8): 1023–1030.
11. Jenkins GJS, D'Souza FR, Suzen SH, Eltahir ZS, James SA, Parry JM, et al. Deoxycholic acid at neutral and acid pH, is genotoxic to oesophageal cells through the induction of ROS: The potential role of anti-oxidants in Barrett's oesophagus. *Carcinogenesis*. 2007; 28(1):136–142.
12. Liu L, Ergun G, Ertan A, Woods K, Sachs I, Younes M. Detection of oxidative DNA damage in oesophageal biopsies of patients with reflux symptoms and normal pH monitoring. *Aliment Pharmacol Ther*. 2003;18(7):693–698.
13. Jenkins GJS, Harries K, Doak SH, Wilmes A, Griffiths AP, Baxter JN, et al. The bile acid deoxycholic acid (DCA) at neutral pH activates NF-kappaB and induces IL-8 expression in oesophageal cells in vitro. *Carcinogenesis*. 2004;25(3):317–323.
14. Huo X, Juergens S, Zhang X, Rezaei D, Yu C, Strauch ED, et al. Deoxycholic acid causes DNA damage while inducing apoptotic resistance through NF-\kappa\B activation in benign Barrett's epithelial cells. *Am J Physiol Gastrointest Liver Physiol*. 2011;301: 278–86.
15. Freund JN, Domon-Dell C, Kedinger M, Duluc I. The Cdx-1 and Cdx-2 homeobox genes in the intestine. *Biochem Cell Biol*. 1998;76(6):957–969.
16. Eda A, Osawa H, Satoh K, Yanaka I, Kihira K, Ishino Y, et al. Aberrant expression of CDX2 in Barrett's epithelium and inflammatory esophageal mucosa. *J Gastroenterol*. 2003;38(1): 14–22.
17. Mutoh H, Sakurai S, Satoh K, Osawa H, Hakamata Y, Takeuchi T, et al. Cdx1 induced intestinal metaplasia in the transgenic mouse stomach: comparative study with Cdx2 transgenic mice. *Gut*. 2004;53(10):1416–1423.
18. Mutoh H, Hakamata Y, Sato K, Eda A, Yanaka I, Honda S, et al. Conversion of gastric mucosa to intestinal metaplasia in Cdx2-expressing transgenic mice. *Biochem Biophys Res Commun*. 2002;294(2):470–479.
19. Silberg DG, Sullivan J, Kang E, Swain GP, Moffett J, Sund NJ, et al. Cdx2 ectopic expression induces gastric intestinal metaplasia in transgenic mice. *Gastroenterology*. 2002;122(3):689-696.
20. Marchetti M, Caliot E, Pringault E. Chronic acid exposure leads to activation of the cdx2 intestinal homeobox gene in a long-term culture of mouse esophageal keratinocytes. *J Cell Sci*. 2003;116 (Pt 8):1429–1436.
21. Kazumori H, Ishihara S, Rumi MAK, Kadowaki Y, Kinoshita Y. Bile acids directly augment caudal related homeobox gene Cdx2 expression in oesophageal keratinocytes in Barrett's epithelium. *Gut*. 2006;55(1):16–25.
22. Debruyne PR, Witek M, Gong L, Birbe R, Chervoneva I, Jin T, et al. Bile acids induce ectopic expression of intestinal guanylyl cyclase C Through nuclear factor-kappaB and Cdx2 in human esophageal cells. *Gastroenterology*. 2006;130(4):1191–1206.
23. Moons LMG, Bax DA, Kuipers EJ, Van Dekken H, Haringsma J, Van Vliet AHM, et al. The homeodomain protein CDX2 is an early marker of Barrett's oesophagus. *J Clin Pathol*. 2004;57(10):1063–1068.
24. Wong NACS, Wilding J, Bartlett S, Liu Y, Warren BF, Piris J, et al. CDX1 is an important molecular mediator of Barrett's metaplasia. *Proc Natl Acad Sci USA*. 2005;102(21):7565–7570.
25. Rahman FB, Kadowaki Y, Ishihara S, Tobita H, Imaoka H, Fukuhara H, et al. Fibroblast-derived HB-EGF promotes Cdx2 expression in esophageal squamous cells. *Lab Invest*. 2010;90(7):1033–1048.
26. Kerkhof M, Bax DA, Moons LMG, van Vuuren AJ, Van Dekken H, Steyerberg EW, et al. Does CDX2 expression predict Barrett's metaplasia in oesophageal columnar epithelium without goblet cells? *Aliment Pharmacol Ther*. 2006;24(11–12):1613–1621.
27. Abdalla SI, Lao-Sirieix P, Novelli MR, Lovat LB, Sanderson IR, Fitzgerald RC. Gastrin-induced cyclooxygenase-2 expression in Barrett's carcinogenesis. *Clin Cancer Res*. 2004;10(14): 4784–4792.
28. Vallb Ohmer D, DeMeester SR, Oh DS, Banki F, Kuramochi H, Shimizu D, et al. Antireflux surgery normalizes cyclooxygenase-2 expression in squamous epithelium of the distal esophagus. *Am J Gastroenterol*. 2006;101(7):1458–1466.
29. Ferguson HR, Wild CP, Anderson LA, Murphy SJ, Johnston BT, Murray LJ, et al. Cyclooxygenase-2 and inducible nitric oxide synthase gene polymorphisms and risk of reflux esophagitis, Barrett's esophagus, and esophageal adenocarcinoma. *Cancer Epidemiol Biomarkers Prev*. 2008;17(3):727–731.
30. Kuramochi H, Vallb Ohmer D, Uchida K, Schneider S, Hamoui N, Shimizu D, et al. Quantitative, tissue-specific analysis of cyclooxygenase gene expression in the pathogenesis of Barrett's adenocarcinoma. *J Gastrointest Surg*. 2004;8(8):1007-16. discussion 1016–7.
31. van der Woude CJ, Jansen PLM, Tiebosch ATGM, Beuving A, Homan M, Kleibeuker JH, et al. Expression of apoptosis-related proteins in Barrett's metaplasia-dysplasia-carcinoma sequence: a switch to a more resistant phenotype. *Hum Pathol*. 2002;33(7): 686–692.

32. Villanacci V, Rossi E, Zambelli C, Galletti A, Cestari R, Missale G, et al. COX-2, CDX2, and CDC2 immunohistochemical assessment for dysplasia-carcinoma progression in Barrett's esophagus. *Dig Liver Dis*. 2007;39(4):305–311.
33. Arber N, Lightdale C, Rotterdam H, Han KH, Sgambato A, Yap E, et al. Increased expression of the cyclin D1 gene in Barrett's esophagus. *Cancer Epidemiol Biomarkers Prev*. 1996;5(6):457–459.
34. Izzo JG, Wu T-T, Wu X, Ensor J, Luthra R, Pan J, et al. Cyclin D1 guanine/adenine 870 polymorphism with altered protein expression is associated with genomic instability and aggressive clinical biology of esophageal adenocarcinoma. *J Clin Oncol*. 2007;25(6): 698–707.
35. Avissar NE, Toia L, Hu Y, Watson TJ, Jones C, Raymond DP, et al. Bile acid alone, or in combination with acid, induces CDX2 expression through activation of the epidermal growth factor receptor (EGFR). *J Gastrointest Surg*. 2009;13(2):212–222.
36. Cronin J, McAdam E, Danikas A, Tselepis C, Griffiths P, Baxter J, et al. Epidermal growth factor receptor (EGFR) is overexpressed in high-grade dysplasia and adenocarcinoma of the esophagus and may represent a biomarker of histological progression in Barrett's esophagus (BE). *Am J Gastroenterol*. 2011;106(1):46–56.
37. al-Kasspooles M, Moore JH, Orringer MB, Beer DG. Amplification and over-expression of the EGFR and erbB-2 genes in human esophageal adenocarcinomas. *Int J Cancer*. 1993;54(2):213–219.
38. Miller CT, Moy JR, Lin L, Schipper M, Normolle D, Brenner DE, et al. Gene amplification in esophageal adenocarcinomas and Barrett's with high-grade dysplasia. *Clin Cancer Res*. 2003;9(13):4819–4825.
39. Sommerer F, Vieth M, Markwarth A, Rohrich K, Vomschloss S, May A, et al. Mutations of BRAF and KRAS2 in the development of Barrett's adenocarcinoma. *Oncogene*. 2004;23(2):554–558.
40. Jankowski J, Coghill G, Hopwood D, Wormsley KG. Oncogenes and onco-suppressor gene in adenocarcinoma of the oesophagus. *Gut*. 1992;33(8):1033–1038.
41. Walch A, Specht K, Bink K, Zitzelsberger H, Braselmann H, Bauer M, et al. Her-2/neu gene amplification, elevated mRNA expression, and protein overexpression in the metaplasia-dysplasia-adenocarcinoma sequence of Barrett's esophagus. *Lab Invest*. 2001;81(6):791–801.
42. Walch A, Bink K, Gais P, Stangl S, Hutzler P, Aubele M, et al. Evaluation of c-erbB-2 overexpression and Her-2/neu gene copy number heterogeneity in Barrett's adenocarcinoma. *Anal Cell Pathol*. 2000;20(1):25–32.
43. Brien TP, Odze RD, Sheehan CE, McKenna BJ, Ross JS. HER-2/neu gene amplification by FISH predicts poor survival in Barrett's esophagus-associated adenocarcinoma. *Hum Pathol*. 2000;31(1):35–39.
44. Bang Y-J, Van Cutsem E, Feyereislova A, Chung HC, Shen L, Sawaki A, et al. Trastuzumab in combination with chemotherapy versus chemotherapy alone for treatment of HER2-positive advanced gastric or gastro-oesophageal junction cancer (ToGA): a phase 3, open-label, randomised controlled trial. *The Lancet*. 2010;376(9742):687–697.
45. Hu Y, Bandla S, Godfrey TE, Tan D, Luketich JD, Pennathur A, et al. HER2 amplification, overexpression and score criteria in esophageal adenocarcinoma. *Mod Pathol*. 2011;24(7):899–907.
46. Muzeau F, Flejou JF, Belghiti J, Thomas G, Hamelin R. Infrequent microsatellite instability in oesophageal cancers. *Br J Cancer*. 1997;75(9):1336–1339.
47. Meltzer SJ, Yin J, Manin B, Rhyu MG, Cottrell J, Hudson E, et al. Microsatellite instability occurs frequently and in both diploid and aneuploid cell populations of Barrett's-associated esophageal adenocarcinomas. *Cancer Res*. 1994;54(13):3379–3382.
48. Keller G, Rotter M, Vogelsang H, Bischoff P, Becker KF, Mueller J, et al. Microsatellite instability in adenocarcinomas of the upper gastrointestinal tract. Relation to clinicopathological data and family history. *Am J Pathol*. 1995;147(3):593–600.
49. Gleeson CM, Sloan JM, McGuigan JA, Ritchie AJ, Weber JL, Russell SE. Ubiquitous somatic alterations at microsatellite alleles occur infrequently in Barrett's-associated esophageal adenocarcinoma. *Cancer Res*. 1996;56(2):259–263.
50. Gu J, Ajani JA, Hawk ET, Ye Y, Lee JH, Bhutani MS, et al. Genome-wide catalogue of chromosomal aberrations in Barrett's esophagus and esophageal adenocarcinoma: a high-density single nucleotide polymorphism array analysis. *Cancer Prev Res (Phila)*. 2010;3(9):1176–1186.
51. Doak SH, Jenkins GJS, Parry EM, D'Souza FR, Griffiths AP, Toffazal N, et al. Chromosome 4 hyperploidy represents an early genetic aberration in premalignant Barrett's oesophagus. *Gut*. 2003;52(5):623–628.
52. Gaj P, Mikula M, Wyrwicz LS, Regula J, Ostrowski J. Barrett's esophagus associates with a variant of IL23R gene. *Acta Biochim Pol*. 2008;55(2):365–369.
53. Moons LMG, Kusters JG, van Delft JHM, Kuipers EJ, Gottschalk R, Geldof H, et al. A pro-inflammatory genotype predisposes to Barrett's esophagus. *Carcinogenesis*. 2008;29(5):926–931.
54. Gough MD, Ackroyd R, Majeed AW, Bird NC. Prediction of malignant potential in reflux disease: are cytokine polymorphisms important? *Am J Gastroenterol*. 2005;100(5):1012–1018.
55. Dvorakova K, Payne CM, Ramsey L, Holubec H, Sampliner R, Dominguez J, et al. Increased expression and secretion of interleukin-6 in patients with Barrett's esophagus. *Clin Cancer Res*. 2004;10(6):2020–2028.
56. Oh DS, DeMeester SR, Vallbohmer D, Mori R, Kuramochi H, Hagen JA, et al. Reduction of interleukin 8 gene expression in reflux esophagitis and Barrett's esophagus with antireflux surgery. *Arch Surg*. 2007;142(6):554–9. discussion 559–60.
57. Fitzgerald RC, Onwuegbusi BA, Bajaj-Elliott M, Saeed IT, Burnham WR, Farthing MJG. Diversity in the oesophageal phenotypic response to gastro-oesophageal reflux: immunological determinants. *Gut*. 2002;50(4):451–459.
58. Zhong Y-QQ, Lin Y, Xu Z. Expression of IFN-γ and IL-4 in the esophageal mucosa of patients with Reflux Esophagitis and Barrett's Esophagus and their relationship with endoscopic and histologic grading. *Dig Dis Sci*. 2011;56:2865–70.
59. Eads CA, Lord RV, Kurumboor SK, Wickramasinghe K, Skinner ML, Long TI, et al. Fields of aberrant CpG island hypermethylation in Barrett's esophagus and associated adenocarcinoma. *Cancer Res*. 2000;60(18):5021–5026.
60. Kawakami K, Brabender J, Lord RV, Groshen S, Greenwald BD, Krasna MJ, et al. Hypermethylated APC DNA in plasma and prognosis of patients with esophageal adenocarcinoma. *J Natl Cancer Inst*. 2000;92(22):1805–1811.
61. Clement G, Braunschweig R, Pasquier N, Bosman FT, Benhattar J. Alterations of the Wnt signaling pathway during the neoplastic progression of Barrett's esophagus. *Oncogene*. 2006;25(21): 3084–3092.
62. Clement G, Braunschweig R, Pasquier N, Bosman FT, Benhattar J. Methylation of APC, TIMP3, and TERT: a new predictive marker to distinguish Barrett's oesophagus patients at risk for malignant transformation. *J Pathol*. 2006;208(1):100–107.
63. Clement G, Guilleret I, He B, Yagui-Beltran A, Lin Y-CC, You L, et al. Epigenetic alteration of the Wnt inhibitory factor-1 promoter occurs early in the carcinogenesis of Barrett's esophagus. *Cancer Sci*. 2008;99(1):46–53.
64. Lee O-JJ, Schneider-Stock R, McChesney PA, Kuester D, Roessner A, Vieth M, et al. Hypermethylation and loss of expression of glutathione peroxidase-3 in Barrett's tumorigenesis. *Neoplasia*. 2005;7(9):854–861.
65. Schulmann K, Sterian A, Berki A, Yin J, Sato F, Xu Y, et al. Inactivation of p16, RUNX3, and HPP1 occurs early in Barrett's-associated neoplastic progression and predicts progression risk. *Oncogene*. 2005;24(25):4138–4148.

66. Hamilton JP, Sato F, Jin Z, Greenwald BD, Ito T, Mori Y, et al. Reprimo methylation is a potential biomarker of Barrett's-Associated esophageal neoplastic progression. *Clin Cancer Res.* 2006;12(22):6637–6642.
67. Onwuegbusi BA, Aitchison A, Chin S-FF, Kranjac T, Mills I, Huang Y, et al. Impaired transforming growth factor beta signalling in Barrett's carcinogenesis due to frequent SMAD4 inactivation. *Gut.* 2006;55(6):764–774.
68. Tischoff I, Hengge UR, Vieth M, Ell C, Stolte M, Weber A, et al. Methylation of SOCS-3 and SOCS-1 in the carcinogenesis of Barrett's adenocarcinoma. *Gut.* 2007;56(8):1047–1053.
69. Kuester D, Dar AA, Moskaluk CC, Krueger S, Meyer F, Hartig R, et al. Early involvement of death-associated protein kinase promoter hypermethylation in the carcinogenesis of Barrett's esophageal adenocarcinoma and its association with clinical progression. *Neoplasia.* 2007;9(3):236–245.
70. Kuester D, El-Rifai W, Peng D, Ruemmele P, Kroeckel I, Peters B, et al. Silencing of MGMT expression by promoter hypermethylation in the metaplasia-dysplasia-carcinoma sequence of Barrett's esophagus. *Cancer Lett.* 2009;275(1):117–126.
71. Abdelatif OM, Chandler FW, Mills LR, McGuire BS, Pantazis CG, Barrett JM. Differential expression of c-myc and H-ras oncogenes in Barrett's epithelium. A study using colorimetric in situ hybridization. *Arch Pathol Lab Med.* 1991;115(9):880–885.
72. Schmidt MK, Meurer L, Volkweis BS, Edelweiss MI, Schirmer CC, Kruel CDP, et al. c-Myc overexpression is strongly associated with metaplasia-dysplasia-adenocarcinoma sequence in the esophagus. *Dis Esophagus.* 2007;20(3):212–216.
73. Sorsdahl K, Casson AG, Troster M, Van Meyel D, Inculet R, Chambers AF. p53 and ras gene expression in human esophageal cancer and Barrett's epithelium: a prospective study. *Cancer Detect Prev.* 1994;18(3):179–185.
74. Trautmann B, Wittekind C, Strobel D, Meixner H, Keymling J, Gossner L, et al. K-ras point mutations are rare events in premalignant forms of Barrett's oesophagus. *Eur J Gastroenterol Hepatol.* 1996;8(8):799–804.
75. Barrett MT, Sanchez CA, Galipeau PC, Neshat K, Emond M, Reid BJ. Allelic loss of 9p21 and mutation of the CDKN2/p16 gene develop as early lesions during neoplastic progression in Barrett's esophagus. *Oncogene.* 1996;13(9):1867–1873.
76. Paulson TG, Galipeau PC, Xu L, Kissel HD, Li X, Blount PL, et al. p16 mutation spectrum in the premalignant condition Barrett's esophagus. *PLoS One.* 2008;3(11):e3809.
77. Wong DJ, Barrett MT, Stoger R, Emond MJ, Reid BJ. p16INK4a promoter is hypermethylated at a high frequency in esophageal adenocarcinomas. *Cancer Res.* 1997;57(13):2619–2622.
78. Bian Y-SS, Osterheld M-CC, Fontolliet C, Bosman FT, Benhattar J. p16 inactivation by methylation of the CDKN2A promoter occurs early during neoplastic progression in Barrett's esophagus. *Gastroenterology.* 2002;122(4):1113–1121.
79. Klump B, Hsieh CJ, Holzmann K, Gregor M, Porschen R. Hypermethylation of the CDKN2/p16 promoter during neoplastic progression in Barrett's esophagus. *Gastroenterology.* 1998;115(6):1381–1386.
80. Wong DJ, Paulson TG, Prevo LJ, Galipeau PC, Longton G, Blount PL, et al. p16(INK4a) lesions are common, early abnormalities that undergo clonal expansion in Barrett's metaplastic epithelium. *Cancer Res.* 2001;61(22):8284–8289.
81. Maley CC, Galipeau PC, Li X, Sanchez CA, Paulson TG, Reid BJ. Selectively advantageous mutations and hitchhikers in neoplasms: p16 lesions are selected in Barrett's esophagus. *Cancer Res.* 2004;64(10):3414–3427.
82. Leedham SJ, Preston SL, McDonald SAC, Elia G, Bhandari P, Poller D, et al. Individual crypt genetic heterogeneity and the origin of metaplastic glandular epithelium in human Barrett's oesophagus. *Gut.* 2008;57(8):1041–1048.
83. Casson AG, Mukhopadhyay T, Cleary KR, Ro JY, Levin B, Roth JA. p53 gene mutations in Barrett's epithelium and esophageal cancer. *Cancer Res.* 1991;51(16):4495–4499.
84. Blount PL, Ramel S, Raskind WH, Haggitt RC, Sanchez CA, Dean PJ, et al. 17p allelic deletions and p53 protein overexpression in Barrett's adenocarcinoma. *Cancer Res.* 1991;51(20): 5482–5486.
85. Hamelin R, Flejou JF, Muzeau F, Potet F, Laurent-Puig P, Fekete F, et al. TP53 gene mutations and p53 protein immunoreactivity in malignant and premalignant Barrett's esophagus. *Gastroenterology.* 1994;107(4):1012–1018.
86. Ramel S, Reid BJ, Sanchez CA, Blount PL, Levine DS, Neshat K, et al. Evaluation of p53 protein expression in Barrett's esophagus by two-parameter flow cytometry. *Gastroenterology.* 1992;102 (4 Pt 1):1220–1228.
87. Younes M, Lebovitz RM, Lechago LV, Lechago J. p53 protein accumulation in Barrett's metaplasia, dysplasia, and carcinoma: a follow-up study. *Gastroenterology.* 1993;105(6):1637–1642.
88. Younes M, Ertan A, Lechago LV, Somoano JR, Lechago J. p53 Protein accumulation is a specific marker of malignant potential in Barrett's metaplasia. *Dig Dis Sci.* 1997;42(4):697–701.
89. Weston AP, Banerjee SK, Sharma P, Tran TM, Richards R, Cherian R. p53 protein overexpression in low grade dysplasia (LGD) in Barrett's esophagus: immunohistochemical marker predictive of progression. *Am J Gastroenterol.* 2001;96(5):1355–1362.
90. Blount PL, Galipeau PC, Sanchez CA, Neshat K, Levine DS, Yin J, et al. 17p allelic losses in diploid cells of patients with Barrett's esophagus who develop aneuploidy. *Cancer Res.* 1994;54(9): 2292–2295.
91. Neshat K, Sanchez CA, Galipeau PC, Blount PL, Levine DS, Joslyn G, et al. p53 mutations in Barrett's adenocarcinoma and high-grade dysplasia. *Gastroenterology.* 1994;106(6):1589–1595.
92. Coggi G, Bosari S, Roncalli M, Graziani D, Bossi P, Viale G, et al. p53 protein accumulation and p53 gene mutation in esophageal carcinoma. A molecular and immunohistochemical study with clinicopathologic correlations. *Cancer.* 1997;79(3):425–432.
93. Doak SH, Jenkins GJS, Parry EM, Griffiths AP, Shah V, Baxter JN, et al. Characterisation of p53 status at the gene, chromosomal and protein levels in oesophageal adenocarcinoma. *Br J Cancer.* 2003;89(9):1729–1735.
94. Vaninetti NM, Geldenhuys L, Porter GA, Risch H, Hainaut P, Guernsey DL, et al. Inducible nitric oxide synthase, nitrotyrosine and p53 mutations in the molecular pathogenesis of Barrett's esophagus and esophageal adenocarcinoma. *Mol Carcinog.* 2008;47(4):275–285.
95. Younes M, Lechago J, Chakraborty S, Ostrowski M, Bridges M, Meriano F, et al. Relationship between dysplasia, p53 protein accumulation, DNA ploidy, and Glut1 overexpression in Barrett metaplasia. *Scand J Gastroenterol.* 2000;35(2):131–137.
96. Reid BJ, Haggitt RC, Rubin CE, Rabinovitch PS. Barrett's esophagus. Correlation between flow cytometry and histology in detection of patients at risk for adenocarcinoma. *Gastroenterology.* 1987;93(1):1–11.
97. Robaszkiewicz M, Hardy E, Volant A, Nousbaum JB, Cauvin JM, Calament G, et al. Flow cytometric analysis of cellular DNA content in Barret's esophagus. A study of 66 cases. *Gastroenterol Clin Biol.* 1991;15(10):703–710.
98. Reid BJ, Blount PL, Rubin CE, Levine DS, Haggitt RC, Rabinovitch PS. Flow-cytometric and histological progression to malignancy in Barrett's esophagus: prospective endoscopic surveillance of a cohort. *Gastroenterology.* 1992;102(4 Pt 1):1212–1219.
99. Menke-Pluymers MB, Mulder AH, Hop WC, van Blankenstein M, Tilanus HW. Dysplasia and aneuploidy as markers of malignant degeneration in Barrett's oesophagus. The Rotterdam Oesophageal Tumour Study Group. *Gut.* 1994;35(10): 1348–1351.

100. Giménez A, Minguela A, Parrilla P, Bermejo J, Pérez D, Molina J, et al. Flow cytometric DNA analysis and p53 protein expression show a good correlation with histologic findings in patients with Barrett's esophagus. *Cancer*. 1998;83(4):641–651.
101. Maley CC, Galipeau PC, Li X, Sanchez CA, Paulson TG, Blount PL, et al. The combination of genetic instability and clonal expansion predicts progression to esophageal adenocarcinoma. *Cancer Res*. 2004;64(20):7629–7633.
102. Galipeau PC, Li X, Blount PL, Maley CC, Sanchez CA, Odze RD, et al. NSAIDs modulate CDKN2A, TP53, and DNA content risk for progression to esophageal adenocarcinoma. *PLoS Med*. 2007;4(2):e67.
103. Wang JS, Guo M, Montgomery EA, Thompson RE, Cosby H, Hicks L, et al. DNA promoter hypermethylation of p16 and APC predicts neoplastic progression in Barrett's esophagus. *Am J Gastroenterol*. 2009;104(9):2153–2160.
104. Jin Z, Cheng Y, Gu W, Zheng Y, Sato F, Mori Y, et al. A multicenter, double-blinded validation study of methylation biomarkers for progression prediction in Barrett's esophagus. *Cancer Res*. 2009;69(10):4112–4115.
105. Yang H, Gu J, Wang KK, Zhang W, Xing J, Chen Z, et al. MicroRNA expression signatures in Barrett's esophagus and esophageal adenocarcinoma. *Clin Cancer Res*. 2009;15(18):5744–5752.

Molecular Pathology of Squamous Carcinomas of the Esophagus

4

Rohinton S. Tarapore and Jonathan P. Katz

Introduction

Esophageal cancer is the eighth most common cancer in the world and ranks sixth as a cause of cancer mortality.[1,2] An estimated 482,300 new esophageal cancer cases and 406,800 deaths occurred worldwide in 2008. Esophageal cancer usually occurs as either esophageal squamous cell carcinoma (ESCC) in the middle or upper one-third of the esophagus or as esophageal adenocarcinoma (EAC) in the lower one-third or at the junction of the esophagus and stomach.[1,2] ESCC is the predominant type of esophageal malignancy in the world, although adenocarcinomas are more prevalent in the USA and other western countries.[3,4] Worldwide, more than 90% of esophageal cancers are ESCC.[5] ESCC develops through a progressive sequence from mild to severe dysplasia, carcinoma in situ, and finally invasive cancer[5–7] (Fig. 4.1). The principal precursor of ESCC is epithelial dysplasia, characterized by accumulation of atypical cells with nuclear hyperchromasia, abnormally clumped chromatin, and loss of polarity.[6,7] Because most esophageal cancer patients have advanced metastatic cancers at the time of diagnosis, only 1 in 5 esophageal cancer patients survive more than 3 years after initial diagnosis.[8,9]

Epidemiology of Esophageal Squamous Cell Carcinoma

The incidence of ESCC shows marked variation in its geographic distribution with the highest rates found in southern and eastern Africa and eastern Asia and the lowest rates observed in western and middle Africa and Central America.[2,5,10–13] The highest risk area, stretching from northern Iran through the central Asian republics to North-Central China is often referred to as the "esophageal cancer belt".[14,15] Areas located in the southern parts of the Taihang mountains on the borders of Henan, Shansi, and Hopei provinces have amongst the highest incidence and mortality rates for ESCC worldwide.[16] The major risk factors for ESCC within these regions are not well understood, but are thought to include poor nutritional status and drinking beverages at higher temperatures.[17–19] In the USA and other developed countries, smoking and excessive alcohol consumption are responsible for approximately 90% of ESCC.[3] Obesity and chronic gastro-esophageal reflux disease (GERD), which triggers Barrett's esophagus, are thought to be the risk factors for EAC but not ESCC in the USA and other Western countries.[3,4]

Risk Factors

Many factors have been investigated in relation to esophageal squamous cell carcinoma. These factors include habits (consumption of alcohol and tobacco), nutritional deficiencies (low intake of fresh fruits and vegetables), infections (*H. pylori*, HPV), predisposing conditions (achalasia, tylosis, poor oral health) and low socioeconomic status (Table 4.1).

Habits

Tobacco Smoke

Cigarette smoke is a contributing factor in the development of several cancers including ESCC.[15,20–24] Numerous studies indicate a 3–6-fold increase in the risk of ESCC among current smokers.[25–29] Smoking cigars or pipes confers a risk similar to cigarette smoke.[25] Chewing betel quid, which often includes tobacco, a common practice in south and south-east

R.S. Tarapore, M.S., Ph.D.
Department of Gastroenterology, University of Pennsylvania, Philadelphia, PA, USA

J.P. Katz, M.D., Ph.D. (✉)
Division of Gastroenterology, University of Pennsylvania, Philadelphia, PA, USA
email: jpkatz@mail.med.upenn.edu

A.R. Sepulveda and J.P. Lynch (eds.), *Molecular Pathology of Neoplastic Gastrointestinal Diseases*, Molecular Pathology Library 7,
DOI 10.1007/978-1-4614-6015-2_4, © Springer Science+Business Media New York 2013

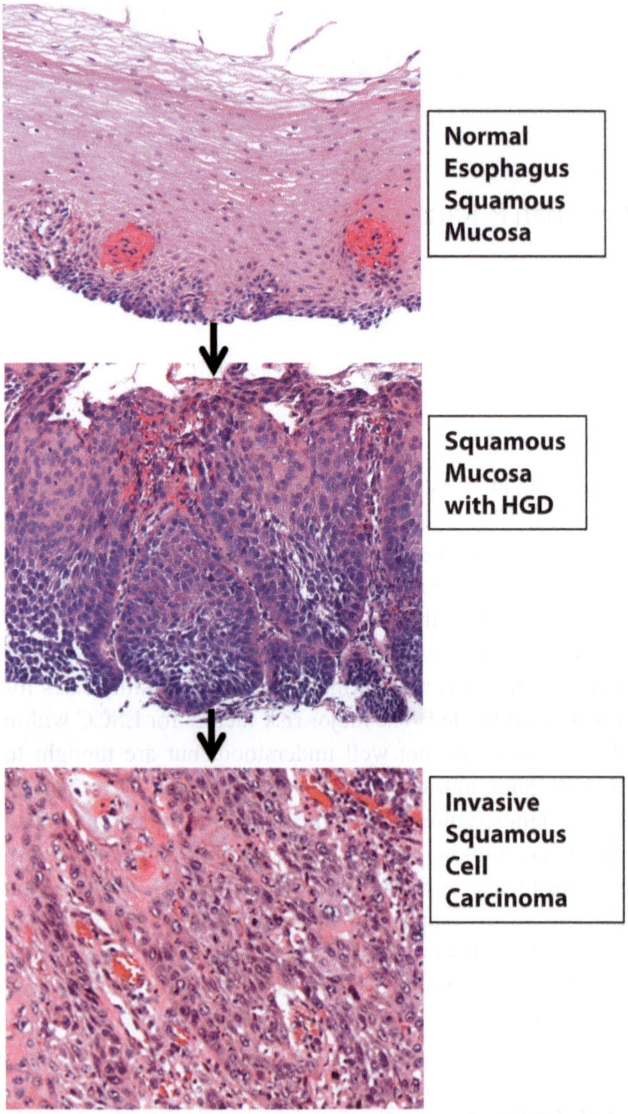

Fig. 4.1 Progression of normal esophageal squamous mucosa to high-grade squamous dysplasia and invasive squamous cell carcinoma (Hematoxylin and Eosin stains). In normal squamous epithelium, the cells mature towards the surface where squamous cells show abundant cytoplasm and small nuclei. In high-grade squamous dysplasia, the epithelial cells show atypical features with increased nuclear to cytoplasmic ratios and loss of the normal maturation pattern towards the surface. However, the epithelial cells remain contained within the epithelial basement membrane. Invasive squamous cell carcinomas are characterized by irregularly shaped islands of tumor cells with increased cytologic atypia and invading into the adjacent tissues. Photomicrograph courtesy of Dr. Antonia Sepulveda

Asia, can also cause ESCC as determined by the International Agency for Research on Cancer (IARC).[30] Cigarette smoke contains more than 2,550 known compounds; greater than 60 have been evaluated by the IARC to be carcinogenic to humans and/or experimental animals.[15,20–24,31–34] Among these carcinogens, exposure to polyaromatic hydrocarbons (PAHs)

Table 4.1 Risk factors for esophageal squamous cell carcinoma

Habits
Tobacco use
Alcohol consumption
Predisposing conditions
Achalasia
Tylosis
Infectious agents
Helicobacter pylori
Human papilloma virus (HPV)
Other
Low intake of fruits and vegetables
Dietary zinc deficiency

such as benzo-a-pyrene and *N*-nitrosamine are considered to be the most significant.[33,34] A strong association between a variety of smoking-induced cancers and these carcinogens exists.[35] The mechanisms underlying their roles in carcinogenesis are believed to be induction of DNA adducts, gene methylation and mutation, and chromosomal translocation in target organs.[20,22,36]

Benzo-a-pyrene undergoes metabolic transformation to electrophilic intermediates like benzo-a-pyrene diol epoxide (BPDE) that react with cellular macromolecules forming DNA adducts (carcinogen metabolites covalently bound to DNA usually at guanine or adenosine residues).[20,37,38] Several studies indicate a permanent mutation in the DNA if DNA adducts escape cellular repair mechanisms.[20,38,39] Cells with damaged DNA may be removed by apoptosis.[40] If a permanent mutation occurs in a critical region, an oncogene may be activated or a tumor suppressor gene deactivated, leading to aberrant cells with loss of normal growth control and migration ultimately leading to cancer.[20,38,39] Several studies have reported a direct association between benzo-a-pyrene exposure and mutations in the *K-RAS* and *p53* genes.[41,42] The major adduct of benzo-a-pyrene produces a G-to-T transversion[43]; the frequency of this transversion is significantly higher in smokers than nonsmokers.[35] Methylated CpG dinucleotides are the preferred sites for G-to-T transversion and the striking sequence specificity of BPDE for producing G-to-T transversion at methylated CpG sequences is similar to the distribution of G-to-T transversion hotspots in cancer patients.[35,41,44]

Alcohol Consumption

Like tobacco use, alcohol consumption is a major risk factor for esophageal squamous cell carcinoma.[21,23] Chronic and excessive consumption of alcohol can impair the body's biochemical metabolism and alter gene expression in target tissues.[45] When used in excessive amounts (3 or more drinks per day), alcohol has almost universally been associated with an elevated risk of ESCC.[27,46–48] While there appears to be no association between alcohol intake and ESCC risk at levels below 170 g/week,[49] above this threshold, a 3% increase in ESCC risk is observed for each additional 10 g/week of alcohol intake. In the human body, ethanol is metabolized by alcohol dehydrogenase resulting in the generation of acetaldehyde which is further metabolized to acetate by aldehyde dehydrogenase. Acetaldehyde is toxic and carcinogenic, inducing gene mutations and inhibiting retinoic acid biosynthesis.[45,50,51] In turn, reduced retinoic acid levels in the cells alter gene expression leading to reduced RAR-β_2 (retinoic acid receptor) expression and increased expression of EGFR, Erk 1/2, AP-1, COX-2.[52,53]

The joint effect of tobacco smoking and alcohol consumption on ESCC is synergistic rather than additive.[54–57] Active smoking plus ethanol challenge results in a sevenfold higher level of salivary acetaldehyde than that in nonsmokers.[58] A classic animal experiment revealed that alcohol acted as a solvent to increase the transportation of benzo-a-pyrene to the esophageal mucosa.[59]

Predisposing Conditions

Achalasia

Achalasia is a motility disorder of the esophagus characterized by aperistalsis in the distal esophagus from loss of LES (lower esophageal sphincter) relaxation. This condition leads to stasis in the esophagus, resulting in increased fermentation of food and a higher risk for esophageal cancer.[60] ESCC is found in 3–7% of achalasia patients,[61] a rate significantly higher than rates in the normal population.[62–65] For example, a long-term study from Sweden shows a tenfold increased risk of both ESCC and EAC in achalasia patients when compared to the rest of the population.[65]

Tylosis

Tylosis, a rare autosomal dominant disease characterized by hyperkeratosis of the squamous epithelia of the esophagus, palms of the hand, and soles of the feet, is associated with ESCC.[66] The early dermatologic manifestation usually begins between 7 and 8 years of age, and approximately 50% of patients will develop ESCC by the age of 45 and 95% by the age of 65.[67,68] Two types of tylosis have been identified: late-onset (type A) tylosis that is associated with high incidence of ESCC; and early-onset (type B) tylosis, which appears to be benign.[69] Using linkage analysis, the tylosis-esophageal cancer gene locus has been mapped to 17q25.[70]

Infectious Agents

Helicobacter pylori

H. pylori infection is a known cause of gastric adenocarcinoma and is associated with EAC.[4] However, no consistent association is observed between *H. pylori* and ESCC. Some studies have reported a twofold increased risk of ESCC with colonization of *H. pylori* in the stomach, while others have found no association or even reduced risk with *H. pylori* colonization.[71,72]

Human Papilloma Virus

Human papilloma virus (HPV) plays an important role in the etiology of epithelial cancers of the cervix, vulva, anus, penis, and oropharyngeal cavity.[73,74] However, despite numerous studies, the role of HPV in the etiology of ESCC remains controversial.[73] While many studies have found no evidence of HPV in esophageal tumors,[75–81] others have found HPV in up to 75% of cancers.[82] The inconsistency of these results could be differences in the study design, geographic variation, or lack of appropriate adjustment for tobacco use and alcohol consumption. Because of these conflicting results, the IARC concluded that "there is inadequate evidence in humans for carcinogenicity of HPV in the esophagus".[73]

Other

Low Intake of Fruits and Vegetables

A low intake of fruits and vegetables has long been considered a possible risk factor for ESCC, and a majority of studies conducted worldwide have found inverse associations between intake of fruits (especially citrus fruits) and the risk of developing esophageal cancer. Recently new cohort studies, carried out in Europe and the USA, have provided additional support for a protective association of both fruit and vegetable intake with esophageal cancer.[83–85] By analyzing the evidence from various studies, the World Cancer Research Fund–American Institute for Cancer Research (WCRF–AICR) concluded that the high intake of fruits and vegetables probably decreases esophageal cancer risk by approximately 20% per 50 g of fruit or vegetable intake per day.[86,87]

Dietary Zinc Deficiency

Dietary zinc deficiency is typically found in those who consume relatively little meat and large quantities of whole grain.[88] This dietary pattern is seen in regions with high rates of ESCC, such as Linzhou, China, which has one of the highest rates in the world with more than 100 cases per 100,000 people annually.[89] Studies of endoscopic biopsy samples demonstrate an inverse relationship between esophageal tissue zinc concentration and ESCC.[90]

Molecular Alterations in Esophageal Squamous Cell Carcinoma

Numerous molecular alterations are associated with the development of ESCC such as altered expression of *p53*, *p16*, *cyclin D1*, *EGFR*, *E-cadherin*, *p27*, *p21*, and others.[5,36,91–95] These changes in gene expression are often correlated with known risk factors in esophageal cancer. In this section, we discuss common genetic and epigenetic alterations in ESCC (see Table 4.2) and their role in the development of ESCC in more detail.

p53

The tumor suppressor p53 maintains genetic stability and DNA repair capacity.[96,97] p53 promotes cell cycle arrest through induction of *p21*[WAF1 98] and induces apoptosis by downregulating *bcl-2* and upregulating *Bax*.[99,100] Wild-type p53 protein plays a crucial role in cell proliferation by arresting the cell cycle in G_1 phase, regulating apoptosis, and suppressing angiogenesis.[101] However, the function of p53 is lost through mutations, as well as by other factors, including overexpression of MDM2 (murine double minute gene 2), which results in increased degradation of p53 or inactivation of p14[ARF], leading to inhibition of cell cycle arrest, DNA repair, and apoptosis.[102] *p53* gene mutations, frequently as point mutations, have been reported in over half of all human cancers[96] and appear to occur at an early stage during esophageal squamous cell carcinogenesis and correlate with tumor progression.[101,103,104] The reported frequency of *p53* gene mutation in esophageal cancer varies widely from 17% to 84%,[105–113] perhaps due to differences in the analytical methods that have been used.[31,101] Dietary carcinogens and habits such as alcohol and tobacco appear to promote *p53* mutations in ESCC, particularly in studies of high risk areas such as China, Southern Brazil, and Taiwan.[96,101,108,114,115] The mutational spectrum of *p53* in esophageal and lung cancers is consistent with the mutation pattern induced by certain polyaromatic hydrocarbons such as benzo-a-pyrene in cigarette smoke.[35,44,116] For example, 40–50% of *p53* gene mutations in Japanese individuals with ESCC are G-to-T transversions, a phenomenon associated with DNA adduct formation by benzo-a-pyrene.[101,117] Among 48 *p53* mutations identified in surgically resected ESCC in Japan between 1995 and 2005 (Table 4.3), transversions are found in 24 (50%), followed by transitions in 14 (29.2%), and frameshifts in 10 (20.8%); similar results are seen in additional studies from China.[108,113] Taken together, these data suggest that *p53* mutation, perhaps as a result of environmental factors, plays a critical role in the multistep process of ESCC.

p16

p16, a tumor suppressor gene located at chromosome 9p21, inhibits the cyclin-dependent kinases Cdk 4 and 6 that bind to cyclin D1 and downregulate the pRb pathway, thereby blocking cell cycle progression from G_1 to S phase.[118] Inactivation of *p16* in human cancers is a frequent event and is associated with homozygous deletion, genetic mutation, or aberrant DNA methylation.[119–121] Loss of the *p16* gene and decreased protein expression occur in the early stage of esophageal carcinogenesis, either by promoter methylation or loss of heterozygosity.[5,36,122] Interestingly, *p16* promoter hypermethylation seems to occur more frequently in heavy drinkers and smokers.[123] While the impact of p16 on patient prognosis is unclear, loss of *p16* expression could result in poor prognosis by inactivation of pRb,[124] and hypermethylation of CpG islands on *p16* may then be a useful biological marker.

Table 4.2 Molecular alterations prevalent in esophageal squamous cell carcinoma

Gene	Chromosome location	Alteration	References
p53	17p13.1	Mutation	Mathew et al[254]
MDM2	12q14.3	Amplification	Shibagaki et al[255]
p21	6p21.2	Polymorphism	Bahl et al[256]
p16	9p21	Hypermethylation	Nie et al[257]
Cyclin D1	11q13	Amplification	Kuwano et al[132], Xu et al[22]
EGFR	4q25	Amplification	Kuwano et al[132]
E-cadherin	16q22.1	Loss of heterozygosity, promoter methylation	Berx et al[187], Si et al[188]

Table 4.3 The mutation spectrum of p53 in ESCC in Japan (adapted from Egashira et al[101])

Type of mutation	Occurrence *n* (%age)
Transition	14 (29.2%)
G:C→A:T	11 (23%)
A:T→G:C	3 (6.3%)
Transversion	24 (50%)
G:C→T:AG:C→C:G	12 (25%)
A:T→T:A	3 (6.3%)
A:T→C:G	5 (10.4%) 4 (8.3%)
Frameshift	10 (20.8%)
Deletion	7 (14.6%)
Insertion	3 (6.3%)
Total	48 (100%)

cyclin D1

Cyclin D1 is the protein product of the *CCND1* gene located on chromosome 11q13 and controls cell cycle progression through the G_1–S checkpoint.[125] Cyclin D1 enhances esophageal squamous cell transformation,[126] and overexpression of cyclin D1 is a common feature of esophageal carcinogenesis, including dysplasia and early cancers, with 23–73% of human ESCC tumor samples exhibiting overexpression of cyclin D1.[127–132] Increased levels of cyclin D1 result from amplification at 11q13, which is observed in several cancers including ESCC.[127–131,133,134] Cyclin D1 overexpression and gene amplification appear to predict poor prognosis in human ESCC patients.[124,131,135–137] A causal relationship between carcinogens found in tobacco smoke and upregulation of *cyclin D1* has been reported in both lung cancer and ESCC,[132] and cigarette smoke extract stimulates cell proliferation and upregulates cyclin D1 expression in various human ESCC cell lines.[138]

EGFR

Epidermal derived growth factor (EGFR), a tyrosine kinase receptor, plays an important role in regulating cell growth and tumorigenesis. Binding of ligands such as epidermal growth factor (EGF) to EGFR triggers a cascade of phosphorylation events in the cytoplasm leading to the activation of downstream targets such as MAPK (mitogen-activated protein kinase) and AP-1 (activator protein 1), nuclear translocation of ERK1/2, and expression of genes like *JUN*, *FOS*, and *COX2*.[139] The net effect is generally induction of cell proliferation, and upregulation of EGFR has been reported in premalignant lesions and ESCC.[5,36,91,94,95] Amplification of *EGFR* is a major mechanism of upregulation and is correlated with the depth of invasion of the tumor, lymph node metastases, and unfavorable prognosis.[140,141] Mutations in *EGFR* exist but are rare.[142]

MAPK Signaling

Mitogen-activated protein kinases (MAPK) are crucial components of signaling cascades that regulate numerous physiological processes in normal tissues and during pathogenesis.[143] There are three major subfamilies of MAPK, the classical extracellular signal-regulated kinases (ERK) and two types of stress-activated MAPK, the c-Jun N-terminal or stress-activated protein kinases (JNK/SAPK) and p38/MAPK14.[144,145] The classical MAPK pathway involves a catalytic series of events triggered by RAS and RAF activation and is important for cell proliferation.[146] Many cancer-associated mutations are found in *RAS* and the serine–threonine kinase *BRAF*,[147,148] and activation of the ERK–MAPK pathway is involved in the progression of various cancers.[149] Mutations in *KRAS* have been reported in various tumors including colon and lung cancers,[150] with approximately 50% of colon cancers containing *KRAS* mutations.[151] Moreover, mutation of *KRAS* is an early event in tumor development.[152] Mutations in *BRAF* are associated with increased kinase activity and may result in constitutive *KRAS* and ERK activation.[153] MAPK is a key downstream mediator of EGFR activation in ESCC,[154] and pharmacologic inhibition of MAPK signaling results in decreased cell proliferation.[154,155]

TGF-β Signaling

Transforming growth factor (TGF-β; TGFB) is a multipotent cytokine that plays an important role in the regulation of apoptosis, differentiation, and cell growth.[156] TGFB is typically anti-inflammatory with a suppressive effect on carcinogenesis under normal conditions. However, many cancers originate from uncontrolled cell growth and differentiation through dysregulation of TGFB signaling.[156] Resistance to TGFB-induced growth inhibition is found in many tumor cells,[157] and, once cellular transformation has occurred, TGFB may promote tumor invasion and metastasis and inhibit immune surveillance.[158] Altered expression of the TGFB mediators SMAD2 and SMAD4 is correlated with tumor progression and poor prognosis in ESCC,[159–162] and, in patients with ESCC, high expression of SMURF2 (a ubiquitin ligase targeting SMAD7[163]) is correlated with ESCC development and poor prognosis.[161]

Retinoic acid and Retinoic Acid Receptors

Retinoids, a group of synthetic vitamin A analogs, can modulate cell growth and differentiation by binding to specific nuclear retinoioic acid receptors (RAR), members of the steroid hormone receptor superfamily.[164] RAR are ligand-activated DNA-binding proteins that modulate gene transcription and are divided into 3 subtypes, α, β, and γ.[165] Retinoic acid

(RA) is growth inhibitory in ESCC cells, and RAR-β is lost early and progressively during esophageal squamous cell carcinogenesis.[53,166–170] Thus many esophageal, lung, and breast cancer cell lines that do not express RAR-β are resistant to retinoid treatment,[53] and restoration of RAR-β_2 suppresses ESCC growth, induces apoptosis, and inhibits tumor formation.[52,139,171] In addition, *RAR*-β_2 is methylated in human cancers, leading to the suggestion that it functions as a tumor suppressor.[53] However, the function of RAR-β is complex, since reduced *RAR*-β_2 expression correlates with increased *RAR*-β_4 expression in ESCC,[172] and induction of *RAR*-β_4 enhances growth of cancer cells that do not express *RAR*-β_2.[173] While the molecular mechanisms of antitumor effects by RA in ESCC are not fully understood, restored sensitivity to RA is associated with suppression of *EGFR*, *ERK1/2*, *AP-1*, and *COX-2*.[139] Interestingly, the induction of cytochrome CYP2E1 by ethanol enhances the degradation of RA which in turn increases the expression of *EGFR*, *ERK1/2*, *AP-1*, and *COX-2*.[53]

Wnt/β-Catenin Signaling

Wnt/β-catenin signaling plays an important role in normal development and stem cell maintenance, whereas its aberrant upregulation is involved in tumorigenesis.[174] In the absence of the Wnt ligand, a large multicomponent complex that includes adenomatous polyposis coli protein (APC), axin, casein kinase 1 (CK1), and glycogen synthase kinase 3β (GSK3β) facilitates the degradation of β-catenin, while binding of Wnt ligand leads to the accumulation of free β-catenin in the cytoplasm, its nuclear translocation, and transcriptional activation of target genes.[175,176] Overexpression of Wnt ligands, mutations in APC, and/or stabilizing β-catenin mutations are commonly associated with constitutively upregulated Wnt signaling and tumor development.[177,178] While studies of Wnt/β-catenin signaling in ESCC are limited, reduced expression of Axin is seen in 47% of ESCC tumor specimens and correlates with tumor progression.[179] Moreover, Wnt/β-catenin signaling may be activated in ESCC,[180] and alterations in β-catenin expression have been identified in ESCC.[181–183]

Cadherins and Catenins

Cadherins are transmembrane glycoproteins that mediate adhesion at intercellular adherens junctions; the intracellular regions of cadherins bind to proteins called catenins.[184] E-cadherin, found mainly in epithelial cells, acts as a mediator for intercellular adhesion, cell polarity, and tissue architecture maintenance,[185] and altered expression and localization of E-cadherin is seen in ESCC, with loss or reduced expression in 43% of patients.[186] Reduction and loss of E-cadherin expression by gene mutation, loss of heterozygosity, and promoter hypermethylation, interrupt intercellular adhesion and correlate with decreased tumor differentiation and increased infiltration and metastasis.[182,183,187,188] Expression of α-catenin, γ-catenin, and p120-catenin is also dysregulated in human ESCC,[183,186] and recently, loss of *p120*-catenin resulted in ESCC in mice, establishing *p120* as a tumor suppressor in ESCC.[189]

Krüppel-Like Factors

Members of the *Krüppel*-like factor (KLF) family of transcription factors are critical regulators of cell proliferation and differentiation during development and tissue homeostasis, as well as in many disease states.[190,191] KLF4, KLF5, and KLF6 have all been shown to have functional roles in proliferation, differentiation, and/or squamous cell carcinogenesis in the esophagus.[192–198] In normal esophageal epithelia, KLF4 is expressed as cells differentiate, with highest levels in the suprabasal layers.[199,200] KLF4 expression is downregulated in ESCC,[201] and in ESCC cells, KLF4 promotes apoptosis and inhibits invasion and represses transcription of the *survivin* gene.[194] Interestingly, microRNA-10b promotes migration and invasion in ESCC cells by directly downregulating *KLF4*. These findings suggest that *KLF4* may function as a tumor suppressor in esophagus, as in stomach and colon.[202,203] KLF5 is expressed predominantly in the proliferative compartments of gastrointestinal epithelia, including in the basal layer of the esophagus.[193,204,205] KLF5 promotes proliferation and migration in nontransformed esophageal keratinocytes,[193,195,196] but in ESCC cells, KLF5 inhibits proliferation and invasion and promotes apoptosis.[194] KLF6, which unlike KLF4 and KLF5 is ubiquitously expressed, coactivates the differentiation marker keratin 4 with KLF4 in esophageal epithelial cells.[192]

microRNAs

microRNAs (miRNAs) are small endogenous, noncoding RNAs which regulate protein expression by repressing gene translation or degrading target mRNAs.[206,207] microRNAs function as both oncogenes or tumor suppressor genes and are involved in a wide variety of biological and pathological processes including cell differentiation, proliferation, apoptosis, and metabolism.[208] Aberrant miRNA levels, specifically an overall downregulation, are observed in many cancers, including ESCC,[209] and the miRNA expression profile of ESCC is distinct from that of EAC. For example, miR-194, miR-192, and miR-200 are significantly upregulated in EAC but not in ESCC,[210] while miR-342 is aberrantly expressed in

ESCC but not EAC.[211] High expression of miR-103, miR-107, and miR-129 in patients with ESCC is associated with poor survival,[210,212] while low expression of miR-21 in ESCC patients correlates with a worse prognosis and poor survival rate.[213] In addition, expression of *RNASEN*, which encodes a key miRNA processing enzyme, correlates with poor prognosis of ESCC.[214] The recent discovery of tumor-derived circulating miRNAs suggests the potential utility for miRNAs as biomarkers or prognostic markers for ESCC.[215,216]

Animal Models to Study ESCC

Animal models are invaluable to understand the molecular pathogenesis of ESCC, from normal to dysplastic states and ultimately cancer. ESCC has been modeled in mice and rats by treatment with N-nitroso compounds, such as N-nitrosomethylbenzylamine (NMBA), or a zinc-deficient diet; in these models, the presence of *p53* deficiency or *cyclin D1* overexpression enhances esophageal squamous cell carcinogenesis.[217–222] The quinoline derivative 4-nitroquinoline-1-oxide (4-NQO) also causes premalignant and malignant squamous lesions of the oral cavity and esophagus, which are increased by *cyclin D1* overexpression.[223,224] Recently, several genetic animal models of ESCC have emerged that recapitulate the human disease process without addition of carcinogen.[189,197,198,225] *Cyclin D1* overexpression in mice produces squamous cell dysplasia of the tongue, esophagus, and forestomach,[226] and in combination with loss of *p53*, null mice produces invasive oral and esophageal squamous cell cancer.[225] Esophageal-specific deletion of *KLF4* results in squamous cell dysplasia and delayed keratinocyte differentiation.[198] Many risk factors for ESCC produce chronic irritation,[5,227] and two recent mouse models, with *KLF4* overexpression or *p120*-catenin deletion, yielded ESCC in the context of chronic inflammation, implicating microenvironment and, possibly, disruption of the esophageal epithelial barrier in the development of ESCC.[189,197] In the case of *KLF4* overexpression, inflammation appears to be mediated by IκB and NFKB activation.

Prevention of Esophageal Squamous Cell Carcinoma

The most obvious approach to the prevention of ESCC is through changes in lifestyle, especially avoiding alcohol and tobacco use, which are the predominant risk factors for ESCC in most parts of the world.[5,228] Additional benefits may be realized by the elimination of high salt foods that may be contaminated with toxins and nitrosamines and the increased consumption of fruits and vegetables, especially in high risk areas for ESCC.[16] Zinc supplementation also be considered, especially in populations at risk for dietary zinc deficiency,[88] as it has been shown to reduce premalignant and malignant lesions in animal models[229,230]; however, the benefits of this zinc supplementation in humans are unclear.[231]

Chemoprevention may have particular relevance in areas of the world where exposure to carcinogens is high. An important component in the chemoprevention of ESCC is that of blocking the progression of premalignant lesions to malignant squamous cell carcinoma.[232] Mechanistically, chemopreventive agents can be either "blocking" or "suppressing".[233] Blocking agents act at the initiation stage of carcinogenesis to influence the metabolism of carcinogens, thereby reducing damage to cellular DNA. Suppressing agents act during tumor promotion or progression to alter cellular processes such as proliferation, apoptosis, differentiation, and invasion.[16] Dietary administration of ellagic acid, a naturally occurring polyphenol, or diallyl sulfide, a component of garlic, inhibits NMBA-mediated ESCC in rats by stimulating Phase II detoxifying enzymes.[234–237] Curcumin, a polyphenol derived from the roots of *Curcumin longa*, inhibits both the initiation and postinitiation stages of NMBA-induced esophageal tumorigenesis by reducing cytochrome CYP2B1 in the rat esophagus to inhibit NMBA activation[238,239]; curcumin also inhibits protein kinase C, EGFR, and IκB.[240] Isothiocyanates are an effective group of anti-initiating agents.[241,242] Phenyl isothiocyanide (PEITC), found in many cruciferous vegetables like cauliflower, cabbage, Brussel sprouts, watercress, is a potent inhibitor of the metabolic activation of nitrosamine carcinogens and DNA methylation both in vitro and in vivo[243]; dietary administration of PEITC can completely inhibit NMBA-induced esophageal tumorigenesis in rats.[244]

Individuals who possess dysplastic lesions that can progress to ESCC are a major subject population for chemoprevention[5,16]; thus an effective chemopreventive agent for human ESCC should possess significant inhibitory activity when administered after tumor initiation. However, few single compounds have been found to effectively inhibit promotion and progression stages following NMBA-mediated tumorigenesis in rat esophagus. PEITC and EA are highly effective anti-initiation agents but have only a modest effect on esophageal tumorigenesis when administered postinitiation.[245,246] Decaffeinated green tea and black tea are effective after tumor initiation by NMBA but only when given at very high concentrations.[247] When given in the diet, the synthetic, selective iNOS inhibitor 1,4-phenylene-bis-(1,2-ethanediyl) bis-isothiourea (PBIT) and the COX2 selective inhibitor L-748706 reduce tumor incidence and multiplicity in the rat esophagus; L-748706 was effective only when it reduced PGE2 levels in preneoplastic esophageal tissues to levels found in normal esophagus.[248] Both the COX2 inhibitor JTE-522 and the natural phenol resveratrol also inhibit tumor development in NMBA-treated rat esophagus by reducing PGE2 levels.[249,250] CPT-11 (irinotecan hydrochloride), a potent anticancer drug for gastric and colorectal cancers, exhibits antiprogression effects by reducing cell proliferation rate in NMBA-exposed squamous epithelium and preneoplastic lesions.[251] Finally, treatment of *cyclin D1* overexpressing, *p53*-deficient mice with a nonsteroidal anti-inflammatory drug sulindac markedly decreased progression of esophageal lesions to severe dysplasia.[225]

Conclusions/Future Directions

Esophageal cancer remains an aggressive and lethal disease and, despite advances in surgical techniques, radiotherapy and chemotherapy, the 5-year survival rate for ESCC has not improved substantially in the past several decades.[252,253] Several preventive approaches can be easily implemented, such as lifestyle changes (avoidance of tobacco and alcohol use) and improved nutrition (consumption of fresh fruits and vegetables, decreased intake of salty foods, and elimination of pickled vegetables). The advent of new animal models should aid in understanding the molecular mechanisms, pathogenesis, prevention, and treatment of ESCC. Still, there remains an urgent need to better define the signaling pathways dysregulated in ESCC and to discover novel biomarkers for malignant progression and patient prognosis. Identification of additional risk factors for ESCC will provide further insights into esophageal cancer development. With the use of effective molecular biomarkers, a more precise risk prediction will be available to detect early and curable lesions, and new targeted therapies may then be implemented to reduce the incidence and mortality of ESCC.

References

1. Jemal A, Bray F, Center MM, Ferlay J, Ward E, Forman D. Global cancer statistics. *CA Cancer J Clin*. 2011;61(2):69–90.
2. Jemal A, Center MM, DeSantis C, Ward EM. Global patterns of cancer incidence and mortality rates and trends. *Cancer Epidemiol Biomarkers Prev*. 2010;19(8):1893–1907.
3. Engel LS, Chow WH, Vaughan TL, et al. Population attributable risks of esophageal and gastric cancers. *J Natl Cancer Inst*. 2003;95(18):1404–1413.
4. Kamangar F, Chow WH, Abnet CC, Dawsey SM. Environmental causes of esophageal cancer. *Gastroenterol Clin North Am*. 2009;38(1):27–57.
5. Stoner GD, Gupta A. Etiology and chemoprevention of esophageal squamous cell carcinoma. *Carcinogenesis*. 2001;22(11): 1737–1746.
6. Anani PA, Gardiol D, Savary M, Monnier P. An extensive morphological and comparative study of clinically early and obvious squamous cell carcinoma of the esophagus. *Pathol Res Pract*. 1991;187(2–3):214–219.
7. Kuwano H, Watanabe M, Sadanaga N, Ikebe M, Mori M, Sugimachi K. Squamous epithelial dysplasia associated with squamous cell carcinoma of the esophagus. *Cancer Lett*. 1993;72(3):141–147.
8. Polednak AP. Trends in survival for both histologic types of esophageal cancer in US surveillance, epidemiology and end results areas. *Int J Cancer*. 2003;105(1):98–100.
9. Younes M, Henson DE, Ertan A, Miller CC. Incidence and survival trends of esophageal carcinoma in the United States: racial and gender differences by histological type. *Scand J Gastroenterol*. 2002;37(12):1359–1365.
10. Rose EF. Esophageal cancer in the Transkei: 1955–69. *J Natl Cancer Inst*. 1973;51(1):7–16.
11. Schottenfeld D. Epidemiology of cancer of the esophagus. *Semin Oncol*. 1984;11(2):92–100.
12. Sons HU. Etiologic and epidemiologic factors of carcinoma of the esophagus. *Surg Gynecol Obstet*. 1987;165(2):183–190.
13. Yang CS. Research on esophageal cancer in China: a review. *Cancer Res*. 1980;40(8 Pt 1):2633–2644.
14. Gholipour C, Shalchi RA, Abbasi M. A histopathological study of esophageal cancer on the western side of the Caspian littoral from 1994 to 2003. *Dis Esophagus*. 2008;21(4):322–327.
15. Tran GD, Sun XD, Abnet CC, et al. Prospective study of risk factors for esophageal and gastric cancers in the Linxian general population trial cohort in China. *Int J Cancer*. 2005;113(3):456–463.
16. Stoner GD, Wang LS, Chen T. Chemoprevention of esophageal squamous cell carcinoma. *Toxicol Appl Pharmacol*. 2007;224(3): 337–349.
17. Islami F, Boffetta P, Ren JS, Pedoeim L, Khatib D, Kamangar F. High-temperature beverages and foods and esophageal cancer risk–a systematic review. *Int J Cancer*. 2009;125(3):491–524.
18. Islami F, Pourshams A, Nasrollahzadeh D, et al. Tea drinking habits and oesophageal cancer in a high risk area in northern Iran: population based case-control study. *BMJ*. 2009;338:b929.
19. Wu M, Liu AM, Kampman E, et al. Green tea drinking, high tea temperature and esophageal cancer in high- and low-risk areas of Jiangsu Province, China: a population-based case-control study. *Int J Cancer*. 2009;124(8):1907–1913.
20. Hecht SS. Cigarette smoking: cancer risks, carcinogens, and mechanisms. *Langenbecks Arch Surg*. 2006;391(6):603–613.
21. Gammon MD, Schoenberg JB, Ahsan H, et al. Tobacco, alcohol, and socioeconomic status and adenocarcinomas of the esophagus and gastric cardia. *J Natl Cancer Inst*. 1997;89(17):1277–1284.
22. Xu XC. Risk factors and gene expression in esophageal cancer. *Methods Mol Biol*. 2009;471:335–360.
23. Zhang ZF, Kurtz RC, Sun M, et al. Adenocarcinomas of the esophagus and gastric cardia: medical conditions, tobacco, alcohol, and socioeconomic factors. *Cancer Epidemiol Biomarkers Prev*. 1996;5(10):761–768.
24. Zhang ZF, Kurtz RC, Yu GP, et al. Adenocarcinomas of the esophagus and gastric cardia: the role of diet. *Nutr Cancer*. 1997; 27(3):298–309.
25. Carstensen JM, Pershagen G, Eklund G. Mortality in relation to cigarette and pipe smoking: 16 years' observation of 25,000 Swedish men. *J Epidemiol Community Health*. 1987;41(2): 166–172.
26. Doll R, Peto R, Wheatley K, Gray R, Sutherland I. Mortality in relation to smoking: 40 years' observations on male British doctors. *BMJ*. 1994;309(6959):901–911.
27. Freedman ND, Abnet CC, Leitzmann MF, et al. A prospective study of tobacco, alcohol, and the risk of esophageal and gastric cancer subtypes. *Am J Epidemiol*. 2007;165(12):1424–1433.
28. Ishikawa A, Kuriyama S, Tsubono Y, et al. Smoking, alcohol drinking, green tea consumption and the risk of esophageal cancer in Japanese men. *J Epidemiol*. 2006;16(5):185–192.
29. McLaughlin JK, Hrubec Z, Blot WJ, Fraumeni JF Jr. Smoking and cancer mortality among U.S. veterans: a 26-year follow-up. *Int J Cancer*. 1995;60(2):190–193.
30. Betel-quid and areca-nut chewing and some areca-nut derived nitrosamines. *IARC Monogr Eval Carcinog Risks Hum*. 2004;85:1–334.

31. Toh Y, Oki E, Ohgaki K, et al. Alcohol drinking, cigarette smoking, and the development of squamous cell carcinoma of the esophagus: molecular mechanisms of carcinogenesis. *Int J Clin Oncol*. 2010;15(2):135–144.
32. Hecht SS, Hoffmann D. N-nitroso compounds and tobacco-induced cancers in man. *IARC Sci Publ*. 1991;105:54–61.
33. Khalili H, Zhang FJ, Harvey RG, Dipple A. Mutagenicity of benzo[a]pyrene-deoxyadenosine adducts in a sequence context derived from the p53 gene. *Mutat Res*. 2000;465(1–2):39–44.
34. MacLeod MC, Evans FE, Lay J, et al. Identification of a novel, N7-deoxyguanosine adduct as the major DNA adduct formed by a non-bay-region diol epoxide of benzo[a]pyrene with low mutagenic potential. *Biochemistry*. 1994;33(10):2977–2987.
35. Pfeifer GP, Denissenko MF, Olivier M, Tretyakova N, Hecht SS, Hainaut P. Tobacco smoke carcinogens, DNA damage and p53 mutations in smoking-associated cancers. *Oncogene*. 2002; 21(48):7435–7451.
36. Mandard AM, Hainaut P, Hollstein M. Genetic steps in the development of squamous cell carcinoma of the esophagus. *Mutat Res*. 2000;462(2–3):335–342.
37. Osborne MR. Sequence specificity in the reaction of benzopyrene diol epoxide with DNA. *Chem Biol Interact*. 1990;75(2): 131–140.
38. Zhang FJ, Cortez C, Harvey RG. New synthetic approaches to polycyclic aromatic hydrocarbons and their carcinogenic oxidized metabolites: derivatives of benzo[s]picene, benzo[rst]pentaphene, and dibenzo[b, def]chrysene. *J Org Chem*. 2000;65(13): 3952–3960.
39. Bartsch H. DNA adducts in human carcinogenesis: etiological relevance and structure-activity relationship. *Mutat Res*. 1996;340 (2–3):67–79.
40. Venkatachalam S, Denissenko MF, Alvi N, Wani AA. Rapid activation of apoptosis in human promyelocytic leukemic cells by (+/-)-anti-benzo[a]pyrene diol epoxide induced DNA damage. *Biochem Biophys Res Commun*. 1993;197(2):722–729.
41. Denissenko MF, Pao A, Tang M, Pfeifer GP. Preferential formation of benzo[a]pyrene adducts at lung cancer mutational hotspots in P53. *Science*. 1996;274(5286):430–432.
42. Mass MJ, Jeffers AJ, Ross JA, et al. Ki-ras oncogene mutations in tumors and DNA adducts formed by benz[j]aceanthrylene and benzo[a]pyrene in the lungs of strain A/J mice. *Mol Carcinog*. 1993;8(3):186–192.
43. Kozack R, Seo KY, Jelinsky SA, Loechler EL. Toward an understanding of the role of DNA adduct conformation in defining mutagenic mechanism based on studies of the major adduct (formed at N(2)-dG) of the potent environmental carcinogen, benzo[a]pyrene. *Mutat Res*. 2000;450(1–2):41–59.
44. Pfeifer GP, Besaratinia A. Mutational spectra of human cancer. *Hum Genet*. 2009;125(5–6):493–506.
45. Wang XD. Alcohol, vitamin A, and cancer. *Alcohol*. 2005;35(3): 251–258.
46. Boffetta P, Garfinkel L. Alcohol drinking and mortality among men enrolled in an American Cancer Society prospective study. *Epidemiology*. 1990;1(5):342–348.
47. Brown LM, Hoover R, Silverman D, et al. Excess incidence of squamous cell esophageal cancer among US Black men: role of social class and other risk factors. *Am J Epidemiol*. 2001;153(2): 114–122.
48. Brown LM, Hoover RN, Greenberg RS, et al. Are racial differences in squamous cell esophageal cancer explained by alcohol and tobacco use? *J Natl Cancer Inst*. 1994;86(17):1340–1345.
49. Pandeya N, Williams G, Green AC, Webb PM, Whiteman DC. Alcohol consumption and the risks of adenocarcinoma and squamous cell carcinoma of the esophagus. *Gastroenterology*. 2009;136(4):1215–1224. e1211–1212.
50. Shiraishi-Yokoyama H, Yokoyama H, Matsumoto M, Imaeda H, Hibi T. Acetaldehyde inhibits the formation of retinoic acid from retinal in the rat esophagus. *Scand J Gastroenterol*. 2006;41(1): 80–86.
51. Wang XD, Liu C, Chung J, Stickel F, Seitz HK, Russell RM. Chronic alcohol intake reduces retinoic acid concentration and enhances AP-1 (c-Jun and c-Fos) expression in rat liver. *Hepatology*. 1998;28(3):744–750.
52. Li M, Song S, Lippman SM, et al. Induction of retinoic acid receptor-beta suppresses cyclooxygenase-2 expression in esophageal cancer cells. *Oncogene*. 2002;21(3):411–418.
53. Xu XC. Tumor-suppressive activity of retinoic acid receptor-beta in cancer. *Cancer Lett*. 2007;253(1):14–24.
54. Castellsague X, Munoz N, De Stefani E, et al. Independent and joint effects of tobacco smoking and alcohol drinking on the risk of esophageal cancer in men and women. *Int J Cancer*. 1999; 82(5):657–664.
55. Kinjo Y, Cui Y, Akiba S, et al. Mortality risks of oesophageal cancer associated with hot tea, alcohol, tobacco and diet in Japan. *J Epidemiol*. 1998;8(4):235–243.
56. Lee CH, Wu DC, Lee JM, et al. Carcinogenetic impact of alcohol intake on squamous cell carcinoma risk of the oesophagus in relation to tobacco smoking. *Eur J Cancer*. 2007;43(7): 1188–1199.
57. Morita M, Kumashiro R, Kubo N, et al. Alcohol drinking, cigarette smoking, and the development of squamous cell carcinoma of the esophagus: epidemiology, clinical findings, and prevention. *Int J Clin Oncol*. 2010;15(2):126–134.
58. Salaspuro V, Salaspuro M. Synergistic effect of alcohol drinking and smoking on in vivo acetaldehyde concentration in saliva. *Int J Cancer*. 2004;111(4):480–483.
59. Kuratsune M, Kohchi S, Horie A. Carcinogenesis in the Esophagus. I. Penetration of Benzo(a) Pyrene and other hydrocarbons into the esophageal mucosa. *Gann*. 1965;56:177–187.
60. Leeuwenburgh I, Haringsma J, Van Dekken H, Scholten P, Siersema PD, Kuipers EJ. Long-term risk of oesophagitis, Barrett's oesophagus and oesophageal cancer in achalasia patients. *Scand J Gastroenterol*. 2006;243(Suppl):7–10.
61. Carter R, Brewer LA III. Achalasia and esophageal carcinoma. Studies in early diagnosis for improved surgical management. *Am J Surg*. 1975;130(2):114–120.
62. Meijssen MA, Tilanus HW, van Blankenstein M, Hop WC, Ong GL. Achalasia complicated by oesophageal squamous cell carcinoma: a prospective study in 195 patients. *Gut*. 1992;33(2): 155–158.
63. Streitz JM Jr, Ellis FH Jr, Gibb SP, Heatley GM. Achalasia and squamous cell carcinoma of the esophagus: analysis of 241 patients. *Ann Thorac Surg*. 1995;59(6):1604–1609.
64. Wychulis AR, Woolam GL, Andersen HA, Ellis FH Jr. Achalasia and carcinoma of the esophagus. *JAMA*. 1971;215(10): 1638–1641.
65. Zendehdel K, Nyren O, Edberg A, Ye W. Risk of esophageal adenocarcinoma in achalasia patients, a retrospective cohort study in Sweden. *Am J Gastroenterol*. 2011;106:57–61.
66. Robertson EV, Jankowski JA. Genetics of gastroesophageal cancer: paradigms, paradoxes, and prognostic utility. *Am J Gastroenterol*. 2008;103(2):443–449.
67. Marger RS, Marger D. Carcinoma of the esophagus and tylosis. A lethal genetic combination. *Cancer*. 1993;72(1):17–19.
68. Messmann H. Squamous cell cancer of the oesophagus. *Best Pract Res Clin Gastroenterol*. 2001;15(2):249–265.
69. Maillefer RH, Greydanus MP. To B or not to B: is tylosis B truly benign? Two North American genealogies. *Am J Gastroenterol*. 1999;94(3):829–834.
70. Risk JM, Field EA, Field JK, et al. Tylosis oesophageal cancer mapped. *Nat Genet*. 1994;8(4):319–321.
71. El-Omar EM, Rabkin CS, Gammon MD, et al. Increased risk of noncardia gastric cancer associated with proinflammatory cytokine gene polymorphisms. *Gastroenterology*. 2003;124(5):1193–1201.

72. Wang Z, Tang L, Sun G, et al. Etiological study of esophageal squamous cell carcinoma in an endemic region: a population-based case control study in Huaian, China. *BMC Cancer.* 2006;6:287.
73. IARC Working Group on the Evaluation of Carcinogenic Risks to Humans. Human papillomaviruses. *IARC Monogr Eval Carcinog Risks Hum.* 2007;90:1–636.
74. Gillison ML, Shah KV. Chapter 9: Role of mucosal human papillomavirus in nongenital cancers. *J Natl Cancer Inst Monogr.* 2003;31:57–65.
75. Benamouzig R, Jullian E, Chang F, et al. Absence of human papillomavirus DNA detected by polymerase chain reaction in French patients with esophageal carcinoma. *Gastroenterology.* 1995; 109(6):1876–1881.
76. Koh JS, Lee SS, Baek HJ, Kim YI. No association of high-risk human papillomavirus with esophageal squamous cell carcinomas among Koreans, as determined by polymerase chain reaction. *Dis Esophagus.* 2008;21(2):114–117.
77. Kok TC, Nooter K, Tjong AHSP, Smits HL, Ter Schegget JT. No evidence of known types of human papillomavirus in squamous cell cancer of the oesophagus in a low-risk area. Rotterdam Oesophageal Tumour Study Group. *Eur J Cancer.* 1997; 33(11):1865–1868.
78. Poljak M, Cerar A, Seme K. Human papillomavirus infection in esophageal carcinomas: a study of 121 lesions using multiple broad-spectrum polymerase chain reactions and literature review. *Hum Pathol.* 1998;29(3):266–271.
79. Saegusa M, Hashimura M, Takano Y, Ohbu M, Okayasu I. Absence of human papillomavirus genomic sequences detected by the polymerase chain reaction in oesophageal and gastric carcinomas in Japan. *Mol Pathol.* 1997;50(2):101–104.
80. Talamini G, Capelli P, Zamboni G, et al. Alcohol, smoking and papillomavirus infection as risk factors for esophageal squamous-cell papilloma and esophageal squamous-cell carcinoma in Italy. *Int J Cancer.* 2000;86(6):874–878.
81. White RE, Mungatana C, Mutuma G, et al. Absence of human papillomavirus in esophageal carcinomas from southwestern Kenya. *Dis Esophagus.* 2005;18(1):28–30.
82. Yao PF, Li GC, Li J, et al. Evidence of human papilloma virus infection and its epidemiology in esophageal squamous cell carcinoma. *World J Gastroenterol.* 2006;12(9):1352–1355.
83. Freedman ND, Park Y, Subar AF, et al. Fruit and vegetable intake and esophageal cancer in a large prospective cohort study. *Int J Cancer.* 2007;121(12):2753–2760.
84. Gonzalez CA, Pera G, Agudo A, et al. Fruit and vegetable intake and the risk of stomach and oesophagus adenocarcinoma in the European Prospective Investigation into Cancer and Nutrition (EPIC-EURGAST). *Int J Cancer.* 2006;118(10):2559–2566.
85. Yamaji T, Inoue M, Sasazuki S, et al. Fruit and vegetable consumption and squamous cell carcinoma of the esophagus in Japan: the JPHC study. *Int J Cancer.* 2008;123(8):1935–1940.
86. Glade MJ. Food, nutrition, and the prevention of cancer: a global perspective. American Institute for Cancer Research/World Cancer Research Fund, American Institute for Cancer Research, 1997. *Nutrition.* 1999;15(6):523–526.
87. Wiseman M. The second World Cancer Research Fund/American Institute for Cancer Research expert report. Food, nutrition, physical activity, and the prevention of cancer: a global perspective. *Proc Nutr Soc.* 2008;67(3):253–256.
88. Lonnerdal B. Dietary factors influencing zinc absorption. *J Nutr.* 2000;130(5S Suppl):1378S–1383S.
89. Ke L. Mortality and incidence trends from esophagus cancer in selected geographic areas of China circa 1970–90. *Int J Cancer.* 2002;102(3):271–274.
90. Abnet CC, Lai B, Qiao YL, et al. Zinc concentration in esophageal biopsy specimens measured by X-ray fluorescence and esophageal cancer risk. *J Natl Cancer Inst.* 2005;97(4):301–306.
91. Chen X, Yang CS. Esophageal adenocarcinoma: a review and perspectives on the mechanism of carcinogenesis and chemoprevention. *Carcinogenesis.* 2001;22(8):1119–1129.
92. Koppert LB, Wijnhoven BP, van Dekken H, Tilanus HW, Dinjens WN. The molecular biology of esophageal adenocarcinoma. *J Surg Oncol.* 2005;92(3):169–190.
93. Lagarde SM, ten Kate FJ, Richel DJ, Offerhaus GJ, van Lanschot JJ. Molecular prognostic factors in adenocarcinoma of the esophagus and gastroesophageal junction. *Ann Surg Oncol.* 2007;14(2): 977–991.
94. Reid BJ, Blount PL, Rabinovitch PS. Biomarkers in Barrett's esophagus. *Gastrointest Endosc Clin N Am.* 2003;13(2):369–397.
95. Spechler SJ. Barrett's esophagus: a molecular perspective. *Curr Gastroenterol Rep.* 2005;7(3):177–181.
96. Hollstein M, Sidransky D, Vogelstein B, Harris CC. p53 mutations in human cancers. *Science.* 1991;253(5015):49–53.
97. Olivier M, Eeles R, Hollstein M, Khan MA, Harris CC, Hainaut P. The IARC TP53 database: new online mutation analysis and recommendations to users. *Hum Mutat.* 2002;19(6):607–614.
98. el-Deiry WS, Tokino T, Velculescu VE, et al. WAF1, a potential mediator of p53 tumor suppression. *Cell.* 1993;75(4):817–825.
99. Miyashita T, Krajewski S, Krajewska M, et al. Tumor suppressor p53 is a regulator of bcl-2 and bax gene expression in vitro and in vivo. *Oncogene.* 1994;9(6):1799–1805.
100. Oltvai ZN, Milliman CL, Korsmeyer SJ. Bcl-2 heterodimerizes in vivo with a conserved homolog, Bax, that accelerates programmed cell death. *Cell.* 1993;74(4):609–619.
101. Egashira A, Morita M, Kakeji Y, et al. p53 gene mutations in esophageal squamous cell carcinoma and their relevance to etiology and pathogenesis: results in Japan and comparisons with other countries. *Cancer Sci.* 2007;98(8):1152–1156.
102. Haupt Y, Maya R, Kazaz A, Oren M. Mdm2 promotes the rapid degradation of p53. *Nature.* 1997;387(6630):296–299.
103. Parenti AR, Rugge M, Frizzera E, et al. p53 overexpression in the multistep process of esophageal carcinogenesis. *Am J Surg Pathol.* 1995;19(12):1418–1422.
104. Hollstein M, Hergenhahn M, Yang Q, Bartsch H, Wang ZQ, Hainaut P. New approaches to understanding p53 gene tumor mutation spectra. *Mutat Res.* 1999;431(2):199–209.
105. Gamieldien W, Victor TC, Mugwanya D, et al. p53 and p16/CDKN2 gene mutations in esophageal tumors from a high-incidence area in South Africa. *Int J Cancer.* 1998;78(5):544–549.
106. Goan YG, Chang HC, Hsu HK, Chou YP, Cheng JT. Risk of p53 gene mutation in esophageal squamous cell carcinoma and habit of betel quid chewing in Taiwanese. *Cancer Sci.* 2005;96(11): 758–765.
107. Hattori K, Kajiyama Y, Tsurumaru M. Mutation of the p53 gene predicts lymph node metastases in Japanese patients with esophageal carcinoma: DNA and immunohistochemical analyses. *Dis Esophagus.* 2003;16(4):301–306.
108. Hu N, Huang J, Emmert-Buck MR, et al. Frequent inactivation of the TP53 gene in esophageal squamous cell carcinoma from a high-risk population in China. *Clin Cancer Res.* 2001;7(4):883–891.
109. Ribeiro U Jr, Finkelstein SD, Safatle-Ribeiro AV, et al. p53 sequence analysis predicts treatment response and outcome of patients with esophageal carcinoma. *Cancer.* 1998;83(1):7–18.
110. Robert V, Michel P, Flaman JM, et al. High frequency in esophageal cancers of p53 alterations inactivating the regulation of genes involved in cell cycle and apoptosis. *Carcinogenesis.* 2000;21(4): 563–565.
111. Sepehr A, Taniere P, Martel-Planche G, et al. Distinct pattern of TP53 mutations in squamous cell carcinoma of the esophagus in Iran. *Oncogene.* 2001;20(50):7368–7374.
112. Shi ST, Yang GY, Wang LD, et al. Role of p53 gene mutations in human esophageal carcinogenesis: results from immunohistochemical and mutation analyses of carcinomas and nearby non-cancerous lesions. *Carcinogenesis.* 1999;20(4):591–597.

113. Wang LD, Zhou FY, Li XM, et al. Genome-wide association study of esophageal squamous cell carcinoma in Chinese subjects identifies susceptibility loci at PLCE1 and C20orf54. *Nat Genet.* 2010;42(9):759–763.
114. Greenblatt MS, Bennett WP, Hollstein M, Harris CC. Mutations in the p53 tumor suppressor gene: clues to cancer etiology and molecular pathogenesis. *Cancer Res.* 1994;54(18):4855–4878.
115. Putz A, Hartmann AA, Fontes PR, et al. TP53 mutation pattern of esophageal squamous cell carcinomas in a high risk area (Southern Brazil): role of life style factors. *Int J Cancer.* 2002;98(1):99–105.
116. Liu Z, Muehlbauer KR, Schmeiser HH, Hergenhahn M, Belharazem D, Hollstein MC. p53 mutations in benzo(a)pyrene-exposed human p53 knock-in murine fibroblasts correlate with p53 mutations in human lung tumors. *Cancer Res.* 2005;65(7): 2583–2587.
117. Oki E, Zhao Y, Yoshida R, et al. The difference in p53 mutations between cancers of the upper and lower gastrointestinal tract. *Digestion.* 2009;79(Suppl 1):33–39.
118. Belinsky SA. Silencing of genes by promoter hypermethylation: key event in rodent and human lung cancer. *Carcinogenesis.* 2005;26(9):1481–1487.
119. Nobori T, Miura K, Wu DJ, Lois A, Takabayashi K, Carson DA. Deletions of the cyclin-dependent kinase-4 inhibitor gene in multiple human cancers. *Nature.* 1994;368(6473):753–756.
120. Okamoto A, Demetrick DJ, Spillare EA, et al. Mutations and altered expression of p16INK4 in human cancer. *Proc Natl Acad Sci USA.* 1994;91(23):11045–11049.
121. Herman JG, Merlo A, Mao L, et al. Inactivation of the CDKN2/p16/MTS1 gene is frequently associated with aberrant DNA methylation in all common human cancers. *Cancer Res.* 1995; 55(20):4525–4530.
122. Tokugawa T, Sugihara H, Tani T, Hattori T. Modes of silencing of p16 in development of esophageal squamous cell carcinoma. *Cancer Res.* 2002;62(17):4938–4944.
123. Ito S, Ohga T, Saeki H, et al. Promoter hypermethylation and quantitative expression analysis of CDKN2A (p14ARF and p16INK4a) gene in esophageal squamous cell carcinoma. *Anticancer Res.* 2007;27(5A):3345–3353.
124. Takeuchi H, Ozawa S, Ando N, et al. Altered p16/MTS1/CDKN2 and cyclin D1/PRAD-1 gene expression is associated with the prognosis of squamous cell carcinoma of the esophagus. *Clin Cancer Res.* 1997;3(12 Pt 1):2229–2236.
125. Motokura T, Bloom T, Kim HG, et al. A novel cyclin encoded by a bcl1-linked candidate oncogene. *Nature.* 1991;350(6318):512–515.
126. Watanabe M, Kuwano H, Tanaka S, Toh Y, Masuda H, Sugimachi K. A significant morphological transformation is recognized in human esophageal cancer cells with an amplification/overexpression of the cyclin D1 gene. *Int J Oncol.* 1999;15(6):1103–1108.
127. Adelaide J, Monges G, Derderian C, Seitz JF, Birnbaum D. Oesophageal cancer and amplification of the human cyclin D gene CCND1/PRAD1. *Br J Cancer.* 1995;71(1):64–68.
128. Nakagawa H, Zukerberg L, Togawa K, Meltzer SJ, Nishihara T, Rustgi AK. Human cyclin D1 oncogene and esophageal squamous cell carcinoma. *Cancer.* 1995;76(4):541–549.
129. Shamma A, Doki Y, Shiozaki H, et al. Cyclin D1 overexpression in esophageal dysplasia: a possible biomarker for carcinogenesis of esophageal squamous cell carcinoma. *Int J Oncol.* 2000;16(2): 261–266.
130. Shamma A, Doki Y, Shiozaki H, et al. Effect of cyclin D1 and associated proteins on proliferation of esophageal squamous cell carcinoma. *Int J Oncol.* 1998;13(3):455–460.
131. Shinozaki H, Ozawa S, Ando N, et al. Cyclin D1 amplification as a new predictive classification for squamous cell carcinoma of the esophagus, adding gene information. *Clin Cancer Res.* 1996;2(7):1155–1161.
132. Kuwano H, Kato H, Miyazaki T, et al. Genetic alterations in esophageal cancer. *Surg Today.* 2005;35(1):7–18.
133. Gaudray P, Szepetowski P, Escot C, Birnbaum D, Theillet C. DNA amplification at 11q13 in human cancer: from complexity to perplexity. *Mutat Res.* 1992;276(3):317–328.
134. Tsuruta H, Sakamoto H, Onda M, Terada M. Amplification and overexpression of EXP1 and EXP2/Cyclin D1 genes in human esophageal carcinomas. *Biochem Biophys Res Commun.* 1993;196(3):1529–1536.
135. Naitoh H, Shibata J, Kawaguchi A, Kodama M, Hattori T. Overexpression and localization of cyclin D1 mRNA and antigen in esophageal cancer. *Am J Pathol.* 1995;146(5):1161–1169.
136. Takeuchi H, Ozawa S, Ando N, Kitagawa Y, Ueda M, Kitajima M. Cell-cycle regulators and the Ki-67 labeling index can predict the response to chemoradiotherapy and the survival of patients with locally advanced squamous cell carcinoma of the esophagus. *Ann Surg Oncol.* 2003;10(7):792–800.
137. Sarbia M, Stahl M, Fink U, et al. Prognostic significance of cyclin D1 in esophageal squamous cell carcinoma patients treated with surgery alone or combined therapy modalities. *Int J Cancer.* 1999;84(1):86–91.
138. Hu H, Zhang S, Zhu S. Influence of aspirin and cigarette smoke extract on the expression of cyclin D1 and effects of cell cycle in esophageal squamous cell carcinoma cell line. *Dis Esophagus.* 2009;22(4):310–316.
139. Song S, Lippman SM, Zou Y, Ye X, Ajani JA, Xu XC. Induction of cyclooxygenase-2 by benzo[a]pyrene diol epoxide through inhibition of retinoic acid receptor-beta 2 expression. *Oncogene.* 2005;24(56):8268–8276.
140. Hanawa M, Suzuki S, Dobashi Y, et al. EGFR protein overexpression and gene amplification in squamous cell carcinomas of the esophagus. *Int J Cancer.* 2006;118(5):1173–1180.
141. Kitagawa Y, Ueda M, Ando N, Ozawa S, Shimizu N, Kitajima M. Further evidence for prognostic significance of epidermal growth factor receptor gene amplification in patients with esophageal squamous cell carcinoma. *Clin Cancer Res.* 1996;2(5):909–914.
142. Sudo T, Mimori K, Nagahara H, et al. Identification of EGFR mutations in esophageal cancer. *Eur J Surg Oncol.* 2007;33(1): 44–48.
143. Wang X, Tournier C. Regulation of cellular functions by the ERK5 signalling pathway. *Cell Signal.* 2006;18(6):753–760.
144. Dong C, Davis RJ, Flavell RA. MAP kinases in the immune response. *Annu Rev Immunol.* 2002;20:55–72.
145. Fang JY, Richardson BC. The MAPK signalling pathways and colorectal cancer. *Lancet Oncol.* 2005;6(5):322–327.
146. Troppmair J, Bruder JT, Munoz H, et al. Mitogen-activated protein kinase/extracellular signal-regulated protein kinase activation by oncogenes, serum, and 12-O-tetradecanoylphorbol-13-acetate requires Raf and is necessary for transformation. *J Biol Chem.* 1994;269(9):7030–7035.
147. Dhillon AS, Hagan S, Rath O, Kolch W. MAP kinase signalling pathways in cancer. *Oncogene.* 2007;26(22):3279–3290.
148. Boutros T, Chevet E, Metrakos P. Mitogen-activated protein (MAP) kinase/MAP kinase phosphatase regulation: roles in cell growth, death, and cancer. *Pharmacol Rev.* 2008;60(3):261–310.
149. Wang X, Wang Q, Hu W, Evers BM. Regulation of phorbol ester-mediated TRAF1 induction in human colon cancer cells through a PKC/RAF/ERK/NF-kappaB-dependent pathway. *Oncogene.* 2004;23(10):1885–1895.
150. Schubbert S, Shannon K, Bollag G. Hyperactive Ras in developmental disorders and cancer. *Nat Rev Cancer.* 2007;7(4):295–308.
151. Malumbres M, Barbacid M. RAS oncogenes: the first 30 years. *Nat Rev Cancer.* 2003;3(6):459–465.
152. Bos JL, Fearon ER, Hamilton SR, et al. Prevalence of ras gene mutations in human colorectal cancers. *Nature.* 1987;327(6120): 293–297.
153. Wan PT, Garnett MJ, Roe SM, et al. Mechanism of activation of the RAF-ERK signaling pathway by oncogenic mutations of B-RAF. *Cell.* 2004;116(6):855–867.

154. Morgan S, Grandis JR. ErbB receptors in the biology and pathology of the aerodigestive tract. *Exp Cell Res*. 2009;315(4): 572–582.
155. Ako E, Yamashita Y, Ohira M, et al. The pan-erbB tyrosine kinase inhibitor CI-1033 inhibits human esophageal cancer cells in vitro and in vivo. *Oncol Rep*. 2007;17(4):887–893.
156. Hong S, Lee HJ, Kim SJ, Hahm KB. Connection between inflammation and carcinogenesis in gastrointestinal tract: focus on TGF-beta signaling. *World J Gastroenterol*. 2010;16(17): 2080–2093.
157. Miyazono K, Suzuki H, Imamura T. Regulation of TGF-beta signaling and its roles in progression of tumors. *Cancer Sci*. 2003;94(3):230–234.
158. Markowitz SD, Roberts AB. Tumor suppressor activity of the TGF-beta pathway in human cancers. *Cytokine Growth Factor Rev*. 1996;7(1):93–102.
159. Fukuchi M, Masuda N, Miyazaki T, et al. Decreased Smad4 expression in the transforming growth factor-beta signaling pathway during progression of esophageal squamous cell carcinoma. *Cancer*. 2002;95(4):737–743.
160. Natsugoe S, Xiangming C, Matsumoto M, et al. Smad4 and transforming growth factor beta1 expression in patients with squamous cell carcinoma of the esophagus. *Clin Cancer Res*. 2002;8(6):1838–1842.
161. Fukuchi M, Fukai Y, Masuda N, et al. High-level expression of the Smad ubiquitin ligase Smurf2 correlates with poor prognosis in patients with esophageal squamous cell carcinoma. *Cancer Res*. 2002;62(24):7162–7165.
162. Fukai Y, Fukuchi M, Masuda N, et al. Reduced expression of transforming growth factor-beta receptors is an unfavorable prognostic factor in human esophageal squamous cell carcinoma. *Int J Cancer*. 2003;104(2):161–166.
163. Kavsak P, Rasmussen RK, Causing CG, et al. Smad7 Binds to Smurf2 to Form an E3 Ubiquitin Ligase that Targets the TGF[beta] Receptor for Degradation. *Mol Cell*. 2000;6(6):1365–1375.
164. Lotan R. Effects of vitamin A and its analogs (retinoids) on normal and neoplastic cells. *Biochim Biophys Acta*. 1980;605(1): 33–91.
165. Chambon P. A decade of molecular biology of retinoic acid receptors. *FASEB J*. 1996;10(9):940–954.
166. Qiu H, Zhang W, El-Naggar AK, et al. Loss of retinoic acid receptor-beta expression is an early event during esophageal carcinogenesis. *Am J Pathol*. 1999;155(5):1519–1523.
167. Kuroki T, Trapasso F, Yendamuri S, et al. Allele loss and promoter hypermethylation of VHL, RAR-beta, RASSF1A, and FHIT tumor suppressor genes on chromosome 3p in esophageal squamous cell carcinoma. *Cancer Res*. 2003;63(13):3724–3728.
168. Su H, Hu N, Shih J, et al. Gene expression analysis of esophageal squamous cell carcinoma reveals consistent molecular profiles related to a family history of upper gastrointestinal cancer. *Cancer Res*. 2003;63(14):3872–3876.
169. Liu ZM, Ding F, Guo MZ, Zhang LY, Wu M, Liu ZH. Downregulation of retinoic acid receptor-beta(2) expression is linked to aberrant methylation in esophageal squamous cell carcinoma cell lines. *World J Gastroenterol*. 2004;10(6):771–775.
170. Wang Y, Fang MZ, Liao J, et al. Hypermethylation-associated inactivation of retinoic acid receptor beta in human esophageal squamous cell carcinoma. *Clin Cancer Res*. 2003;9(14): 5257–5263.
171. Mariette C, Finzi L, Piessen G, Van Seuningen I, Triboulet JP. Esophageal carcinoma: prognostic differences between squamous cell carcinoma and adenocarcinoma. *World J Surg*. 2005;29(1): 39–45.
172. Xu XC, Lee JJ, Wu TT, Hoque A, Ajani JA, Lippman SM. Increased retinoic acid receptor-beta4 correlates in vivo with reduced retinoic acid receptor-beta2 in esophageal squamous cell carcinoma. *Cancer Epidemiol Biomarkers Prev*. 2005;14(4): 826–829.
173. Song S, Guan B, Men T, Hoque A, Lotan R, Xu XC. Antitumor effect of retinoic acid receptor-beta2 associated with suppression of cyclooxygenase-2. *Cancer Prev Res (Phila)*. 2009;2(3): 274–280.
174. Clevers H. Wnt/[beta]-Catenin signaling in development and disease. *Cell*. 2006;127(3):469–480.
175. Moon RT, Kohn AD, De Ferrari GV, Kaykas A. WNT and beta-catenin signalling: diseases and therapies. *Nat Rev Genet*. 2004;5(9):691–701.
176. Elcheva I, Tarapore RS, Bhatia N, Spiegelman VS. Overexpression of mRNA-binding protein CRD-BP in malignant melanomas. *Oncogene*. 2008;27(37):5069–5074.
177. Tarapore RS, Siddiqui IA, Saleem M, Adhami VM, Spiegelman VS, Mukhtar H. Specific targeting of Wnt/beta-catenin signaling in human melanoma cells by a dietary triterpene lupeol. *Carcinogenesis*. 2010;31(10):1844–1853.
178. Lustig B, Behrens J. The Wnt signaling pathway and its role in tumor development. *J Cancer Res Clin Oncol*. 2003;129(4):199–221.
179. Li AF, Hsu PK, Tzao C, et al. Reduced axin protein expression is associated with a poor prognosis in patients with squamous cell carcinoma of esophagus. *Ann Surg Oncol*. 2009;16(9):2486–2493.
180. Wang W, Xue L, Liu H, Wang P, Xu P, Cai Y. Aberrant changes of Wnt2/Beta-catenin signaling pathway induced by sodium nitroprusside in human esophageal squamous cell carcinoma cell lines. *Cancer Investig*. 2010;28(3):230–241.
181. Situ DR, Hu Y, Zhu ZH, Wang J, Long H, Rong TH. Prognostic relevance of beta-catenin expression in T2-3N0M0 esophageal squamous cell carcinoma. *World J Gastroenterol*. 2010;16(41): 5195–5202.
182. Zhao XJ, Li H, Chen H, et al. Expression of e-cadherin and beta-catenin in human esophageal squamous cell carcinoma: relationships with prognosis. *World J Gastroenterol*. 2003;9(2):225–232.
183. Lin YC, Wu MY, Li DR, Wu XY, Zheng RM. Prognostic and clinicopathological features of E-cadherin, alpha-catenin, beta-catenin, gamma-catenin and cyclin D1 expression in human esophageal squamous cell carcinoma. *World J Gastroenterol*. 2004;10(22):3235–3239.
184. Shapiro L, Weis WI. Structure and biochemistry of cadherins and catenins. *Cold Spring Harb Perspect Biol*. 2009;1(3):a003053.
185. van Roy F, Berx G. The cell-cell adhesion molecule E-cadherin. *Cell Mol Life Sci*. 2008;65(23):3756–3788.
186. Chung Y, Lam AK, Luk JM, et al. Altered E-cadherin expression and p120 catenin localization in esophageal squamous cell carcinoma. *Ann Surg Oncol*. 2007;14(11):3260–3267.
187. Berx G, Becker KF, Hofler H, van Roy F. Mutations of the human E-cadherin (CDH1) gene. *Hum Mutat*. 1998;12(4):226–237.
188. Si HX, Tsao SW, Lam KY, et al. E-cadherin expression is commonly downregulated by CpG island hypermethylation in esophageal carcinoma cells. *Cancer Lett*. 2001;173(1):71–78.
189. Stairs DB, Bayne LJ, Rhoades B, et al. Deletion of p120-catenin results in a tumor microenvironment with inflammation and cancer that establishes it as a tumor suppressor gene. *Cancer Cell*. 2011;19(4):470–483.
190. McConnell BB, Ghaleb AM, Nandan MO, Yang VW. The diverse functions of *Krüppel*-like factors 4 and 5 in epithelial biology and pathobiology. *Bioessays*. 2007;29(6):549–557.
191. Tetreault M, Katz JP. *Krüppel*-like factors in gastrointestinal tract development and differentiation. In: Nagai R, Friedman SL, Kasuga M, eds. *The biology of Krüppel-like factors*. Tokyo: Springer; 2009:107–120.
192. Okano J, Opitz OG, Nakagawa H, Jenkins TD, Friedman SL, Rustgi AK. The Kruppel-like transcriptional factors Zf9 and GKLF coactivate the human keratin 4 promoter and physically interact. *FEBS Lett*. 2000;473(1):95–100.

193. Goldstein BG, Chao HH, Yang Y, Yermolina YA, Tobias JW, Katz JP. Overexpression of Kruppel-like factor 5 in esophageal epithelia in vivo leads to increased proliferation in basal but not suprabasal cells. *Am J Physiol Gastrointest Liver Physiol.* 2007;292(6):G1784–1792.
194. Yang Y, Goldstein BG, Chao HH, Katz JP. KLF4 and KLF5 regulate proliferation, apoptosis and invasion in esophageal cancer cells. *Cancer Biol Ther.* 2005;4(11):1216–1221.
195. Yang Y, Goldstein BG, Nakagawa H, Katz JP. Kruppel-like factor 5 activates MEK/ERK signaling via EGFR in primary squamous epithelial cells. *FASEB J.* 2007;21(2):543–550.
196. Yang Y, Tetreault MP, Yermolina YA, Goldstein BG, Katz JP. Kruppel-like factor 5 controls keratinocyte migration via the integrin-linked kinase. *J Biol Chem.* 2008;283(27):18812–18820.
197. Tetreault MP, Wang ML, Yang Y, et al. Klf4 overexpression activates epithelial cytokines and inflammation-mediated esophageal squamous cell cancer in mice. *Gastroenterology.* 2010;139(6): 2124–2134.
198. Tetreault MP, Yang Y, Travis J, et al. Esophageal squamous cell dysplasia and delayed differentiation with deletion of *Krüppel-like* factor 4 in murine esophagus. *Gastroenterology.* 2010; 139(1):171–181.
199. Garrett-Sinha LA, Eberspaecher H, Seldin MF, de Crombrugghe B. A gene for a novel zinc-finger protein expressed in differentiated epithelial cells and transiently in certain mesenchymal cells. *J Biol Chem.* 1996;271(49):31384–31390.
200. Shields JM, Christy RJ, Yang VW. Identification and characterization of a gene encoding a gut-enriched Kruppel-like factor expressed during growth arrest. *J Biol Chem.* 1996;271(33): 20009–20017.
201. Wang N, Liu ZH, Ding F, Wang XQ, Zhou CN, Wu M. Down-regulation of gut-enriched *Krüppel*-like factor expression in esophageal cancer. *World J Gastroenterol.* 2002;8(6):966–970.
202. Zhao W, Hisamuddin IM, Nandan MO, Babbin BA, Lamb NE, Yang VW. Identification of Kruppel-like factor 4 as a potential tumor suppressor gene in colorectal cancer. *Oncogene.* 2004;23(2): 395–402.
203. Wei D, Gong W, Kanai M, et al. Drastic down-regulation of Kruppel-like factor 4 expression is critical in human gastric cancer development and progression. *Cancer Res.* 2005;65(7): 2746–2754.
204. Ohnishi S, Laub F, Matsumoto N, et al. Developmental expression of the mouse gene coding for the Kruppel-like transcription factor KLF5. *Dev Dyn.* 2000;217(4):421–429.
205. Conkright MD, Wani MA, Anderson KP, Lingrel JB. A gene encoding an intestinal-enriched member of the Kruppel-like factor family expressed in intestinal epithelial cells. *Nucl Acids Res.* 1999;27(5):1263–1270.
206. Siomi H, Siomi MC. On the road to reading the RNA-interference code. *Nature.* 2009;457(7228):396–404.
207. Rana TM. Illuminating the silence: understanding the structure and function of small RNAs. *Nat Rev Mol Cell Biol.* 2007;8(1): 23–36.
208. Zhang B, Pan X, Cobb GP, Anderson TA. microRNAs as oncogenes and tumor suppressors. *Dev Biol.* 2007;302(1):1–12.
209. Matsushima K, Isomoto H, Kohno S, Nakao K. MicroRNAs and esophageal squamous cell carcinoma. *Digestion.* 2010;82(3): 138–144.
210. Ogawa R, Ishiguro H, Kuwabara Y, et al. Expression profiling of micro-RNAs in human esophageal squamous cell carcinoma using RT-PCR. *Med Mol Morphol.* 2009;42(2):102–109.
211. Lee KH, Goan YG, Hsiao M, et al. MicroRNA-373 (miR-373) post-transcriptionally regulates large tumor suppressor, homolog 2 (LATS2) and stimulates proliferation in human esophageal cancer. *Exp Cell Res.* 2009;315(15):2529–2538.
212. Guo Y, Chen Z, Zhang L, et al. Distinctive microRNA profiles relating to patient survival in esophageal squamous cell carcinoma. *Cancer Res.* 2008;68(1):26–33.
213. Mathe EA, Nguyen GH, Bowman ED, et al. MicroRNA expression in squamous cell carcinoma and adenocarcinoma of the esophagus: associations with survival. *Clin Cancer Res.* 2009;15(19):6192–6200.
214. Sugito N, Ishiguro H, Kuwabara Y, et al. RNASEN regulates cell proliferation and affects survival in esophageal cancer patients. *Clin Cancer Res.* 2006;12(24):7322–7328.
215. Mitchell PS, Parkin RK, Kroh EM, et al. Circulating microRNAs as stable blood-based markers for cancer detection. *Proc Natl Acad Sci USA.* 2008;105(30):10513–10518.
216. Zhou SL, Wang LD. Circulating microRNAs: novel biomarkers for esophageal cancer. *World J Gastroenterol.* 2010;16(19):2348–2354.
217. Fong LYY, Li J-X, Farber JL, Magee PN. Cell proliferation and esophageal carcinogenesis in the zinc-deficient rat. *Carcinogenesis.* 1996;17(9):1841–1848.
218. Fong LY, Ishii H, Nguyen VT, et al. p53 deficiency accelerates induction and progression of esophageal and forestomach tumors in zinc-deficient mice. *Cancer Res.* 2003;63(1):186–195.
219. Fong LY, Magee PN. Dietary zinc deficiency enhances esophageal cell proliferation and N-nitrosomethylbenzylamine (NMBA)-induced esophageal tumor incidence in C57BL/6 mouse. *Cancer Lett.* 1999;143(1):63–69.
220. Gurski RR, Schirmer CC, Kruel CR, Komlos F, Kruel CD, Edelweiss MI. Induction of esophageal carcinogenesis by diethylnitrosamine and assessment of the promoting effect of ethanol and N-nitrosonornicotine: experimental model in mice. *Dis Esophagus.* 1999;12(2):99–105.
221. Jenkins TD, Mueller A, Odze R, et al. Cyclin D1 overexpression combined with N-nitrosomethylbenzylamine increases dysplasia and cellular proliferation in murine esophageal squamous epithelium. *Oncogene.* 1999;18(1):59–66.
222. Fong LYY, Jiang Y, Farber JL. Zinc deficiency potentiates induction and progression of lingual and esophageal tumors in p53-deficient mice. *Carcinogenesis.* 2006;27(7):1489–1496.
223. Tang XH, Knudsen B, Bemis D, Tickoo S, Gudas LJ. Oral cavity and esophageal carcinogenesis modeled in carcinogen-treated mice. *Clin Cancer Res.* 2004;10(1 Pt 1):301–313.
224. Wilkey JF, Buchberger G, Saucier K, et al. Cyclin D1 overexpression increases susceptibility to 4-nitroquinoline-1-oxide-induced dysplasia and neoplasia in murine squamous oral epithelium. *Mol Carcinog.* 2009;48(9):853–861.
225. Opitz OG, Harada H, Suliman Y, et al. A mouse model of human oral-esophageal cancer. *J Clin Invest.* 2002;110(6):761–769.
226. Nakagawa H, Wang TC, Zukerberg L, et al. The targeting of the *cyclin D1* oncogene by an Epstein-Barr virus promoter in transgenic mice causes dysplasia in the tongue, esophagus and forestomach. *Oncogene.* 1997;14(10):1185–1190.
227. Enzinger PC, Mayer RJ. Esophageal cancer. *N Engl J Med.* 2003;349(23):2241–2252.
228. Morita M, Kumashiro R, Kubo N, et al. Alcohol drinking, cigarette smoking, and the development of squamous cell carcinoma of the esophagus: epidemiology, clinical findings, and prevention. *Int J Clin Oncol.* 2010;15(2):126–134.
229. Fong LYY, Jiang Y, Rawahneh ML, et al. Zinc supplementation suppresses 4-nitroquinoline 1-oxide-induced rat oral carcinogenesis. *Carcinogenesis.* 2011;32(4):554–560.
230. Taccioli C, Wan S-G, Liu C-G, et al. Zinc replenishment reverses overexpression of the proinflammatory mediator S100A8 and esophageal preneoplasia in the rat. *Gastroenterology.* 2009;136(3): 953–966.
231. Munoz N, Wahrendorf J, Bang LJ, et al. No effect of riboflavine, retinol, and zinc on prevalence of precancerous lesions of oesoph-

agus. Randomised double-blind intervention study in high-risk population of China. *Lancet*. 1985;2(8447):111–114.
232. Wang GQ, Abnet CC, Shen Q, et al. Histological precursors of oesophageal squamous cell carcinoma: results from a 13 year prospective follow up study in a high risk population. *Gut*. 2005;54(2):187–192.
233. Wattenberg LW. Chemoprevention of cancer. *Cancer Res*. 1985; 45(1):1–8.
234. Barch DH, Fox CC. Dietary ellagic acid reduces the esophageal microsomal metabolism of methylbenzylnitrosamine. *Cancer Lett*. 1989;44(1):39–44.
235. Mandal S, Stoner GD. Inhibition of N-nitrosobenzylmethylamine-induced esophageal tumorigenesis in rats by ellagic acid. *Carcinogenesis*. 1990;11(1):55–61.
236. Brady JF, Li DC, Ishizaki H, Yang CS. Effect of diallyl sulfide on rat liver microsomal nitrosamine metabolism and other monooxygenase activities. *Cancer Res*. 1988;48(21):5937–5940.
237. Wargovich MJ, Woods C, Eng VW, Stephens LC, Gray K. Chemoprevention of N-nitrosomethylbenzylamine-induced esophageal cancer in rats by the naturally occurring thioether, diallyl sulfide. *Cancer Res*. 1988;48(23):6872–6875.
238. Mori Y, Tatematsu K, Koide A, Sugie S, Tanaka T, Mori H. Modification by curcumin of mutagenic activation of carcinogenic N-nitrosamines by extrahepatic cytochromes P-450 2B1 and 2E1 in rats. *Cancer Sci*. 2006;97(9):896–904.
239. Ushida J, Sugie S, Kawabata K, et al. Chemopreventive effect of curcumin on N-nitrosomethylbenzylamine-induced esophageal carcinogenesis in rats. *Jpn J Cancer Res*. 2000;91(9):893–898.
240. Lin JK. Suppression of protein kinase C and nuclear oncogene expression as possible action mechanisms of cancer chemoprevention by Curcumin. *Arch Pharm Res*. 2004;27(7):683–692.
241. Hecht SS. Chemoprevention by isothiocyanates. *J Cell Biochem Suppl*. 1995;22:195–209.
242. Hecht SS. Inhibition of carcinogenesis by isothiocyanates. *Drug Metab Rev*. 2000;32(3–4):395–411.
243. Carlson DG, Daxenbichler ME, VanEtten CH, Tookey HL, Williams PH. Glucosinolates in crucifer vegetables: turnips and rutabagas. *J Agric Food Chem*. 1981;29(6):1235–1239.
244. Stoner GD, Morrissey DT, Heur YH, Daniel EM, Galati AJ, Wagner SA. Inhibitory effects of phenethyl isothiocyanate on N-nitrosobenzylmethylamine carcinogenesis in the rat esophagus. *Cancer Res*. 1991;51(8):2063–2068.
245. Siglin JC, Barch DH, Stoner GD. Effects of dietary phenethyl isothiocyanate, ellagic acid, sulindac and calcium on the induction and progression of N-nitrosomethylbenzylamine-induced esophageal carcinogenesis in rats. *Carcinogenesis*. 1995;16(5): 1101–1106.
246. Hu G, Han C, Wild CP, Hall J, Chen J. Lack of effects of selenium on N-nitrosomethylbenzylamine-induced tumorigenesis, DNA methylation, and oncogene expression in rats and mice. *Nutr Cancer*. 1992;18(3):287–295.
247. Wang ZY, Wang LD, Lee MJ, et al. Inhibition of N-nitrosomethylbenzylamine-induced esophageal tumorigenesis in rats by green and black tea. *Carcinogenesis*. 1995;16(9): 2143–2148.
248. Chen T, Nines RG, Peschke SM, Kresty LA, Stoner GD. Chemopreventive effects of a selective nitric oxide synthase inhibitor on carcinogen-induced rat esophageal tumorigenesis. *Cancer Res*. 2004;64(10):3714–3717.
249. Li Z, Shimada Y, Kawabe A, et al. Suppression of N-nitrosomethylbenzylamine (NMBA)-induced esophageal tumorigenesis in F344 rats by JTE-522, a selective COX-2 inhibitor. *Carcinogenesis*. 2001;22(4):547–551.
250. Li ZG, Hong T, Shimada Y, et al. Suppression of N-nitrosomethylbenzylamine (NMBA)-induced esophageal tumorigenesis in F344 rats by resveratrol. *Carcinogenesis*. 2002;23(9): 1531–1536.
251. Fujiwara Y, Osugi H, Morimura K, et al. Suppressive effect of CPT-11 on rat esophageal tumorigenesis induced by N-nitrosomethylbenzylamine. *Oncol Rep*. 2004;12(6):1169–1176.
252. Okines A, Sharma B, Cunningham D. Perioperative management of esophageal cancer. *Nat Rev Clin Oncol*. 2010;7(4): 231–238.
253. Quiros RM, Bui CL. Multidisciplinary approach to esophageal and gastric cancer. *Surg Clin North Am*. 2009;89(1):79–96.
254. Mathew R, Arora S, Khanna R, et al. Alterations in p53 and pRb pathways and their prognostic significance in oesophageal cancer. *Eur J Cancer*. 2002;38(6):832–841.
255. Shibagaki I, Tanaka H, Shimada Y, et al. p53 mutation, murine double minute 2 amplification, and human papillomavirus infection are frequently involved but not associated with each other in esophageal squamous cell carcinoma. *Clin Cancer Res*. 1995 Jul;1(7):769–773.
256. Bahl R, Arora S, Nath N, et al. Novel polymorphism in p21(waf1/cip1) cyclin dependent kinase inhibitor gene: association with human esophageal cancer. *Oncogene*. 2000 Jan 20;19(3): 323–328.
257. Nie Y, Liao J, Zhao X, et al. Detection of multiple gene hypermethylation in the development of esophageal squamous cell carcinoma. *Carcinogenesis*. 2002 Oct;23(10):1713–1720.

Molecular Mechanisms and Pathology of Gastric Carcinogenesis: Sporadic Cancers

5

Shuko Harada and Antonia R. Sepulveda

Introduction

Gastric carcinoma (GC) is the most frequent malignancy arising in the stomach and represents the fourth most frequent cancer worldwide.[1,2] In the United States, approximately 21,000 new cases of gastric cancer are diagnosed each year.[1,3] The frequency of cancers of the distal stomach has been dropping in Western countries whereas the numbers of adenocarcinoma of the gastric cardia and gastroesophageal junction (GEJ) have markedly increased.[4] About 1.4 million cancer cases involving the GEJ and stomach are diagnosed each year with 1.1 million attributed deaths worldwide.[2]

Significant advances that have contributed to unraveling the underlying mechanisms of gastric carcinogenesis include: (a) Identification of *Helicobacter pylori* gastritis as a major factor in gastric cancer development and subsequent studies characterizing the complex molecular alterations in gastric mucosa induced by *H. pylori* infection; (b) Identification of inherited forms of gastric cancer, discussed in Chap. 6; and (c) Comprehensive genome-wide molecular studies combined with hypothesis-driven research that have given greater insights into the molecular mechanisms of development and progression of gastric cancers, providing molecular approaches for gastric cancer classification and identification of genes and specific pathways potentially amenable to personalized targeted therapies. Furthermore, there are several factors known to play a role in gastric cancer development including host genetic susceptibility and carcinogens present in specific diets or associated with smoking that work together with other factors such as the cellular injury caused by chronic gastritis to enhance the risk of gastric cancer.[5–8]

S. Harada, M.D.
Department of Pathology, University of Albama at Brimingham, Birmingham, AL 35243, USA
e-mail: sharada1@uab.edu

A.R. Sepulveda, M.D., Ph.D. (✉)
Department of Pathology & Cell Biology, Columbia University, 630 W 168th Street, VC-14 RM 212, New York, NY 10032, USA
e-mail: as4400@columbia.edu

Classifications of Gastric Cancer

Gastric cancers can be divided into distinct subtypes based on: differential mechanisms of neoplastic initiation and underlying risk factors (such as inherited vs. sporadic) and different histopathologic and molecular phenotypes that can be further stratified by prognosis or into groups potentially amenable to individualized targeted therapies. The subgroup classifications of gastric cancer have potential implications for cancer prevention, surveillance, conventional surgical and chemotherapeutic regimen approaches, and selection for targeted personalized therapies (Table 5.1).

The pathologic classification of gastric cancer used in clinical practice is based on a combination of morphologic features to establish a morphologic pattern (tubular, papillary, mucinous, and poorly cohesive which includes signet ring cell type carcinoma) as proposed in the 2010 WHO classification, grade of differentiation into well, moderately, and poorly differentiated tumors, depth of tumor invasion, lymph node status, and other features detailed in the AJCC (7th Edition) publication, which allow for tumor staging.[9,10] The Lauren classification reported in 1965 has been widely used in studies of gastric adenocarcinomas, separating gastric cancers into the intestinal, diffuse, and mixed types, based on the tumor morphologic features.[11–13] Mechanistically, gastric cancers currently fall into three main groups: (1) sporadic adenocarcinomas with multifactorial underlying mechanisms (approximately >80% of all cases of GC); (2) gastric cancers associated with Epstein–Barr infection (approximately <10% of all cases of GC); and (3) familial gastric cancer, including hereditary diffuse gastric cancer (HDGC) (approximately <10% of all GC cases).

A.R. Sepulveda and J.P. Lynch (eds.), *Molecular Pathology of Neoplastic Gastrointestinal Diseases*, Molecular Pathology Library 7, DOI 10.1007/978-1-4614-6015-2_5, © Springer Science+Business Media New York 2013

Table 5.1 Clinical utility of gastric cancer subgroup classifications

Classification	Approaches	Clinical utility
Morphology and pathologic stage	Histopathological evaluation of surgical resection specimens	TNM staging: selection of surgical and conventional therapy
Mechanistic: *H. pylori*, EBV, HDGC[a]	Histopathological evaluation of biopsy or surgical resection	Prevention and surveillance
Molecular profiling	Molecular testing	Diagnosis, targeted therapy selection, and prognostic information

[a]The definitive diagnosis of HDGC requires germline testing for inherited mutations (Chap. 6)

Table 5.2 Cell surface receptor inhibitors and potential targeted therapies for gastric and GEJ cancers[16]

Inhibitor-type	Drug
EGFR antibody	Cetuximab; panitumumab
EGFR tyrosine kinase inhibitors	Gefitinib; erlotinib
HER2-R antibody	Trastuzumab
EGF/HER2-R	Lapatinib
VEGF-R antibody	Bevacizumab
VEGF-R tyrosine kinase inhibitors	Vatalanib

Biomarker development for gastric cancers aims several goals:

1. Identification of molecular biomarkers of cancer risk for inherited and sporadic forms of gastric cancer. Presently, molecular tools can be used for the assessment of HDGC risk in individuals with suspicious history through identification of *ECAD* (*CDH1*) gene mutation carriers (Chap. 6). Further, identification of molecular alterations associated with a field defect in the background stomach before cancer develops such as in the mucosa of patients positive for *H. pylori* infection may provide information regarding the risk of developing sporadic type gastric cancer. Among the molecular subtypes of gastric cancer are the large group of tumors characterized by the chromosomal instability pathway (CIN), while a smaller proportion of tumors develop through the microsatellite instability pathway (MSI), and/or the CpG island methylator phenotype pathway, reviewed in.[14]
2. Identification of molecular markers that can be used in combination with pathologic, clinical, and imaging data to establish the diagnosis and identify clinically relevant GC subtypes.
   (a) Identification of molecular markers to help with the selection of best therapeutic interventions, both at the level of conventional and targeted therapies. For example, molecular classifications of GC offer some promise for potentially guiding conventional chemotherapy.[15] Current targeted therapies in gastric cancer are discussed in Chap. 2, with emphasis on the use of *HER2/ErbB2* in advanced gastric and GE junction adenocarcinomas. Clinical trials are under way (Table 5.2) to evaluate the potential application of multiple agents for targeted therapies.[16]
   (b) Additionally, studies aim the characterization of molecular markers that might predict metastatic potential and tumor recurrence.

Role of *H. pylori* in Gastric Carcinogenesis

Helicobacter pylori bacteria were recognized as the main agent of chronic gastritis and ulcers by Warren and Marshal,[17,18] and later studies revealed an association with gastric cancer,[19,20] leading to the classification of *H. pylori* as a human carcinogen.[21] The attributable risk of gastric cancer related to *H. pylori* infection in the population has been estimated to be 75%.[20]

The chronic nature of *H. pylori* gastritis is relevant to the carcinogenic potential of this infection, resulting in a long-term interaction of the bacteria and inflammatory mediators with epithelial cells, with accumulation of mutations, epigenetic modifications, and deregulation of cell function that may ultimately lead to neoplasia. Therefore, *H. pylori* infection plays a critical role during the initiating steps of gastric cancer.

H. pylori infection is usually acquired at young age and results in variable symptoms and complications related to the potential development of gastric and duodenal ulcers, gastric cancer, and extranodal marginal zone B-cell lymphoma of mucosa-associated lymphoid tissue (MALT-Lymphoma).[22–26] Cure of *H. pylori* infection requires eradication with anti-*H. pylori* therapy.[27–29] Gastric cancer develops several decades after acquisition of the infection, following progressive mucosal damage secondary to chronic gastritis.[30,31]

Histologically, *H. pylori* gastritis is characterized by a combination of chronic and acute inflammation of the gastric mucosa. There is progressive damage of gastric glands that results in mucosal atrophy manifested by loss of the oxyntic glands in the gastric body/fundus, loss of mucous glands in the antrum, and replacement of normal gastric glands by intestinal metaplasia, overall resulting in a picture of atrophic gastritis, with potential development of dysplasia and carcinoma in some patients (Fig. 5.1).[19,31–33] Extensive gastritis and mucosal atrophy in the gastric body and fundus result in hypochlorhydria, which creates an environment that allows for overgrowth of a number of bacteria that may

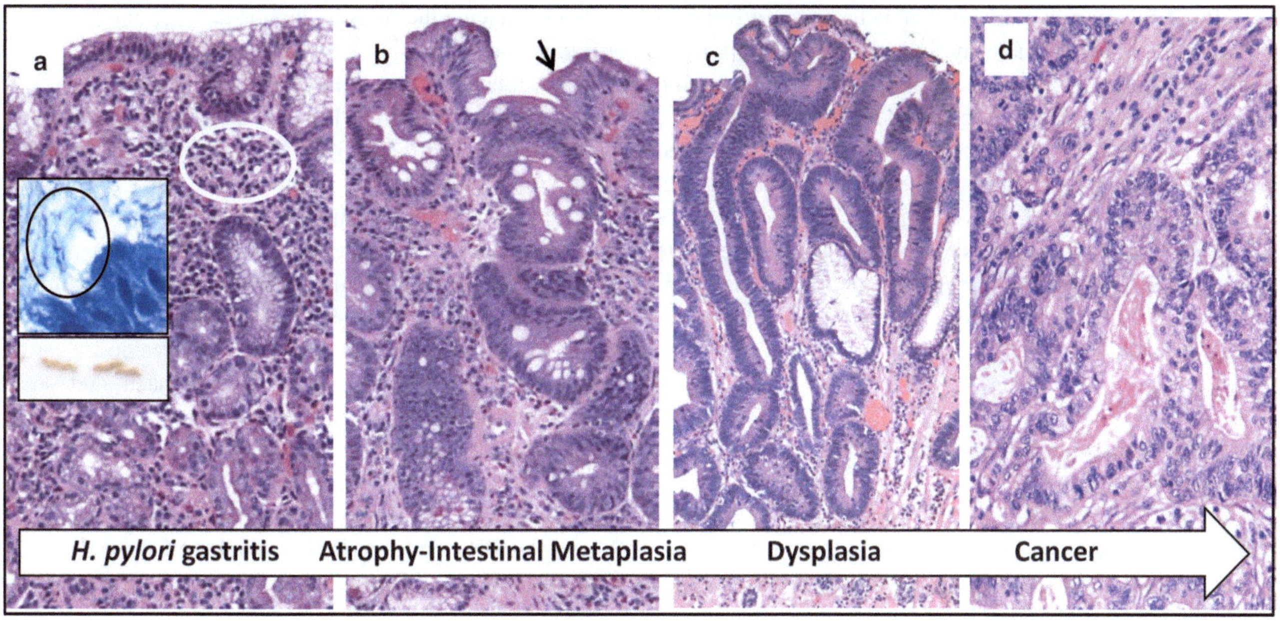

Fig. 5.1 Stomach pathology of *H. pylori*-associated gastric carcinogenesis. (**a**) *H. pylori* gastritis with characteristic inflammation in the lamina propria of gastric mucosa (*white circle*), demonstrated by H&E stain (original magnification ×200). The *upper inset* shows *H. pylori* bacteria stained with Thiazine stain (*blue*), while the *lower inset* demonstrates *H. pylori* by immunohistochemistry (original magnification of inset ×400). (**b**) Intestinal metaplasia (exemplified by the area indicated by the *arrow*) with resulting gastric gland atrophy (atrophic gastritis). (**c**) Progression of gastric epithelium to dysplasia/adenoma. (**d**) Invasive moderately differentiated adenocarcinoma (intestinal type adenocarcinoma). Hematoxylin & Eosin stains original magnification ×200 (**b**, **c**, **d**)

increase carcinogenic activity in the stomach through the conversion of nitrites to carcinogenic nitroso-N compounds.[34,35] *H. pylori*-associated pangastritis (involving both the body/fundus and antrum) is frequently seen in family relatives of gastric cancer patients, which may contribute to gastric cancer clustering in some families.[36] The histologic changes that precede gastric cancer, including intestinal metaplasia, represent pre-neoplastic epithelial changes in gastric carcinogenesis and have been shown to carry numerous genomic, epigenetic, and functional changes that can also be detected in cancer tissues.[8,37–45] Therefore, characterization of molecular alterations in the background mucosa before patients develop GC may offer an opportunity to identify patterns associated with increased risk of gastric cancer development.

The cancers arising in the inflammatory background of *H. pylori*-associated chronic gastritis are most commonly of intestinal type, which are predominantly well to moderately differentiated adenocarcinomas (Fig. 5.1), but diffuse type adenocarcinomas which are poorly cohesive and poorly differentiated and may include a variable component with signet ring cell features also occur in association with *H. pylori*.[46–48]

Helicobacter infection of several animal models, including Mongolian gerbils and mice, results in development of gastritis as well as other *Helicobacter*-associated gastric diseases, including intestinal metaplasia, dysplasia, and gastric cancer.[49–54]

Role of Stem cells in *H. pylori*-Associated Gastric Cancer Development

Gastric stem cells provide the capacity for renewal of all cell lineages of gastric epithelium. The molecular markers that identify epithelial stem cells in the oxyntic mucosa of gastric body and in the antrum appear to be different, consistent with the different cellular lineages that constitute gastric glands in these two different areas of the stomach.[55] In the antrum, the leucine-rich repeat containing G protein-coupled receptor Lgr5, an orphan G protein-coupled receptor and a Wnt target gene, was shown to be expressed in adult stem cells in the stomach and intestinal epithelium in mice.[56] Barker et al[56] showed that Lgr5 was expressed at the base of the gastric glands and that Lgr5-positive cells had the capacity of self-renewal and could build long-lived gastric antral units in vivo, thus meeting the criteria for stem cells.[57] Further, Lgr5 was shown to mark epithelial stem cells in human gastric antrum.[58,59] In the oxyntic mucosa, trefoil factor family 2 (TFF2) was reported in progenitors for mucous neck, parietal, and zymogen-producing cells.[60] Another marker of progenitor cells in oxyntic mucosa may be doublecortin-like kinase (Dclk1).[61] Other putative gastric stem cell markers are ADAM17, CD44, and Musashi-1.[57,58,62] Bone marrow derived stem cells may contribute to the gastric stem cell pool in chronic gastritis and *H. pylori*-associated neoplastic progression.[53,63] It has been postulated that the engrafted bone marrow derived stem cells may not follow a normal differentiation pathway and could undergo uncontrolled replication, progressive loss of differentiation, and neoplastic behavior.[53,63–65] Recent studies reported that the Lgr5-positive epithelial stem cell (LPECs) pool is expanded in *H. pylori*-associated gastritis in the antrum of patients with GC. In GC patients with active *H. pylori* infection, LPECs may be more susceptible to DNA damage than Lgr5-negative epithelial cells, suggesting that *H. pylori* infection may contribute to GC risk by affecting epithelial stem cells in the human stomach.[59]

H. pylori Virulence Factors in Gastric Carcinogenesis

Studies have shown that a number of *H. pylori* virulence factors play a role in determining the patterns of disease associated with infection.[66,67] These virulence factors include the vacuolating cytotoxin (VacA), cytotoxin-associated antigen A (CagA) proteins,[68,69] and *babA*,[70] among others. *H. pylori* strains characterized by the presence of babA, cagA, and vacAs1 have been reported to be associated with duodenal ulcer and gastric adenocarcinoma in Western populations.[71] The VacA toxin affects T and B lymphocytes and contributes to the ability of *H. pylori* to establish persistent chronic gastritis.[72] The CagA protein is encoded by the *cagA* gene, one of the genes that constitute the Cag pathogenicity island which encodes a type IV secretion system.[69,73] *H. pylori* strains carrying a *cagA* gene have been shown to have a stronger association with gastric cancer,[66,74] and specific structural variants of CagA have a stronger association with gastric cancer. The CagA type C strains were associated with more severe degrees of atrophic gastritis and gastric cancer.[75] *H. pylori* strains with phosphorylation at the EPYIA site of CagA proteins are more common in East Asia than in Western countries, which may contribute to the increased incidence of gastric cancer in East Asia.[69,76] There are several mechanisms by which CagA affects epithelial cells and may contribute to gastric cancer development.[69] CagA protein is injected from the bacterium into gastric epithelial cells via the type IV secretion system and then interacts with several intracellular signaling molecules in both tyrosine phosphorylation dependent and independent manners.[69] Once in the epithelial cell CagA undergoes tyrosine phosphorylation by the epithelial cell Src protein and other signaling molecules at the EPIYA sites and binds Src homology 2 domain containing tyrosine phosphatase (SHP2), deregulating the phosphatase activity.[69]

CagA-positive *H. pylori* were also shown to induce higher levels of interleukin-8 (IL-8) as compared to CagA-negative strains, with enhanced inflammation of the gastric mucosa,[77,78] further enhancing the risk of genomic damage and neoplastic development.

CagA-related intracellular signaling potentially affects multiple cellular functions. For example, recent studies show that methylation of the MGMT (O (6)-methylguanine-DNA methyltransferase) DNA repair gene was significantly associated with CagA-positive *H. pylori* strains associated with chronic gastritis, suggesting a role for CagA-positive *H. pylori*-mediated effects in epigenetic regulation.[79] Studies in mice carrying a transgenic *cagA* gene showed gastric epithelial hyperplasia and some mice developed gastric polyps and adenocarcinomas of the stomach and small intestine,[80] further supporting a role for CagA in gastric carcinogenesis.

Susceptibility to *H. pylori*-Associated Gastric Cancer and Host Genetics

Although it is clear that development of GC is multifactorial and requires interaction with host susceptibility genetic factors, to date, few well-defined susceptibility factors have been confirmed. Inflammation-related host genetic susceptibility factors include the pro-inflammatory gene polymorphisms in *IL-1beta* and *IL-1RN* (receptor antagonist) genes, which have shown to increase the risk of hypochlorhydria, gastric atrophy, gastric cancer, and neoplastic precursors in *H. pylori*-infected individuals.[81–84]

Molecular Mechanisms of *H. pylori*-Associated Gastric Carcinogenesis

H. pylori infection results in alterations in cellular signaling, and altered proliferation and apoptosis of gastric epithelial cells.[85,86] Overtime, *H. pylori* infection leads to mutations, epigenetic, microRNA, and gene expression changes that underlie and define gastric carcinogenesis, occurring from early stages of *H. pylori* gastritis throughout the progression from pre-neoplastic to neoplastic lesions.[8]

Mutations in Gastric Carcinogenesis

The types of mutations and mechanisms of mutagenesis in gastric carcinogenesis are multiple and include microsatellite instability (MSI)-type mutations resulting from altered DNA mismatch repair, point mutations, and genomic instability including loss of heterozygosity (LOH), gene amplifications, insertion and deletion type mutations, and chromosomal losses and duplications. These genomic lesions accumulate during the steps of gastric carcinogenesis in cells representing intestinal metaplasia, dysplasia/adenoma, and adenocarcinoma.[87] Mucosal atrophy and hypochlorhydria which are associated with long-standing chronic gastritis may enhance the action of environmental carcinogens in the stomach, with increased likelihood of mutagenesis.

Mutations of *TP53* and *APC* genes can be detected in intestinal metaplasia and gastric dysplasia.[88–91] As in other cancers, *TP53* mutations (in exons 5–8) characterized by G:C to A:T transitions are detected in gastric neoplasia.[90,92] *APC* mutations, including stop codon and frameshift mutations, were reported in 46% and 5q allelic loss in 33% of informative cases of gastric adenomas[93] and *APC* mutations were found in 45% of cancers.[94] *KRAS* mutations in codon 12 are rare in gastric carcinogenesis and were reported in 14% of cases with atrophic gastritis, and in less than 10% of adenomas, dysplasia, and carcinomas.[95,96] The spectrum of mutations in gastric cancer has been explored by massive parallel sequencing approaches. A study by Wang et al reported whole exome sequencing data in gastric cancer as compared to matching non-neoplastic tissue and determined the molecular pathways most frequently revealing gene mutations.[97] Chromatin modification and cell junction pathways showed the most significant enrichment of mutated genes. Mutations were found in members of the SWI–SNF complex (*ARID1A*, *PBRM1*, and *SMARCC1*), ISWI complex (*SMARCA1*), and NuRD complex (*CHD3*, *CGD4*, and *MBD2*), and other genes encoding histone-modifying proteins (*SIRT1* and *SETD2*), affecting 59% of gastric cancers.[97] Overall, 59% of gastric cancers had mutations in genes involved in cell adhesion, including *CHD1*. Genes involved in cell cycle regulation including *TP53*, *PTEN*, and *TTK* were mutated in 77% of gastric cancers. Other signaling pathways frequently mutated in gastric cancers included the Wnt-BMP-TGF-beta, axon guidance, MAPK, DNA replication, focal adhesion, ERBB, ATR-BRCA, and Rb pathways.[97] Another study also using exome sequencing found that cell adhesion was the pathway most enriched for mutations.[98] *TP53* was mutated in 66.7%, and *PIK3CA* and *ARID1A* were mutated in 20% of gastric cancers.[98] Frequent mutations in chromatin remodeling genes (*ARID1A*, *MLL3*, and *MLL*) were found in 47% of gastric cancers.[98] *ARID1A* mutations were associated with *PIK3CA* mutations and microsatellite instability.[98]

The mechanisms through which *H. pylori*-associated gastritis results in mutagenesis and deregulation of the molecular program of gastric epithelial cells are multiple. *H. pylori* infection leads to increased DNA damage of epithelial cells due to oxidative stress caused by reactive oxygen species (ROS), and reactive nitrogen species (RNS) generated by inflammatory cells as well as by gastric epithelial cells after activation by *H. pylori*.[99] In addition to the increased production of ROS, there is limited availability of oxygen radical scavengers, such as glutathione and glutathione-S-transferase during *H. pylori* gastritis, which may contribute to higher levels of oxygen radicals in the mucosa of infected patients.[100] Gastric mucosa with *H. pylori* gastritis and pre-neoplastic lesions such as intestinal metaplasia and gastric atrophy was shown to have increased levels of DNA 8-hydroxydeoxyguanosine (8OHdG), a marker for oxidative DNA damage.[101,102] Notably, the levels of 8OHdG in the gastric mucosa significantly decreased after cure of *H. pylori* infection.[101,102] Mutations associated with oxidative damage include point mutations in genes such as the tumor suppressor *TP53*, GTPase *KRAS*, and other genes involved in gastric carcinogenesis.[90] Epithelial expression of the activation-induced cytidine deaminase (AID) in *H. pylori* gastritis may induce C/G to T/A transitions by its cytidine deaminase activity.[103]

Specific deficiencies of DNA repair functions during *H. pylori* gastritis also contribute to *H. pylori*-associated mutagenesis.[8,79,104,105] Altered DNA repair mechanisms include those involved in DNA mismatch repair as well as other proteins that primarily repair DNA lesions induced by oxidative and nitrosative stress, such as MGMT and polymorphic glycosylase (OGG1). The DNA mismatch repair proteins are required for the repair of DNA replication-associated sequence errors (reviewed in Chaps. 1, 7, and 8). Several studies have reported a role for DNA mismatch repair deficiency in mutation accumulation during *H. pylori* infection.[37,59,79,104,106] DNA mismatch repair deficiency leads to frameshift mutagenesis which can alter the coding region of genes, as well as repetitive regions known as short tandem repeats or microsatellite regions, with resulting microsatellite instability.[107] High levels of microsatellite instability (MSI-H) correlate well with loss of DNA mismatch repair function in tissues.[107] Microsatellite instability can be detected in chronic gastritis and intestinal metaplasia from patients with gastric cancer, indicating that MSI can occur in pre-neoplastic mucosa.[37,87,108–111] For example, a study of microsatellite instability in the stepwise gastritis cancer sequence reported MSI in chronic gastritis (13% of cases), intestinal metaplasia (20% of cases), dysplasias (25% of cases), and gastric cancers (38% of cases), consistent with a role for DNA MMR deficiency in *H. pylori*-associated gastric carcinogenesis.[112] Interestingly, identical MSI patterns were observed in some cases at the stage of gastritis several years before the diagnosis of adenocarcinoma.[113] Consistent with the role of *H. pylori* on DNA mismatch repair deficiency in gastric carcinogenesis, several studies reported that patients with MSI-positive tumors showed a significantly higher frequency of active *H. pylori* infection.[37,114,115] Using a co-culture in vitro system, gastric cell lines exposed to *H. pylori* expressed reduced levels of DNA mismatch repair proteins MLH1 and MSH2,[106] and these changes were associated with increased mutagenesis of a reporter vector, including MSI-type frameshift mutations as well as point mutations.[104]

High level of MSI (MSI-H), defined as MSI detected in greater than 30% microsatellite marker loci tested[116], is associated with loss of expression and promoter hypermethylation of the MLH1 DNA mismatch repair gene in gastric adenomas and cancers.[116–119] MSI has been reported in 17–35% of gastric adenomas,[93,113,120] and in 17–59% of gastric carcinomas.[37,93,96,113,120–123] Gastric cancers with MSI-H may carry frameshift mutations that may affect the function of cancer-related genes, such as *BAX*, *IGFRII*, *TGFβRII*, *MSH3*, and *MSH6*.[110,124–127] In MSI-H adenomas, frameshift mutations of *TGFβRII* were detected in 38–88% of the cases, *BAX* in 13%, *MSH3* in 13%, and E2F-4 gene in 50% of the cases.[128,129]

Other DNA repair proteins are involved in the correction of oxidative stress-associated mutations during *H. pylori* infection such as repair of 8-OHdG by polymorphic glycosylase (OGG1). A gene polymorphism that may affect the function of OGG1 was reported frequently in patients with intestinal metaplasia and gastric cancer, suggesting that deficient OGG1 function may contribute to increased mutagenesis during gastric carcinogenesis.[130]The DNA repair protein MGMT can remove O (6)alkylG DNA adducts. In the absence of functional MGMT these adducts are not removed and mispair with T during DNA replication, resulting in G-to-A mutations. *MGMT* promoter methylation has been reported in various stages of gastric carcinogenesis, suggesting a role for this DNA repair protein in gastric cancer development.[131] Hypermethylation of the *MGMT* gene and reduced levels of MGMT proteins in the gastric epithelium, particularly in patients infected with CagA-positive strains, occur during *H. pylori* gastritis. Further, *MGMT* promoter methylation was shown to be partially reversible after eradication of *H. pylori* infection. Overall, these studies indicate that MGMT-dependent DNA repair is disrupted during *H. pylori* gastritis, likely contributing to higher levels of mutagenesis in *H. pylori*-infected gastric mucosa.[79]

Alterations of Epigenetic Gene Regulation in Gastric Carcinogenesis

Gene regulation mediated by epigenetic modification such as CpG methylation occurs early in gastric carcinogenesis, affecting genes such as *MLH1*, p14, p15, p16, E-cadherin, *RUNX3*, thrombospondin-1 (*THBS1*), tissue inhibitor of metalloproteinase 3 (*TIMP-3*), *COX-2*, and *MGMT*.[8,38–45] Methylation of these and a number of other genes is associated with chronic inflammation in the gastric mucosa.[132] Proinflammatory interleukin-1-beta polymorphisms were shown to be associated with CpG island methylation of target genes such as the E-cadherin gene.[133,134] Interestingly, CpG methylation of the gastric mucosa has been shown to be partially reversible after eradication of *H. pylori* infection.[44,79,135]

Gene Expression Changes in Gastric Carcinogenesis

Unique patterns of gene expression that characterize the stepwise lesions of gastric carcinogenesis have been reported leading to the identification of specific expression profiles that characterize gastritis, intestinal metaplasia, and subtypes of gastric adenocarcinoma, including GC groups with differing prognosis.[15,136–145] Studies have reported signatures that can differentiate between normal and cancer samples, with intestinal metaplasia showing gene expression signatures close to adenocarcinoma; however, these approaches have not shown to be robust enough for routine clinical practice.[145,146] Recently, Tan et al used expression microarrays to identify subtypes of gastric cancer predictive of survival and response to chemotherapy,[15] through comparison of gene expression patterns in established GC cell lines and primary gastric cancer tissues. Two intrinsic tumor cell types were identified with 171 differentially expressed genes. The concordance between the Lauren classification into intestinal type and diffuse type was 64%.[15] These data are consistent with earlier studies where gastric mucins were used for classification of gastric cancer, showing that diffuse type gastric tumors may indeed express intestinal mucin phenotypes.[47] Gastric cancers with intestinal type molecular patterns but showing diffuse type histology had improved survival compared to gastric cancers with diffuse type molecular patterns but showing intestinal type histology.[15]

Role of MicroRNAs in Gastric Carcinogenesis

MicroRNAs (miRNAs) are small noncoding RNAs that regulate gene expression at the posttranscriptional level. MicroRNAs have been shown to be involved in *H. pylori*-associated diseases.[147] Increased expression of miR-21 was detected in *H. pylori*-infected gastric mucosa, as compared to noninfected tissue,[148] while *miR-218-2* was downregulated,[149] and most gastric cancers overexpress miR-21.[150] MicroRNA-378 showed 87.5% sensitivity and 70.73% specificity in discriminating GC patients from healthy controls. The expression levels of five serum miRNAs (miR-1, miR-20a, miR-27a, miR-34, and miR-423-5p) were shown to correlate with tumor stage.[151] MicroR-204 downregulation was shown to represent a novel mechanism for aberrant Ras activation in gastric carcinogenesis.[152] A total of 24 miRNAs with a more than twofold change were differentially expressed between normal gastric tissue and GC. Of these, 22 miRNAs (miR-223, miR-106b, miR-147, miR-34a, miR-130b*, miR-106a, miR-18a, miR-17, miR-98, miR-616*, miR-181a-2*, miR-185, miR-1259, miR-601, miR-196a*, miR-221*, miR-302f, miR-340*, miR-337-3p, miR-520c-3p, miR-575, and miR-138) were significantly upregulated in GC, whereas miR-638 and miR-378 were significantly downregulated in GC compared to normal gastric tissue.[153]

Epstein–Barr Virus-Associated Gastric Cancer

Epstein–Barr Virus (EBV) is a member of the herpesvirus family. EBV is an enveloped virus that contains a double-stranded DNA. EBV was discovered in 1964 by electron microscopy of Burkitt's lymphoma tumor cells.[154] In 1968, EBV was identified as the causative agent of infectious mononucleosis.[155] EBV is widespread throughout the world, and more than 90% of adults in any country are seropositive against EBV viral capsid antigen (EBV-VCA).[156] While the vast majority of EBV infections remain asymptomatic, a small portion of EBV-infected individuals develop hematopoietic, epithelial, or mesenchymal tumors. These tumors include Burkitt's lymphoma, Hodgkin's lymphoma, nasopharyngeal lymphoepithelioma, and a small subset of gastric carcinomas.

The presence of EBV in a patient with gastric cancer was first reported in a case of undifferentiated gastric carcinoma with intense lymphoid infiltration, resembling nasopharyngeal lymphoepithelioma.[157] Subsequently, Shibata and Weiss reported that EBV sequences were detected in 16% of typical gastric adenocarcinoma cases in the United States by polymerase chain reaction (PCR) and in situ hybridization techniques.[158] The prevalence of EBV-associated gastric carcinoma has been reported, ranging from 1.3% to 20.1% in different countries.[159] EBV-associated GC has several characteristic clinicopathological features. These include a male predominance, high incidence of EBV in both lymphoepithelial carcinoma and remnant gastric cancers, and high incidence in the gastric cardia and body. A meta-analysis revealed that the frequency of EBV-associated GC among all gastric cancers was about 9% and these tumors generally showed the diffuse histologic type.[159,160] There was no significant association between EBV-associated GC and the tumor depth, lymph node metastasis, or the clinical stage.[159]

Virology and Molecular Biology of EBV

EBV is transmitted from host to host via saliva and preferentially infects B lymphocytes through the binding of the major viral envelope glycoprotein gp350 to the CD21 cell surface receptor. In addition, glycoprotein gp42 binds to human leukocyte antigen (HLA) class II molecules as a co-receptor.[161] Binding to CD21 and MHC class II results in CD19- and MHC class II-associated src and syk tyrosine kinase activations. EBV is endocytosed, the EBV envelope fuses with an endocytic vesicle membrane, and capsids are released into the cytoplasm.[159] EBV has the unique ability to transform resting B cells into lifelong, latently infected lymphoblastoid cell lines (LCLs). Primary epithelial cells are also relatively resistant to infection, whereas some epithelial cell lines, including the HEK 293 gastric carcinoma cell line[162], can be infected. The latent cycle (lysogenic) programs are those that do not result in production of virions. A very limited, distinct set of viral proteins are produced during the latent cycle of infection. These include six EBV nuclear antigens: EBNAs 1, 2, 3A, 3B, and 3C and leader protein (LP), three latent membrane proteins (LMPs 1, 2A, and 2B), and the EBV non-polyadenylated (noncoding) RNAs (EBERs).[161] The latent cycle is classified into three patterns, Latency I, II, and III based on the expression pattern of viral latent gens.

EBNA1 is expressed in all virus-infected cells and its role is maintenance and replication of the episomal EBV genome.[159] In contrast, EBNA2 and EBNA-LP play a crucial role in transformation via transcriptional activation of cellular genes such as CD23 and key viral genes LMP1 and LMP2A.[161] LMP1 is the main transformation protein of EBV. LMP1 constitutively activates the tumor necrosis factor receptor (TNFR) superfamily and several signaling pathways in a ligand-independent manner.[159] In addition to the latent proteins, two small non-polyadenylated, uncapped, noncoding nuclear RNAs, EBER1 and EBER2, are expressed abundantly in nearly all latently infected cells.[159] EBERs bind to certain nucleoprotein particles, enabling binding to PKR (dsRNA-dependent serine/threonine protein kinase), thus inhibiting its function.[159] However, the exact mechanism(s) by which EBERs initiate effects on cell growth or survival remain unclear.

A group of abundantly expressed RNAs that are encoded by the *Bam*HIA region of the EBV genome were originally identified in nasopharyngeal carcinoma (NPC), and subsequently found in other EBV-associated malignancies such as Burkitt's lymphoma and Hodgkin's lymphoma. These transcripts are commonly referred as *Bam*HIA rightward transcripts (BARTs) or complementary-strand transcripts (CSTs).[163] One of the transcripts that is generated from *Bam*HIA region is BARF1, which encodes a 31 kDa protein and was originally identified as an early antigen expressed by induction of the EBV lytic cycle. BARF1 is expressed as a latent protein in EBV-associated NPC and gastric carcinoma.[164,165]

Clinicopathological Characteristics of EBV-Associated Gastric Cancer

Association of EBV with gastric cancer is detected in almost all lymphoepithelioma-like gastric carcinomas (LELCs). The prevalence of EBV-associated gastric carcinoma has been reported, ranging from 1.3% to 20.1% in different countries, and meta-analyses revealed EBV detected in about

9% of the cases.[159,160] Most studies showed no evidence of age dependence of EBV-associated GC frequency, but reported clear male predominance.[166] EBV-associated GC is detected more in cardia and body and less in the gastric antrum, whereas *H. pylori* infection-associated cancers are typically associated with antral location. Histologically, there are two types of EBV-associated GC: lymphoepithelioma-like and ordinary type of gastric carcinoma.[155,156] The latter generally shows a diffuse histological type. EBV-positive early gastric carcinoma shows a unique "lace pattern" morphology of branching and/or anastomosing structures with lymphocytic infiltration in and around the carcinoma.[167] EBV-associated GC appears to have gastric mucin expression and low expression of intestinal type mucin MUC2.[168] A study using tight-junction protein claudin expression profiling has showed that the claudin expression pattern in EBV-associated GC corresponds to that of normal gastric epithelium in adults and fetuses, with more CLDN18 and less CLDN3.[169] These results indicate that EBV-associated GC preserves well the nature of the cells of origin and may undergo distinct carcinogenic mechanisms, differing from EBV-negative gastric cancers.

The Role of EBV in Gastric Carcinogenesis

The role of EBV in gastric carcinogenesis is supported by the observation that EBV genomes are specifically present in the tumor cells, but not in surrounding lymphocytes, normal stromal cells, and normal gastric mucosa.[158] In addition, analysis of fusion terminal repeats (TR) by Southern blot demonstrated monoclonal EBV in an episomal form without integration into the host genome, and monoclonal EBV was still present in submucosal invasion and further advanced carcinoma.[170,171] This monoclonal proliferation of EBV-associated GC has strongly suggested that EBV infects the gastric mucosa before neoplastic transformation and is involved in the early stage of gastric carcinogenesis.

How EBV infection is established in stomach mucosa is not completely understood. Entry of EBV into the cells requires CD21. However, CD21 expression is very low or nonexistent on the gastric epithelial cell surface. Therefore, direct cell-to-cell contact between gastric epithelial cells and lymphocytes with EBV is thought to be the main route.[172] It is speculated that EBV infection to the gastric epithelium is related to the damage of gastric mucosa because the background of gastric mucosa in EBV-associated GC is characterized by atrophic gastritis and lymphocyte infiltration,[173] and gastric remnant cancers have high incidence of EBER positivity (27.1%) demonstrated by in situ hybridization.[174] EBV-carrying lymphocytes may be recruited to the damaged or regenerative gastric mucosa, increasing the chance of direct contact with epithelial cells.

Molecular Pathways of EBV-Associated Gastric Cancer

EBV-associated GCs display a restricted pattern of EBV latent gene expression, including EBERs, EBNA1, LMP2A, BARTs, and BARF1, but not EBNA2 and LMP1.[171,175] Another EBV gene BARF1, which has transforming and immortalizing capabilities, is shown to be expressed in EBV-associated GC.[165] Because BARF1 exerts immortalizing effects on human epithelial cells in vitro and EBV-associated GCs lack the expression of LMP1, the major known EBV oncogene, it is thought that the BARF1 gene might act as the viral oncogene in EBV-associated GCs.

The tumor suppressor gene *TP53* is frequently inactivated in gastric carcinoma by loss of heterozygosity (LOH), missense mutations, and frameshift deletions. Ojima and colleagues[176] examined p53 protein immunoexpression in EBV-positive and EBV-negative gastric cancers. Overexpression of p53 protein was demonstrated in only 8.4% of EBV-positive gastric cancers compared with 34.4% of EBV-negative cases. However, a study by Leung et al[177] found that all EBV-associated GC in the study showed weak to moderate p53 expression, characterized by heterogeneous intensity, suggesting a non-mutational mechanism of p53 upregulation.

Loss of cell cycle regulation is one of the major features of tumor cells. The *CDKN2A* gene product, p16/IKN4a, plays a crucial role in preventing inappropriate cell proliferation. EBV infection was significantly associated with loss of p16 expression.[178] Subsequently, Kang et al reported that EBV-associated GCs have p16/INK4a increased CpG methylation compared to EBV-negative GCs.[179] In addition, aberrant methylation of many more genes including *PTEN*, *RASSF1A*, *GSTP1*, *MGMT*, and *MINT2* was shown in EBV-associated GC.[179] Therefore, it appears that epigenetic silencing of these genes is associated with the development of EBV-associated GCs.

The mechanism involved in aberrant CpG methylation in EBV-associated GC is not known. One possible connection could be overexpression of DNA methyltransferase 1 (DNMT1) protein.[180] LMP1, which is known to play a major role in transformation, directly activated *DNMT1-P1* promoter through c-Jun NH2-terminal kinase signaling.[181] However, LMP1 is not expressed in EBV-associated GCs. Therefore, Fukayama et al hypothesized that LMP2A rather than LMP1 may play a major role in gastric carcinogenesis. Using gastric cancer cell lines in culture such as MKN-1, they showed that LMP2A activates NF-Kappa-B signaling and increases *DNMT-1* expression and CpG methylation of the *PTEN* promoter.[182] These findings suggest that LMP2A may play a major role in the development of EBV-associated GC.

E-cadherin is also an important protein in carcinogenesis of the stomach. Some studies have shown that the abnormality of E-cadherin gene expression caused by aberrant methylation of the E-cadherin gene promoter was closely associated with the development of EBV-associated gastric carcinomas.[183] Recently, the expression of miR-200 family was shown to be decreased in EBV-associated GC, as compared to expression in EBV-negative carcinoma.[184] Downregulation of miR-200 was also seen in the gastric carcinoma cell line (MKN74) infected with recombinant EBV, and this was accompanied with loss of cell adhesion, reduction of E-cadherin expression, and upregulation of *ZEB1* and *ZEB2*.[182] Transfection of MKN74 cells with BARF0, EBNA1, and LMP2A resulted in a decrease of primary precursor of miR-200, pri-miR-200, whereas transfection with EBV-encoded small RNA (EBER) did not.[184] These findings suggest that all the latency type I genes have a synergetic effect on the downregulation of the miR-200 family, in turn leading to reduced E-cadherin expression, which may be a crucial step in the carcinogenesis of EBV-associated GC.

Gastric Cancer Treatment Approaches

Tumor resection is the only potentially curative option for gastric cancer and is recommended for stages Tis-T3N0-N2M0 or T4N0M0.[185] For tumors not amenable to surgical curative resection, including locally advanced, recurrent, or metastatic cancers, a number of chemotherapy regimens can be used. However, 5-year survival rates for advanced gastric and GEJ cancers are disappointingly low at 20–50% for stages II–III and 5–10% for stage IV tumors.[9] A number of agents that target specific molecules in cancer-related pathways have become available or are being tested in patients with gastric and GEJ carcinomas, offering promising new therapeutic approaches.

Molecular Classification of Gastric Cancer and Personalized Cancer Therapies

Attempts at the clinical use of molecular classifications for GC have been based on combinations of immunohistochemistry and in situ hybridization, proteomics, gene and microRNA expression profiles, and the mutational and epigenetic spectrum in cancer tissues. However, applications of molecular classification algorithms in clinical practice have been limited given the difficulties in obtaining reproducible results in different laboratories, in particular when different testing approaches such as different microarray platforms are used. Improved test performance for tumor classification may be achieved by using a multiplexed small number of classifier genes, subsequent to the initial discovery phase utilizing arrays with large genomic coverage. For example, massive parallel sequencing also known as deep sequencing, used to sequence the coding regions of 384 genes belonging to various pathways known to be altered in other gastrointestinal cancers, revealed genetic alterations in the WNT, Hedgehog, cell cycle, DNA damage, and epithelial-to-mesenchymal transition pathways, suggesting that targeted therapies approved or in clinical development for gastric carcinoma may be of benefit to approximately 22% of the patients studied.[186] However, additional validation in subsets of clinical samples and using specific combinations of limited gene targets will be needed before clinically relevant testing can be offered in routine practice.

As described in Chap. 2 anti-*HER2/ErbB2* therapies are being used in clinical practice for targeted treatment of gastric and GEJ adenocarcinomas. A number of agents that target specific molecules in cancer-related pathways have become available and are being tested in patients with gastric and GEJ carcinomas (Table 5.2) and their potential cellular targets for personalized therapies in gastric cancers are reviewed below.

Cell Surface Receptor Inhibitors: EGFR Family

Current available therapies may target the EGFR pathways (Chaps. 2 and 8) through inhibition of the EGFR using two different mechanisms: (1) inhibition of the EGFR via monoclonal antibodies (i.e., cetuximab, panitumumab, trastuzumab) or (2) tyrosine kinase inhibitors (i.e., gefitinib, erlotinib).

HER2 (HER2/neu, ErbB-2) targeted therapies: As reviewed in Chap. 2 overexpression and amplification of *HER2* have been described in gastric and GEJ adenocarcinomas,[187,188] and *HER2/ErbB* represents a possible target for therapy in advanced gastric cancer currently used in clinical practice.

EGFR (HER1; erbB1) targeted therapy: Cetuximab is a recombinant chimeric IgG1 monoclonal antibody that binds specifically to the extracellular domain of EGFR and competitively inhibits the binding of EGF and other ligands such as TGF-alpha. Cetuximab also mediates antibody-dependent cell cycle toxicity. Cetuximab is currently approved for patients with advanced colorectal and head and neck cancers.[189] Several ongoing phase III trials are evaluating cetuximab in combination with other chemotherapy agents for patients with advanced gastric and GEJ cancers. In contrast to colorectal cancer, in gastric cancers, the presence of a K-ras mutation (13.3%) was not associated with either progression-free survival or overall survival in patients receiving cetuximab therapy.[190,191,192]

Notably, the EGFR tyrosine kinase inhibitors have shown minimal evidence of efficacy in gastric carcinomas.[16]

Anti-angiogenic Agents

Tumor-associated angiogenesis requires a number of pro-angiogenic factors, among which vascular endothelial growth factors (VEGF family A–D) play a key role in vasculogenesis and angiogenesis. A number of anti-angiogenic agents for gastric and GEJ tumors have been investigated or are undergoing clinical trials.[16] Bevacizumab is a chimeric monoclonal antibody that binds the VEGF receptor and prevents the interaction of VEGF to its receptors (Flt1 and KDR) on the surface of endothelial cells. Clinical data of bevacizumab therapy in patients with advanced gastric or GEJ cancer are promising but are still limited. Another approach to inhibit the VEGF pathway uses tyrosine kinase inhibitors directed against the receptors of VEGF (Flt1 and KDR). There are several compounds available, some specifically targeting VEGF receptors, such as PTK787/ZK222584 (Vatalanib), and others that inhibit both the VEGF receptors and other tyrosine kinase receptors such as sunitinib and sorafenib (Table 5.2).

Other Targeted Therapies for Gastric and GEJ Cancers

A large number of specific inhibitors of molecular targets in gastric and GEJ cancer pathways are in the early stages of clinical trials or have only been evaluated in preclinical studies. Among these agents are the insulin-like growth factor-I receptor (IGF-IR) inhibitors, fibroblast growth factor (FGF) receptor inhibitors, c-Met signaling pathway inhibitors, and cell cycle-associated drug targets including Aurora kinase inhibitors, polo-like kinase inhibitors, and cyclin-dependent kinase (cdk) inhibitors.

Inhibition of cancer-associated epigenetic changes offers another approach for targeted tumor treatments. Histone deacetylase (HDAC) inhibitors are being investigated given the potential to re-express tumor suppressor genes silenced by hypermethylation in cancer cells.

Other agents being considered for targeted therapies in gastric and GEJ cancers include heat shock protein 90 (HS90) inhibitors, ubiquitin-proteasome pathway inhibitors, PI3K/Akt/mTOR pathway inhibitors, and matrix metalloproteinase (MMP) inhibitors.

Therapeutic Approaches for EBV-Associated GC

Since EBV genes play an essential role in the development of cancer, molecules interfering with the functions of these genes may be an important tool to treat EBV-associated malignancies. Strategies to inhibit virus-induced tumorigenesis include antiviral and antitumor molecules, gene therapy approaches, immune-based therapies, and epigenetic approaches. Many studies and clinical trials were undertaken for EBV-associated other malignancies, such as Burkitt's lymphoma, Hodgkin's disease, and nasopharyngeal carcinoma, and some of them are promising.

One approach is the induction of EBV lytic cycle, leading to expression of a much larger number of viral proteins, which may serve as potential therapeutic targets. A recent study[193] reported that one of the HDAC inhibitors suberoylanilide hydroxamic acid is a potent lytic cycle inducer in EBV-positive gastric carcinoma cells. Fu et al[194] pretreated the proteasome inhibitor bortezomib to activate viral thymidine kinase, coupled with radiolabeled substrates to specifically target tumor cells that express viral thymidine kinase. Another approach is to disrupt epigenetic silencing by demethylating agents, such as 5-azacytidine (5-AC). This approach should have a particular merit in EBV-associated GC as methylation of tumor suppressor genes is a key abnormality. A recent phase I study of 5-AC in combination with a HDAC inhibitor sodium phenylbutyrate in patients with refractory solid tumors failed to show a clinical benefit.[195] Further studies are warranted in order to investigate these reagents as a possible therapeutic approach.

More focused approaches are to abrogate the functions of specific EBV proteins. Since EBNA1 is expressed in all EBV-associated tumors, blocking EBNAs is a potential target. Blocking the trans-activating function of EBNA2 using short peptides inhibited cell proliferation in cultured B cells.[196] Suppression of EBNA1 by RNAi inhibited growth of EBV-positive extranodal nasal-type NK cell lymphoma.[197] These results suggest EBNAs as potential novel therapeutic targets.

There are two general approaches to treat tumors based on immune-response: adoptive immunotherapies, in which preformed cells or antibodies are passively transferred to patients, and active immunotherapy, in which an immunogen is administered to stimulate a response from the patient's immune system.[198] Although extensive studies have been performed on immunotherapy for EBV-associated tumors, studies in GC are limited. Okugawa et al[199] investigated the feasibility of immunotherapy for EBV-associated GC by inducing cytotoxic T lymphocytes (CTLs) from peripheral blood lymphocytes using antigen-presenting cells (APCs) such as an autologous lymphoblastoid cell line (LCL) and LMP2-derived peptide-pulsed dendritic cells (DCs). T cells induced by peptide-loaded DCs and autologous LCL efficiently lysed peptide-pulsed targets and successfully induced CTL response against EBV-associated GC cells.

References

1. Parkin DM, Bray F, Ferlay J, Pisani P. Global cancer statistics, 2002. *CA Cancer J Clin.* 2005;55:74–108.
2. Kamangar F, Dores GM, Anderson WF. Patterns of cancer incidence, mortality, and prevalence across five continents: defining priorities to reduce cancer disparities in different geographic regions of the world. *J Clin Oncol.* 2006;24:2137–50.
3. Howlader N, Noone AM, Krapcho M, et al., eds. *SEER Cancer Statistics Review, 1975–2009 (Vintage 2009 Populations).* Bethesda, MD: National Cancer Institute; 2012.
4. Brown LM, Devesa SS, Chow WH. Incidence of adenocarcinoma of the esophagus among white Americans by sex, stage, and age. *J Natl Cancer Inst.* 2008;100:1184–7.
5. Palli D. Epidemiology of gastric cancer: an evaluation of available evidence. *J Gastroenterol.* 2000;35(Suppl 12):84–9.
6. Sriamporn S, Setiawan V, Pisani P, et al. Gastric cancer: the roles of diet, alcohol drinking, smoking and *Helicobacter pylori* in Northeastern Thailand. *Asian Pac J Cancer Prev.* 2002;3: 345–352.
7. Brenner H, Arndt V, Bode G, Stegmaier C, Ziegler H, Stumer T. Risk of gastric cancer among smokers infected with *Helicobacter pylori. Int J Cancer.* 2002;98:446–9.
8. Gologan A, Graham DY, Sepulveda AR. Molecular markers in *Helicobacter pylori*-associated gastric carcinogenesis. *Clin Lab Med.* 2005;25:197–222.
9. Edge S, Byrd D, Compton C, Fritz A, Greene F, Trotti A III. *Stomach. AJCC Cancer Staging manual.* 7th ed. NY: Springer; 2010:117–126.
10. Bosman F, Carneiro F, Hruban R, Theise N. *Tumours of the stomach. WHO classification of tumors of the digestive system.* Lyon: IARC; 2010:46–80.
11. Lauren P. The two histological main types of gastric carcinoma: diffuse and so-called intestinal-type carcinoma an attempt at a histo-clinical classification. *Acta Pathol et Microbiol Scandinav.* 1965;64:31–49.
12. Watanabe H, Jass JR, Sobin LH. *Histological typing of esophageal and gastric tumors. WHO International Classification of Tumors.* 2nd ed. Berlin: Springer; 1990.
13. Greene F, Page D, Fleming I, et al. *AJCC cancer staging manual.* 6th ed. New York: Springer-Verlag; 2002.
14. Sepulveda A, Aisner D. Molecular Basis of Diseases of the Gastrointestinal Tract. In: Coleman WB, Tsongalis GJ, eds. *Molecular pathology: the molecular basis of human disease.* Academic Press; 2009:365–393.
15. Tan IB, Ivanova T, Lim KH, et al. Intrinsic subtypes of gastric cancer, based on gene expression pattern, predict survival and respond differently to chemotherapy. *Gastroenterology.* 2011;141:476–85. 485 e1–11.
16. Arkenau HT. Gastric cancer in the era of molecularly targeted agents: current drug development strategies. *J Cancer Res Clin Oncol.* 2009;135:855–66.
17. Warren JR, Marshall B. Unidentified curved bacilli on gastric epithelium in active chronic gastritis. *Lancet.* 1983;1:1273–1275.
18. Marshall BJ. *Helicobacter pylori*: the etiologic agent for peptic ulcer. *JAMA.* 1995;274:1064–1066.
19. Parsonnet J, Friedman GD, Vandersteen DP, et al. *Helicobacter pylori* and the risk of gastric carcinoma. *N Eng J Med.* 1991;325:1127–1131.
20. Herrera V, Parsonnet J. *Helicobacter pylori* and gastric adenocarcinoma. *Clin Microbiol Infect.* 2009;15:971–6.
21. International Agency for Research of Cancer. Shistosomes, liver flukes and *Helicobacter pylori. IARC Monogr Eval Carcinog Risks Hum.* 1994;61:1–241.
22. Kusters JG, van Vliet AH, Kuipers EJ. Pathogenesis of *Helicobacter pylori* infection. *Clin Microbiol Rev.* 2006;19: 449–90.
23. Isaacson PG, Spencer J. Gastric lymphoma and *Helicobacter pylori.* Important Adv Oncol 1996:111–21.
24. Bouzourene H, Haefliger T, Delacretaz F, Saraga E. The role of *Helicobacter pylori* in primary gastric MALT lymphoma. *Histopathology.* 1999;34:118–23.
25. Sepulveda A, Goyal A. Helicobacter and gastric neoplasms. In: Tan DaL G, ed. *Advances in surgical pathology: gastric cancer.* Philadelphia: Lippincott Williams and Wilkins; 2011:22–37.
26. Makola D, Peura DA, Crowe SE. *Helicobacter pylori* infection and related gastrointestinal diseases. *J Clin Gastroenterol.* 2007;41:548–58.
27. Goodman KJ, Correa P. The transmission of *Helicobacter pylori.* A critical review of the evidence. *Int J Epidemiol.* 1995;24:875–87.
28. Malfertheiner P, Megraud F, O'Morain C, et al. Current concepts in the management of *Helicobacter pylori* infection: the Maastricht III Consensus Report. *Gut.* 2007;56:772–81.
29. Chey WD, Wong BC. American College of Gastroenterology guideline on the management of *Helicobacter pylori* infection. *Am J Gastroenterol.* 2007;102:1808–25.
30. Asaka M, Sugiyama T, Nobuta A, Kato M, Takeda H, Graham DY. Atrophic gastritis and intestinal metaplasia in Japan: results of a large multicenter study. *Helicobacter.* 2001;6:294–9.
31. Correa P. *Helicobacter pylori* and gastric carcinogenesis. *Am J Surg Pathol.* 1995;19:S37-S43.
32. Nomura A, Stemmermann GN, Chyou PH, Kato I, Perez GI, Blaser MJ. *Helicobacter pylori* infection and gastric carcinoma among Japanese Americans in Hawaii. *N Engl J Med.* 1991;325:1132–1136.
33. Dixon MF. Histological responses to *Helicobacter pylori* infection: gastritis, atrophy and preneoplasia. *Baillieres Clin Gastroenterol.* 1995;9:467–86.
34. Recavarren-Arce S, Leon-Barua R, Cok J, et al. *Helicobacter pylori* and progressive gastric pathology that predisposes to gastric cancer. *Scand J Gastroenterol Suppl.* 1991;181:51–7.
35. Kodama K, Sumii K, Kawano M, et al. Gastric juice nitrite and vitamin C in patients with gastric cancer and atrophic gastritis: is low acidity solely responsible for cancer risk? *Eur J Gastroenterol Hepatol.* 2003;15:987–93.
36. Sepulveda A, Peterson LE, Shelton J, Gutierrez O, Graham DY. Histological patterns of gastritis in *H. pylori*-infected individuals with a family history of gastric cancer. *Am J Gastroenterol.* 2002;97:1365–70.
37. Leung WK, Kim JJ, Kim JG, Graham DY, Sepulveda AR. Microsatellite instability in gastric intestinal metaplasia in patients with and without gastric cancer. *Am J Pathol.* 2000;156: 537–43.
38. Toyota M, Ahuja N, Suzuki H, et al. Aberrant methylation in gastric cancer associated with the CpG island methylator phenotype. *Cancer Res.* 1999;59:5438–42.
39. Kang GH, Shim YH, Jung HY, Kim WH, Ro JY, Rhyu MG. CpG island methylation in premalignant stages of gastric carcinoma. *Cancer Res.* 2001;61:2847–51.
40. To KF, Leung WK, Lee TL, et al. Promoter hypermethylation of tumor-related genes in gastric intestinal metaplasia of patients with and without gastric cancer. *Int J Cancer.* 2002; 102:623–8.
41. Waki T, Tamura G, Sato M, Terashima M, Nishizuka S, Motoyama T. Promoter methylation status of DAP-kinase and RUNX3 genes in neoplastic and non-neoplastic gastric epithelia. *Cancer Sci.* 2003;94:360–4.
42. Kang GH, Lee S, Kim JS, Jung HY. Profile of aberrant CpG island methylation along the multistep pathway of gastric carcinogenesis. *Lab Invest.* 2003;83:635–41.

43. Lee JH, Park SJ, Abraham SC, et al. Frequent CpG island methylation in precursor lesions and early gastric adenocarcinomas. *Oncogene*. 2004;23:4646–54.
44. Sepulveda AR, Jones D, Ogino S, et al. CpG methylation analysis–current status of clinical assays and potential applications in molecular diagnostics: a report of the Association for Molecular Pathology. *J Mol Diagn*. 2009;11:266–78.
45. Mikata R, Yokosuka O, Fukai K, et al. Analysis of genes upregulated by the demethylating agent 5-aza-2′-deoxycytidine in gastric cancer cell lines. *Int J Cancer*. 2006;119:1616–22.
46. Huang JQ, Sridhar S, Chen Y, Hunt RH. Meta-analysis of the relationship between *Helicobacter pylori* seropositivity and gastric cancer. *Gastroenterology*. 1998;114:1169–79.
47. Sepulveda AR, Wu L, Ota H, et al. Molecular identification of main cellular lineages as a tool for the classification of gastric cancer. *Hum Pathol*. 2000;31:566–74.
48. Uemura N, Okamoto S, Yamamoto S, et al. *Helicobacter pylori* infection and the development of gastric cancer. *N Engl J Med*. 2001;345:784–9.
49. Watanabe T, Tada M, Nagai H, Sasaki S, Nakao M. *Helicobacter pylori* infection induces gastric cancer in mongolian gerbils. *Gastroenterology*. 1998;115:642–8.
50. Sugiyama A, Maruta F, Ikeno T, et al. *Helicobacter pylori* infection enhances N-methyl-N-nitrosourea-induced stomach carcinogenesis in the Mongolian gerbil. *Cancer Res*. 1998;58:2067–9.
51. Honda S, Fujioka T, Tokieda M, Satoh R, Nishizono A, Nasu M. Development of *Helicobacter pylori*-induced gastric carcinoma in Mongolian gerbils. *Cancer Res*. 1998;58:4255–9.
52. Shimizu N, Inada K, Nakanishi H, et al. *Helicobacter pylori* infection enhances glandular stomach carcinogenesis in Mongolian gerbils treated with chemical carcinogens. *Carcinogenesis*. 1999;20:669–76.
53. Houghton J, Stoicov C, Nomura S, et al. Gastric cancer originating from bone marrow-derived cells. *Science*. 2004;306:1568–71.
54. Franco AT, Johnston E, Krishna U, et al. Regulation of gastric carcinogenesis by *Helicobacter pylori* virulence factors. *Cancer Res*. 2008;68:379–87.
55. Mills JC, Shivdasani RA. Gastric epithelial stem cells. *Gastroenterology*. 2011;140:412–24.
56. Barker N, Huch M, Kujala P, et al. Lgr5(+ve) stem cells drive self-renewal in the stomach and build long-lived gastric units in vitro. *Cell Stem Cell*. 2010;6:25–36.
57. Qiao XT, Gumucio DL. Current molecular markers for gastric progenitor cells and gastric cancer stem cells. *J Gastroenterol*. 2011;46:855–65.
58. Simon E, Petke D, Boger C, et al. The spatial distribution of LGR5+ cells correlates with gastric cancer progression. *PLoS One*. 2012;7:e35486.
59. Uehara T, Ma D, Yao Y, Lynch JP, N. M, Ziober A, Feldman M, Ota H, Sepulveda AR. *H. pylori* infection is associated with DNA damage of Lgr5-positive epithelial stem cells in the stomach of patients with gastric cancer. Dig Dis Sci 2012. (Epub ahead of print).
60. Quante M, Marrache F, Goldenring JR, Wang TC. TFF2 mRNA transcript expression marks a gland progenitor cell of the gastric oxyntic mucosa. *Gastroenterology*. 2010;139:2018–2027. e2.
61. May R, Sureban SM, Hoang N, et al. Doublecortin and CaM kinase-like-1 and leucine-rich-repeat-containing G-protein-coupled receptor mark quiescent and cycling intestinal stem cells, respectively. *Stem Cells*. 2009;27:2571–9.
62. Takaishi S, Okumura T, Tu S, et al. Identification of gastric cancer stem cells using the cell surface marker CD44. *Stem Cells*. 2009;27:1006–20.
63. Correa P, Houghton J. Carcinogenesis of *Helicobacter pylori*. *Gastroenterology*. 2007;133:659–72.
64. Giannakis M, Chen SL, Karam SM, Engstrand L, Gordon JI. *Helicobacter pylori* evolution during progression from chronic atrophic gastritis to gastric cancer and its impact on gastric stem cells. *Proc Natl Acad Sci USA*. 2008;105:4358–63.
65. Katoh M. Dysregulation of stem cell signaling network due to germline mutation, SNP, *Helicobacter pylori* infection, epigenetic change and genetic alteration in gastric cancer. *Cancer Biol Ther*. 2007;6:832–9.
66. Wen S, Moss SF. *Helicobacter pylori* virulence factors in gastric carcinogenesis. *Cancer Lett*. 2009;282:1–8.
67. Mascellino MT, Margani M, Oliva A. *Helicobacter pylori*: determinant and markers of virulence. *Dis Markers*. 2009;27:137–56.
68. Cover TL, Blanke SR. *Helicobacter pylori* VacA, a paradigm for toxin multifunctionality. *Nat Rev Microbiol*. 2005;3:320–32.
69. Handa O, Naito Y, Yoshikawa T. CagA protein of *Helicobacter pylori*: a hijacker of gastric epithelial cell signaling. *Biochem Pharmacol*. 2007;73:1697–702.
70. Rad R, Gerhard M, Lang R, et al. The *Helicobacter pylori* blood group antigen-binding adhesin facilitates bacterial colonization and augments a nonspecific immune response. *J Immunol*. 2002;168:3033–41.
71. Gerhard M, Lehn N, Neumayer N, et al. Clinical relevance of the *Helicobacter pylori* gene for blood-group antigen-binding adhesin. *Proc Natl Acad Sci USA*. 1999;96:12778–83.
72. Torres VJ, VanCompernolle SE, Sundrud MS, Unutmaz D, Cover TL. *Helicobacter pylori* vacuolating cytotoxin inhibits activation-induced proliferation of human T and B lymphocyte subsets. *J Immunol*. 2007;179:5433–40.
73. Censini S, Lange C, Xiang Z, et al. cag, a pathogenicity island of *Helicobacter pylori*, encodes type I-specific and disease-associated virulence factors. *Proc Natl Acad Sci USA*. 1996;93:14648–53.
74. Parsonnet J, Friedman GD, Orentreich N, Vogelman H. Risk for gastric cancer in people with CagA positive or CagA negative *Helicobacter pylori* infection [see comments]. *Gut*. 1997;40: 297–301.
75. Yamaoka Y, Kodama T, Kashima K, Graham DY, Sepulveda AR. Variants of the 3' region of the cagA gene in *Helicobacter pylori* isolates from patients with different H. pylori-associated diseases. *J Clin Microbiol*. 1998;36:2258–63.
76. Hatakeyama M, Higashi H. *Helicobacter pylori* CagA: a new paradigm for bacterial carcinogenesis. *Cancer Sci*. 2005;96:835–43.
77. Crabtree JE, Wyatt JI, Trejdosiewicz LK, et al. Interleukin-8 expression in *Helicobacter pylori* infected, normal, and neoplastic gastroduodenal mucosa. *J Clin Pathol*. 1994;47:61–6.
78. Crabtree JE, Covacci A, Farmery SM, et al. *Helicobacter pylori* induced interleukin-8 expression in gastric epithelial cells is associated with CagA positive phenotype. *J Clin Pathol*. 1995;48: 41–5.
79. Sepulveda AR, Yao Y, Yan W, et al. CpG methylation and reduced expression of O6-methylguanine DNA methyltransferase is associated with *Helicobacter pylori* infection. *Gastroenterology*. 2010;138:1836–44.
80. Ohnishi N, Yuasa H, Tanaka S, et al. Transgenic expression of *Helicobacter pylori* CagA induces gastrointestinal and hematopoietic neoplasms in mouse. *Proc Natl Acad Sci USA*. 2008;105:1003–8.
81. El-Omar EM, Carrington M, Chow WH, et al. Interleukin-1 polymorphisms associated with increased risk of gastric cancer. *Nature*. 2000;404:398–402.
82. El-Omar EM, Rabkin CS, Gammon MD, et al. Increased risk of noncardia gastric cancer associated with proinflammatory cytokine gene polymorphisms. *Gastroenterology*. 2003;124:1193–201.
83. El-Omar EM. Role of host genes in sporadic gastric cancer. *Best Pract Res Clin Gastroenterol*. 2006;20:675–86.
84. Machado JC, Figueiredo C, Canedo P, et al. A proinflammatory genetic profile increases the risk for chronic atrophic gastritis and gastric carcinoma. *Gastroenterology*. 2003;125:364–71.

85. Peek RM Jr, Wirth HP, Moss SF, et al. *Helicobacter pylori* alters gastric epithelial cell cycle events and gastrin secretion in Mongolian gerbils. *Gastroenterology*. 2000;118:48–59.
86. Chattopadhyay R, Bhattacharyya A, Crowe SE. Dual regulation by apurinic/apyrimidinic endonuclease-1 inhibits gastric epithelial cell apoptosis during *Helicobacter pylori* infection. *Cancer Res*. 2010;70:2799–808.
87. Kobayashi K, Okamoto T, Takayama S, Akiyama M, Ohno T, Yamada H. Genetic instability in intestinal metaplasia is a frequent event leading to well-differentiated early adenocarcinoma of the stomach. *Eur J Cancer*. 2000;36:1113–9.
88. Correa P, Shiao Y-H. Phenotypic and genotypic events in gastric carcinogenesis. *Cancer Res*. 1994;54(Supplement): 1941–1943.
89. Nakatsuru S, Yanagisawa A, Furukawa Y, et al. Somatic mutations of the APC gene in precancerous lesion of the stomach. *Hum Mol Genet*. 1993;2:1463–5.
90. Shiao YH, Rugge M, Correa P, Lehmann HP, Scheer WD. p53 alteration in gastric precancerous lesions. *Am J Pathol*. 1994; 144:511–7.
91. Imatani A, Sasano H, Asaki S, et al. Analysis of p53 abnormalities in endoscopic gastric biopsies. *Anticancer Res*. 1996;16: 2049–56.
92. Maesawa C, Tamura G, Suzuki Y, et al. The sequential accumulation of genetic alterations characteristic of the colorectal adenoma-carcinoma sequence does not occur between gastric adenoma and adenocarcinoma. *J Pathol*. 1995;176:249–58.
93. Abraham SC, Park SJ, Lee JH, Mugartegui L, Wu TT. Genetic alterations in gastric adenomas of intestinal and foveolar phenotypes. *Mod Pathol*. 2003;16:786–95.
94. Lee HS, Choi SI, Lee HK, et al. Distinct clinical features and outcomes of gastric cancers with microsatellite instability. *Mod Pathol*. 2002;15:632–40.
95. Hunt JD, Mera R, Strimas A, et al. KRAS mutations are not predictive for progression of preneoplastic gastric lesions. *Cancer Epidemiol Biomarkers Prev*. 2001;10:79–80.
96. Lee JH, Abraham SC, Kim HS, et al. Inverse relationship between APC gene mutation in gastric adenomas and development of adenocarcinoma. *Am J Pathol*. 2002;161:611–8.
97. Wang K, Kan J, Yuen ST, et al. Exome sequencing identifies frequent mutation of ARID1A in molecular subtypes of gastric cancer. *Nat Genet*. 2011;43:1219–23.
98. Zang ZJ, Cutcutache I, Poon SL, et al. Exome sequencing of gastric adenocarcinoma identifies recurrent somatic mutations in cell adhesion and chromatin remodeling genes. *Nat Genet*. 2012;44: 570–4.
99. Shimada T, Watanabe N, Hiraishi H, Terano A. Redox regulation of interleukin-8 expression in MKN28 cells. *Dig Dis Sci*. 1999;44:266–73.
100. Verhulst ML, van Oijen AH, Roelofs HM, Peters WH, Jansen JB. Antral glutathione concentration and glutathione S-transferase activity in patients with and without *Helicobacter pylori*. *Dig Dis Sci*. 2000;45:629–32.
101. Farinati F, Cardin R, Degan P, et al. Oxidative DNA damage accumulation in gastric carcinogenesis. *Gut*. 1998;42:351–6.
102. Hahm KB, Lee KJ, Choi SY, et al. Possibility of chemoprevention by the eradication of *Helicobacter pylori*: oxidative DNA damage and apoptosis in *H. pylori* infection. *Am J Gastroenterol*. 1997;92:1853–7.
103. Chiba T, Marusawa H. A novel mechanism for inflammation-associated carcinogenesis; an important role of activation-induced cytidine deaminase (AID) in mutation induction. *J Mol Med (Berl)*. 2009;87:1023–7.
104. Yao Y, Tao H, Park DI, Sepulveda JL, Sepulveda AR. Demonstration and characterization of mutations induced by *Helicobacter pylori* organisms in gastric epithelial cells. *Helicobacter*. 2006;11:272–86.
105. Park DI, Park SH, Kim SH, et al. Effect of *Helicobacter pylori* infection on the expression of DNA mismatch repair protein. *Helicobacter*. 2005;10:179–84.
106. Kim JJ, Tao H, Carloni E, Leung WK, Graham DY, Sepulveda AR. *Helicobacter pylori* impairs DNA mismatch repair in gastric epithelial cells. *Gastroenterology*. 2002;123:542–53.
107. Umar A. Lynch syndrome (HNPCC) and microsatellite instability. *Dis Markers*. 2004;20:179–80.
108. Semba S, Yokozaki H, Yamamoto S, Yasui W, Tahara E. Microsatellite instability in precancerous lesions and adenocarcinomas of the stomach. *Cancer*. 1996;77:1620–7.
109. Hamamoto T, Yokozaki H, Semba S, et al. Altered microsatellites in incomplete-type intestinal metaplasia adjacent to primary gastric cancers. *J Clin Pathol*. 1997;50:841–6.
110. Ottini L, Palli D, Falchetti M, et al. Microsatellite instability in gastric cancer is associated with tumor location and family history in a high-risk population from Tuscany. *Cancer Res*. 1997;57:4523–9.
111. Fang DC, Jass JR, Wang DX, Zhou XD, Luo YH, Young J. Infrequent loss of heterozygosity of APC/MCC and DCC genes in gastric cancer showing DNA microsatellite instability. *J Clin Pathol*. 1999;52:504–8.
112. Ling XL, Fang DC, Wang RQ, Yang SM, Fang L. Mitochondrial microsatellite instability in gastric cancer and its precancerous lesions. *World J Gastroenterol*. 2004;10:800–3.
113. Kashiwagi K, Watanabe M, Ezaki T, et al. Clinical usefulness of microsatellite instability for the prediction of gastric adenoma or adenocarcinoma in patients with chronic gastritis. *Br J Cancer*. 2000;82:1814–8.
114. Wu MS, Lee CW, Shun CT, et al. Clinicopathological significance of altered loci of replication error and microsatellite instability-associated mutations in gastric cancer. *Cancer Res*. 1998;58:1494–7.
115. Wu MS, Lee CW, Shun CT, et al. Distinct clinicopathologic and genetic profiles in sporadic gastric cancer with different mutator phenotypes. *Genes Chromosomes Cancer*. 2000;27:403–11.
116. Umar A, Boland CR, Terdiman JP, et al. Revised Bethesda Guidelines for hereditary nonpolyposis colorectal cancer (Lynch syndrome) and microsatellite instability. *J Natl Cancer Inst*. 2004;96:261–8.
117. Baek MJ, Kang H, Kim SE, et al. Expression of hMLH1 is inactivated in the gastric adenomas with enhanced microsatellite instability. *Br J Cancer*. 2001;85:1147–52.
118. Fleisher AS, Esteller M, Tamura G, et al. Hypermethylation of the hMLH1 gene promoter is associated with microsatellite instability in early human gastric neoplasia. *Oncogene*. 2001;20: 329–35.
119. Edmonston TB, Cuesta KH, Burkholder S, et al. Colorectal carcinomas with high microsatellite instability: defining a distinct immunologic and molecular entity with respect to prognostic markers. *Hum Pathol*. 2000;31:1506–14.
120. Kim SS, Bhang CS, Min KO, et al. p53 mutations and microsatellite instabilities in the subtype of intestinal metaplasia of the stomach. *J Korean Med Sci*. 2002;17:490–6.
121. Hayden JD, Martin IG, Cawkwell L, Quirke P. The role of microsatellite instability in gastric carcinoma. *Gut*. 1998;42:300–3.
122. Strickler JG, Zheng J, Shu Q, Burgart LJ, Alberts SR, Shibata D. p53 mutations and microsatellite instability in sporadic gastric cancer: when guardians fail. *Cancer Res*. 1994;54:4750–5.
123. Sepulveda AR, Santos AC, Yamaoka Y, et al. Marked differences in the frequency of microsatellite instability in gastric cancer from different countries. *Am J Gastroenterol*. 1999;94:3034–8.
124. Yamamoto H, Sawai H, Perucho M. Frameshift somatic mutations in gastrointestinal cancer of the microsatellite mutator phenotype. *Cancer Res*. 1997;57:4420–6.
125. Shinmura K, Tani M, Isogaki J, Wang Y, Sugimura H, Yokota J. RER phenotype and its associated mutations in familial gastric cancer. *Carcinogenesis*. 1998;19:247–51.

126. Myeroff LL, Parsons R, Kim SJ, et al. A transforming growth factor beta receptor type II gene mutation common in colon and gastric but rare in endometrial cancers with microsatellite instability. *Cancer Res*. 1995;55:5545–7.
127. Chung YJ, Park SW, Song JM, et al. Evidence of genetic progression in human gastric carcinomas with microsatellite instability. *Oncogene*. 1997;15:1719–26.
128. Kim JJ, Baek MJ, Kim L, et al. Accumulated frameshift mutations at coding nucleotide repeats during the progression of gastric carcinoma with microsatellite instability. *Lab Invest*. 1999;79: 1113–20.
129. Kim HS, Woo DK, Bae SI, Kim YI, Kim WH. Microsatellite instability in the adenoma-carcinoma sequence of the stomach. *Lab Invest*. 2000;80:57–64.
130. Farinati F, Cardin R, Bortolami M, et al. Oxidative DNA damage in gastric cancer: CagA status and OGG1 gene polymorphism. *Int J Cancer*. 2008;123:51–5.
131. Park TJ, Han SU, Cho YK, Paik WK, Kim YB, Lim IK. Methylation of O(6)-methylguanine-DNA methyltransferase gene is associated significantly with K-ras mutation, lymph node invasion, tumor staging, and disease free survival in patients with gastric carcinoma. *Cancer*. 2001;92:2760–8.
132. Kang GH, Lee HJ, Hwang KS, Lee S, Kim JH, Kim JS. Aberrant CpG island hypermethylation of chronic gastritis, in relation to aging, gender, intestinal metaplasia, and chronic inflammation. *Am J Pathol*. 2003;163:1551–6.
133. Chan AO, Chu KM, Huang C, et al. Association between *Helicobacter pylori* infection and interleukin 1beta polymorphism predispose to CpG island methylation in gastric cancer. *Gut*. 2007;56:595–7.
134. Qian X, Huang C, Cho CH, Hui WM, Rashid A, Chan AO. E-cadherin promoter hypermethylation induced by interleukin-1beta treatment or *H. pylori* infection in human gastric cancer cell lines. *Cancer Lett*. 2008;263:107–13.
135. Chan AO, Peng JZ, Lam SK, et al. Eradication of *Helicobacter pylori* infection reverses E-cadherin promoter hypermethylation. *Gut*. 2006;55:463–8.
136. Hasegawa S, Furukawa Y, Li M, et al. Genome-wide analysis of gene expression in intestinal-type gastric cancers using a complementary DNA microarray representing 23,040 genes. *Cancer Res*. 2002;62:7012–7.
137. Hippo Y, Taniguchi H, Tsutsumi S, et al. Global gene expression analysis of gastric cancer by oligonucleotide microarrays. *Cancer Res*. 2002;62:233–40.
138. Lee S, Baek M, Yang H, et al. Identification of genes differentially expressed between gastric cancers and normal gastric mucosa with cDNA microarrays. *Cancer Lett*. 2002;184:197–206.
139. Kim B, Bang S, Lee S, et al. Expression profiling and subtype-specific expression of stomach cancer. *Cancer Res*. 2003;63: 8248–55.
140. Wu MS, Lin YS, Chang YT, Shun CT, Lin MT, Lin JT. Gene expression profiling of gastric cancer by microarray combined with laser capture microdissection. *World J Gastroenterol*. 2005;11:7405–12.
141. Kim SY, Kim JH, Lee HS, et al. Meta- and gene set analysis of stomach cancer gene expression data. *Mol Cells*. 2007;24:200–9.
142. Myllykangas S, Junnila S, Kokkola A, et al. Integrated gene copy number and expression microarray analysis of gastric cancer highlights potential target genes. *Int J Cancer*. 2008;123:817–25.
143. Boussioutas A, Li H, Liu J, et al. Distinctive patterns of gene expression in premalignant gastric mucosa and gastric cancer. *Cancer Res*. 2003;63:2569–77.
144. Jinawath N, Furukawa Y, Hasegawa S, et al. Comparison of gene-expression profiles between diffuse- and intestinal-type gastric cancers using a genome-wide cDNA microarray. *Oncogene*. 2004;23:6830–44.
145. Meireles SI, Cristo EB, Carvalho AF, et al. Molecular classifiers for gastric cancer and nonmalignant diseases of the gastric mucosa. *Cancer Res*. 2004;64:1255–65.
146. Meireles SI, Carvalho AF, Hirata R, et al. Differentially expressed genes in gastric tumors identified by cDNA array. *Cancer Lett*. 2003;190:199–211.
147. Belair C, Darfeuille F, Staedel C. *Helicobacter pylori* and gastric cancer: possible role of microRNAs in this intimate relationship. *Clin Microbiol Infect*. 2009;15:806–12.
148. Zhang Z, Li Z, Gao C, et al. miR-21 plays a pivotal role in gastric cancer pathogenesis and progression. *Lab Invest*. 2008;88:1358–66.
149. Volinia S, Calin GA, Liu CG, et al. A microRNA expression signature of human solid tumors defines cancer gene targets. *Proc Natl Acad Sci USA*. 2006;103:2257–61.
150. Chan SH, Wu CW, Li AF, Chi CW, Lin WC. miR-21 microRNA expression in human gastric carcinomas and its clinical association. *Anticancer Res*. 2008;28:907–11.
151. Liu R, Zhang C, Hu Z, et al. A five-microRNA signature identified from genome-wide serum microRNA expression profiling serves as a fingerprint for gastric cancer diagnosis. *Eur J Cancer*. 2011;47:784–91.
152. Lam EK, Wang X, Shin VY, et al. A microRNA contribution to aberrant Ras activation in gastric cancer. *Am J Transl Res*. 2011;3:209–18.
153. Yao Y, Suo AL, Li ZF, et al. MicroRNA profiling of human gastric cancer. *Mol Med Report*. 2009;2:963–70.
154. Epstein MA, Achong BG, Barr YM. Virus particles in cultured lymphoblasts from Burkitt's Lymphoma. *Lancet*. 1964;1:702–3.
155. Henle G, Henle W, Diehl V. Relation of Burkitt's tumor-associated herpes-ytpe virus to infectious mononucleosis. *Proc Natl Acad Sci USA*. 1968;59:94–101.
156. Rickinson A, Kieff E. Epstein–Barr virus. In: Knipe D, Howley P, eds. *Fields virology*. 5th ed. Philadelphia: Lippincott Williams & Wilkins; 2007:2604–2701.
157. Shibata D, Tokunaga M, Uemura Y, Sato E, Tanaka S, Weiss LM. Association of Epstein-Barr virus with undifferentiated gastric carcinomas with intense lymphoid infiltration Lymphoepithelioma-like carcinoma. *Am J Pathol*. 1991;139:469–74.
158. Shibata D, Weiss LM. Epstein-Barr virus-associated gastric adenocarcinoma. *Am J Pathol*. 1992;140:769–74.
159. Lee JH, Kim SH, Han SH, An JS, Lee ES, Kim YS. Clinicopathological and molecular characteristics of Epstein-Barr virus-associated gastric carcinoma: a meta-analysis. *J Gastroenterol Hepatol*. 2009;24:354–65.
160. Murphy G, Pfeiffer R, Camargo MC, Rabkin CS. Meta-analysis shows that prevalence of Epstein-Barr virus-positive gastric cancer differs based on sex and anatomic location. *Gastroenterology*. 2009;137:824–33.
161. Young LS, Rickinson AB. Epstein-Barr virus: 40 years on. *Nat Rev Cancer*. 2004;4:757–68.
162. Yoshiyama H, Imai S, Shimizu N, Takada K. Epstein-Barr virus infection of human gastric carcinoma cells: implication of the existence of a new virus receptor different from CD21. *J Virol*. 1997;71:5688–91.
163. Smith PR, de Jesus O, Turner D, et al. Structure and coding content of CST (BART) family RNAs of Epstein-Barr virus. *J Virol*. 2000;74:3082–92.
164. Decaussin G, Sbih-Lammali F, de Turenne-Tessier M, Bouguermouh A, Ooka T. Expression of BARF1 gene encoded by Epstein-Barr virus in nasopharyngeal carcinoma biopsies. *Cancer Res*. 2000;60:5584–8.
165. zur Hausen A, Brink AA, Craanen ME, Middeldorp JM, Meijer CJ, van den Brule AJ. Unique transcription pattern of Epstein-Barr virus (EBV) in EBV-carrying gastric adenocarcinomas: expression of the transforming BARF1 gene. *Cancer Res*. 2000;60:2745–8.

166. Akiba S, Koriyama C, Herrera-Goepfert R, Eizuru Y. Epstein-Barr virus associated gastric carcinoma: epidemiological and clinicopathological features. *Cancer Sci.* 2008;99:195–201.
167. Uemura Y, Tokunaga M, Arikawa J, et al. A unique morphology of Epstein-Barr virus-related early gastric carcinoma. *Cancer Epidemiol Biomarkers Prev.* 1994;3:607–11.
168. Hirano N, Tsukamoto T, Mizoshita T, et al. Down regulation of gastric and intestinal phenotypic expression in Epstein-Barr virus-associated stomach cancers. *Histol Histopathol.* 2007;22: 641–9.
169. Shinozaki A, Ushiku T, Morikawa T, et al. Epstein-Barr virus-associated gastric carcinoma: a distinct carcinoma of gastric phenotype by claudin expression profiling. *J Histochem Cytochem.* 2009;57:775–85.
170. Fukayama M. Epstein-Barr virus and gastric carcinoma. *Pathol Int.* 2010;60:337–50.
171. Imai S, Koizumi S, Sugiura M, et al. Gastric carcinoma: monoclonal epithelial malignant cells expressing Epstein-Barr virus latent infection protein. *Proc Natl Acad Sci USA.* 1994;91:9131–5.
172. Imai S, Nishikawa J, Takada K. Cell-to-cell contact as an efficient mode of Epstein-Barr virus infection of diverse human epithelial cells. *J Virol.* 1998;72:4371–8.
173. Yanai H, Murakami T, Yoshiyama H, et al. Epstein-Barr virus-associated gastric carcinoma and atrophic gastritis. *J Clin Gastroenterol.* 1999;29:39–43.
174. Yamamoto N, Tokunaga M, Uemura Y, et al. Epstein-Barr virus and gastric remnant cancer. *Cancer.* 1994;74:805–9.
175. Fukayama M, Hayashi Y, Iwasaki Y, et al. Epstein-Barr virus-associated gastric carcinoma and Epstein-Barr virus infection of the stomach. *Lab Invest.* 1994;71:73–81.
176. Ojima H, Fukuda T, Nakajima T, Nagamachi Y. Infrequent overexpression of p53 protein in Epstein-Barr virus-associated gastric carcinomas. *Jpn J Cancer Res.* 1997;88:262–6.
177. Leung SY, Chau KY, Yuen ST, Chu KM, Branicki FJ, Chung LP. p53 overexpression is different in Epstein-Barr virus-associated and Epstein-Barr virus-negative carcinoma. *Histopathology.* 1998;33:311–7.
178. Schneider BG, Gulley ML, Eagan P, Bravo JC, Mera R, Geradts J. Loss of p16/CDKN2A tumor suppressor protein in gastric adenocarcinoma is associated with Epstein-Barr virus and anatomic location in the body of the stomach. *Hum Pathol.* 2000;31:45–50.
179. Kang GH, Lee S, Kim WH, et al. Epstein-barr virus-positive gastric carcinoma demonstrates frequent aberrant methylation of multiple genes and constitutes CpG island methylator phenotype-positive gastric carcinoma. *Am J Pathol.* 2002;160:787–94.
180. Etoh T, Kanai Y, Ushijima S. al. e. Increased DNA methyltransferase 1 (DNMT1) protein expression correlates significantly with poorer tumor differentiation and frequent DNA hypermethylation of multiple CpG islands in gastric cancers. *Am J Pathol.* 2004;164:689–699.
181. Tsai CL, Li HP, Lu YJ, et al. Activation of DNA methyltransferase 1 by EBV LMP1 Involves c-Jun NH(2)-terminal kinase signaling. *Cancer Res.* 2006;66:11668–76.
182. Hino R, Uozaki H, Murakami N, et al. Activation of DNA methyltransferase 1 by EBV latent membrane protein 2A leads to promoter hypermethylation of PTEN gene in gastric carcinoma. *Cancer Res.* 2009;69:2766–74.
183. Sudo M, Chong JM, Sakuma K, et al. Promoter hypermethylation of E-cadherin and its abnormal expression in Epstein-Barr virus-associated gastric carcinoma. *Int J Cancer.* 2004;109:194–9.
184. Shinozaki A, Sakatani T, Ushiku T, et al. Downregulation of microRNA-200 in EBV-associated gastric carcinoma. *Cancer Res.* 2010;70:4719–27.
185. Van Cutsem E, Van de Velde C, Roth A, et al. Expert opinion on management of gastric and gastro-oesophageal junction adenocarcinoma on behalf of the European Organisation for Research and Treatment of Cancer (EORTC)-gastrointestinal cancer group. *Eur J Cancer.* 2008;44:182–94.
186. Holbrook JD, Parker JS, Gallagher KT, et al. Deep sequencing of gastric carcinoma reveals somatic mutations relevant to personalized medicine. *J Transl Med.* 2011;9:119.
187. Tanner M, Hollmen M, Junttila TT, et al. Amplification of HER-2 in gastric carcinoma: association with Topoisomerase IIalpha gene amplification, intestinal type, poor prognosis and sensitivity to trastuzumab. *Ann Oncol.* 2005;16:273–8.
188. Gravalos C, Jimeno A. HER2 in gastric cancer: a new prognostic factor and a novel therapeutic target. *Ann Oncol.* 2008;19: 1523–9.
189. Saltz LB, Meropol NJ, Loehrer PJ Sr, Needle MN, Kopit J, Mayer RJ. Phase II trial of cetuximab in patients with refractory colorectal cancer that expresses the epidermal growth factor receptor. *J Clin Oncol.* 2004;22:1201–8.
190. Park SR, Kook MC, Choi IJ, et al. Predictive factors for the efficacy of cetuximab plus chemotherapy as salvage therapy in metastatic gastric cancer patients. *Cancer Chemother Pharmacol.* 2010;65:579–87.
191. De Roock W, Piessevaux H, De Schutter J, et al. KRAS wild-type state predicts survival and is associated to early radiological response in metastatic colorectal cancer treated with cetuximab. *Ann Oncol.* 2008;19:508–15.
192. Allegra CJ, Jessup JM, Somerfield MR, et al. American Society of Clinical Oncology provisional clinical opinion: testing for KRAS gene mutations in patients with metastatic colorectal carcinoma to predict response to anti-epidermal growth factor receptor monoclonal antibody therapy. *J Clin Oncol.* 2009;27:2091–6.
193. Hui KF, Chiang AK. Suberoylanilide hydroxamic acid induces viral lytic cycle in Epstein-Barr virus-positive epithelial malignancies and mediates enhanced cell death. *Int J Cancer.* 2010;126:2479–89.
194. Fu DX, Tanhehco Y, Chen J, et al. Bortezomib-induced enzyme-targeted radiation therapy in herpesvirus-associated tumors. *Nat Med.* 2008;14:1118–22.
195. Lin J, Gilbert J, Rudek MA, et al. A phase I dose-finding study of 5-azacytidine in combination with sodium phenylbutyrate in patients with refractory solid tumors. *Clin Cancer Res.* 2009;15:6241–9.
196. Farrell CJ, Lee JM, Shin EC, Cebrat M, Cole PA, Hayward SD. Inhibition of Epstein-Barr virus-induced growth proliferation by a nuclear antigen EBNA2-TAT peptide. *Proc Natl Acad Sci USA.* 2004;101:4625–30.
197. Ian MX, Lan SZ, Cheng ZF, Dan H, Qiong LH. Suppression of EBNA1 expression inhibits growth of EBV-positive NK/T cell lymphoma cells. *Cancer Biol Ther.* 2008;7:1602–6.
198. De Paoli P. Novel virally targeted therapies of EBV-associated tumors. *Curr Cancer Drug Targets.* 2008;8:591–6.
199. Okugawa K, Itoh T, Kawashima I, et al. Recognition of Epstein-Barr virus-associated gastric carcinoma cells by cytotoxic T lymphocytes induced in vitro with autologous lymphoblastoid cell line and LMP2-derived, HLA-A24-restricted 9-mer peptide. *Oncol Rep.* 2004;12:725–31.

Hereditary Diffuse Gastric Cancer and Other Gastric Cancers Associated with Hereditary Predisposition Syndromes

6

Fátima Carneiro, Carla Oliveira, and Raquel Seruca

Introduction

Gastric cancer is a heterogeneous and highly prevalent disease, being the fourth most common cancer and the second leading cause of cancer-associated death worldwide.[1] There are two main types of gastric carcinoma—diffuse and intestinal—which display different clinicopathologic profiles and often occur in distinct epidemiologic settings.[2] The new WHO Classification of Tumors of the Digestive System highlights the heterogeneity of gastric carcinoma, individualizing poorly cohesive carcinomas (including signet ring cell carcinoma and other variants) and tubular and papillary carcinomas (roughly corresponding to diffuse and intestinal carcinomas, respectively) as well as mixed and mucinous carcinomas.[3]

Intestinal carcinoma is more prevalent in elderly persons, of the masculine gender, whereas diffuse carcinoma tends to occur in younger individuals, mainly females, and frequently depicts hereditary conditioning. The incidence of intestinal carcinomas is steadily decreasing in most countries, in contrast to diffuse carcinomas whose incidence is quite stable or even increasing.[4,5]

Most cases of gastric cancer are sporadic, although descriptions of clustering of multiple gastric cancer cases in the same family are also present in the literature.[6,7]

F. Carneiro, M.D., Ph.D. (✉)
Department of Pathology and Cancer Genetics Group, Institute of Molecular Pathology and Immunology of the University of Porto and Centro Hospitalar São João/Medical Faculty of the University of Porto, Porto, Portugal
e-mail: fcarneiro@ipatimup.pt

C. Oliveira, Ph.D. • R. Seruca, M.D., Ph.D.
Cancer Genetics Group, Institute of Molecular Pathology and Immunology of the University of Porto and Medical Faculty of the University of Porto, Porto, Portugal

In 1998, Guilford et al[8] identified an inherited cancer syndrome designated as Hereditary Diffuse Gastric Cancer (HDGC), described below.

Hereditary Diffuse Gastric Cancer and E-cadherin gene

Definition

It is now established that 1–3% of gastric cancers arise as a result of inherited gastric cancer predisposition syndromes.[9-11]

In 1998, Guilford et al reported three Maori kindred with early-onset, multigenerational, diffuse gastric cancer, in which germline mutations of the E-cadherin (*CDH1*) gene were identified by genetic linkage analysis and mutation screening.[8] These findings led to the identification of a new inherited cancer syndrome designated as Hereditary Diffuse Gastric Cancer (HDGC) [MIM #137215].[8] Shortly afterwards, families from other ethnicities were identified sharing similar features.[12-14]

The *CDH1* gene [MIM +192090] localizes in the long arm of chromosome 16, comprises 16 exons transcribed into a 4.5 kb mRNA, and encodes for E-cadherin[15] (Fig. 6.1). The 135 kDa precursor polypeptide, which also encloses a short signal peptide, undergoes cleavage resulting in a 120 kDa mature transmembrane glycoprotein[16] consisting of a large extracellular domain, and smaller transmembrane and cytoplasmic domains.[17] The extracellular domain of E-cadherin plays a key role in the correct folding and homo- and hetero-dimerization of the proteins, as well as in the adhesion mechanism itself. The cytoplasmic domain of the protein interacts with the catenins [α (alpha), β (beta), γ (gamma), p120ctn] indirectly influencing the actin cytoskeleton organization.[18,19] E-cadherin is a transmembrane calcium dependent protein that is predominantly expressed at the basolateral membrane of epithelial cells, where it exerts primarily cell–cell adhesion and invasion suppression functions.[20]

A.R. Sepulveda and J.P. Lynch (eds.), *Molecular Pathology of Neoplastic Gastrointestinal Diseases*, Molecular Pathology Library 7, DOI 10.1007/978-1-4614-6015-2_6, © Springer Science+Business Media New York 2013

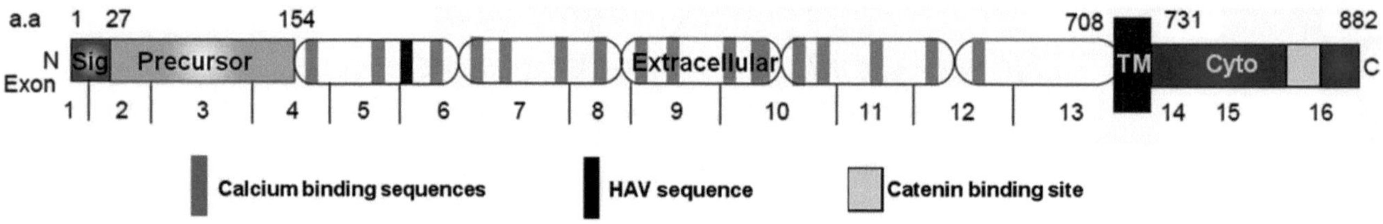

Fig. 6.1 Schematic structure of the *CDH1* gene and protein. The immature form of E-cadherin is 882 amino acids long encoded by 16 exons. After cleavage of the signal (Sig) and precursor peptides, the 728 amino acids mature form of the protein is generated and comprises a long extracellular domain with five E-cadherin repeats (EC-repeats), a small transmembrane (TM), and a cytoplasmic (Cyto) domain. The amino acid numbering (a.a) is marked on top of the image and the exon numbering (Exon) is marked underneath

Table 6.1 Criteria for testing for *CDH1* mutation: updated recommendations from the International Gastric Cancer Linkage Consortium (IGCLC)[a]

1. Two or more documented cases of gastric cancer in first-degree relatives, with at least one documented case of diffuse gastric cancer diagnosed before the age of 50 years
2. Three or more cases of documented diffuse gastric cancer in first- or second-degree relatives, independent of age of onset
3. Diffuse gastric cancer before the age of 40 years without a family history
4. Families with diagnoses of both diffuse gastric cancer and lobular breast cancer, with one case before the age of 50 years

[a]In addition, in cases where expert pathologists detect carcinoma in situ carcinoma adjacent to diffuse-type gastric cancer, genetic testing should be considered since this is rarely, if ever, seen in sporadic cases

Clinical Criteria

On the basis of clinical criteria, the International Gastric Cancer Linkage Consortium (IGCLC) defined in 1999 families with the HDGC syndrome as those fulfilling one of the following features[21]:

1. Two or more documented cases of diffuse gastric cancer in first- or second-degree relatives, with at least one diagnosed before the age of 50
2. Three or more cases of documented diffuse gastric cancer in 1st/2nd-degree relatives, independent of age of onset

According to the criteria of the IGCLC, families with aggregation of gastric cancer and an index case with diffuse gastric cancer, but not fulfilling the IGCLC criteria for HDGC, are coined as familial diffuse gastric cancer (FDGC).[21] The designation of familial gastric cancer (FGC) is used for cases with familial aggregation of gastric cancer in which the histopathology of the tumors is unknown. Additionally, families with aggregation of intestinal carcinomas are designated familial intestinal gastric cancer.[21,22]

Full screening of the *CDH1* gene (genetic testing) is recommended in an individual fulfilling the HDGC criteria as defined above. The criteria for genetic testing were updated in 2010[23] and are shown in Table 6.1. The updated recommendations include broadening of *CDH1* testing criteria such that histological confirmation of diffuse gastric criteria is only required for one family member, inclusion of individuals with diffuse gastric cancer before the age of 40 years without a family history, and inclusion of individuals and families with diagnoses of both diffuse gastric cancer and lobular breast cancer, with one case before the age of 50 years.[23]

From the above descriptions it is clear that the definition of HDCG is based mainly on clinical features (according to the IGCLC) while, according to the criteria adopted by the New Zealand group, the designation of HDGC should be restricted to cases in which *CDH1* gene germline mutations have been identified.[8,14] The IGCLC definition for HDGC will be used in this chapter.[21,23]

Genetic Counseling and Screening

Genetic counseling is the first and a key step in the management of HDGC. This counseling should be made by experts in clinical genetics with a solid training in oncology. This combination of expertise allows the best evaluation of the clinical situation to the proband and guarantees to design the most adequate surveillance program to the patient and offspring. The genetic counseling process should be complemented by interviews with a group of experts in distinct clinical areas, namely gastroenterology, gastric surgery, and nutrition and with a solid support of molecular pathology and advanced imaging.[23]

The genetic evaluation should include a careful (3-generation) family pedigree and the histopathological confirmation of diffuse gastric cancer diagnoses or precursor lesions in the proband. During genetic counseling session it is mandatory that the genetic counselor has an open discussion of lifetime risks of diffuse gastric (updated to >80% in both men and women by age 80)[23] and other associated cancers, namely lobular breast cancer in women (updated to 60% in women by age 80).[23] An informed discussion should be carried about the limitations of the genetic testing, and the clear restrictions of the screening methods for early detection of cancer in positive mutation carriers, due to the pathophysiology of this type of cancer (see next section). Whenever genetic testing is recommended (after genetic counseling), informed consent is mandatory and all laboratory tests should be initiated in the affected proband. The criteria for *CDH1* genetic testing were discussed in the previous section.

The recommended youngest age to offer testing to relatives at risk is not well established. Rare cases of clinically significant diffuse gastric cancer have been reported before the age of 18, but the overall risk of diffuse gastric cancer before the age of 20 is very low.[24,25] The IGCLC agreed that consideration of genetic testing can begin at the age of consent (16/18 years), but that the testing of family members less than 18 years should consider the earliest age of cancer onset in HDGC families from the local population and the psychological, emotional, and physical health of the individual and their family.[23]

In order to offer the most advanced genetic test as possible, clinical geneticist should refer patient samples to reference centers able to conduct the most recent methodologies for the screening of genetic alterations associated with HDGC families. (See next sections for details in *CDH1* alterations associated with HDGC.) To begin with, DNA and RNA should be extracted from a blood sample of the referred proband. In case there are clear limitations of access, this type of biological material, RNA and DNA from paraffin-embedded tissue, can be considered as an alternative (despite obvious technical restrictions) to assure a comprehensive laboratory analysis and a complete detection of all types of alterations described so far in HDGC families.

Direct sequencing of all intron and exon boundaries of *CDH1* gene should be performed as the first step. In case a germline missense mutation is found, other complementary studies should be offered. This is the case of *CDH1* missense mutations' functional assessment, which should be performed in international reference centers recognized for this type of work. IPATIMUP (Institute of molecular Pathology and Immunology of the University of Porto) is such a center and is available for this type of analysis. (See details in next section.) Another important issue related with assessment of mutation functional relevance is to determine whether an apparently common missense mutation or an intronic variant in the vicinity of the splice site (five nucleotides or more up- or downstream) is an uncovered splice-site mutation. In this case, several bioinformatic tools may be used to predict the impact of such mutations in inducing cryptic splicing, but proof can only be made if RNA from the mutation carrier is available to be analyzed. Kaurah et al[26] have used a minigene approach that also proved to be very useful in predicting the impact in splicing, whenever patients' RNA is not available.

In 2009, Oliveira et al described for the first time large genomic deletions of *CDH1* in apparently mutation-negative HDGC families.[27] Since then, it was recommended that in HDGC families with undetectable *CDH1* germline mutations by conventional direct sequencing methods, the screening of large *CDH1* deletions should be performed with multiplex ligation dependent probe amplification (MLPA) or alternative methods (array comparative genomic hybridization (CGH), using high-quality DNA extracted from a blood sample of the proband.[27]

Very recently, using a single-nucleotide primer extension-based procedure, the same group of researchers described *CDH1* downregulation by *CDH1* allele-specific expression (ASE) imbalance in HDGC families.[28] Monoallelic *CDH1* expression or high allelic expression imbalance (AI) was present in about 70% of apparently *CDH1*-negative HDGC probands, implicating the *CDH1 locus* in the majority of apparently mutation-negative HDGC families. Germline mutations, deletions, and promoter hypermethylation were found in probands displaying high *CDH1* AI, validating this methodology as a valuable screening approach recommended in all families that fulfill the criteria for *CDH1* testing in the frame of HDGC.[28]

This type of analysis requires good quality RNA; thus a blood sample as starting material for this test should be recommended.

Pathology

Macroscopy

Macroscopic features differ in stomachs from asymptomatic *CDH1* mutation carriers submitted to prophylactic gastrectomy and index cases with HDGC. In the former, stomachs nearly always appear normal to the naked eye, there is no mass lesion, and slicing shows normal mucosal thickness.[29-31] In some apparently normal stomachs, subtle pale areas are visible on standard white-light endoscopy,[32] and close inspection may show white patches that after formalin fixation correspond to intramucosal signet ring cell (diffuse) carcinoma.

Most index cases with HDGC present with cancers that are indistinguishable from sporadic diffuse gastric cancer, often with linitis plastica, which can involve all topographic regions within the stomach.

Microscopy (Precursor Lesions)

Systematic complete mapping of total gastrectomies from asymptomatic carriers of *CDH1* mutations show microscopic, usually multiple, *foci* of intramucosal (T1a) signet ring cell (diffuse) carcinoma in almost all cases.[25,29-31,33-36] Individual *foci* of intramucosal (T1a) signet ring cell (diffuse) carcinoma are small, ranging from 0.1 mm to 10 mm (Fig. 6.2). In North American and European families, microscopic *foci* of intramucosal carcinoma were not restricted to any topographic region in the stomach: *foci* were identified from cardia to pre-pyloric region, without evidence of antral

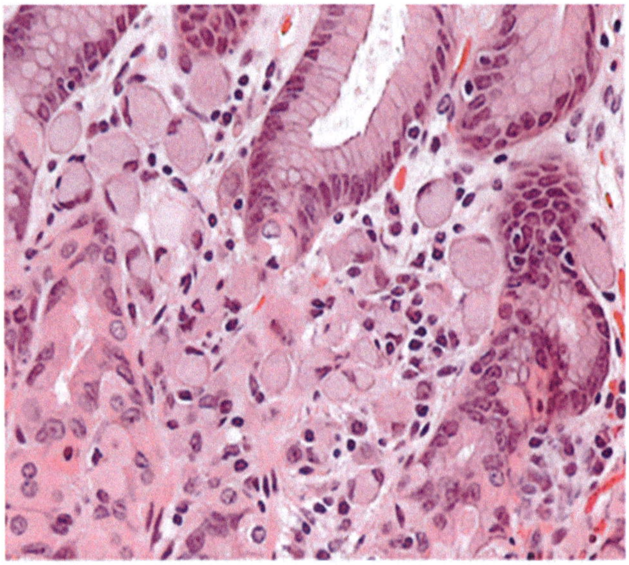

Fig. 6.2 Invasive *focus* of T1a intramucosal signet ring cell (diffuse) carcinoma

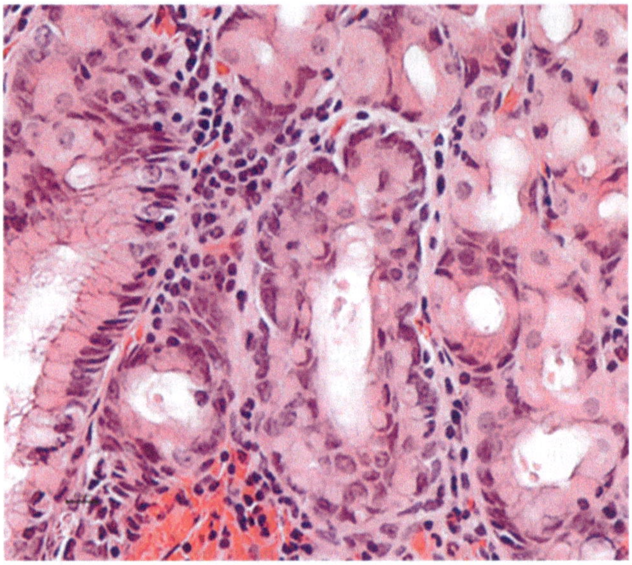

Fig. 6.3 Signet ring cell carcinoma in situ

clustering.[29,33,35,37] In a series of eight cases reported by Rogers et al,[31] 70% of the total *foci* were localized in the proximal 1/3 of the stomach. In another series from United Kingdom[35] the highest number of *foci* was observed in the fundus (44.7%) followed by the body (40.2%). In New Zealand Maori families, a predilection was observed for the occurrence of early invasive carcinomas for the distal stomach and the body-antral transitional zone.[25,30] Reasons for the different anatomical localization of the cancer *foci* in the aforementioned studies remain to be clarified, although both background genetics and environmental factors are probable contributing factors.

As all regions of the gastric mucosa can be affected, pathological examination of the resected specimen should include confirmation of the presence of a complete cuff of proximal squamous esophageal mucosa and distal duodenal mucosa.

As precursors of the invasive cancers, two distinct types of lesions were identified in prophylactic gastrectomies: (1) in situ signet ring cell carcinoma, corresponding to the presence of signet ring cells within basal membrane, generally with hyperchromatic and depolarized nuclei (Fig. 6.3), and (2) pagetoid spread of signet ring cells below the preserved epithelium of glands/foveolae (Fig. 6.4).[29]

Strictly following criteria for the identification of these precursors will diminish the risk of over-diagnosing nonspecific changes and distinguish precursors from mimics of signet ring cells in situ, including telescoped normal glands. Confirmation of carcinoma in situ (Tis) by an independent histopathologist with experience in this area is strongly recommended.

On the basis of the findings in prophylactic gastrectomies, a model for the development of diffuse gastric cancer in ger-

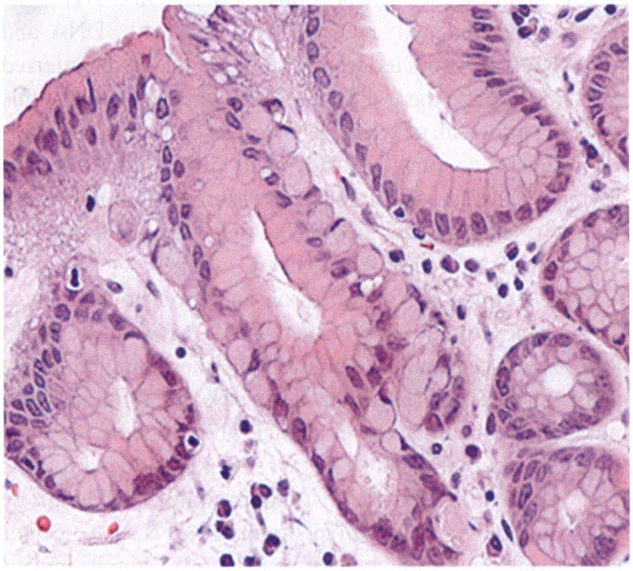

Fig. 6.4 Pagetoid spread of signet ring cells

mline *CDH1* deleterious mutation carriers was proposed[22,29], encompassing the following lesions: mild non-atrophic gastritis, in situ signet ring cell carcinoma, pagetoid spread of signet ring cells, and invasive carcinoma. E-cadherin immunoexpression was shown to be reduced or absent in early invasive gastric carcinomas (T1a), contrasting with the normal membranous E-cadherin expression in adjacent non-neoplastic mucosa, in keeping with a clonal origin of the cancer *foci*. However, one should be aware that E-cadherin may be expressed at the cell membrane of neoplastic cells (reduced intensity and/or dotted pattern) as well as in the cytoplasm.[38] In in situ carcinomas and pagetoid spread

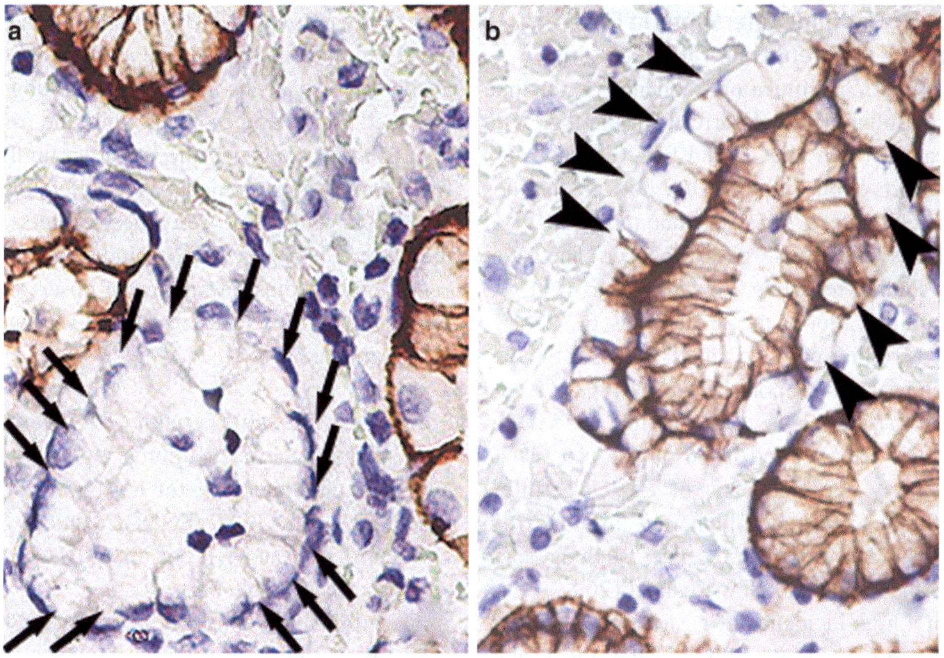

Fig. 6.5 Absence of E-cadherin expression as shown by immunohistochemistry. (**a**) Signet ring cell carcinoma in situ (delimited by *arrows*). (**b**) Pagetoid spread of signet ring cells (*arrow heads*)

lesions, E-cadherin immunoexpression was also shown to be reduced or absent (Fig. 6.5).[29]

Background changes in the gastric mucosa of prophylactic gastrectomy specimen encompass mild chronic gastritis, foveolar hyperplasia, and tufting of surface epithelium (Oliveira et al[39]). Occasionally, an inflammatory granulomatous reaction is observed. In almost all prophylactic gastrectomies studied so far, intestinal metaplasia and *Helicobacter pylori* infection are absent, namely in families from North America and Europe.

Genetic Susceptibility

CDH1 Germline Alterations

Heterozygous germline alterations in *CDH1* are the only germline genetic defect associated with HDGC.[8,12,39] This germline defect has also been reported in a few early-onset gastric cancer (EOGC) patients who developed tumors with partial or complete diffuse histology (EODGC),[40] as well as in two families with hereditary Lobular Breast Cancer (LBC) without gastric cancer involvement (see sections below).[41,42]

Overall, around 40% of HDGC families selected on the basis of established clinical criteria harbor *CDH1* germline alterations. So far, 120 families/probands (111 HDGC, 7 EODGC, 2 LBC) have been described to harbor *CDH1* germline alterations.[27,28,43] The most frequently found *CDH1* germline alterations are point and small frameshift mutations, which occur in approximately 93% of positive families, but other alterations have also been described such as large deletions in approximately 5% of the cases, germline promoter methylation in ~1% and in-frame deletion also in ~1% of the cases.[27,28,43]

In total, 99 different germline *CDH1* alterations have been described in the 120 probands. Fifteen of the 99 (15.2%) alterations have recurrently appeared in several families, suggesting that *CDH1*-associated HDGC can either arise from a common ancestor[26,27] or be the result of a mutation hotspot. More specifically, a third of all HDGC families (36/120 = 30%), described so far in the literature, either display a shared ancestor as proved at least for 12 of them (carrying four mutations and a large deletion)[26,27] or carry a hotspot mutation.

The frequency of *CDH1* germline alterations is highly variable between countries with different incidences of gastric cancer.[26,27,39,44-47] These data raise the (still) unanswered question on the criteria to be applied for regions with low incidence (North America or North Europe) and high incidence of gastric cancer (Japan, Korea, Portugal, etc.). In the latter, familial clustering of gastric cancer may reflect the cumulative effect of environmental risk factors (virulent *Helicobacter pylori* strains) and genetic susceptibility of the individuals associated with low-penetrance genes.[48,49] These two risk factors are thought to be responsible for a high prevalence of gastric cancer and clustering in families in the absence of germline mutations of high-penetrance genes such as *CDH1*.

Frequency of *CDH1* Germline Alterations in Different Clinical Settings and Different Geographic Origins

A study assessing the *CDH1* mutation frequency (at the time the only *CDH1* germline defect described) in families with diffuse gastric cancer (both HDGC and FDGC)[22] analyzed separately case reports of one or two *CDH1* positive families and studies on screening of *CDH1* germline mutations in at least three families with diffuse gastric cancer. The latter encompassed 23 studies, reporting 267 families: 151 HDGC and 116 FDGC families. Among the 267 families, 62 (23.2%) harbored *CDH1* germline point or small frameshift mutations, the frequency varying upon the family type (HDGC versus FDGC): *CDH1* mutations were identified in 46 out of 151 HDGC families (30.5%) and in 16 out of 116 FDGC (13.8%). Interestingly, the frequency of *CDH1* germline mutations was found to be much higher in families from regions with low incidence of gastric cancer, such as North America and North Europe and New Zealand (26.8%) than in countries with a high incidence of gastric cancer (Japan, Korea, and South Europe) (13.0%). In the latter, most families may well represent the aggregation of gastric cancer cases associated with environmental factors, rather than with a *CDH1* germline defect.

A more recent study[27] analyzed probands either fulfilling clinical criteria for HDGC ($n = 160$) or probands from families that did not meet the above testing criteria (FDGC families, $n = 123$) that were referred to five different centers (University of British Columbia, Vancouver, Canada; Institute of Molecular Pathology and Immunology, University of Porto, Porto, Portugal; Department of Human Pathology and Oncology, Section of Surgical Oncology, Translational Research Laboratory, University of Siena, Italy; Institute of Pathology, Technische Universität München, Munich, Germany; Department of Oncology, University of Cambridge, Cambridge, UK). This study analyzed not only *CDH1* point or small frameshift mutations but also large rearrangements of the *CDH1 locus*. Among HDGC probands, 45.6% (73/160) displayed *CDH1* germline alterations (41.8% point or small frameshift mutations and 3.8% large deletions) while, among FDGC probands, 5.7% (7/123) carried *CDH1* mutations but not large deletions. Similarly to the above-mentioned report, it was verified that in low incidence countries, namely in the North America, Canada, UK, and Holland, the frequency of germline *CDH1* alterations described was 51.6%, whilst in moderate (Germany) and high (Portugal and Italy) incidence countries, the frequency of alterations was 25% and 22.2%, respectively. In the latter, no large deletions of the *CDH1* were described.[27]

The differences between these two studies are related with the type of data available as well as with the type of alterations analyzed. In the first,[22] a literature search was done which was limited by the information made available in each paper and only point and small frameshift mutations were known to cause HDGC, while in the second one,[27] all the family information as well as all mutation data was made available for analysis and *CDH1* rearrangements were also analyzed. On the other hand, while the first report encloses data from all studies in the literature until 2007, and therefore from all geographic areas reported, the second encloses data from only five reference centers until 2008 and, therefore, a less wide dataset. Independently of these differences, both studies reveal similar observations for mutation frequency both in different clinical settings and in different geographic areas.

Frequency, Site, and Type of *CDH1* Germline Alterations

This section encloses a summary of all the currently available data in the literature for 120 families/probands, encompassing 111 HDGC, 7 EODGC, and 2 LBC in terms of frequency, site, and type of all *CDH1* germline alterations ever described (Table 6.2).

Germline alterations are not restricted to specific *CDH1* gene or E-cadherin protein domains, being distributed throughout the coding, splice-site sequences, and UTRs (5′- and 3′-untranslated regions) of the gene as well as throughout all protein functional domains [Fig. 6.6, panel A (gene) and B (protein)].

Small frameshift insertions and deletions, which occur in one-third of all families described so far, are the most frequent mutation type found in *CDH1*-associated families, followed by splice-site mutations that occur in one-fourth and nonsense and missense mutations both occurring in 19.2% of the families. Large deletions account for 5% of all families, while in-frame deletions and germline promoter methylation are very rare events, accounting for less than 2% of *CDH1*-associated families (Fig. 6.7).

In terms of the predicted impact of all these alterations in the protein structure and function, 80% of the families encompass alterations that potentially result in protein truncation or even complete lack of expression due to hypermethylation and complete or partial deletion of the promoter region of the gene. The remaining 20% of the alterations are not expected to lead to protein loss of expression as their impact is expected to change or remove a single amino acid, in the case of missense mutations or in-frame deletion, respectively (Fig. 6.7).

CDH1 Germline Allelic Imbalance

Most diffuse gastric cancers, occurring in *CDH1* germline mutation carriers, display abnormal or absent E-cadherin protein expression.[69] Interestingly, independently of harboring a germline *CDH1* alteration, tumors from HDGC families display similar abnormal E-cadherin expression patterns. Therefore, it is plausible to hypothesize that other *CDH1* germline genetic and epigenetic defects could be the cause of diffuse gastric cancer clustering in families that remain

Table 6.2 *CDH1* germline mutations described to date

Reference	Mutations in families ($N=120$)	Independent mutation ($N=99$)	Gene domain	Protein domain	Mutation type	Mutation effect	Clinical criteria	Recurrent mutation ($n=15$)	Families with recurrent mutations ($n=36$)
Pinheiro et al[28]	Promoter methylation	Promoter methylation	Promoter	Na	Methylation	Non-expressing	HDGC		
Oliveira et al[27]	Del ex1-2_ 193 593 bp	Del ex1-2_193 593 bp	chr16:67193822-67387415	Signal	Large deletion	Non-expressing	HDGC	Yes	Yes
Oliveira et al[27]	Del ex1-2_ 193 593 bp		chr16:67193822-67387415	Signal	Large deletion	Non-expressing	HDGC		Yes
Oliveira et al[27]	Del 5′-UTR-ex1_150bp	Del 5′-UTR-ex1_150bp	chr16:67328695-67328844	Signal	Large deletion	Non-expressing	HDGC		
Oliveira et al[27]	Del 5′-UTR-ex1_5671bp	Del 5′-UTR-ex1_5671bp	chr16:67324886-67330557	Signal	Large deletion	Non-expressing	HDGC		
Guilford et al[43]	2T>C	2T>C	EXON 1	Signal	Nonsense	Truncating	HDGC		
Suriano et al[45]	3G>C	3G>C	EXON 1	Signal	Nonsense	Truncating	HDGC		
Bacani et al[50]	*41delT*	*41delT*	*EXON 1*	*Signal*	*Frameshift_del*	*Truncating*	*EODGC*		
Oliveira et al[51]	45insT	45insT	EXON 1	Signal	Frameshift_ins	Truncating	HDGC		
Guilford et al[43]	46insTGC	46insTGC	EXON 1	Signal	In-frame insertion	In-frame insertion	HDGC		
More et al[52]	49-2A>C	49-2A>C	INTRON 1	Signal	Splice-site	Truncating	HDGC		
Richards et al[13]	49-2A>G	49-2A>G	INTRON 1	Signal	Splice-site	Truncating	HDGC	Yes	Yes
Moran et al[53]	49-2A>G		INTRON 1	Signal	Splice-site	Truncating	HDGC		Yes
Humar et al[54]	53delC	53delC	EXON 2	Signal	Frameshift_del	Truncating	HDGC		
Richards et al[13]	59G>A	59G>A	EXON 2	Signal	Nonsense	Truncating	HDGC		
Guilford et al[14]	70G>T	70G>T	EXON 2	Signal	Nonsense	Truncating	HDGC		
Shinmura et al[55]	185G>T	185G>T	EXON 3	Signal	Missense	Missense	HDGC		
Suriano et al[45]	187C>T	187C>T	EXON 3	Precursor	Nonsense	Truncating	HDGC	Yes	Yes
Gayther et al[12]	187C>T		EXON 3	Precursor	Nonsense	Truncating	HDGC		Yes
Guilford et al[14]	190C>T	190C>T	EXON 3	Precursor	Nonsense	Truncating	HDGC		
Dussaulx-Garin et al[56]	283C>T	283C>T	EXON 3	Precursor	Nonsense	Truncating	HDGC	Yes	Yes
Kaurah et al[26]	283C>T		EXON 3	Precursor	Nonsense	Truncating	HDGC		Yes
More et al[52]	353C>G	353C>G	EXON 3	Precursor	Missense	Missense	HDGC		
Keller et al[57]	372-377delC	372-377delC	EXON 3	Precursor	Frameshift_del	Truncating	HDGC		
Brooks-Wilson et al[58]	382delC	382delC	EXON 3	Precursor	Frameshift_del	Truncating	HDGC		
Masciari et al[41]	517insA	517insA	EXON 4	Precursor	Frameshift_ins	Truncating	LBC		
Frebourg et al[59]	531+2T>A	531+2T>A	INTRON 4	Precursor	Splice-site	Truncating	HDGC		
Brooks-Wilson et al[58]	531+1G>A	531+1G>A	INTRON 4	Precursor	Splice-site	Truncating	HDGC		
Guilford et al[14]	586G>T	586G>T	EXON 5	Extracell	Nonsense	Truncating	HDGC		
Mateus et al[60]	*641T>C*	*641T>C*	*EXON 5*	*Extracell*	*Missense*	*Missense*	*EODGC*		
Brooks-Wilson et al[58]	687+1G>A	687+1G>A	INTRON 5	Extracell	Splice-site	Truncating	HDGC		
More et al[52]	715G>A	715G>A	EXON 6	Extracell	Splice-site	Truncating	HDGC	Yes	Yes
Kaurah et al[26]	715G>A		EXON 6	Extracell	Splice-site	Truncating	HDGC		Yes

(continued)

Table 6.2 (continued)

Reference	Mutations in families ($N=120$)	Independent mutation ($N=99$)	Gene domain	Protein domain	Mutation type	Mutation effect	Clinical criteria	Recurrent mutation ($n=15$)	Families with recurrent mutations ($n=36$)
Yoon et al[61]	731A>G	731A>G	EXON 6	Extracell	Missense	Missense	HDGC		
Guilford et al[43]	753insG	753insG	EXON 6	Extracell	Frameshift_ins	Truncating	HDGC		
Kaurah et al[26]	808T>G	808T>G	EXON 6	Extracell	Missense	Missense	HDGC		
Oliveira et al[51]	832G>A	832G>A	EXON 6	Extracell	Splice-site	Truncating	HDGC		
Rogers et al[31]	833-2A>G	833-2A>G	INTRON 6	Extracell	Splice-site	Truncating	HDGC		
Brooks-Wilson et al[58]	892G>A	892G>A	EXON 7	Extracell	Missense	Missense	HDGC		
Jonsson et al[62]	1003C>T	1003C>T	EXON 7	Extracell	Nonsense	Truncating	HDGC	Yes	Yes
Suriano et al[45]	1003C>T		EXON 7	Extracell	Nonsense	Truncating	HDGC		Yes
Huntsman, unpublished	1003C>T		EXON 7	Extracell	Nonsense	Truncating	HDGC		Yes
Guilford et al[8]	1008G>T	1008G>T	EXON 7	Extracell	Splice-site	Truncating	HDGC		
Oliveira et al[51]	1018A>G	1018A>G	EXON 8	Extracell	Missense	Missense	HDGC	Yes	Yes
Kaurah et al[26]	1018A>G		EXON 8	Extracell	Missense	Missense	HDGC		Yes
Guilford et al[43]	1023T>G	1023T>G	EXON 8	Extracell	Nonsense	Truncating	HDGC		
Suriano et al[45]	*1063del*	*1063del*	*EXON 8*	*Extracell*	*Frameshift_del*	*Truncating*	*EODGC*		
Brooks-Wilson et al[58]	1064insT	1064insT	EXON 8	Extracell	Frameshift_ins	Truncating	HDGC		
More et al[52]	1107delC	1107delC	EXON 8	Extracell	Frameshift_del	Truncating	HDGC		
Roviello et al[63]	1118C>T	1118C>T	EXON 8	Extracell	Missense	Missense	HDGC		
Oliveira et al[38]	1135del8ins5	1135del8ins5	EXON 8	Extracell	Splice-site	Truncating	HDGC		
Frebourg et al[59]	1137G>A	1137G>A	EXON 8	Extracell	Splice-site	Truncating	HDGC	Yes	Yes
Kaurah et al[26]	1137G>A		EXON 8	Extracell	Splice-site	Truncating	HDGC		Yes
More et al[52]	1137G>A		EXON 8	Extracell	Splice-site	Truncating	HDGC		Yes
Guilford et al[14]	1137+1G>A	1137+1G>A	INTRON 8	Extracell	Splice-site	Truncating	HDGC		
Brooks-Wilson et al[58]	1212delC	1212delC	EXON 9	Extracell	Frameshift_del	Truncating	HDGC		
Brooks-Wilson et al[58]	*1225T>C*[a]	*1225T>C*	*EXON 9*	*Extracell*	*Missense*	*Missense*	*EODGC*		
Wang et al[47]	1243A>C	1243A>C	EXON 9	Extracell	Missense	Missense	HDGC	Yes	Yes
Wang et al[47]	1243A>C		EXON 9	Extracell	Missense	Missense	HDGC		Yes
Suriano et al[45]	*1285C>T*	*1285C>T*	*EXON 9*	*Extracell*	*Missense*	*Missense*	*EODGC*		
Mayrbaeurl et al[64]	1302_1303insA, 1306_1307delTT	1302_1303insA, 1306_1307delTT	EXON 9	Extracell	Frameshift ins_del	Truncating	HDGC		
More et al[52]	1391delTC	1391delTC	EXON 10	Extracell	Frameshift_del	Truncating	HDGC		
More et al[52]	1397delTC	1397delTC	EXON 10	Extracell	Frameshift_del	Truncating	HDGC	Yes	Yes
Kaurah et al[26]	1397delTC		EXON 10	Extracell	Frameshift_del	Truncating	HDGC		Yes
Yoon et al[61]	1460T>C	1460T>C	EXON 10	Extracell	Missense	Missense	HDGC		
Barber et al[65]	1466insC	1466insC	EXON 10	Extracell	Frameshift_ins	Truncating	HDGC		
Oliveira et al[51]	1472insA	1472insA	EXON 10	Extracell	Frameshift_ins	Truncating	HDGC		
Brooks-Wilson et al[58]	1476delAG	1476delAG	EXON 10	Extracell	Frameshift_del	Truncating	HDGC		
Guilford et al[14]	*1487del7*	*1487del7*	*EXON 10*	*Extracell*	*Frameshift_del*	*Truncating*	*EODGC*		

Kaurah et al[26]	1507C>T	1507C>T	EXON 10	Extracell	Nonsense	Truncating	HDGC		
Humar et al[54]	1565+1G>T	1565+1G>T	INTRON 10	Extracell	Splice-site	Truncating	HDGC		
Schrader et al[42]	1565+1G>A	1565+1G>A	INTRON 10	Extracell	Splice-site	Truncating	LBC		
Rogers et al[31]	1565+2insT	1565+2insT	INTRON 10	Extracell	Splice-site	Truncating	HDGC		
Keller, unpublished	1587insT	1587insT	EXON 11	Extracell	Frameshift_ins	Truncating	HDGC		
Guilford et al[14]	1588insC	1588insC	EXON 11	Extracell	Frameshift_ins	Truncating	HDGC		
Rodriguez-Sanjuan et al[66]	1610delC	1610delC	EXON 11	Extracell	Frameshift_del	Truncating	HDGC		
Keller et al[67]	*1619insG*	*1619insG*	*EXON 11*	*Extracell*	*Frameshift_ins*	*Truncating*	*EODGC*		
Kaurah et al[26]	1682insA	1682insA	EXON 11	Extracell	Frameshift_ins	Truncating	HDGC		
Humar et al[54]	1710delT	1710delT	EXON 11	Extracell	Frameshift_del	Truncating	HDGC		
Brooks-Wilson et al[58]	1711insG	1711insG	EXON 11	Extracell	Frameshift_ins	Truncating	HDGC		
Brooks-Wilson et al[58]	1711+5G>A	1711+5G>A	INTRON 11	Extracell	Splice-site	Truncating	HDGC		
Brooks-Wilson et al[58]	1779insC	1779insC	EXON 12	Extracell	Frameshift_ins	Truncating	HDGC		
Gayther et al[12]	1792C>T	1792C>T	EXON 12	Extracell	Nonsense	Truncating	HDGC	Yes	Yes
Humar et al[54]	1792C>T		EXON 12	Extracell	Nonsense	Truncating	HDGC		Yes
Suriano et al[45]	1792C>T		EXON 12	Extracell	Nonsense	Truncating	HDGC		Yes
Keller unpublished	1792C>T		EXON 12	Extracell	Nonsense	Truncating	HDGC		Yes
Kaurah et al[26]	1795A>T	1795A>T	EXON 12	Extracell	Missense	Missense	HDGC		
Kaurah et al[26]	1876T>A	1876T>A	EXON 12	Extracell	Missense	Missense	HDGC		
Suriano et al[68]	1901C>T[b]	1901C>T	EXON 12	Extracell	Splice-site	Truncating	HDGC	Yes	Yes
More et al[52]	1901C>T		EXON 12	Extracell	Splice-site	Truncating	HDGC		Yes
Oliveira et al[44]	1901C>T		EXON 12	Extracell	Splice-site	Truncating	HDGC		Yes
Kaurah et al[26]	1901C>T		EXON 12	Extracell	Splice-site	Truncating	HDGC		Yes
Kaurah et al[26]	1913G>A	1913G>A	EXON 12	Extracell	Nonsense	Truncating	HDGC		
Unpublished	2061insTG	2061insTG	EXON 13	Extracell	Frameshift_ins	Truncating	HDGC		
Brooks-Wilson et al[58]	2064delTG	2064delTG	EXON 13	Extracell	Frameshift_del	Truncating	HDGC	Yes	Yes
Kaurah et al[26]	2064delTG		EXON 13	Extracell	Frameshift_del	Truncating	HDGC		Yes
Guilford et al[8]	2095C>T	2095C>T	EXON 13	Extracell	Nonsense	Truncating	HDGC		
Suriano et al[45]	2161C>G	2161C>G	EXON 13	Transmemb	Missense	Missense	HDGC		
Kaurah et al[26]	2164+5G>A	2164+5G>A	INTRON 13	Transmemb	Splice-site	Truncating	HDGC		
Oliveira et al[27]	Del ex14-16	Del ex14-16	Exon 14-16_ chr16:67416845-67424923	Cytoplasm	Large deletion	Truncating	HDGC		
Brooks-Wilson et al[58]	2195G>A	2195G>A	EXON 14	Cytoplasm	Splice-site	Truncating	HDGC	Yes	Yes
Kaurah et al[26]	2195G>A		EXON 14	Cytoplasm	Splice-site	Truncating	HDGC		Yes
Oliveira et al[69]	2195G>A		EXON 14	Cytoplasm	Splice-site	Truncating	HDGC		Yes
Kaurah et al[26]	2245C>T	2245C>T	EXON 14	Cytoplasm	Missense	Missense	HDGC		
Simoes-Correia et al[70]	2269G>A	2269G>A	EXON 14	Cytoplasm	Missense	Missense	HDGC		
Ghaffari et al[71]	2275G>T	2275G>T	EXON 14	Cytoplasm	Nonsense	Truncating	HDGC		
Suriano et al[45]	2276delG	2276delG	EXON 14	Cytoplasm	Frameshift_del	Truncating	HDGC		

(continued)

Table 6.2 (continued)

Reference	Mutations in families ($N=120$)	Independent mutation ($N=99$)	Gene domain	Protein domain	Mutation type	Mutation effect	Clinical criteria	Recurrent mutation ($n=15$)	Families with recurrent mutations ($n=36$)
Guilford et al[43]	2287G>T	2287G>T	EXON 14	Cytoplasm	Nonsense	Truncating	HDGC		
Humar et al[54]	2295+5G>A	2295+5G>A	INTRON 14	Cytoplasm	Splice-site	Truncating	HDGC		
Brooks-Wilson et al[58]	2310delC	2310delC	EXON 15	Cytoplasm	Frameshift_del	Truncating	HDGC		
Kaurah et al[26]	2329G>A	2329G>A	EXON 15	Cytoplasm	Missense	Missense	HDGC		
Kaurah et al[26]	2343A>T	2343A>T	EXON 15	Cytoplasm	Missense	Missense	HDGC		
Guilford et al[8]	2382-2386insC	2382-2386insC	EXON 15	Cytoplasm	Frameshift_ins	Truncating	HDGC		
Rogers et al[31]	2395delC	2395delC	EXON 15	Cytoplasm	Frameshift_del	Truncating	HDGC		
Keller et al[67]	2396C>G	2396C>G	EXON 15	Cytoplasm	Missense	Missense	HDGC		
Kaurah et al[26]	2398delC[c]	2398delC	EXON 15	Cytoplasm	Frameshift_del	Truncating	HDGC	Yes	Yes
Caron et al[72]	2399delG	2399delG	EXON 15	Cytoplasm	Frameshift_del	Truncating	HDGC		
More et al[52]	2440-6C>G	2440-6C>G	INTRON 15	Cytoplasm	Splice-site	Truncating	HDGC		
Yabuta et al[46]	2494G>A	2494G>A	EXON 16	Cytoplasm	Missense	Missense	HDGC		
Oliveira et al[27]	Del ex16_828bp	Del ex16_828bp	EXON 16_3′-UTR_ chr16:67424298-67425126	Cytoplasm	Large deletion	Truncating	HDGC		

Note: EODGC, are depicted in italic; LBC, Lobular breast cancer underlined

[a]This proband was considered EOGC, but it developed diffuse gastric cancer at age 51

[b]Mutation 1901C>T was initially described in a proband apparently without family history, nevertheless it was demonstrated later by Kaurah et al[26] that this individual shared an haplotype with the family described by Oliveira et al,[44] therefore it was herein re-classified as HDGC

[c]This mutation was reported in the same paper regarding four families and considered as a founder mutation. For the sake of simplicity, all familial cases in which mutations were identified are referred in this table as HDGC

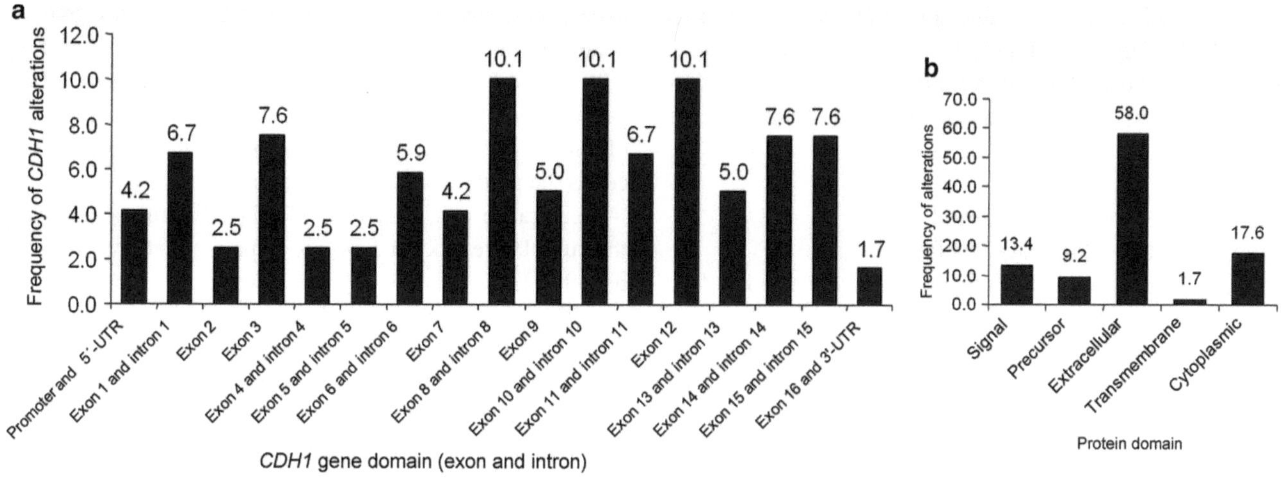

Fig. 6.6 Frequency of *CDH1* alterations in the gene domains (**a**) and in the protein domains (**b**). On top of each bar is represented the percentage of families carrying *CDH1* mutations in domain

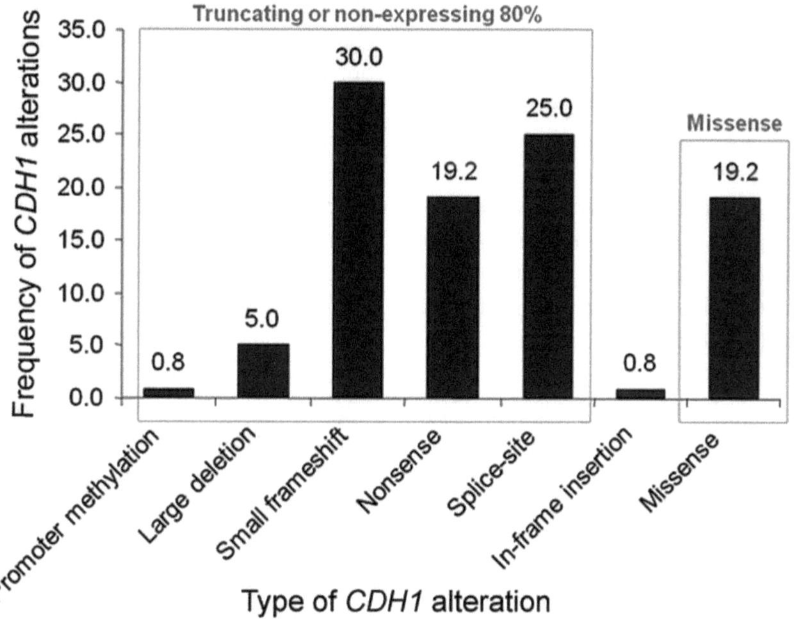

Fig. 6.7 Type of *CDH1* alterations in HDGC families. Each bar represents the percentage of families with a certain type of molecular alteration. Truncating or mutations leading to lack of E-cadherin protein expressing are surrounded by the *left square*. Missense mutations are surrounded by the *right square*

genetically unexplained. To address this issue, Pinheiro et al searched for germline *CDH1* allele-specific expression imbalance (AI) in HDGC patients who tested negative for *CDH1* germline alterations.[28]

The analysis of germline RNA extracted from the blood of 21 cancer-free individuals and 22 HDGC probands (5 *CDH1* mutation carriers and 17 *CDH1* negative) revealed that both *CDH1* alleles from cancer-free individuals displayed equivalent expression levels, whereas monoallelic *CDH1* expression or high allelic expression imbalance (AI) was present in 80% of *CDH1* mutant and 70.6% of *CDH1*-negative HDGC probands. Germline deletions and promoter hypermethylation were found in 25% of probands displaying high *CDH1* AI, proving that this feature was in fact pinpointing *CDH1* germline inactivating mechanisms. Given that germline *CDH1* AI is highly frequent among *CDH1* alteration-negative probands and not seen in cancer-free individuals, this phenomenon (AI) emerges as a powerful tool to prescreen HDGC patients. In fact, high *CDH1* AI determination provides a simple, cost-effective, and efficient tool to perceive indirectly changes of *CDH1* expression that escape detection in genomic DNA-based screenings. More importantly, these observations implicate the *CDH1* locus in the majority of mutation-negative HDGC families.

When considering the values of *CDH1* AI as part of the overall germline alterations affecting the *CDH1* gene in HDGC, the percentage of families caused by alterations related to *CDH1* is approximately 80% and not 40%, as previously mentioned (see previous sections).

CDH1-Associated Syndromes

Cleft Lip with or Without Cleft Palate

In 2006, two families (one from Brazil and another from France) were reported to encompass several patients affected with diffuse gastric cancer and, additionally, some family members were concomitantly affected with congenital midline malformations. In both families, there was an association of *CDH1* germline mutations with diffuse gastric cancers and cleft lip, with or without cleft palate (CLP).[59]

In the French family, six members were affected with diffuse gastric cancer and four patients had also a cleft lip with or without cleft palate. In the Brazilian family, the proband and her father had diffuse gastric cancer, one sister had cleft lip and one brother had congenital scalp aplasia cutis and partial acrania. In the Brazilian family, members affected with midline malformations were both carriers of germline *CDH1* mutation but had no clinical evidence of gastric cancer at the time of diagnosis.

In both families, RT-PCR analysis of *CDH1* and sequencing analysis was performed in all affect members with and without cancer. The amplified cDNA demonstrated that in both HDGC families the *CDH1* germline mutations induced complex aberrant splicing leading to various aberrant transcripts.

In the French family, two distinct aberrant transcripts were found: (1) a complete retention of intron 4 resulting in a premature stop codon within intron 4 and (2) an in-frame deletion of exon 4, resulting from the activation of an exonic cryptic donor splicing site in all cases affected.

In the Brazilian family, the screening of the *CDH1* gene revealed a germline mutation in exon 8 (1137G>A) in the four members affected either with cancer or with congenital malformations, also generating several aberrant transcripts, one of which was an in-frame deletion that removes extracellular cadherin repeat domains involved in cell–cell adhesion.

These two families draw the attention to the role of cell adhesion molecules, such as E-cadherin, for the craniofacial morphogenesis and to the alterations of the E-cadherin pathway in the genesis of midline congenital malformations such as lip and palate clefting.

Hereditary Lobular Breast Cancer

In HDGC families, LBC is the second most frequent type of neoplasia.[23,24] In 1999, it was reported the first case of histologically defined LBC in association with HDGC.[57] Since then, several other HDGC families with associated breast cancer were reported.[26,45,51] These observations led to efforts to determine whether *CDH1* was a breast cancer susceptibility gene. For that purpose, two series of LBC families lacking *BRCA1* and *BRCA 2* gene mutations were screened for *CDH1* germline mutations.[41,42] Two *CDH1* germline mutations (Table 6.2) were identified in two families having breast cancer as the predominant cancer diagnosis.

Penetrance data based on 11 HDGC families estimated the cumulative risk for LBC for female mutation carriers to be 39% (95% CI, 12–84%) by 80 years of age.[24] More recently, an estimated cumulative risk of breast cancer for females by the age of 75 years was reported as 52% (95% CI, 29–94%), on the basis of the analysis of four predominantly gastric cancer pedigrees from Newfoundland with the 2398delC *CDH1* founder mutation.[26]

At this time, it seems reasonable to conclude that not only *BRCA1* and *BRCA2* mutation carriers are at risk of developing LBC, but also two other groups of women are at increased risk for LBC: women carrying a known *CDH1* mutation and belonging to HDGC families, and women from families with clustering of diffuse gastric cancer in whom no *CDH1* mutation has been identified yet.

Other Candidate Genes

A percentage of HDGC families screened worldwide remain genetically unexplained and the concern related with the management of these *CDH1*-negative gastric cancer families persists. Since linkage mapping is only feasible in the few families of sufficient size, strategies to identify novel genes will rely on screening of candidate genes. Tumor suppressor genes commonly inactivated in sporadic gastric cancers or implicated in gastric cancer development in experimental models represent putative susceptibility genes for familial gastric cancer. Examples of such candidate genes are *RUNX3*, *HPP1*, *CASP10*, *SMAD4*, *MET*, and *DSG2*.

RUNX3 was found to be causally related to gastric cancer development in Runx3/Pebp2alphaC null mouse model.[73] *HPP1* encodes a cell surface receptor with multiple roles in cell growth, maturation, and adhesion, and was shown to be frequently inactivated by promoter hypermethylation in gastric cancer.[74] *CASP10* is mutated in a small proportion of sporadic gastric cancers and in vitro expression studies showed that cells carrying *CASP10* mutations have impairment of apoptosis.[75] *SMAD4,* a tumor suppressor gene, encodes a transcription factor that binds to specific DNA sequences. In *SMAD4* heterozygous mice, the presence of *foci* of signet ring cell (diffuse) carcinoma in the stomach was shown.[76]

Sixty-five Portuguese and German families (HDGC families negative for *CDH1* germline mutations and FDGC/FGC families) proved to be negative for mutations in all aforementioned genes.[44,67] Despite the small number of families analyzed, these studies discourage further mutation screening of these genes.

Taking into account the biology of E-cadherin, obvious candidate genes for mutations are those encoding E-cadherin binding partners within the adhesion complex, namely the catenins [α (alpha), β (beta), γ (gamma), p120ctn]. The assessment of the mutational *status* of these genes in the setting of *CDH1*-negative HDGC disclosed no germline mutations, suggesting that catenins are also not major susceptibility genes in HDGC.[77]

MET gene recently emerged as a putative gene involved in familial gastric cancer development. The receptor tyrosine kinase encoded by *MET* transduces motility, proliferation, and morphogenic signals in epithelial cells under the effect of its ligand, the hepatocyte growth factor/scatter factor (HGF/SF).[78] *MET* germline mutations occur in patients with hereditary papillary renal carcinoma (HPRC) and somatic overexpression of MET was found in gastric carcinomas.[79] Lee et al described the first germline *MET* mutation in a Korean patient with intestinal gastric cancer (no family history was available).[80] This mutation (P1009S) localizes at the juxtamembrane domain and was not previously described in HPRC patients. In order to disclose the role of *MET* in familial gastric cancer, Kim et al[81] screened for *MET* germline mutations in a series of 21 Korean families negative for *CDH1* mutations. These authors found that one of 21 probands, with metastatic diffuse gastric cancer and without papillary renal carcinoma, harbored a missense mutation (P791L) localized in a highly conserved residue of the extracellular domain of MET.[81] Two asymptomatic siblings carried the same *MET* alteration.

Both P1009S and P791L localize to upstream sites (juxtamembrane and extracellular domains, respectively), while *MET* mutations associated with HPRC or sporadic papillary renal carcinomas localize to the tyrosine kinase domain suggesting different pathogenic mechanisms for *MET*-induced gastric and papillary renal carcinomas. It was hypothesized that *MET* mutations in gastric cancers may affect dimerization/oligomerization of MET molecules on the cell surface while *MET* missense mutations in HPRC alter the protein conformation, leading to constitutive activation of the MET protein in the absence of the ligand.[81]

Chen et al suggested that *MET* mutations might be specific to people of Asian or Korean ancestry, because no *MET* germline mutations were found in 18 white or Indian gastric cancer kindred.[82] However, although all *MET* germline mutations found in gastric cancer patients to date have been associated with Koreans, further investigation is required to determine the ethnic specificity of these mutations and the true relationship between *MET* and familial gastric cancer.

A cell adhesion molecule with functional similarity to E-cadherin is desmoglein 2 (dsg2), a major component of the desmosomes. Biedermann et al[83] searched for *DSG2* germline mutations in 31 familial gastric cancer patients without *CDH1* germline mutations, and found one germline missense variant leading to a nonconservative amino acid change in a patient with diffuse gastric cancer.[83] Despite this finding, given the unclear pathogenic effect of this mutation these authors claimed that their results rule out *DSG2* as a major gastric cancer predisposition gene.[83]

Molecular Pathology

CDH1 Second-Hit Inactivating Mechanisms

Heterozygous carriers of *CDH1* germline mutations bear in their genomes a single functional *CDH1* allele which apparently produces sufficient amount of protein in the stomach of these patients, to maintain all normal E-cadherin-dependent functions, for at least 2 decades of life. The inactivation of the wild-type allele, by a 2nd-hit molecular mechanism, leads to biallelic inactivation of the *CDH1* gene and determines diffuse gastric cancer development.[38, 65, 84, 85] The initial reports addressing the type and frequency of *CDH1* 2nd hits in HDGC tumors indicated *CDH1* promoter hypermethylation as the most common 2nd-hit mechanism of inactivation,[65, 84, 85] while a second mutation and deletion (LOH or intragenic deletions)[38, 65, 84] were less frequently identified. As a consequence, *CDH1* promoter hypermethylation has been suggested as the basis for development of early detection tools as well as for chemoprophylaxis in unaffected *CDH1* mutation carriers.[86] Moreover, HDGC patients with clinical disease and displaying *CDH1* promoter hypermethylation as a 2nd hit, in their neoplastic lesions, would probably benefit from the administration of drugs leading to the reversion of *CDH1* promoter methylated state. Among many anticancer drugs directed to targeted or molecular therapies, "epigenetic drugs" constitute an attractive possibility for disease control, because they inhibit histone deacetylases (HDAC) and DNA methyltransferases, leading to gene re-expression. Therefore, HDAC inhibitors and DNA demethylating agents emerge, in this view, as attractive drugs to use in combination with classical chemotherapy agents. Such a strategy would nevertheless imply the definitive proof that hypermethylation was the most common mechanism of *CDH1* wild-type allele inactivation in HDGC neoplastic lesions, and the unique mechanism in different neoplastic lesions developing in the same patient.

In all above-mentioned studies, a single neoplastic lesion was investigated *per* HDGC patient, which constitutes a drawback since HDGC is a disease characterized by multiple and apparently unrelated tumor *foci*, scattered in the stomach of mutation carriers.[29, 33] To overcome this problem, Oliveira et al performed a systematic study to quantify the different *CDH1* 2nd hits occurring in neoplastic lesions from HDGC patients.[69] Somatic *CDH1* epigenetic and genetic alterations were detected in lesions from 80% of HDGC families and in 75% of all lesions analyzed. Promoter hypermethylation was found in 32.1%, LOH in 25%, both alterations in 17.9%, and no alterations in 25%. Half of the *CDH1* 2nd hits in primary tumors were epigenetic modifications, whereas in metastases the most frequent 2nd hit was LOH (58.3%).[69] Different neoplastic lesions from the same patient frequently displayed distinct 2nd-hit mechanisms.[69] Different 2nd-hit mechanisms were also detected in the same tumor sample. This study was critical to elucidate the mechanism(s) underlying multifocal HDGC in both the stomach and lymph node metastases.[69] Because of the heterogeneity of these alterations in neoplastic lesions and the plasticity of hypermethylated promoters during tumor initiation and progression, drugs targeting only epigenetic alterations may be less effective than initially predicted, particularly in patients with metastatic HDGC.

c-Src kinase Activation in Early Hereditary Diffuse Gastric Cancer

The earliest known manifestation of HDGC is the accumulation of multiple microscopic *foci* of signet ring cells confined to the mucosa of *CDH1* germline mutation carriers.[29,33] To understand the general mechanisms underlying early HDGC development, Humar et al analyzed samples from various stages of hereditary and sporadic DGC.[87] These authors assumed that the progression from early HDGC to advanced HDGC was mediated by the acquisition of Epithelial to Mesenchymal (EMT) features by neoplastic cells of early HDGC. The kinase c-Src, a well-characterized EMT inducer,[88,89] was not expressed in the small early HDGC *foci*.[87] On the contrary, strong expression of the protein was observed in large intramucosal HDGC lesions with poorly differentiated cells, as well as in cells invading the *muscularis mucosae*.[87] Moreover, fibronectin (a downstream target of c-Src kinase) was also strongly expressed in carcinoma cells invading beyond the mucosa, consistent with the acquisition of EMT features. Furthermore, P-Fak and P-Stat3 were expressed in poorly differentiated cells located deep to the intramucosal signet ring cells and correlated also with the expression of active c-Src.[87]

Based on these data, Humar et al suggested that a successful therapeutic strategy for patients with early HDGC would be the prevention of the EMT by c-Src antagonists, particularly because c-Src is overexpressed in proliferating, poorly differentiated cells of diffuse gastric carcinoma.[87]

In an in vitro model established to analyze genotype–phenotype associations between *CDH1* missense mutations and cell motility, it was verified that cells expressing extracellular E-cadherin mutants exhibited increased activation of c-Src kinase, reenforcing the above-mentioned findings.[60]

CD44 Overexpression

Most HDGC early lesions remain undetected with currently used diagnostic tools and this limitation in cancer detection supports prophylactic gastrectomy as the only reliable medical approach to prevent disease progression in *CDH1* mutation carriers belonging to HDGC families. The identification of molecules expressed de novo in HDGC neoplastic cells would represent a major finding for early screening and therapeutic intervention.

Recently, CD44v6 overexpression was observed along the process of malignant transformation of gastric mucosa, from gastric premalignant (complete and incomplete intestinal metaplasia, low- and high-grade dysplasia) to malignant lesions (gastric cancer-derived cell lines and advanced gastric cancers).[90] Moreover, it was observed that CD44v6 overexpression in E-cadherin-negative tumors developed in *CDH1* germline mutation carriers from HDGC families.[90]

CD44 is a ubiquitously expressed cell surface receptor that undergoes extensive alternative splicing generating highly restrict and highly specific variable isoforms, unlike the canonical CD44s isoform.[91] CD44v6 isoform has been shown to have a role as a *major* cellular matrix adhesion molecule that leads to the activation of several signaling pathways associated with cancer progression.

These results raised the hypothesis of using CD44v6 as a biomarker for the identification of premalignant and malignant lesions prior to resection procedures and, eventually, as a target for therapy.[90]

Animal Models and Cell Culture Models of Disease

CDH1+/– mice

CDH1+/– mice have been generated to carry a heterozygous *CDH1* mutation.[92] In the homozygous state, the mutation affects preimplantation development severely, but the availability of viable mice carrying the *CDH1* mutation in a heterozygous state represents a powerful tool to analyze the role of E-cadherin in tumor progression. This system was later used to promote gastric carcinogenesis either in *CDH1*+/– and in wild-type (wt) mice using *N*-methyl-*N*-nitrosourea (MNU).[93] In this model, intramucosal signet ring cell (diffuse) carcinoma developed much more frequently in *CDH1*+/– mice than in wt mice. The murine signet ring cell (diffuse) carcinoma resembled the human early HDGC *foci* in that they were hypoproliferative and had reduced membrane localization of E-cadherin and its interacting junctional proteins. Together, these findings provided compelling evidence for a deficiency in cell-to-cell adhesion being sufficient to initiate diffuse gastric cancer in the absence of hyperproliferation.

CHO Cell Lines Stably Expressing *CDH1* Mutations

Most germline *CDH1* mutations identified to date in HDGC patients are truncating, as the produced mutant mRNAs encompassing premature termination codons (PTC). These

PTC containing transcripts are commonly downregulated by the mRNA nonsense-mediated decay (NMD) system, a mechanism of mRNA surveillance.[94] In case these mRNAs escape NMD, they lead to the generation of premature termination of translation and production of truncated proteins.

A group of *CDH1* germline mutations, which occur in about 20% of the HDGC families and also in EOGC patients, are of the missense type and, in contrast to truncating mutations, their pathogenicity is not straightforward, therefore constituting a problem in terms of genetic counseling.[60,68,95-97]

An additional problem related to HDGC families carrying *CDH1* missense mutations is related to disease penetrance. In contrast to *CDH1* germline truncating mutations, for which 80% disease penetrance is estimated, missense mutations display a low-penetrance phenotype, with only a few mutation carriers being affected within pedigrees.[24,97]

This, together with the fact that these HDGC families are usually very small so that very few individuals are available for testing, has not allowed segregation analysis within *CDH1* germline missense mutations families. Lacking this clinical information, which constitutes a limiting step to infer the pathogenic significance of missense mutations, it was suggested that the significance of missense mutations in *CDH1* should be assessed in at least four affected members in combination with functional and transcript analysis to look for activation of cryptic splice sites.[98] However, in some cases this type of analysis is impossible to accomplish due to the lack of biological material.

To circumvent this limitation, a working model was developed to classify the significance of missense *CDH1* mutations, based on the information collected on the co-segregation of the mutation within pedigrees, the frequency in healthy control population, the recurrence in independent families, and functional in vitro and in silico data.[97] This model allowed the classification of *CDH1* missense variants into two distinct groups: neutral variants and mutations, thus providing an important tool that can ultimately improve the genetic counseling offered to the carriers of germline *CDH1* missense variants.[97]

As reference laboratory of the International Gastric Cancer Linkage Consortium, IPATIMUP has been involved in the functional characterization of new HDGC-associated *CDH1* germline missense mutations, aiming at revealing their pathogenicity, using in silico and in vitro assays. The in silico analysis included the estimation of the degree of conservation within species of the mutated site, the impact of the mutation on the protein structure, and its effect on splicing.

To functionally characterize the different *CDH1* missense mutations identified, cell lines stably expressing each of the *CDH1* missense mutations, as well as the wt human *CDH1*, have been established by site-direct mutagenesis and transduced into the mammalian E-cadherin-negative CHO (Chinese Hamster Ovary) cell line. E-cadherin function is currently evaluated in vitro by assessing its two main functions, cell–cell adhesion establishment and cell invasion suppression. Slow aggregation in soft agar and Matrigel invasion assays, two good assays proposed by Boterberg et al,[99] are performed in cells expressing different *CDH1* missense mutants in comparison to cells expressing WT *CDH1*. Cells expressing in vitro pathogenic *CDH1* missense mutations commonly fail to aggregate and are able to invade, in contrast to cells expressing the wt protein, which form strong compact cell aggregates and are unable to invade the Matrigel matrix. In all tested missense mutations that proved to be pathogenic, cell–cell adhesion was proven to be inversely correlated with the capacity of cells to invade, confirming the role of E-cadherin in both cell–cell adhesion and suppression of invasion. Taken together, the functional assays performed so far showed that mutations T118R, L214P, G239R, A298T, T340A, P373L, A634V, R749W, E757K, E781D, P799R, and V832M exhibit strong loss of function, supporting their pathogenic role in vivo.[60,97]

To understand if the loss of function of the above-mentioned *CDH1* mutants was related to differences in E-cadherin expression, both western-blot and immunofluorescence analysis of E-cadherin were performed. With the exception of mutants R749W and E757K, all the other mutants expressed E-cadherin at levels similar to those observed for wt *CDH1* expressing cells.[70] These results are of clinical importance since they show that immunohistochemistry is not a valuable screening method to unravel the pathogenic significance of *CDH1* missense mutants in most cases. Moreover, immunofluorescence analysis revealed that the protein is correctly located at the cell membrane, indicating that the loss of function of these mutants is neither due to abnormal expression, nor to mislocalization of the protein.

In the case of the *CDH1* missense juxtamembrane domain mutants, R749W and E757K, both display reduced total and surface expression (60% and 25%, respectively), due to Endoplasmic Reticulum-Associated Degradation (ERAD).[70]

Besides the critical importance of these in vitro functional studies for the genetic counseling of HDGC families, the distinct stable cell lines harboring the set of missense mutations, now available at Seruca's group at IPATIMUP, represent a unique resource to identify, among the signaling pathways activated by E-cadherin, those critical for cell invasion, aggregation, and motility and thus to be able to spot new therapeutic targets for medical intervention in E-cadherin-dependent cancer, sporadic or hereditary (see section below).

The above-mentioned in vitro systems using cell lines stably expressing distinct *CDH1* missense mutants have provided evidence for an association between the specific location of each mutation in the *CDH1* gene and cell phenotype.[60,70,100,101]

Cells harboring extracellular domain mutations L214P, G239R, A298T, T340A, and P373L were significantly more motile (2- to 3-fold increase) than cells expressing wt allele. Mutations in the so-called juxtamembrane domain of E-cadherin (R749W and E757K), which is a particular region of the intracellular E-cadherin domain, rendered cells significantly more motile (2- to 2.5-fold increase) than the ones expressing wt E-cadherin. However, this migratory behavior was not observed for cells expressing other *CDH1* mutations, namely one mutation that affects the precursor region of the protein, a region that is normally cleaved to generate the mature protein, and mutations localized in the intracellular domain (E781D, P799R, and V832M). Interestingly, all stable mutant cells lines exhibit enhanced cell motility mediated through *RAS* homolog gene pathway (RhoA) activation and present high EGFR activation.[60,102]

In contrast, the *CDH1* intracellular mutations do not lose the ability to suppress EGFR and do not respond to EGF by acquiring a motile behavior. Interestingly, it was verified that the intracellular V832M mutation adjacent to the β-catenin-binding domain hampers cell motility by destabilizing the E-cadherin/β-catenin junctional complex.[95,103]

Although these differences were verified mainly using in vitro models, one can hypothesize that patients harboring *CDH1* mutations in the distinct domains of the protein may have a distinct disease progression (i.e., E-cadherin-mediated cell motility may increase metastatic potential of some tumor cells).

Treatment

Prophylactic Gastrectomy

Stomachs removed from germline *CDH1* deleterious mutation carriers have constituted an extremely useful tool to understand the morphologic steps underlying the development of HDGC, encompassing prophylactic (biopsy-negative cases) and curative (biopsy-positive cases) total gastrectomies. Currently, there is information available from 96 total gastrectomies in the setting of HDGC, corresponding to published reports[25,29-33,35-37,72,104-111] and unpublished observations. Seventy three of these gastrectomies were systematically studied according to a research protocol, and 70 (96%) displayed one or multiple *foci* of intramucosal signet ring cell (diffuse) carcinoma (number of *foci* varying from 1 to 318). In two out of the three cases in which intramucosal (T1a) carcinomas were not identified, tiny *foci* of in situ signet ring cell carcinoma were observed (unpublished observations). Additionally, three other publications reported prophylactic gastrectomies performed in *CDH1* germline mutation carriers in which cancer was not identified.[108,111,112] Two of these publications did not provide detailed data on the protocol used for the study of the surgical specimens.[108,111] The case reported in the third study[112] was later submitted to a detailed analysis according to a research protocol and shown to be positive for early invasive carcinoma (four *foci*).[35] Similar findings had been previously reported by Lewis et al.[104]

On the basis of these observations, unless total sampling of the whole stomachs is performed, the diagnosis of intramucosal cancers cannot be excluded. Actually, one of us (FC) had the opportunity to see in consultation several prophylactic gastrectomies, originally reported as negative for cancer, in which the detailed microscopic study of the whole length of gastric mucosa (after complete embedding of the whole stomach) revealed the presence of *foci* of early invasive signet ring cell carcinomas in all cases (data not published).

Since the analysis of gastrectomy specimens shows that microscopic *foci* of signet ring cell (diffuse) carcinoma are almost universally present in *CDH1* mutation carriers and since the penetrance of HDGC is >80%, surgery should be strongly considered whenever an at-risk family member is found to have a *CDH1* pathogenic mutation. However, the timing of the gastrectomy is debatable. Available evidence suggests that the intramucosal signet ring cell (diffuse) carcinomas have an indolent growth and may remain latent, without progression, for unknown periods of time, most probably due to the fact that they have a low proliferative index.[65] However, with our current lack of knowledge on the behavior of intramucosal signet ring cancer cells, it is recommended that if they are detected on endoscopic biopsies, the patient should be advised to undergo a curative total gastrectomy regardless of age, although it is rare that endoscopy would be recommended before 16 years of age. Carriers of pathogenic *CDH1* mutations with normal gastric biopsies should be advised to undergo prophylactic total gastrectomy once the genetic testing results are known and once individuals are older than 20 years.[25] Patients under the age of 40 who develop symptomatic invasive diffuse gastric carcinoma have a poor prognosis with as few as 10% having early and curable disease.[113] There are now reports showing that pregnancy can be carried to full term following a prophylactic gastrectomy[114] and individuals are able to return to full-time work including manual workers.

Potential Molecular Targets

At initial diagnosis, most HDGC probands present an advanced disease stage with a high risk of relapse after surgical treatment. The high prevalence of incurable disease produces a heavy burden on patients' care which has a huge effect on healthcare resources.

For a long time, the consequences of E-cadherin loss of function have been seen as a structural cell–cell adhesion disruption rather than as a loss of E-cadherin-dependent regulatory events. However, E-cadherin acts indeed as a cell membrane receptor,[115,116] and many signaling molecules have been reported to interact with E-cadherin, namely the Receptor Tyrosine Kinases (RTKs), which have been found to localize also at the basolateral membrane of epithelial cells.[117,118]

RTK activity in resting normal cells is tightly controlled, but RTKs can become potent oncoproteins. Of notice, the Epidermal Growth Factor Receptor (EGFR) has been reported to be involved in a bidirectional cross talk with E-cadherin.[119]

Using an in vitro model, Seruca's group demonstrated that there is a tight regulation of E-cadherin–EGFR and E-cadherin–HER2 heterodimers.[60,102] Moreover, recently they showed also, using in vitro assays, that cancer-associated E-cadherin alterations (extracellular mutations or complete loss) modify the stability of E-cadherin/EGFR heterodimer leading to the activation of EGFR downstream targets, namely increased RhoA activation. This effect on EGFR–RhoA activation mediated by altered E-cadherin was shown to be reverted upon EGFR pharmacological inhibition.[102]

Epidermal Growth Factor Receptor (EGFR) and HER2 are members of the HER family of receptors. Abnormal activation of HER in transformed cells is involved in the development and progression of many human cancers. HER receptors are important targets for therapeutic intervention, namely in non-small cell lung cancer (NSCLC), in colorectal and breast carcinomas, and in pancreatic adenocarcinomas. Thus, one can hypothesize that EGFR or HER2 inhibitors can be used in the treatment of gastric cancer, not only in patients harboring tumors with EGFR/HER2 alterations, namely amplification and/or mutation, but also in patients with tumors with E-cadherin deregulation.

Since EGFR and HER2 inhibitors are already commercially available and used in clinical practice in other tumor models, testing these drugs as new therapeutic tools for gastric cancer associated with E-cadherin is a clinical challenge.

E-cadherin and Tumor Cell Survival

Cell survival depends on signals from the environment, such as those provided by adhesion molecules that mediate contacts between cells or between cells and the extracellular matrix.[120] If these interactions are disrupted, the cells are programmed to die.[121-123]

E-cadherin, besides its role in cell–cell adhesion, is involved in the regulation of programmed cell death.[124] This was shown also using an in vitro model, in which mutational loss of functional E-cadherin renders cells more resistant to apoptotic stimuli.[125] Cell lines stably expressing *CDH1* mutants are capable not only to invade but also to survive and grow in the absence of contact with other cells in a "hostile" environment.[125] The apoptotic stimulus used in this in vitro study was taxol, a drug widely used in the treatment of advanced cancers, including epithelial tumors harboring *CDH1* dysfunction. Importantly, these results question the effectiveness of such treatment in these types of tumors and highlight the need for further research on the subject in order to find alternative therapeutic strategies.

It was also demonstrated the existence of an interplay between E-cadherin and the anti-apoptotic factor bcl-2, supporting the hypothesis that E-cadherin is more than a simple mediator of cell contact and adhesion but is also involved in the control of programmed cell death and thus has a dual role in cancer development.

Early-Onset Diffuse Gastric Cancer

Definition

Early-onset gastric cancer (EOGC) is defined as any gastric cancer presenting at the age of 45 or earlier, and represents approximately 10% of all patients with stomach cancer with reported frequencies varying between 2.7% and 15%, according to different populations studied.[113] Gastric cancer patients younger than 40–45 years old are believed to develop gastric cancer involving molecular pathways different from those of patients with sporadic carcinomas that occur later in life.[113,126,127] Gastric cancer occurring in patients younger than 30 years is very rare (1.1–1.6%) and most of EOGCs are diagnosed in patients older than 35.[128,129] Gastric cancers diagnosed before 20 years of age are exceptional and current literature is limited to a small number of cases.[130,131]

Early-onset diffuse gastric cancer (EODGC) is part of the EOGC setting, but its most frequent presentation occurs in HDGC families, where most family members develop diffuse gastric cancer at young age, before 45 years old.[22] Guilford et al reported the first young patient with apparently sporadic diffuse gastric cancer, carrying a *CDH1* germline mutation.[14]

The age of onset has been used in several types of hereditary cancer syndromes to recruit patients without a family history for genetic screening, as these isolated patients represent putative carriers of de novo germline mutations.

Clinical and Pathological Features of EOGC

From the clinicopathologic stand point, EOGC preferentially occur in female gender presenting tumors with diffuse histology, multifocal appearance, proximal location, and poor outcome. In EOGC patients, the advanced stage at the time of diagnosis remains a clinical burden due to the poor long-term survival.[40]

Etiological factors of EOGC remain unknown as environmental agents represent a *minor* component and therefore a high impact of genetic causes is predicted. *CDH1* germline mutations in well-documented diffuse EOGC cases remain the only germline genetic defect described in this type of patients.

Positive family history of gastric cancer has been reported in about 10% of young patients with diffuse histotype of gastric cancer[132] and therefore these patients are frequently considered strong candidates to be part of HDGC families. In such cases, families should be offered genetic counseling and should be tested for the presence of germline alterations at the *CDH1* gene.

CDH1 Germline Sequence Variants in EOGC

Several authors identified *CDH1* germline alterations in apparently sporadic EOGC, always presenting diffuse or mixed histotype. The largest series of diffuse EOGC screened for *CDH1* germline mutations was reported by Bacani et al[50] who identified eight germline sequence variants in 81 (9.9%) patients younger than 50 years, in the Central-East Ontario region, Canada, a region of low incidence of gastric cancer.[50] Suriano et al[68] described also a large series of 54 diffuse or mixed type EOGC patients for which five (9.3%) germline sequence variants were reported.

To date, 264 apparently sporadic diffuse or mixed EOGC patients, aged 51 years or less, have been screened for the presence of *CDH1* germline sequence variants (Table 6.3). From these 264 EOGC cases, 19 (7.2%) carried *CDH1* constitutional germline sequence variants, but only 2.3% (6/264) of them did in fact represent variants with a proven potentially deleterious effect (Table 6.3). This predicted pathogenicity was based on the type of mutation (frameshift) or on the results obtained from in vitro functional analysis. Tumors from EOGC mutation carriers invariably presented partial (mixed) or complete diffuse histology and occurred in patients younger than 35 years old. Based on these and other similar observations, germline *CDH1* mutation screening is now recommended for patients with these characteristics.[23]

Gastric Cancers Associated with Other Hereditary Predisposition Syndromes

Lynch Syndrome

Lynch syndrome (previously referred to as Hereditary Nonpolyposis Colorectal Cancer (HNPCC) [MIM #120435]) is an autosomal dominantly inherited disorder of cancer susceptibility with high penetrance (80–85%)[135] and is one of the most common inherited cancer syndromes in humans. Lynch syndrome occurs in about 2–4% of all colorectal cancer cases and is caused by a mutation in one of the mismatch repair (MMR) genes: *MLH1*, *MSH2*, *MSH6*, or *PMS2*. Lynch syndrome is also associated with various types of extracolonic malignancies and, in this case, is commonly referred as Lynch syndrome II. In Lynch syndrome II there is a high risk of non-colonic malignancies within the digestive system, affecting the stomach, small intestine, pancreas, and biliary tree. Until recently, the incidence of gastric cancer in Lynch syndrome II remained unclear depending largely on the rate of gastric cancer itself within the population under analysis.[136,137] However, Capelle et al[138] determined recently the incidence of gastric cancer in a large series of Lynch syndrome mutation carriers (known and putative) and found that standardized incidence ratio of gastric cancer was 3.4 (95% confidence interval, 2.1–5.2).[138] To have a correct estimation of gastric cancer risk in Lynch syndrome, the authors evaluated 2,014 mutation carriers and found gastric tumors only in 32 cases (1.6%) and, in one family with Lynch syndrome II, four cases of gastric cancer were diagnosed.[138] In this study, gastric cancer occurred more frequently in males than in females (1.9:1) with a lifetime risk of 8.0% in males versus 5.3% in females, but this difference is likely to be related to the fact that males are already at a higher risk of developing gastric cancer due to lifestyle habits.[138] In Lynch syndrome, gastric cancer is diagnosed at 45 years of age or older in the majority of the cases (87.5%) at a median age of 55 years (range, 27–82 years), the intestinal-type gastric adenocarcinoma being the most commonly reported.

Concerning the association between the types of germline defects in mismatch repair genes associated with gastric cancer, in the study reported by Capelle et al[138] none of the 378 *MSH6* carriers developed gastric cancer. In contrast, in patients with germline defects of *MLH1* or *MSH2*, there was a risk for gastric cancer development, 4.8% and 9%, respectively. Due to this genotype–phenotype association, surveillance gastroscopy for Lynch syndrome patients carrying an *MLH1* or *MSH2* mutation should be considered.[138]

A hallmark of the Lynch syndrome is the presence of microsatellite instability (MSI) in the tumors and it is mandatory to search for this molecular biomarker in cases of gastric cancer occurring in the setting of suspected Lynch syndrome, before offering germline mutation screen of *MSH2* and *MLH1* defects.[139,140]

Interestingly, in "pure" familial gastric cancer (FGC) no MMR gene mutations have yet been identified.[141] However, a subset of these families is putatively linked to "non-classic" MMR defects. This hypothesis is based on the fact that MSI tumors have been identified in families with aggregation of gastric cancer only.[141,142]

Recently, Leite et al[141] analyzed a series of gastric cancer families presenting at least one gastric cancer case aged less than 50 years old, excluding familial cases belonging to families

Table 6.3 Geographic, clinical and molecular features of EOGC

Reference	Total EOGC screened, *n* (age setting)	*CDH1* sequence variants (%)	Ethnicity	Histotype	Age onset	Population frequency	*CDH1* sequence variant	Mutation type	Gene position	Predicted protein change	Predicted pathogenicity
Guilford et al[14]	1	1	*New Zealand*	*Diffuse*	*31*	*Nd*	*1487del7*	*Frameshift*	*Exon 10*	*PTC_556*	*Yes*
Suriano et al[68]	54[a] (age≤51)	5 (7.6%)	Africa/USA	Diffuse	43	1%	1849G>A	Missense	Exon 12	Ala617Thr	No
			Africa/USA	Diffuse	43	1%	1849G>A	Missense	Exon 12	Ala617Thr	No
			Portugal	*Diffuse*	*30*	*0%*	*1901C>T*[b,c]	*Missense/splice-site*	*Exon 12*	*Ala634Val*	*Yes*
			England	Diffuse	51	0%	532-18C>T	Intronic	Intron 4	Nd	No
			Portugal	Mixed	42	0%	532-18C>T	Intronic	Intron 4	Nd	No
Suriano et al[45]	10 (age≤35)	2 (20%)	*USA*	*Diffuse*	*27*	*Nd*	*1285C>T*	*Missense*	*Exon 9*	*Pro429Ser*	*Yes*
			USA	*Diffuse*	*27*	*Nd*	*1063delT*	*Frameshift*	*Exon 8*	*PTC_355*	*Yes*
Keller et al[67]	15 (age≤45)	1 (6.7%)	*Europe*	*Diffuse*	*29*	*Nd*	*1619_1620insG*	*Frameshift*	*Exon 11*	*PTC_546*	*Yes*
Bacani et al[50]	81 (age<50)	8 (9.9%)	USA	Diffuse	Na	Nd	−117G>A	5'-UTR substitution	Promotor	Nd	Nd
			USA	Diffuse	Na	3.9%	−71C>G	5'-UTR substitution	Promotor	Nd	Nd
			Europe/USA	*Diffuse*	*30*	*Nd*	*41delT*	*Frameshift*	*Exon 1*	*PTC_55*	*Yes*
			USA	Diffuse	Na	0%	48-5G>C	Intronic	Intron 1	Nd	Nd
			USA	Diffuse	Na	Nd	48-15C>G	Intronic	Intron 1	Nd	Nd
			USA	Diffuse	Na	Nd	387+26C>T	Intronic	Intron 3	Nd	Nd
			USA	Diffuse	Na	Nd	2295+53G>A	Intronic	Intron 14	Nd	Nd
			USA	Diffuse	Na	Nd	2439+31G>A	Intronic	Intron 15	Nd	Nd
Corso et al[40]	21 (age≤50)	2 (8.9%)	Italy	Diffuse	50	0%	−63C>A	5'-UTR substitution	Promotor	Nd	Nd
			Italy	Diffuse	45	0.4%	670C>T	Missense	Exon 5	Arg224Cys	No
Saito et al[133]	9 (age<35)	–	Japan	Diffuse	<35	–	–	–	–	–	–
Brooks-Wilson et al[58]	9 (age<50)	–	USA	Diffuse	<50	–	–	–	–	–	–
Zhang et al[134]	24 (age<50)	–	China	Unknown	<50	–	–	–	–	–	–
Carvalho et al[126]	40 (age<45)	–	Europe and USA	21 diffuse 9 mixed	<45	–	–	–	–	–	–
Total	264	19 (7.2%)	–	–	–	–	–	–	–	–	6/264 (2.3%)

Abbreviations: PTC premature termination codon, *Na* not available, *Nd* not determined

[a]The whole series encompassed 66 EOGC cases, from which only 54 were of diffuse or mixed histology; *Italic*, predicted pathogenicity based on mutation type (frameshift) or in vitro functional analysis

[b]This mutation also generates a cryptic splice-site at the site of the missense change leading to the generation of premature termination at codon 653

[c]The EOGC proband carrying this mutation was later found to share an haplotype with another family described in reference[44]

harboring *CDH1* alterations (HDGC) and families with criteria of Lynch syndrome.[141] In these families, females were significantly more affected than in the sporadic setting, but the reason behind this finding (a higher female–male ratio) remains unknown. To disclose the mechanism underlying these cases of familial clustering of gastric cancer, MSI was searched for, the *status* and frequency of *MLH1* promoter methylation were analyzed, and MMR gene mutations were screened in selected cases: 71.4% of the MSI gastric cancer families harbored somatic *MLH1* promoter hypermethylation. Gene rearrangements at *MLH1* and *MSH2* genes, as well as germline methylation of the *MLH1* promoter, were searched for in the probands of two gastric cancer families with tumors lacking *MLH1* immunoexpression. At least in these two cases, no germline alterations were detected that could explain familial aggregation of early-onset MSI gastric cancer.

Li–Fraumeni Syndrome

Li and Fraumeni reported a familial cancer syndrome characterized by autosomal dominant inheritance and early onset of tumors, multiple tumors within an individual, and multiple affected family members, which is denominated as Li–Fraumeni syndrome (LFS) [MIM #151623].[143,144] In contrast to other inherited cancer syndromes, which are predominantly characterized by site-specific cancers, LFS families present with a variety of tumor types. The most common types are soft tissue sarcomas and osteosarcomas, breast cancer, brain tumors, leukemia, and adrenocortical carcinoma. Other less frequent tumors include melanoma and carcinomas of the lung, pancreas, cervix, and prostate. Classic LFS is defined as a proband with a sarcoma before the age of 45 years and a first-degree relative age <45 years with any cancer and one additional first- or second-degree relative in the same lineage with any cancer age <45 years or a sarcoma at any age. Gastric cancer can occur in some affected LFS families, both of intestinal and diffuse types.

To date, germline *TP53* mutations have been identified in approximately 70–75% of LFS families fulfilling the classic criteria.[145-147] In most tumors, both alleles are altered—one by inherited mutation, and the other by somatic loss of the wild-type allele.[148] Very recently, it was demonstrated that the functional effects of particular mutations, polymorphisms in *TP53* or in regulators such as *MDM2*, variations in DNA copy number, and variations in telomere length have a strong impact on individual risk and on tumor patterns.[149]

In two families (one Portuguese and one German) with heavy history of gastric cancer and lacking *CDH1* germline mutations, *TP53* germline mutations were found.[44,67] The Portuguese family had been misclassified in clinical terms as familial gastric cancer (FGC) and not as a Li–Fraumeni family and thus proposed at first for *CDH1* and not *TP53* screening. Cases like this should draw the attention of genetic counselors for the possibility that a minority of apparent FGC cases can be explained by *TP53* germline mutations leading to a distinct clinical follow-up.

Somatic alterations of *TP53* have been found in more than 60% of gastric carcinomas and can be of the diverse type: missense mutations, frameshift, deletions, or LOH. Some studies showed that the frequency of *TP53* mutations in early and advanced intestinal type gastric cancer was similar to that observed in advanced diffuse carcinomas (around 40% in all cases), while *TP53* mutations rarely occurred in early diffuse gastric cancers.[150-154]

CHEK2 gene in long arm of chromosome 22 was recently implicated as a tumor suppressor gene and a second predisposing *locus* for LFS.[155] The role of *CHEK2* mutations has been somewhat controversial due to the presence of related genes on various other chromosomes in the human genome.[155]

A third Li–Fraumeni syndrome predisposition *locus* was assigned to human chromosome 1q23.[156]

Familial Adenomatosis Polyposis

Familial adenomatous polyposis (FAP) [MIM #175100] is a rare hereditary syndrome characterized by multiple colorectal polyps and early development of colorectal cancer.[157,158] Although FAP uniformly involves the large bowel, it is often significantly confounded by extracolonic cancers including gastric cancer.[159-161] An attenuated form of FAP, called attenuated FAP, has been distinguished from classic FAP.[162]

The syndrome, when inherited in an autosomal dominant manner, is caused by germline mutations in the adenomatous polyposis coli (*APC*) gene, which is a tumor suppressor gene located on the long arm of chromosome 5 (5q21–22).[163,164] This gene plays a central role in the development and homeostasis of the intestine and many other tissues. Recently another polyposis gene has been identified, the *MUTYH* gene, in which biallelic mutations cause an autosomal recessive pattern of inheritance.[165] This form of polyposis is usually referred to as *MUTYH*-associated polyposis (MAP).[166] Gastric cancer does not seem to belong to the extracolonic tumor spectrum in *MUTYH*-associated polyposis.[167]

Both adenomas and fundic gland polyps develop in the stomach in the setting of FAP.[158] Fundic gland polyposis is the most common gastric lesion in FAP. In the general population, these polyps are considered benign and have no malignant potential. However, in FAP patients, fundic gland polyps have been occasionally recognized as precursor lesions from which invasive cancer may develop.[168,169] Fundic gland polyps are common in familial adenomatous polyposis and attenuated familial adenomatous polyposis and, if voluminous, may interfere with effective endoscopic gastric cancer surveillance.[161]

Cowden Syndrome

Cowden syndrome [MIM #158350] comprises a heterogeneous group of disorders, some of them considered to be pathognomonic like mucocutaneous lesions, and macrocephaly.

Up to now, the only gene identified to cause Cowden disease is the phosphatase and tensin homolog (*PTEN*).

PTEN mutation carriers usually develop clinical features by their second decade of life, but the age of onset can vary depending on the clinical presentation of the disease. Mutation carriers are at an increased risk to develop benign and malignant tumors of the breast, endometrium, and thyroid. The first description of gastric involvement in Cowden disease was reported by Weinstock and Kawanishi.[170]

Hamartomatous polyps throughout the gastrointestinal tract can be found in more than 60% of Cowden patients, in association or not with ganglioneuromas and lipomatous and inflammatory polyps.

The risk of gastric carcinoma development in Cowden syndrome is not well established; thus the National Comprehensive Cancer Network (NCCN) does not provide specific guidelines for endoscopic screening of the gastrointestinal tract in this syndrome. In fact, very rare cases of gastric carcinomas have been reported in the literature.

PTEN-associated cancers, namely gastric cancer, show somatic loss of PTEN protein whereas the surrounding non-neoplastic tissue retains PTEN immunoexpression. This was clearly reported in a gastric cancer patient belonging to a Cowden's family presenting a germline *PTEN* mutation (Gly293X), reinforcing the role of this technique as a complementary assay in the case of a suspect individual.[171]

Peutz–Jeghers Syndrome

Peutz–Jeghers syndrome (PJS) [MIM #175200] is characterized by the association of gastrointestinal polyposis and mucocutaneous pigmentation.[172]

The *sine qua non* of the diagnosis of PJS is the hamartomatous gastrointestinal polyp characterized histopathologically by the unique finding of mucosa with interdigitating smooth-muscle bundles in a characteristic branching tree appearance.[173]

A working definition of PJS was suggested by Giardiello et al[174] and further defined in a recent consensus meeting.[175] In a single individual, a clinical diagnosis of PJS may be made when any one of the following is present: (1) Two or more histologically confirmed PJ polyps; (2) Any number of PJ polyps detected in one individual who has a family history of PJS in close relative(s); (3) Characteristic mucocutaneous pigmentation in an individual who has a family history of PJS in close relative(s); and (4) Any number of PJ polyps in an individual who also has characteristic mucocutaneous pigmentation.

PJS is an autosomal dominant inherited disorder associated with increased cancer risk, in particular breast and gastrointestinal cancers, including gastric cancer.[176, 177] In a recent systematic PubMed search, it was found that the most common malignancy was colorectal cancer, followed by breast, small bowel, gastric, and pancreatic cancers, the lifetime risk for any cancer varying between 37% and 93%.[178]

Germline mutations in the gene *STK11* (*LKB1*) have been identified as a cause of Peutz–Jeghers syndrome.[179, 180] Mutations in this gene account for most cases of PJS, being detected in nearly all individuals who have a positive family history and approximately 90% of individuals who have no family history of PJS.[172] However, identification in a PJS patient of a germline mutation in the gene coding for smooth-muscle myosin (*MYH11*) suggests it cannot be ruled out completely that alterations in genes other than STK11/LKB1 may be responsible for this disease.[181]

References

1. Globocan 2008. http://globocan.iarc.fr. Accessed November 12, 2010.
2. Laurén P. The two histological main types of gastric carcinoma: diffuse and so-called intestinal-type carcinoma. An attempt at a histo-clinical classification. *Acta Pathol Microbiol Scand.* 1965;64:31–49.
3. Lauwers GY, Carneiro F, Graham DY, Curado M-P, Franceschi S, Montgomery E, Tatematsu M, Hattori T. Gastric carcinoma. In: Bosman FT, Carneiro F, Hruban RH, Theise ND, eds. *WHO Classification of Tumours of the Digestive System.* 4th ed. IARC: Lyon; 2010:48–58.
4. Henson DE, Dittus C, Younes M, et al. Differential trends in the intestinal and diffuse types of gastric carcinoma in the United States, 1973–2000: increase in the signet ring cell type. *Arch Pathol Lab Med.* 2004;128:765–770.
5. Miyahara R, Niwa Y, Matsuura T, et al. Prevalence and prognosis of gastric cancer detected by screening in a large Japanese population: data from a single institute over 30 years. *J Gastroenterol Hepatol.* 2007;22:1435–1442.
6. Ekstrom AM, Serafini M, Nyren O, et al. Dietary antioxidant intake and the risk of cardia cancer and noncardia cancer of the intestinal and diffuse types: a population-based case–control study in Sweden. *Int J Cancer.* 2000;87:133–140.
7. Palli D, Galli M, Caporaso NE, et al. Family history and risk of stomach cancer in Italy. *Cancer Epidemiol Biomarkers Prev.* 1994;3:15–18.
8. Guilford P, Hopkins J, Harraway J, et al. E-cadherin germline mutations in familial gastric cancer. *Nature.* 1998;392:402–405.
9. Vasen HF, Wijnen JT, Menko FH, et al. Cancer risk in families with hereditary nonpolyposis colorectal cancer diagnosed by mutation analysis. *Gastroenterology.* 1996;110:1020–1027.
10. Varley JM, McGown G, Thorncroft M, et al. An extended Li-Fraumeni kindred with gastric carcinoma and a codon 175 mutation in TP53. *J Med Genet.* 1995;32:942–945.
11. La Vecchia C, Negri E, Franceschi S, et al. Family history and the risk of stomach and colorectal cancer. *Cancer.* 1992;70:50–55.
12. Gayther SA, Gorringe KL, Ramus SJ, et al. Identification of germline E-cadherin mutations in gastric cancer families of European origin. *Cancer Res.* 1998;58:4086–4089.
13. Richards FM, McKee SA, Rajpar MH, et al. Germline E-cadherin gene (*CDH1*) mutations predispose to familial gastric cancer and colorectal cancer. *Hum Mol Genet.* 1999;8:607–610.

14. Guilford PJ, Hopkins JB, Grady WM, et al. E-cadherin germline mutations define an inherited cancer syndrome dominated by diffuse gastric cancer. *Hum Mutat.* 1999;14:249–255.
15. Berx G, Cleton-Jansen AM, Nollet F, et al. E-cadherin is a tumour/invasion suppressor gene mutated in human lobular breast cancers. *EMBO J.* 1995;14:6107–115.
16. Shore EM, Nelson WJ. Biosynthesis of the cell adhesion molecule uvomorulin (E-cadherin) in Madin-Darby canine kidney epithelial cells. *J Biol Chem.* 1991;266:19672–19680.
17. Ringwald M, Schuh R, Vestweber D, et al. The structure of cell adhesion molecule uvomorulin. Insights into the molecular mechanism of Ca2+–dependent cell adhesion. The. *EMBO J.* 1987;6:3647–3653.
18. Blaschuk OW, Sullivan R, David S, et al. Identification of a cadherin cell adhesion recognition sequence. *Dev Biol.* 1990;39:227–229.
19. Polakis P. Wnt signaling and cancer. *Genes Dev.* 2000;14:1837–1851.
20. Nagar B, Overduin M, Ikura M, et al. Structural basis of calcium-induced E-cadherin rigidification and dimerization. *Nature.* 1996;380:360–364.
21. Caldas C, Carneiro F, Lynch HT, et al. Familial gastric cancer: overview and guidelines for management. *J Med Genet.* 1999;36:873–880.
22. Carneiro F, Oliveira C, Suriano G, et al. Molecular pathology of familial gastric cancer, with an emphasis on Hereditary Diffuse Gastric Cancer (HDGC). *J Clin Pathol.* 2008;61:25–30.
23. Fitzgerald RC, Hardwick R, Huntsman D, et al. on behalf of the International Gastric Cancer Linkage Consortium. Hereditary diffuse gastric cancer: updated consensus guidelines for clinical management and directions for future research. *J Med Genet.* 2010;47:436–444.
24. Pharoah PD, Guilford P, Caldas C. International Gastric Cancer Linkage Consortium. Incidence of gastric cancer and breast cancer in *CDH1* (E-cadherin) mutation carriers from hereditary diffuse gastric cancer families. *Gastroenterology.* 2001;121:1348–1353.
25. Blair V, Martin I, Shaw D, et al. Hereditary diffuse gastric cancer: diagnosis and management. *Clin Gastroenterol Hepatol.* 2006;4:262–275.
26. Kaurah P, MacMillan A, Boyd N, et al. Founder and recurrent *CDH1* mutations in families with hereditary diffuse gastric cancer. *JAMA.* 2007;297:2360–2372.
27. Oliveira C, Senz J, Kaurah P, et al. Germline *CDH1* deletions in hereditary diffuse gastric cancer families. *Hum Mol Genet.* 2009;18:1545–1555.
28. Pinheiro H, Bordeira-Carriço R, Seixas S, et al. Allele-specific *CDH1* downregulation and hereditary diffuse gastric cancer. *Hum Mol Genet.* 2010;19:943–952.
29. Carneiro F, Huntsman DG, Smyrk TC, et al. Model of the early development of diffuse gastric cancer in E-cadherin mutation carriers and its implications for patient screening. *J Pathol.* 2004;203:681–687.
30. Charlton A, Blair V, Shaw D, et al. Hereditary diffuse gastric cancer: predominance of multiple *foci* of signet ring cell carcinoma in distal stomach and transitional zone. *Gut.* 2004;53:814–820.
31. Rogers WM, Dobo E, Norton JA, et al. Risk-reducing total gastrectomy for germline mutations in E-cadherin (*CDH1*): pathologic fi ndings with clinical implications. *Am J Surg Pathol.* 2008;32:799–809.
32. Shaw D, Blair V, Framp A, et al. Chromoendoscopic surveillance in hereditary diffuse gastric cancer: an alternative to prophylactic gastrectomy? *Gut.* 2005;54:461–468.
33. Huntsman DG, Carneiro F, Lewis FR, et al. Early gastric cancer in young, asymptomatic carriers of germ-line *E-cadherin* mutations. *N Engl J Med.* 2001;344:1904–1909.
34. Norton JA, Ham CM, Van Dam J, et al. *CDH1* truncating mutations in the Ecadherin gene: an indication for total gastrectomy to treat hereditary diffuse gastric cancer. *Ann Surg.* 2007;245:873–879.
35. Barber M, Save V, Carneiro F, et al. Histopathological and molecular analysis of gastrectomy specimens from hereditary diffuse gastric cancer patients has implications for endoscopic surveillance of individuals at risk. *J Pathol.* 2008;216:286–294.
36. Hebbard PC, MacMillan A, Huntsman D, et al. Prophylactic total gastrectomy (PTG) for hereditary diffuse gastric cancer (HDGC): the Newfoundland experience with 23 patients. *Ann Surg Oncol.* 2009;16:1890–1895.
37. Chun YS, Lindor NM, Smyrk TC, et al. Germline *E-cadherin* gene mutations: is prophylactic total gastrectomy indicated? *Cancer.* 2001;92:181–187.
38. Oliveira C, de Bruin J, Nabais S, et al. Intragenic deletion of *CDH1* as the inactivating mechanism of the wild-type allele in a HDGC tumour. *Oncogene.* 2004;23:2236–2240.
39. Oliveira C, Seruca R, Carneiro F. Genetics, pathology, and clinics of familial gastric cancer. *Int J Surg Pathol.* 2006;14:21–33.
40. Corso G, Pedrazzani C, Pinheiro H, et al. E-cadherin genetic screening and clinico-pathologic characteristics of early onset gastric cancer. *Eur J Cancer.* 2010;47:631–639.
41. Masciari S, Larsson N, Senz J, et al. Germline E-cadherin mutations in familial lobular breast cancer. *J Med Genet.* 2007;44:726–731.
42. Schrader KA, Masciari S, Boyd N, et al. Hereditary diffuse gastric cancer: association with lobular breast cancer. *Fam Cancer.* 2008;7:73–82.
43. Guilford P, Humar B, Blair V. Hereditary diffuse gastric cancer: translation of *CDH1* germline mutations into clinical practice. *Gastric Cancer.* 2010;13:1–10.
44. Oliveira C, Ferreira P, Nabais S, et al. E-Cadherin (*CDH1*) and TP53 rather than SMAD4 and Caspase-10 germline mutations contribute to genetic predisposition in Portuguese gastric cancer patients. *Eur J Cancer.* 2004;40:1897–1903.
45. Suriano G, Yew S, Ferreira P, et al. Characterization of a recurrent germ line mutation of the Ecadherin gene: implications for genetic testing and clinical management. *Clin Cancer Res.* 2005;11:5401–5409.
46. Yabuta T, Shinmura K, Tani M, et al. E-cadherin gene variants in gastric cancer families whose probands are diagnosed with diffuse gastric cancer. *Int J Cancer.* 2002;101:434–441.
47. Wang Y, Song JP, Ikeda M, et al. Ile-Leu substitution (I415L) in germline E-cadherin gene (*CDH1*) in Japanese familial gastric cancer. *Jpn J Clin Oncol.* 2003;33:17–20.
48. Figueiredo C, Machado JC, Pharoah P, et al. *Helicobacter pylori* and interleukin 1 genotyping: an opportunity to identify high-risk individuals for gastric carcinoma. *J Natl Cancer Inst.* 2002;94:1680–1687.
49. Machado JC, Figueiredo C, Canedo P, et al. A proinflammatory genetic profile increases the risk for chronic atrophic gastritis and gastric carcinoma. *Gastroenterology.* 2003;125:364–371.
50. Bacani JT, Soares M, Zwingerman R, et al. *CDH1*/E-cadherin germline mutations in early-onset gastric cancer. *J Med Genet.* 2006;43:867–872.
51. Oliveira C, Bordin MC, Grehan N, et al. Screening E-cadherin in gastric cancer families reveals germline mutations only in hereditary diffuse gastric cancer kindred. *Hum Mutat.* 2002;19:510–517.
52. More H, Humar B, Weber W, et al. Identification of seven novel germline mutations in the human E-cadherin (*CDH1*) gene. *Hum Mutat.* 2007;28:203–211.
53. Moran CJ, Joyce M, McAnena OJ. *CDH1* associated gastric cancer: a report of a family and review of the literature. *Eur J Surg Oncol.* 2005;31:259–264.
54. Humar B, Toro T, Graziano F, et al. Novel germline *CDH1* mutations in hereditary diffuse gastric cancer families. *Hum Mutat.* 2002;19:518–525.
55. Shinmura K, Kohno T, Takahashi M, et al. Familial gastric cancer: clinicopathological characteristics, RER phenotype and germline p53 and E-cadherin mutations. *Carcinogenesis.* 999;20:1127–1131.

56. Dussaulx-Garin L, Blayau M, Pagenault M, et al. A new mutation of E-cadherin gene in familial gastric linitis plastica cancer with extra-digestive dissemination. *Eur J Gastroenterol Hepatol.* 2001;13:711–715.
57. Keller G, Vogelsang H, Becker I, et al. Diffuse type gastric and lobular breast carcinoma in a familial gastric cancer patient with an E-cadherin germline mutation. *Am J Pathol.* 1999;155:337–342.
58. Brooks-Wilson AR, Kaurah P, Suriano G, et al. Germline E-cadherin mutations in hereditary diffuse gastric cancer: assessment of 42 new families and review of genetic screening criteria. *J Med Genet.* 2004;41:508–517.
59. Frebourg T, Oliveira C, Hochain P, et al. Cleft lip/palate and *CDH1*/E-cadherin mutations in families with hereditary diffuse gastric cancer. *J Med Genet.* 2006;43:138–142.
60. Mateus AR, Simoes-Correia J, Figueiredo J, et al. E-cadherin mutations and cell motility: a genotype-phenotype correlation. *Exp Cell Res.* 2009;315:1393–1402.
61. Yoon K, Ku J, Yang H, et al. Germline mutations of E-cadherin gene in Korean familial gastric cancer patients. *J Hum Genet.* 1999;44:177–180.
62. Jonsson BA, Bergh A, Stattin P, et al. Germline mutations in E-cadherin do not explain association of hereditary prostate cancer, gastric cancer and breast cancer. *Int J Cancer.* 2002;98: 838–843.
63. Roviello F, Corso G, Pedrazzani C, et al. Hereditary diffuse gastric cancer and E-cadherin: description of the first germline mutation in an Italian family. *Eur J Surg Oncol.* 2007;33:448–451.
64. Mayrbaeurl B, Keller G, Schauer W, et al. Germline mutation of the E-cadherin gene in three sibling cases with advanced gastric cancer: clinical consequences for the other family members. *Eur J Gastroenterol Hepatol.* 2010;22:306–310.
65. Barber M, Murrell A, Ito Y, et al. Mechanisms and sequelae of E-cadherin silencing in hereditary diffuse gastric cancer. *J Pathol.* 2008;216:295–306.
66. Rodriguez-Sanjuan JC, Fontalba A, Mayorga M, et al. A novel mutation in the E-cadherin gene in the fi rst family with hereditary diffuse gastric cancer reported in Spain. *Eur J Surg Oncol.* 2006;32:1110–1113.
67. Keller G, Vogelsang H, Becker I, et al. Germline mutations of the E-cadherin (*CDH1*) and TP53 genes, rather than of RUNX3 and HPP1, contribute to genetic predisposition in German gastric cancer patients. *J Med Genet.* 2004;41:e89.
68. Suriano G, Oliveira C, Ferreira P, et al. Identification of *CDH1* germline missense mutations associated with functional inactivation of the E-cadherin protein in young gastric cancer probands. *Hum Mol Genet.* 2003;12:575–582.
69. Oliveira C, Sousa S, Pinheiro H, et al. Quantification of epigenetic and genetic second hits in *CDH1* during hereditary diffuse gastric cancer syndrome progression. *Gastroenterology.* 009;136:2137–2148.
70. Simões-Correia J, Figueiredo J, Oliveira C, et al. Endoplasmic reticulum quality control: a new mechanism of E-cadherin regulation and its implication in cancer. *Hum Mol Genet.* 2008;17: 3566–3576.
71. Ghaffari SR, Dastan J, Rafati M, et al. Novel human pathological mutations. Gene symbol: *CDH1*. Disease: gastric cancer. *Hum Genet.* 2009;125:337.
72. Caron O, Schielke A, Svrcek M, et al. Usefulness of prophylactic gastrectomy in a novel large hereditary diffuse gastric cancer (HDGC) family. *Am J Gastroenterol.* 2008;103:2160–2161.
73. Li QL, Ito K, Sakakura C, et al. Causal relationship between the loss of RUNX3 expression and gastric cancer. *Cell.* 2002;109: 113–124.
74. Shibata DM, Sato F, Mori Y, et al. Hypermethylation of HPP1 is associated with hMLH1 hypermethylation in gastric adenocarcinomas. *Cancer Res.* 2002;62:5637–5640.
75. Park WS, Lee JH, Shin MS, et al. Inactivating mutations of the caspase-10 gene in gastric cancer. *Oncogene.* 2002;21:2919–2925.
76. Takaku K, Miyoshi H, Matsunaga A, et al. Gastric and duodenal polyps in Smad4 (Dpc4) knockout mice. *Cancer Res.* 1999;59: 6113–6117.
77. Lynch HT, Grady W, Suriano G, et al. Gastric cancer: new genetic developments. *J Surg Oncol.* 2005;90:114–33.
78. Duh FM, Scherer SW, Tsui LC, et al. Gene structure of the human MET proto-oncogene. *Oncogene.* 1997;15:1583–1586.
79. Nakajima M, Sawada H, Yamada Y, et al. The prognostic significance of amplification and overexpression of c-met and c-erb B-2 in human gastric carcinomas. *Cancer.* 1999;85:1894–1902.
80. Lee JH, Han SU, Cho H, et al. A novel germ line juxtamembrane Met mutation in human gastric cancer. *Oncogene.* 2000;19:4947–4953.
81. Kim I-J, Park J-H, Kang HC, et al. A novel germline mutation in the MET extracellular domain in a Korean patient with the diffuse type of familial gastric cancer. *J Med Genet.* 2003;40:97.
82. Chen JD, Kearns S, Porter T, et al. *MET* mutation and familial gastric cancer. *J Med Genet.* 2001;38:e26.
83. Biedermann K, Vogelsang H, Becker I, et al. Desmoglein 2 is expressed abnormally rather than mutated in familial and sporadic gastric cancer. *J Pathol.* 2005;207:199–206.
84. Grady WM, Willis J, Guilford PJ, et al. Methylation of the *CDH1* promoter as the second genetic hit in hereditary diffuse gastric cancer. *Nat Genet.* 2000;26:16–17.
85. Corso G, Roviello F, Paredes J, et al. Characterization of the P373L E-cadherin germline missense mutation and implication for clinical management. *Eur J Surg Oncol.* 2007;33:1061–1067.
86. Humar B, Guilford P. Hereditary diffuse gastric cancer and lost cell polarity: a short path to cancer. *Future Oncol.* 2008;4:229–239.
87. Humar B, Fukuzawa R, Blair V, et al. Destabilized adhesion in the gastric proliferative zone and c-Src kinase activation mark the development of early diffuse gastric cancer. *Cancer Res.* 2007; 67:2480–2489.
88. Avizienyte E, Frame MC. Src and FAK signalling controls adhesion fate and the epithelial-to-mesenchymaltransition. *Curr Opin Cell Biol.* 2005;17:542–547.
89. Gionti E, Capasso O, Capasso O, Cancedda R. The culture of chick embryo chondrocytes and the controlof their differentiated functions in vitro. Transformation by rous sarcoma virus induces a switch in the collagen type synthesis and enhances fibronectin expression. *J Biol Chem.* 1983;258:7190–7194.
90. da Cunha CB, Oliveira C, Wen X, et al. De novo expression of CD44 variants in sporadic and hereditary gastric cancer. *Lab Invest.* 2010;90:1604–1614.
91. Ponta H, Wainwright D, Herrlich P. Molecules in focus The CD44 protein family. *Int J Biochem Cell Biol.* 1998;30:299–305.
92. Riethmacher D, Brinkmann V, Birchmeier C. A targeted mutation in the mouse E-cadherin gene results in defective preimplantation development. *Proc Natl Acad Sci.* 1995;92:855–859.
93. Humar B, Blair V, Charlton A, et al. E-cadherin deficiency initiates gastric signet-ring cell carcinoma in mice and man. *Cancer Res.* 2009;69:2050–2056.
94. Karam R, Carvalho J, Bruno I, et al. The NMD mRNA surveillance pathway downregulates aberrant E-cadherin transcripts in gastric cancer cells and in *CDH1* mutation carriers. *Oncogene.* 2008;27:4255–4260.
95. Suriano G, Mulholland D, de Wever O, et al. The intracellular E-cadherin germline mutation V832 M lacks the ability to mediate cell-cell adhesion and to suppress invasion. *Oncogene.* 2003;22:5716–5719.
96. Suriano G, Ferreira P, Mateus AR, et al. Genetics of hereditary diffuse gastric cancer: progress and future challenges. *Future Oncol.* 2006;2:363–370.
97. Suriano G, Seixas S, Rocha J, Seruca R. A model to infer the pathogenic significance of *CDH1* germline missense variants. *J Mol Med.* 2006;84:1023–1031.
98. Fitzgerald RC, Caldas C. Clinical implications of E-cadherin associated hereditary diffuse gastric cancer. *Gut.* 2004;53:775–778.

99. Boterberg T, Vennekens KM, Thienpont M, et al. Internalization of the E-cadherin/catenin complex and scattering of human mammary carcinoma cells MCF-7/AZ after treatment with conditioned medium from human skin squamous carcinoma cells COLO 16. *Cell Adhes Commun*. 2000;7:299–310.
100. Suriano G, Oliveira MJ, Huntsman D, et al. E-cadherin germline missense mutations and cell phenotype: evidence for the independence of cell invasion on the motile capabilities of the cells. *Hum Mol Genet*. 2003;12:3007–3016.
101. Pereira PS, Teixeira A, Pinho S, et al. E-cadherin missense mutations, associated with hereditary diffuse gastric cancer (HDGC) syndrome, display distinct invasive behaviors and genetic interactions with the Wnt and Notch pathways in Drosophila epithelia. *Hum Mol Genet*. 2006;15:1704–1712.
102. Mateus AR, Seruca R, Machado JC, et al. EGFR regulates RhoA-GTP dependent cell motility in E-cadherin mutant cells. *Hum Mol Genet*. 2007;16:1639–1647.
103. Bajpai S, Correia J, Feng Y, et al. {alpha}-Catenin mediates initial E-cadherin-dependent cell-cell recognition and subsequent bond strengthening. *Proc Natl Acad Sci USA*. 2008;105:18331–18336.
104. Lewis FR, Mellinger JD, Hayashi A, et al. Prophylactic total gastrectomy for familial gastric cancer. *Surgery*. 2001;130:612–619.
105. van Kouwen MC, Drenth JP, Oyen WJ, et al. [18 F]Fluoro-2-deoxy-D-glucose positron emission tomography detects gastric carcinoma in an early stage in an asymptomatic *E-cadherin* mutation carrier. *Clin Cancer Res*. 2004;10:6456–6459.
106. Oliveira C, Moreira H, Seruca R, et al. Role of pathology in the identification of Hereditary Diffuse Gastric Cancer: Report of a Portuguese family. *Virchows Arch*. 2005;446:181–184.
107. Oelschlager BK, Yigit T, Kaufman JA, Pellegrini CA. Hereditary diffuse gastric cancer. *Med Gen Med*. 2005;7:16.
108. Newman EA, Mulholland MW. Prophylactic gastrectomy for hereditary diffuse gastric cancer syndrome. *J Am Coll Surg*. 2006;202:612–617.
109. Francis WP, Rodrigues DM, Perez NE, et al. Prophylactic laparoscopic-assisted total gastrectomy for hereditary diffuse gastric cancer. *JSLS*. 2007;11:142–147.
110. Chung D, Yoon S, Lauwers G, et al. A women with a family history of gastric and breast cancer. *N Engl J Med*. 2007;357:283–291.
111. Lynch HT, Kaurah P, Wirtzfeld D, et al. Hereditary diffuse gastric cancer: diagnosis, genetic counseling, and prophylactic total gastrectomy. *Cancer*. 2008;112:2655–2663.
112. Gaya DR, Stuart RC, McKee RF, et al. E-cadherin mutation-associated diffuse gastric adenocarcinoma: penetrance and non-penetrance. *Eur J Gastroenterol Hepatol*. 2005;17:1425–1428.
113. Koea JB, Karpeh MS, Brennan MF. Gastric cancer in young 524 patients: demographic, clinicopathological, and prognostic 525 factors in 92 patients. *Ann Surg Oncol*. 2000;7:346–351.
114. Kaurah P, Fitzgerald R, Dwerryhouse S, Huntsman DG. Pregnancy after prophylactic total gastrectomy. *Fam Cancer*. 2010;9:331–334.
115. Mareel M, Leroy A. Clinical, cellular, and molecular aspects of cancer invasion. *Physiol Rev*. 2003;83:337–376.
116. Yap AS, Kovacs EM. Direct cadherin-activated cell signaling: a view from the plasma membrane. *J Cell Biol*. 2003;160:11–16.
117. Crepaldi T, Pollack AL, Prat M, et al. Targeting of the SF/HGF receptor to the basolateral domain of polarized epithelial cells. *J Cell Biol*. 1994;125:313–320.
118. Hoschuetzky H, Aberle H, Kemler R. Beta-catenin mediates the interaction of the cadherin-catenin complex with epidermal growth factor receptor. *J Cell Biol*. 1994;127:1375–1380.
119. Qian X, Karpova T, Sheppard AM, et al. E-cadherin-mediated adhesion inhibits ligand-dependent activation of diverse receptor tyrosine kinases. *EMBO J*. 2004;23:1739–1748.
120. Comoglio PM, Boccaccio C, Trusolino L. Interactions between growth factor receptors and adhesion molecules: breaking the rules. *Curr Opin Cell Biol*. 2003;15:565–571.
121. Hermiston ML, Gordon JI. In vivo analysis of cadherin function in the mouse intestinal epithelium: essential roles in adhesion, maintenance of differentiation, and regulation of programmed cell death. *J Cell Biol*. 1995;129:489–506.
122. Ruoslahti E, Reed JC. Anchorage dependence, integrins, and apoptosis. *Cell*. 1994;77:477–478.
123. Frisch SM, Ruoslahti E. Integrins and anoikis. *Curr Opin Cell Biol*. 1997;9:701–706.
124. Hirata K, Ajiki T, Okazaki T, et al. Frequent occurrence of abnormal E-cadherin/beta-catenin protein expression in advanced gallbladder cancers and its association with decreased apoptosis. *Oncology*. 2006;71:102–110.
125. Ferreira P, Oliveira MJ, Beraldi E, et al. Loss of functional E-cadherin renders cells more resistant to the apoptotic agent taxol *in vitro*. *Exp Cell Res*. 2005;310:99–104.
126. Carvalho R, Milne AN, van Rees BP, et al. Early-onset gastric carcinomas display molecular characteristics distinct from gastric carcinomas occurring at a later age. *J Pathol*. 2004;204:75–83.
127. Milne AN, Carvalho R, Morsink FM, et al. Early-onset gastric cancers have a different molecular expression profile than conventional gastric cancers. *Mod Pathol*. 2006;19:564–572.
128. Mori M, Sugimachi K, Ohiwa T, et al. Early gastric carcinoma in Japanese patients under 30 years of age. *Br J Surg*. 1985;72:289–291.
129. Nakamura T, Yao T, Niho Y, Tsuneyoshi M. A clinicopathological study in young patients with gastric carcinoma. *J Surg Oncol*. 1999;71:214–219.
130. Ramos de la Medina A, Salgado-Nesme N, Torres-Villalobos G, Medina-Franco H. Clinicopathologic characteristics of gastric cancer in a young patient population. *J Gastrointest Surg*. 2004;8:240–244.
131. McGill TW, Downey EC, Westbrook J, et al. Gastric carcinoma in children. *J Pediatr Surg*. 1993;28:1620–1621.
132. Kokkola A, Sipponen P. Gastric carcinoma in young adults. *Hepatogastroenterology*. 2001;48:1552–1555.
133. Saito A, Kanai Y, Maesawa C, et al. Disruption of E-cadherin-mediated cell adhesion systems in gastric cancers in young patients. *Jpn J Cancer Res*. 1999;90:993–999.
134. Zhang Y, Liu X, Fan Y, et al. Germline mutations and polymorphic variants in MMR, E-cadherin and MYH genes associated with familial gastric cancer in Jiangsu of China. *Int J Cancer*. 2006;119:2592–2596.
135. de la Chapelle A. Genetic predisposition to colorectal cancer. *Nat Rev Cancer*. 2004;4:769–780.
136. Gruber SB. New development in Lynch syndrome (hereditary nonpolyposis colorectal cancer) and Mismatch repair gene testing. *Gastroenterology*. 2006;130:577–587.
137. Lynch HT, Smyrk TC, Watson P, et al. Genetics, natural history tumor spectrum, and pathology of hereditary non-polyposis colorectal cancer. An update review. *Gastroenterology*. 1993;104:1535–1549.
138. Capelle LG, Van Grieken NC, Lingsma HF, et al. Risk and epidemiological time trends of gastric cancer in Lynch syndrome carriers in the Netherlands. *Gastroenterology*. 2010;138:487–492.
139. Aaltonen LA, Peltomaki P, Leach FS, et al. Clues to the pathogenesis of familial colorectal cancer. *Science*. 1993;260:812–816.
140. Liu B, Parsons R, Papadopoulos N, et al. Analysis of mismatch repair genes in hereditary non-polyposis colorectal cancer patients. *Nat Med*. 1996;2:169–174.
141. Leite M, Corso G, Sousa S, et al. MSI phenotype and MMR alterations in familial and sporadic gastric cancer. *Int J Cancer*. 2010;128:1606–13.
142. Oliveira C, Suriano G, Ferreira P, et al. Genetic screening for familial gastric cancer. *Hered Cancer Clin Pract*. 2004;2:51–64.
143. Li FP, Fraumeni JF Jr. Rhabdomyosarcoma in children: epidemiologic study and identification of a familial cancer syndrome. *J Natl Cancer Inst*. 1969;43:1365–173.

144. Li FP, Fraumeni JF Jr. Soft-tissue sarcomas, breast cancer, and other neoplasms. A familial syndrome? *Ann Intern Med.* 1969;71:747–752.
145. Birch JM, Hartley AL, Tricker KJ, et al. Prevalence and diversity of constitutional mutations in the p53 gene among 21 Li-Fraumeni families. *Cancer Res.* 1994;54:1298–1304.
146. Frebourg T, Barbier N, Yan YX, et al. Germ-line p53 mutations in 15 families with Li-Fraumeni syndrome. *Am J Hum Genet.* 1995;56:608–615.
147. MacGeoch C, Turner G, Bobrow LG, et al. Heterogeneity in Li-Fraumeni families: p53 mutation analysis and immunohistochemical staining. *J Med Genet.* 1995;32:186–190.
148. Olivier M, Eeles R, Hollstein M, et al. The IARC TP53 database: new online mutation analysis and recommendations to users. *Hum Mutat.* 2002;19:607–614.
149. Palmero EI, Achatz MI, Ashton-Prolla P, et al. Tumor protein 53 mutations and inherited cancer: beyond Li-Fraumeni syndrome. *Curr Opin Oncol.* 2010;22:64–69.
150. Fenoglio-Preiser CM, Wang J, Stemmermann GN, Noffsinger A. TP53 and gastric carcinoma: a review. *Hum Mutat.* 2003;21:258–270.
151. Gomyo Y, Osaki M, Kaibara N, Ito H. Numerical aberration and point mutation of p53 gene in human gastric intestinal metaplasia and well-differentiated adenocarcinoma: analysis by fluorescence in situ hybridization (FISH) and PCR-SSCP. *Int J Cancer.* 1996;66:594–599.
152. Seruca R, David L, Holm R, et al. P53 mutations in gastric carcinomas. *Br J Cancer.* 1992;65:708–710.
153. Seruca R, David L, Castedo S, et al. p53 alterations in gastric carcinoma: a study of 56 primary tumors and 204 nodal metastases. *Cancer Genet Cytogenet.* 1994;75:45–50.
154. Seruca R, David L, Sobrinho-Simões M. Relationship between the expression of p53 and the aggressiveness of gastric carcinoma. *J Pathol.* 1997;181:349.
155. Bell DW, Varley JM, Szydlo TE, et al. Heterozygous germ line hCHK2 mutations in Li-Fraumeni syndrome. *Science.* 1999;286: 2528–2531.
156. Bachinski LL, Olufemi SE, Zhou X, et al. Genetic mapping of a third Li–Fraumeni syndrome predisposition locus to human chromosome 1q23. *Cancer Res.* 2005;65:427–431.
157. Lipton L, Tomlinson I. The genetics of FAP and FAP-like syndromes. *Fam Cancer.* 2006;5:221–226.
158. Vasen HF, Möslein G, Alonso A, et al. Guidelines for the clinical management of familial adenomatous polyposis (FAP). *Gut.* 2008;57:704–713.
159. Coffey RJ Jr, Knight CD Jr, van Heerden JA, et al. Gastric adenocarcinoma complicating Gardner's syndrome in a North American woman. *Gastroenterology.* 1985;88:1263–1266.
160. Park JG, Park KJ, Ahn YO, et al. Risk of gastric cancer among Korean familial adenomatous polyposis patients. Report of three cases. *Dis Colon Rectum.* 1992;35:996–998.
161. Lynch HT, Snyder C, Davies JM, et al. FAP, gastric cancer, and genetic counseling featuring children and young adults: a family study and review. *Fam Cancer.* 2010;9:581–588.
162. Knudsen AL, Bisgaard ML, Bulow S. Attenuated familial adenomatous polyposis (AFAP). A review of the literature. *Fam Cancer.* 2003;2:43–55.
163. Groden J, Thliveris A, Samowitz W, et al. Identification and characterization of the familial adenomatous polyposis coli gene. *Cell.* 1991;66:589–600.
164. Burt R, Neklason DW. Genetic testing for inherited colon cancer. *Gastroenterology.* 2005;128:1696–1716.
165. Al-Tassan N, Chmiel NH, Maynard J, et al. Inherited variants of MYH associated with somatic G:CRT: A mutations in colorectal tumors. *Nat Genet.* 2002;30:227–232.
166. Poulsen ML, Bisgaard ML. MUTYH Associated Polyposis (MAP). *Curr Genomics.* 2008;9:420–435.
167. Vogt S, Jones N, Christian D, et al. Expanded extracolonic tumor spectrum in MUTYH-associated polyposis. *Gastroenterology.* 2009;137:1976–1985.
168. Attard TM, Giardiello FM, Argani P, Cuffari C. Fundic gland polyposis with high-grade dysplasia in a child with attenuated familial adenomatous polyposis and familial gastric cancer. *J Pediatr Gastroenterol Nutr.* 2001;32:215–218.
169. Abraham SC, Park SJ, Mugartegui L, et al. Sporadic fundic gland polyps with epithelial dysplasia: evidence for preferential targeting for mutations in the adenomatous polyposis coli gene. *Am J Pathol.* 2002;161:1735–1742.
170. Weinstock JV, Kawanishi H. Gastrointestinal polyposis with orocutaneous hamartomas (Cowden's disease). *Gastroenterology.* 1978;74(5 Pt 1):890–895.
171. Al-Thihli K, Palma L, Marcus V, et al. A case of Cowden's syndrome presenting with gastric carcinomas and gastrointestinal polyposis. *Nat Clin Pract Gastroenterol Hepatol.* 2009;6:184–189.
172. Amos CI, Frazier ML, McGarrity TJ. Peutz Jeghers syndrome. In: Pagon RA, Bird TC, Dolan CR, Stephens K, (eds) GeneReviews [Internet]. Seattle (WA): University of Washington, Seattle; 1993–2001. [updated 2010 Nov 2].
173. Buck JL, Harned RK, Lichtenstein JE, Sobin LH. Peutz-Jeghers syndrome. *Radiographics.* 1992;12:365–378.
174. Giardiello FM, Welsh SB, Hamilton SR, et al. Increased risk of cancer in the Peutz-Jeghers syndrome. *N Engl J Med.* 1987;316:1511–1514.
175. Beggs AD, Latchford AR, Vasen HF, et al. Peutz-Jeghers syndrome: a systematic review and recommendations for management. *Gut.* 2010;59:975–986.
176. Takahashi M, Sakayori M, Takahashi S, et al. A novel germline mutation of the LKB1 gene in a patient with Peutz-Jeghers syndrome with early-onset gastric cancer. *J Gastroenterol.* 2004; 39:1210–1214.
177. Shinmura K, Goto M, Tao H, et al. A novel STK11 germline mutation in two siblings with Peutz-Jeghers syndrome complicated by primary gastric cancer. *Clin Genet.* 2005;67:81–86.
178. van Lier MG, Wagner A, Mathus-Vliegen EM, et al. High cancer risk in Peutz-Jeghers syndrome: a systematic review and surveillance recommendations. *Am J Gastroenterol.* 2010;105:1258–1264.
179. Hemminki A, Markie D, Tomlinson I, et al. A serine/threonine kinase gene defective in Peutz-Jeghers syndrome. *Nature.* 1998;391:184–187.
180. Jenne DE, Reimann H, Nezu J, et al. Peutz-Jeghers syndrome is caused by mutations in a novel serine threonine kinase. *Nat Genet.* 1998;18:38–43.
181. Alhopuro P, Phichith D, Tuupanen S, et al. Unregulated smooth-muscle myosin in human intestinal neoplasia. *Proc Natl Acad Sci USA.* 2008;105:5513–5518.

Cancer Predisposition Syndromes of the Gastrointestinal Tract

7

Ian S. Hagemann and Antonia R. Sepulveda

Introduction

Cancer predisposition syndromes affecting the gastrointestinal (GI) tract represent a small proportion of GI cancers and may arise in the background of a polyposis syndrome (Table 7.1). The molecular mechanisms underlying these syndromes have been instrumental in our understanding of the molecular basis of development and progression of the more frequent counterpart sporadic neoplasms, sharing many common molecular features. Syndromic hereditary cancers can involve any segment of the GI tract but predominantly involve the colon, and the most common cancers are colorectal adenocarcinomas (CRC). The most frequent inheritable GI cancer syndromes are those associated with germline mutations in the DNA mismatch repair (MMR) genes, in which case cancers do not arise in a polyposis background, and those attributed to underlying germline mutations in the *APC* or *MYH* genes in patients who manifest an adenomatous polyposis phenotype in the intestine. In addition to the well-characterized cancer syndromes, there are families with clustering of colon cancer, including patients with colon cancers before age 50, for whom the susceptibility gene loci have not been identified.[1–3]

I.S. Hagemann, M.D., Ph.D.
Department of Pathology and Immunology, Washington University, St. Louis, MO, USA

A.R. Sepulveda, M.D., Ph.D. (✉)
Department of Pathology & Cell Biology, Columbia University, 630 W 168th Street, VC-14 RM 212, New York, NY 10032, USA
e-mail: as4400@columbia.edu

Hereditary Non-Polyposis Colorectal Cancer–Lynch Syndrome

Clinical Features

Hereditary Non-Polyposis Colorectal Cancer, also known as Lynch syndrome (HNPCC/LS) is diagnosed on the basis of a germline mutation in one of the DNA MMR genes that results in deficient DNA mismatch repair (dMMR).[4–6] The deficiency of DNA mismatch repair results in increased mutation accumulation in the genome and higher risk of neoplastic transformation. HNPCC/LS represents an estimated 3–6% of all colorectal cancer cases.[4,7] HNPCC/LS is inherited as an autosomal dominant cancer predisposition syndrome, and is characterized by early onset of colorectal cancers, and increased frequency of cancers in the small bowel, stomach, biliary tract, pancreas, endometrium, ovary, urothelium (urinary bladder, ureter, and renal pelvis), brain, sebaceous gland adenomas, and keratoacanthomas.[5–9] The extra-gastrointestinal neoplasms associated with HNPCC/LS will be described in further detail later in this chapter. Sebaceous gland adenomas and keratoacanthomas are part of the Muir-Torre syndrome, whereas tumors of the brain, usually glioblastomas, occur in the Turcot syndrome.[5,9]

The average age of presentation of colorectal cancer in HNPCC patients is 45 years of age, but the disease can be discovered in older patients.[10,11] Tumors are located in the proximal colon in two-thirds of cases, but can occur in any segment of the gastrointestinal tract.[10,11] Tumors are often multiple or associated with other synchronous or metachronous neoplasms of the HNPCC-cancer spectrum.[5,7,9,10] HNPCC/LS patients are at higher lifetime risk for colorectal cancer than the general population, developing CRC in up to 80% and endometrial carcinoma in up to 60% of mutation carriers.[5]

A.R. Sepulveda and J.P. Lynch (eds.), *Molecular Pathology of Neoplastic Gastrointestinal Diseases*, Molecular Pathology Library 7, DOI 10.1007/978-1-4614-6015-2_7, © Springer Science+Business Media New York 2013

Table 7.1 Polyposis Syndromes of the Gastrointestinal Tract[172,173,180,181,187]

Syndrome	Major clinical features	Risk of CRC cancer	Gene	Gene product function
Familial adenomatous polyposis	>100 colonic adenomas; duodenal and periampullary adenomas; gastric fundic gland polyps	100% lifetime risk for colorectal carcinoma (later age in AFAP)	*APC*	Growth inhibitory: targets beta-catenin for destruction
–Gardner syndrome	FAP and CHRPE, osteomas, desmoid tumors			
–Turcot syndrome	FAP and medulloblastoma			
–Attenuated FAP (AFAP)	>15 but <100 colonic adenomas; other FAP manifestations are less frequent			
MYH-associated polyposis	FAP-like presentation: colonic adenomas; but no APC mutation identifiable	Slight increase in risk of CRC	*MYH*	DNA damage repair
Peutz-Jeghers syndrome	Hamartomatous gastrointestinal polyps; predisposition for multiple extracolonic malignancies	GI and extra-GI malignancies (>90% risk of cancer by 65 years of age)	*STK11*	Serine/threonine kinase
Cowden syndrome	Hamartomatous gastrointestinal polyps: juvenile type polyps, ganglioneuromas, lymphoid hyperplasia, lipomas	Rare GI malignancy	*PTEN*	Protein phosphatase
BRR syndrome	Hamartomatous gastrointestinal polyps: juvenile-type polyps	Rare GI malignancy	*PTEN*	Protein phosphatase
Juvenile polyposis	Hamartomatous gastrointestinal polyposis	Increased risk for colorectal carcinoma	*SMAD4 BMPR1A, ENG*	TGF-beta signaling
Neurofibromatosis type I	Neurofibromas; ganglioneuromas; malignant peripheral nerve sheath tumors	N/A	*NF1*	Negative regulator of Ras oncogene
Multiple endocrine neoplasia type II	Neural polyps: ganglioneuromas, most common in colon and rectum	N/A	*RET*	Proto-oncogene

The polyposis syndromes listed in the table are inherited as Mendelian autosomal dominant disorders, except for MYH-associated polyposis, which is inherited as an autosomal recessive disease. Two-thirds of Turcot syndrome occur in patients with APC gene mutation and one-third in DNA mismatch repair gene mutation (LS). *CHRPE* Congenital hypertrophy of the retinal pigment epithelium, *BRR* Bannayan–Ruvalcaba–Riley syndrome

Pathologic Features

Unique histopathologic features may be seen in colorectal adenocarcinomas with underlying dMMR that suggest the possibility of HNPCC/LS (reviewed in Gologan et al[11,12]), (Fig. 7.1). These features are not specific for HNPCC/LS cancers, and are also seen frequently in sporadic CRC with dMMR, as well as in some tumors that are proficient in DNA MMR.[11,13] Three major histopathologic groups of dMMR colorectal cancers can be recognized (reviewed in Gologan

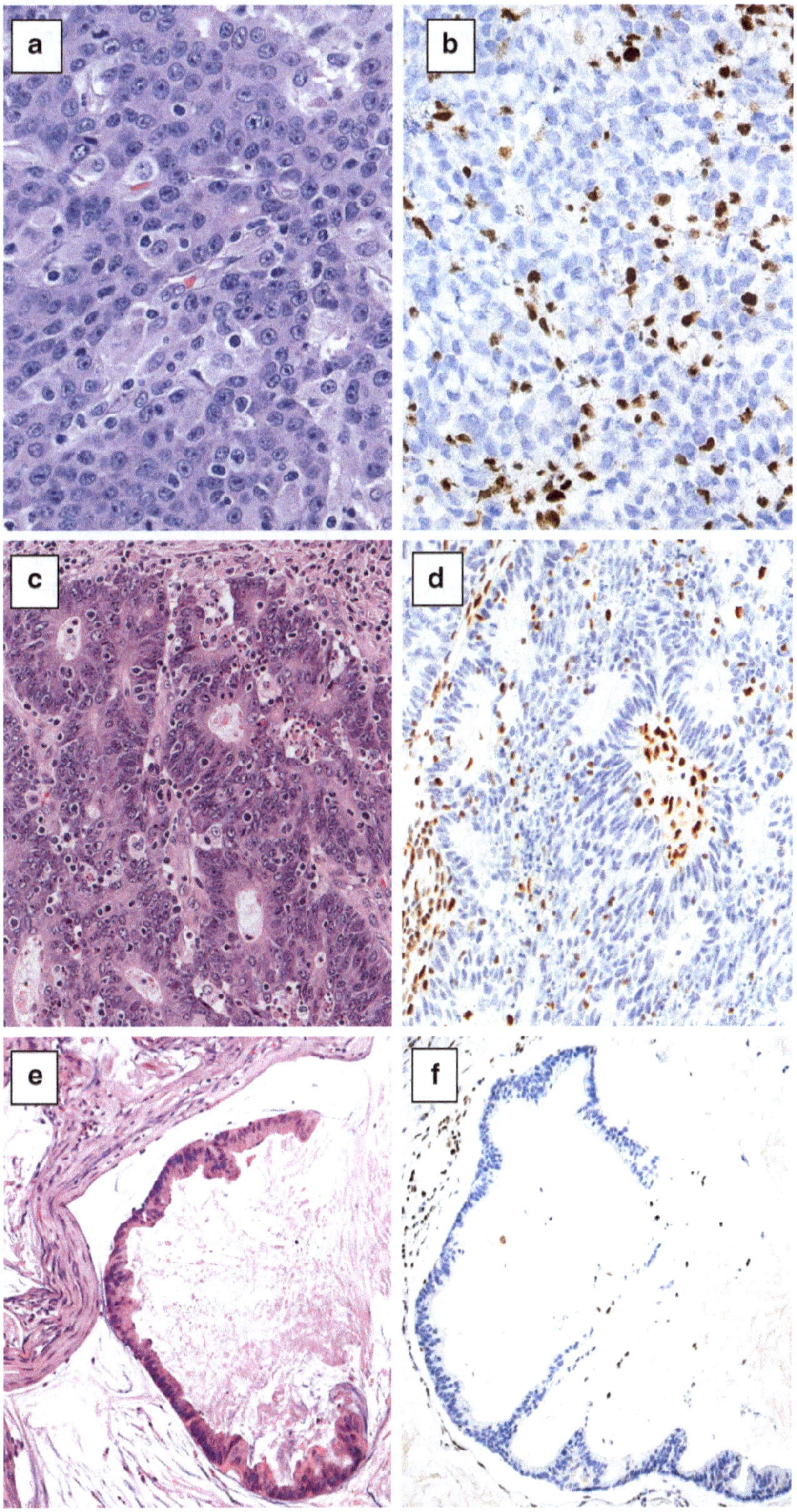

Fig. 7.1 (**a**) Poorly differentiated adenocarcinoma with medullary features, showing prominent TILs; (**b**) Immunohistochemistry for MLH1 shows loss of expression of the protein in tumor cell nuclei, whereas MLH1 remains positive in the nucleus of infiltrating lymphocytes and surrounding stromal cells. (**c**) Moderately differentiated CRC with prominent TILs. (**d**) Immunohistochemistry for MSH2 shows loss of expression in tumor cell nuclei, whereas MSH2 remains positive in the nucleus of infiltrating lymphocytes and surrounding stromal cells. (**e**) Mucinous adenocarcinoma (H&E). (**f**) Immunohistochemistry for MLH1 shows loss of expression in tumor cell nuclei. Original magnifications ×200

et al[12] (Fig. 7.1): (1) poorly differentiated adenocarcinomas, including medullary-type carcinomas, in which the neoplastic epithelium is infiltrated with high numbers of lymphocytes (tumor-infiltrating lymphocytes/TILs), and carcinomas with signet ring cell features; (2) mucinous adenocarcinomas, and (3) well to moderately differentiated adenocarcinomas. The presence of prominent intratumoral lymphocytes, with at least four lymphocytes infiltrating the tumor epithelium in a single 400× microscopic field,[11] is the most predictive histologic finding of dMMR in CRC (Fig. 7.1). TILs may be particularly numerous not only in poorly differentiated cancers but also occur in the other morphologic types of HNPCC/LS-associated cancers. The intratumoral lymphocytes are CD3-positive T cells and most are CD8-positive cytotoxic T lymphocytes. Peritumoral lymphocytic inflammation and lymphoid aggregates forming a Crohn-like reaction are also frequent in carcinomas with dMMR.[11,12,14–18]

Patients with HNPCC/LS typically develop a small number of colonic adenomas of traditional type (tubular or tubulovillous adenomas) at earlier age (mean 42–43, range 24–62 years) as compared to noncarriers of DNA mismatch repair gene mutations.[11,14–16,19–21] Progression from adenoma to invasive adenocarcinoma occurs rapidly, in many patients within less than 3 years, in contrast to an average of 15 years in patients without HNPCC/LS.[19,22] HNPCC/LS adenomas arise most frequently in the proximal colon and often contain high-grade dysplasia.[19,23]

Molecular Mechanisms of Cancer Development and Progression in HNPCC/LS

As introduced in Chap. 1 and further discussed in Chap. 8, deficiencies of DNA mismatch repair have been implicated in the development and progression of CRC in two contexts: (1) in HNPCC/LS patients with inhered DNA MMR gene mutations and (2) in patients with sporadic colorectal cancers, where deficient MMR is nearly always attributed to epigenetic silencing of the DNA MMR MLH1 gene.[24]

The two most frequent genes underlying MMR deficiency in HNPCC/LS are *MLH1* and *MSH2*. Although the reported proportions vary in different studies, HNPPC/LS patients inherit germline mutations affecting the coding regions of *MLH1* (approximately 40%), *MSH2* (approximately 40%), *MSH6* (approximately 10%), and *PMS2* (approximately 5%).[12,25–35] In addition to inherited germline mutations, germline epimutation of the promoter regions of *MLH1* or *MSH2* have been reported in rare cases of HNPCC/LS[35–37] (Table 7.1).

Deficient DNA MMR occurs when both alleles of one of the MMR genes are inactivated. During normal DNA replication, errors such as base mismatches and insertion or deletion loops, especially in repetitive regions, are corrected by the DNA mismatch repair proteins. MMR deficiency allows for replication-associated errors to be propagated in newly synthesized DNA strands (Fig. 7.2). In HNPCC/LS, pathogenic mutations of MMR genes are inherited and are present in constitutional DNA such as is found in peripheral blood; however, dMMR only develops in somatic tissues, especially in colonic epithelium and a few other cellular targets, when a second hit affects the MMR gene and leads to its loss of function. It has been shown that the second hits in HNPCC/LS can be caused by large or small chromosomal deletions or by mitotic recombination-mediated gene conversion, occurring in up to 46% of tumors.[3] Somatic methylation of the promoter of the wild-type allele occurs in some cases, affecting *MLH1* more often than *MSH2*.[3] Somatic point mutations are thought to be the least common second-hit mechanism.[3] The double allelic dMMR leads to a mutational phenotype that affects primarily repetitive nucleotides, known as microsatellite regions, with resulting microsatellite instability (MSI) seen in more than 90% of CRC cases in HNPCC/LS patients[10] (Fig. 7.3), as well as mutations in target genes that may contribute to neoplastic development.

The DNA MMR genes encode the MutS proteins MSH2, MSH3, and MSH6, and the MutL proteins MLH1, PMS1, PMS2, and MLH3[38,39] (Fig. 7.2). In the process of DNA MMR, the MMR proteins form heterodimers (MutS and MutL)[38,40–43] (Fig. 7.2). The MSH2 protein can interact with MSH6, forming the MutS-alpha complex, or with MSH3, forming the MutS-beta complex. MutS-alpha and MutS-beta heterodimers recognize and bind to post-DNA replication mismatched sequences. The MutS-alpha heterodimers are involved in the repair of single base mispairs and small insertion or deletion mispairs, whereas MutS-beta heterodimers primarily are involved in the correction of insertion or deletion mispairs.[44–46] MutL heterodimers bind MutS-alpha or MutS-beta.[38] Of the two possible MutL heterodimers, only MutL-alpha (MLH1 and PMS2) heterodimers are involved in DNA MMR, whereas the MutL-beta heterodimers (MLH1 and PMS1) do not appear to be significantly involved in DNA mismatch repair functions.[47,48] The MMR proteins are stabilized by heterodimerization, and loss of the heterodimer protein(s) may result in their degradation. Since MSH2 and MLH1 have two possible proteins to heterodimerize with (Fig. 7.2), their expression is only lost when their respective genes are primarily inactivated by a mutation or epigenetic silencing. However, MSH6 only heterodimerizes with MSH2, and PMS2 only heterodimerizes with MLH1; thus, loss of MSH6 expression can be secondary to primary loss of MSH2 and loss of PMS2 expression can be secondary to primary loss of MLH1 (Figs. 7.2, 7.4, and 7.5).

The molecular mechanisms that underlie the neoplastic development and progression in HNPCC/LS characterize the so-called microsatellite instability (MSI pathway).[32,49,51]

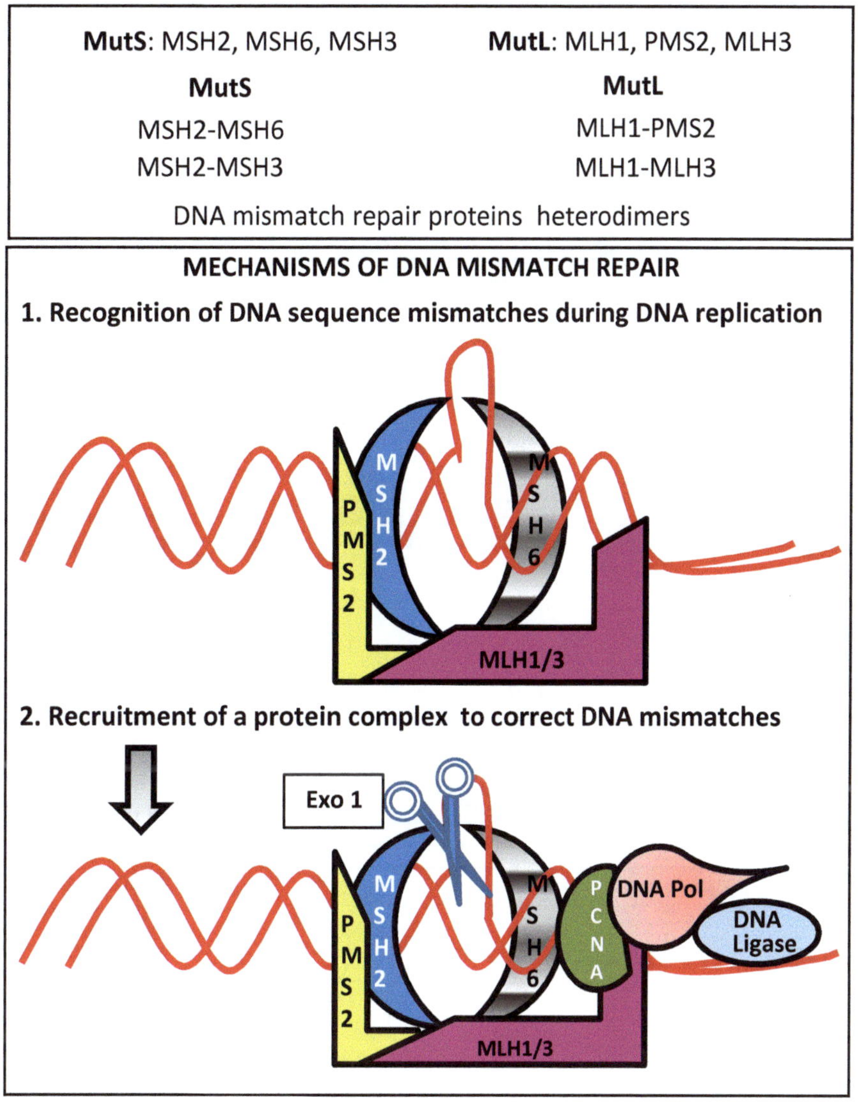

Fig. 7.2 DNA mismatch repair proteins and mechanisms of repair. MutS heterodimers (MSH2/MSH6 or MSH2/MSH3) recognize a DNA strand loop or base mismatch and recruit MutL (MLH1/PMS2) heterodimers to the site. Other molecules required for strand discrimination, helicase, endonuclease activity, resynthesis, and ligation are recruited in the complex with correction and maintenance of the native DNA sequence

As in sporadic MSI-pathway carcinomas, dMMR may lead to accumulation of mutations in cancer-related genes, such as the TGF-beta receptor II, *BAX*, and *MSH6* genes among others, in early pre-neoplastic cell populations as well as during the steps of neoplastic progression.[52] In contrast to sporadic CRC, patients with germline mutations in DNA mismatch repair genes do not carry *BRAF* activating mutations in their tumors.[53] *BRAF* V600E activating mutations have been reported in about 5% of all CRCs, 4–12% of CRC without microsatellite instability (MSS tumors), 40–70% of sporadic CRC with microsatellite instability (MSI-H), but are not seen in HNPCC/LS CRCs which nearly always show MSI-H.[54–56] HNPCC/LS tumors, similar to sporadic CRCs with dMMR, show frequent aberrant nuclear beta-catenin, but aberrant p53 expression, 5q loss of heterozygosity, and *KRAS* mutations are uncommon.[11]

Criteria for Identification of HNPCC/ LS Patients and Molecular Testing Approaches

Historically, the first criteria to identify patients with HNPCC/LS, known as the Amsterdam criteria, were established in the early 1990s, with subsequent revisions.[10,57] Later, more inclusive criteria, known as the Bethesda guidelines were established by a consensus group.[5,35,58–60] According to Amsterdam II Criteria, patients are diagnosed with HNPCC when[10]:

1. The family includes three or more relatives with an HNPCC-associated cancer, verified by pathological examination and:
   (a) One affected patient is a first-degree relative of the other two
   (b) two or more successive generations are affected

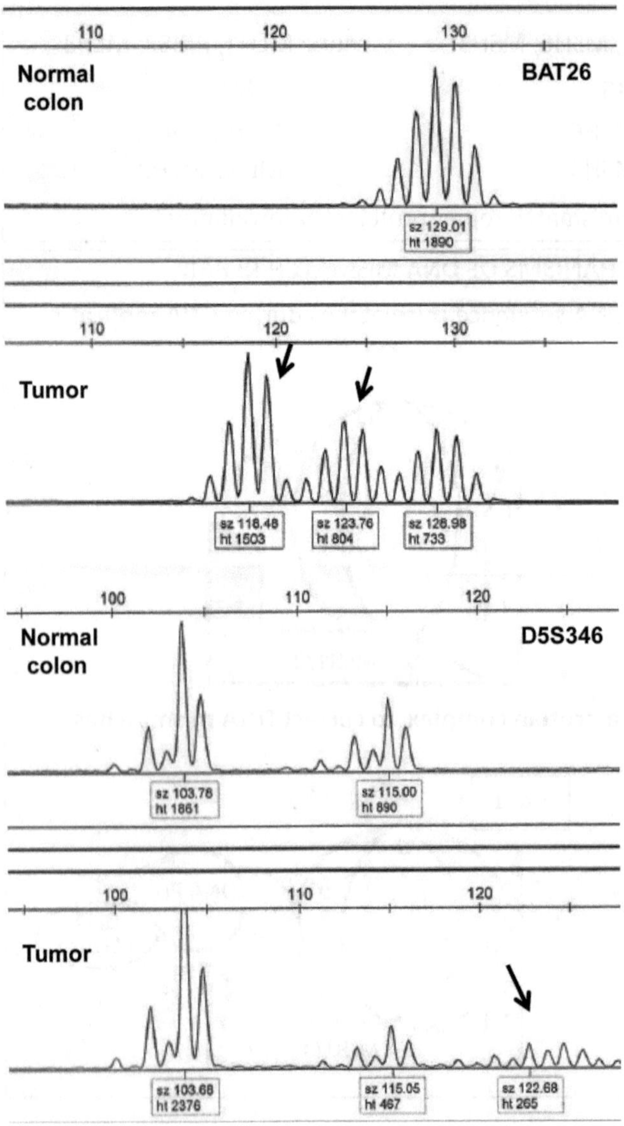

Fig. 7.3 Microsatellite instability detected by amplification of markers of the NCI panel. PCR amplification of the BAT26 locus reveals the appearance of novel alleles (*arrows*), of smaller size, in the tumor DNA as compared to non-neoplastic colonic DNA. The dinucleotide repeat marker D5S346 shows microsatellite instability characterized by a novel allele (*arrow*), of larger size, in the tumor DNA

   (c) cancer in one or more affected relatives is diagnosed before the age of 50 years
   (d) familial adenomatous polyposis is excluded.
2. Alternatively, patients meet one of the following modified Amsterdam criteria:
   (a) Very small families can be considered to have HNPCC with only two colorectal cancers in first-degree relatives if at least 2 generations have cancer and at least one case of CRC was diagnosed by the age of 55 years
   (b) In families with two first-degree relatives affected by colorectal cancer, the presence of a third relative with an unusual early onset neoplasm or endometrial cancer is sufficient
   (c) If an individual is diagnosed before the age of 40 years and does not have a family history that fulfills Amsterdam II or modified Amsterdam criteria, they are still considered as having HNPCC/LS.

The most recently revised Bethesda criteria recommend testing patients to rule out HNPCC/LS if there is one of the following criteria[5,35,59,60]:

1. Patient is diagnosed with colorectal cancer before the age of 50 years.
2. Patient has synchronous or metachronous colorectal cancer and another HNPCC-related tumor [stomach, urinary bladder, ureter and renal pelvis, biliary tract, brain (glioblastoma), sebaceous gland adenomas, keratoacanthomas, and small bowel], regardless of age.
3. Colorectal cancers with histopathologic features suggestive of dMMR–microsatellite instability: abundant tumor infiltrating lymphocytes, Crohn-like lymphocytic reaction, mucinous or signet ring cell differentiation, or medullary growth pattern of poorly differentiated adenocarcinoma, diagnosed before the age of 60 years.
4. Colorectal cancer patient with one or more first-degree relatives with CRC or other HNPCC-related tumors. One of the cancers must have been diagnosed before the age of 50 years.
5. Colorectal cancer patient with two or more relatives with colorectal cancer or other HNPCC-related tumors, regardless of age.

The revised Bethesda guidelines resulted in an increased identification of patients with dMMR as compared to previous guidelines, identifying not only more HNPCC/LS cancers but also more sporadic-type cancers with dMMR.[18] Given recent knowledge of the molecular changes underlying sporadic as compared to HNPCC-associated dMMR cancers, algorithms have been proposed to determine whether a patient has sporadic or HNPCC/LS cancers.[61] Alternatively, as discussed later, universal testing for dMMR of all CRC has been proposed.[3,62–64]

Molecular Testing for HNPCC/LS

The diagnostic workup for dMMR either due to HNPCC/LS or due to sporadic CRC is initiated by testing cancer tissue for DNA for microsatellite instability (MSI) (Fig. 7.3), the functional end point of dMMR, and/or by performing immunohistochemistry (IHC) of tumor tissues for MSH2, MLH1, MSH6, and PMS2 DNA mismatch repair proteins, to evaluate for their preserved (in DNA MMR-proficient tumors) or loss of expression (in deficient DNA MMR) tumor cell nuclei. Usually, CRC tissue is used for testing but other tumors of the HNPCC/LS spectrum, such as endometrial carcinoma, can be used.

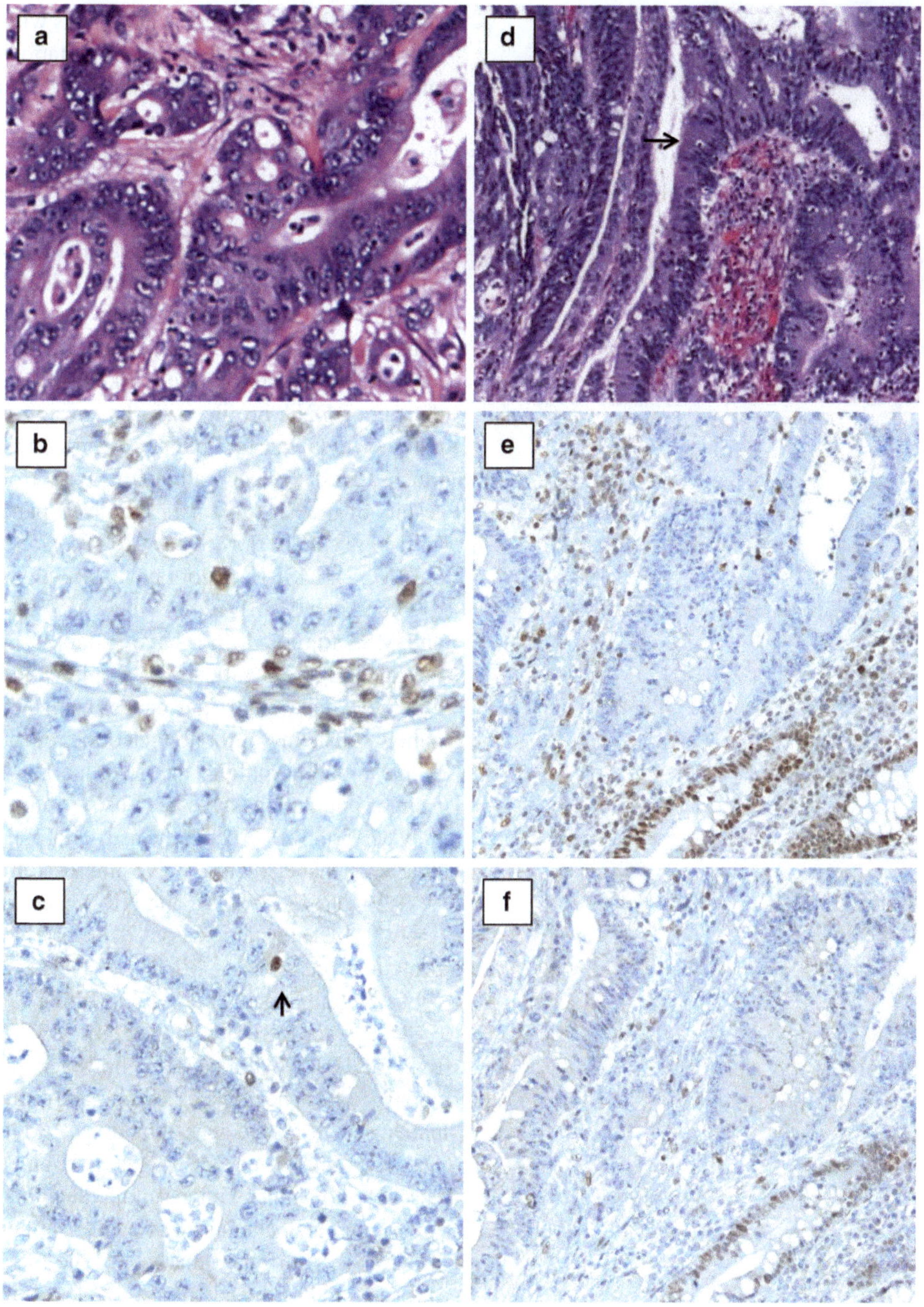

Fig. 7.4 Loss of expression of MLH1 (**b**) or MSH2 (**e**) is associated with loss of their MMR heterodimer proteins PMS2 (**c**) and MSH6 (**f**), respectively, exemplified in these two cases of moderately differentiated colonic adenocarcinoma. Note the prominent TILs in both cases, indicated by the *arrows* (**c** and **d**). Hematoxylin and Eosin stain (**a**) and (**b**).

MSI DNA Test

The DNA-based test to assess for microsatellite instability (MSI) in tumor cells is based on the evaluation of instability in small 100–200 base pair DNA segments that consist of repetitive nucleotides, called microsatellite regions or short tandem repeats (STRs). The nucleotide sequences within the repetitive elements of marker loci used in the MSI test are mononucleotide repeats of adenine $(A)_n$ or cytosine–adenine $(CA)_n$ dinucleotide repeats. During DNA replication these repetitive sequences may undergo variations in length due to DNA strand slippage, leading to increased or reduced length of STRs. In normal cells, proficient DNA MMR proteins are able to correct these replication-associated DNA sequence errors; however, in dMMR cells with loss of function of both

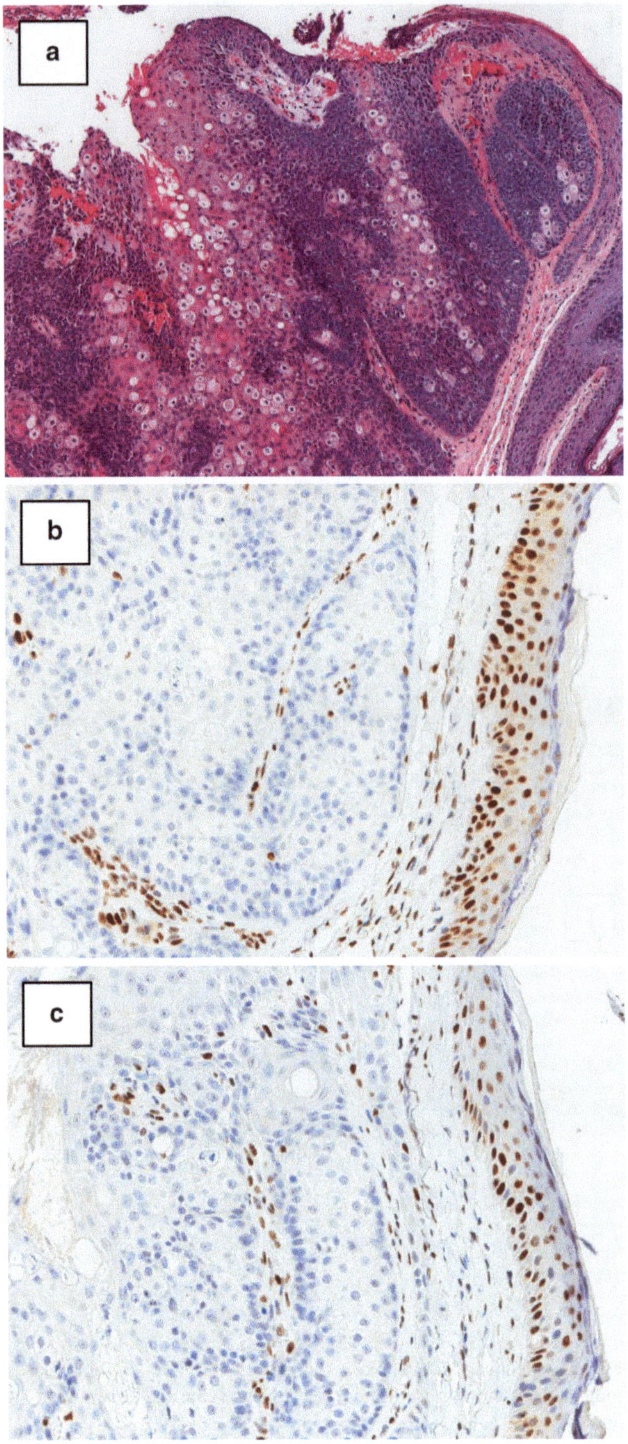

Fig. 7.5 Sebaceous adenoma in a patient with Muir-Torre syndrome (**a**) shows loss of expression of MSH2 (**b**) and MSH6 (**c**), suggestive of germline mutation in *MSH2* and secondary loss of MSH6 due to inability to form stabilizing heterodimers. (**a**) H&E stain, (**b** and **c**) immunohistochemistry

alleles, these mutations persist in the genome of daughter cells and in future cell generations in the tumor. The resulting changes in length of nucleotide repeats are known as microsatellite instability. Therefore, MSI can be detected in cells with dMMR, as occurs in patients with HNPCC/LS and sporadic dMMR cancers, as these mutations are not repaired and persist in the DNA of tumor cells. Tissue sections from formalin-fixed tumor tissue used for routine pathologic diagnosis and embedded in paraffin (FFPE) are adequate for the MSI test. Tumor enrichment by micro or macro-dissection is recommended. One of the most used sets of microsatellite markers was recommended by a NCI consensus group and consists of 5 loci: 2 poly(A) mononucleotide repeat markers (BAT25 and BAT26) and 3 poly(CA) dinucleotide repeat markers (D2S123, D5S346, and D17S250).[35,58] The NCI panel of five microsatellite markers requires comparison of the tumor DNA profile with that of non-neoplastic/normal tissue, which can be obtained from non-neoplastic colonic mucosa and adjacent wall layers, away from the tumor. The results of the MSI test using the NCI panel are reported as MSI-high (MSI-H), MSI-low (MSI-L), or microsatellite stable (MSS). MSI-H tumors have MSI in at least two of the five markers, MSI-L tumors have MSI in only one marker, and MSS tumors do not have instability at any of the five markers. Figure 7.3 illustrates amplification of the microsatellite loci in a colorectal cancer with MSI-H. Alternative panels consisting of mononucleotide repeat markers that are highly monomorphic in the germline DNA of a wide spectrum of populations have been used, with the advantage that they perform well without the use of normal control DNA.[65,66] One such panel includes five microsatellite loci (BAT-25, BAT-26, NR-21, NR-24, and NR-27) providing a pentaplex assay.[66–68] The pentaplex assay data correlate well with MMR protein expression for MLH1, MSH2, and PMS2, but less robustly with MSH6 expression, similar to the NCI panel.

Testing for MSI-H with the DNA MSI test is highly sensitive for HNPCC/LS cancers; however, the test may yield about 5% false negative cases among overall CRC cases from patients with MMR gene mutations.[4] Additionally, the MSI DNA test may detect MSI-H status in only 86% of the CRC cases from patients with germline mutations in MSH6.[4]

Immunohistochemistry of cancer tissues for DNA MMR proteins is a surrogate marker for the MSI status and when informative has the advantage of identifying the underlying deficient DNA mismatch repair gene based on the finding of which MMR protein is primarily lost in tumor cells. Overall, the sensitivity of immunohistochemistry to detect dMMR is about 95%.[4] Limitations of immunohistochemistry result in part from occasional problems with tissue immunoreactivity and interpretation pitfalls.[69] In MLH1-deficient tumors of sporadic type, where the *MLH1* gene is silenced by promoter methylation, IHC shows complete loss of MLH1 expression in tumor cells, and this is accompanied by parallel loss of PMS2, since the latter proteins are unstable in the absence of MLH1.[70] However, IHC may be difficult to interpret in cancers of HNPCC/LS patients with *MLH1* missense mutations that result in nonfunctional protein and MSI-H phenotypes, where the mutant protein may be expressed and retain its immunoreactivity, at least partially, with variable levels of expression of PMS2 in parallel.[70–72] In addition, MSI-H CRCs with preserved or variable expression of MLH1 protein, with associated loss or variably reduced PMS2 in tumor tissue, may represent a germline mutation in *PMS2*. IHC for MSH2 in HNPCC/LS patients with germline mutations in *MSH2* usually cause a complete loss of gene expression in tumor tissues, accompanied by loss of MSH6 protein expression, but IHC heterogeneity has been reported in a rare case.[70] Since both the MSI DNA test and IHC for DNA mismatch repair proteins will miss a small number of tumors in patients with underlying HNPCC/LS, it has been proposed to perform both tests upfront in the evaluation of CRC for potential HNPCC/LS.[73]

Genetic Testing for Constitutional Germline Mutations in DNA MMR Genes

If the tumor tissue reveals MSI-H and/or there is loss of expression of one of the DNA repair proteins by immunohistochemistry, constitutional germline testing should be performed for the gene encoding the deficient protein, after appropriate genetic counseling of the patient. If tissue testing is not feasible, or if there is sufficient clinical evidence of HNPCC/LS, germline analysis of the *MSH2* and/or *MLH1* genes can be done as first line testing.[35,61,74] Mutation analysis can be performed by using a number of approaches, including single-strand conformational polymorphism analysis, denaturing gradient gel electrophoresis analysis, DNA sequencing, monoallelic expression analysis, Southern analysis, and quantitative polymerase chain reaction.[35] Overall, the likelihood of finding a germline mutation in the *MLH1* or *MSH2* genes of patients with colorectal cancers that are not MSI-H is low.[35] The germline mutations that occur in *MSH2* and *MLH1* are widely distributed throughout the two genes. More than 200 pathogenic mutations have been reported in *MLH1* and in *MSH2*.[75]

Two additional tests, *MLH1* methylation and *BRAF* V600E activating mutation assays, may help discriminate between a sporadic MSI-tumor and HNPCC/LS tumor with loss of expression of *MLH1* by immunohistochemistry but an undetected *MLH1* mutation.[61] Using quantitative methylation analysis, HNPCC/LS patients showed no or low level of *MLH1* promoter methylation, in contrast to high levels of methylation (greater than a cutoff value of 18% methylation) in sporadic MSI-cancers.[24] In addition, none of the patients with an unambiguous germline mutation in DNA mismatch repair genes demonstrated *BRAF* activating mutation.[53] If no loss of expression of *MSH2, MLH1, MSH6,* or *PMS2* is seen in MSI-H tumors or if the tumor is MSI-L or MSS but there is clinical suspicion of HNPCC/LS testing for germline constitutional mutations in the DNA MMR genes should be performed.[35,76] Identification of a germline mutation in index cancer patients is important because it confirms the diagnosis of HNPCC/LS and the identified mutation may then be used to screen at risk relatives who may be mutation carriers and benefit from increased colonoscopic surveillance.

After a germline mutation is identified or the patient is diagnosed with HNPCC/LS, relatives should be referred for genetic counseling and testing should be offered. If no mismatch repair gene mutation is found in a proband with an MSI-H tumor and/or a clinical history of HNPCC/LS, the genetic test result is noninformative. The patients and the relatives at-risk should be counseled as if HNPCC/LS was confirmed and high-risk surveillance should be performed.[5,35,61]

Testing dMMR in Adenomas

In HNPCC/LS a significant association was found between MSI-H and high-grade dysplasia in adenomas, with loss of either MLH1 or MSH2 expression.[77] Based on these findings it was recommended that immunohistochemical staining/MSI testing of large adenomas with high-grade dysplasia in young patients (younger than 50 years) may be performed to help identify patients with suspected HNPCC/LS.[19,77]

Universal Testing of CRC for dMMR

During the past two decades, patients who presented with one of the tumors of the HNPCC/LS syndrome, in particular colon cancer, were offered testing for HNPCC/LS following guidelines based on family history (as described by the Amsterdam criteria) or based on a combination of family history, age of presentation, and histopathologic features of the tumor (as described by the Bethesda guidelines). However, more recently, studies have suggested a universal screening approach entailing the evaluation of all diagnosed colorectal cancers for markers of HNPCC/LS regardless of the family history.[3,62,64] One of these studies evaluated more than 1,000 patients with colorectal cancer whose tumors were tested for MSI.[78] Patients with MSI-positive tumors were tested for expression of MMR genes and germline mutations in *MSH2, MLH1, MSH6*, and *PMS2* by genomic sequencing and deletion studies. A mutation causing HNPCC/LS was detected in 23 patients (2.2%), of whom as many as 22% would have been missed if Amsterdam or Bethesda criteria had been used alone. In families that meet strict clinical criteria for HNPCC/LS, germline mutations in *MSH2* or *MLH1* have been found in 45–70% of the families, and overall, germline mutations in these two genes account for 95% of HNPCC/LS cases with an identified mutation.[31,74] These data show that despite extensive testing there is still a significant number of families without an identified germline mutation accounting for HNPCC/LS. It has been proposed that if an individual has a family history that is suggestive of HNPCC/LS, but does not fulfill the Amsterdam criteria, they are considered to represent an HNPCC variant, or familial colorectal cancer type X.[79,80] Further, it was observed that nearly 40–60% of all cases who meet Amsterdam criteria for HNPCC/LS do not have characteristic MMR deficiency or germline mutation in a DNA MMR gene. The age at diagnosis of these MSS familial CRC patients is 6 years older on average and most tumors occur on the left side of the colon.[2] The underlying genetic defect for these tumors is not yet known. Conversely there are also individuals who have tumors with MSI and germline mutation in a DNA MMR gene, but whose family history does not meet the Amsterdam criteria.[3]

In 2010, a consensus recommendation was published, stating that all CRCs should be screened using IHC for the four DNA MMR gene products, or alternatively by MSI, in order to evaluate for HNPCC/LS.[3] Another point raised by this consensus group was that MSI and IHC testing should not be considered genetic tests and should be ordered by appropriate medical personnel as needed for medical care.[3] Further, other investigators in the USA have advocated that all newly diagnosed colorectal and endometrial cancer patients should be screened for HNPCC/LS.[62,81–83] Review of this topic by the Evaluation of Genomic Applications in Prevention and Practice (EGAPP) working group[56] led to the recommendation that all newly diagnosed colorectal cancer patients should be screened for HNPCC/LS to reduce the morbidity and mortality from colorectal cancer in their at-risk unaffected relatives. A cost analysis of several possible screening methods indicated that the most cost-effective approach for screening all newly diagnosed colorectal cancer patients for HNPCC/LS would be to test tumor tissue with IHC followed by genetic testing in patients in whom any MMR protein was absent, after ruling out epigenetic (*MLH1* CpG methylation) causes of protein absence to exclude sporadic dMMR cases.[84] However, as reviewed earlier in this chapter, it should be cautioned that IHC alone will miss a small proportion of MSI-H cancers.[73] A report from the Association for Molecular Pathology proposed a testing strategy combining IHC for the four DNA MMR proteins and MSI DNA test upfront, followed by *BRAF* and *KRAS* mutation testing, serving both the purposes of screening for HNPCC/LS as well as for evaluation for targeted anti-EGFR therapies.[73]

Extra-colonic Neoplasia in Lynch Syndrome

Early-onset colorectal cancer (CRC) is the hallmark of HNPCC/LS, but it has been estimated that extracolonic manifestations may be as common as CRC, particularly in women. MMR germline mutations collectively confer an 80% risk of CRC before age 70 in men and 30–50% in women.[85,86] In comparison, the best characterized of the extracolonic manifestations is early-onset endometrial cancer, which occurs in an estimated 40–60% of at-risk patients.[4,85,87]

Weaker but definite associations[10] have been made between LS and cancers of the ovary, stomach, hepatobiliary tract, and small bowel, transitional cell carcinoma of the ureter and renal pelvis, glioblastoma (Turcot variant of Lynch syndrome), and sebaceous adenoma/carcinoma (Muir-Torre variant of Lynch syndrome).[88]

Breast cancer has often been detected in patients with LS.[89–95] The lifetime (to age 70) risk of breast cancer in LS patient series has been 2.2–5.4%.[87,96] This risk is not convincingly higher than the 7.6% rate seen in the general population,[97] in contrast to the dramatic enrichment seen for most LS-associated tumors.[96] It remains unsettled whether breast cancer is part of the LS spectrum.

While there are no conclusive studies linking LS with other cancers, case reports have suggested potential associations of LS with cancer of the pancreas, adrenal cortical carcinoma,[98] sarcomas (malignant fibrous histiocytoma,[99] rhabdomyosarcoma,[100] liposarcoma[101,102]), prostate cancer,[103] and neurofibromatosis-like features including café-au-lait macules and plexiform neurofibromas.[104]

The prevalence of extracolonic tumors in HNPCC/LS is variable and reflects the incomplete penetrance of the underlying mutation. CRC is relatively more common in *MLH1* germline mutants, while other cancers are more common in *MSH2* mutation.[88] *MSH6* mutation also appears to favor endometrial cancer.[88] *PMS2* mutants tend to present with atypical tumors in childhood.[88]

Endometrial Cancer

Endometrial cancer (EC) is the most common extracolonic manifestation of HNPCC/LS and has been extensively studied and reviewed.[105–110] The cumulative incidence of EC was 60% to age 70 in a study of 183 Finnish women with confirmed MMR mutations,[87] compared with 54% for colorectal cancer in the same population. Other series of women with MMR mutations showed a 42% lifetime risk of EC and 30–54% lifetime risk of CRC.[85,111]

EC becomes all the more salient as a feature of Lynch syndrome when one notes that CRC is less common in women than in men with HNPCC/LS, for whom the lifetime cumulative incidence of CRC is 74–83%.[85,111]

Given that its cumulative incidence approaches or exceeds that of CRC, it is clear that EC may be the sentinel cancer in some Lynch syndrome patients and kindreds. In a series of 111 women meeting Amsterdam criteria and having both CRC and EC, the CRC presented first in 49 (median age of 40), EC presented first in 46 (median age of 45), and the tumors presented simultaneously in 12.[112] When EC presented first in this series, the mean lead time before subsequent development of CRC was 11 years, allowing for follow-up and prevention if the Lynch phenotype is successfully identified.[112] The converse situation, of course, also provides an opportunity for cancer prevention, since Lynch-associated CRC patients have a markedly elevated risk of subsequently developing endometrial cancer (10-year cumulative risk of 23.4% in LS patients, versus 1.6% in patients with sporadic CRC).[113] The reported average lead time from CRC to the second malignancy (usually EC or ovarian carcinoma) was 8 years.[112]

LS-associated EC occurs at a younger age than sporadic cancer, and Lynch syndrome is more common in women presenting with EC at a young age. Functionally significant MMR gene mutations are present in 1.4–2.6% of EC overall,[114,115] but 9% of EC occurring before age 50.[116] Young age at presentation of EC has therefore been proposed as a trigger for further testing, usually either IHC testing for loss of MMR proteins or molecular testing for the MSI phenotype. Importantly, LS patients with EC are less likely than average women to fit the typical clinical profile of EC (obese, nulliparous), given that their tumors arise due to a genetic lesion. Thus, low BMI, family history suggestive of LS, and LS-associated histology (see below) have all been suggested as additional features to prompt further testing.[117] Using age below 50 as the main trigger for further testing would, however, result in low sensitivity for detecting Lynch syndrome. In one study of 562 unselected EC patients, the 13 women with eventual discovery of LS had a mean age of 54.1 years at diagnosis.[82] In another group of 7 women with Lynch syndrome related to inactivating *MSH6* mutations, the mean age at diagnosis was 54.8 years, compared to 64.6 years in the overall population.[118]

There are conflicting data on the prognosis of LS-associated EC, with some studies showing no difference in 5-year survival between LS patients and matched controls.[119–121] Other studies have variously shown either worse[122] or better survival[123] in MSI-H tumors. Taking these data together, it appears to be difficult to demonstrate a significant prognostic difference in LS-associated EC. Its prognostic importance lies, rather, in the likelihood of observing other associated malignancies in the patient and family members.

Pathologic Features

HNPCC/LS-associated endometrial carcinoma has a characteristic morphology.[124–127] Typical features include numerous peritumoral and tumor-infiltrating lymphocytes (TILs). These features related to the inflammatory response are reminiscent of the Crohn-like reaction and dense TILs that are common in MSI-H CRC cases. Both features show a statistically significant association with MSI-H status, but neither of them is sensitive or specific enough to serve as a diagnostic marker.[124] Although there appears to be no specific TIL density that sensitively and specifically identifies MSI-H cases,[125] 40 TILs/10 HPF (using a 400× high-power field) was suggested in one study as an analytically useful cutoff by which to define this feature.

The majority of LS-associated EC is of endometrioid histology, but these endometrioid cases show some propensity to demonstrate a biphasic morphology in which a typical, rather well-differentiated endometrioid adenocarcinoma (FIGO grade 1 or 2) is admixed with an undifferentiated component.[124,125] The resulting "dedifferentiated" carcinoma must, by definition, contain at least 10% of each component. 21% of MSI-H cases showed this phenotype versus 6% of non-MSI-H cases ($p = 0.06$).[124]

LS-associated EC also shows a propensity toward nonendometrioid histology. One series of 23 patients with germline MMR mutations consisted of 57% endometrioid tumors and 43% nonendometrioid ones, while sporadic controls were 96% endometrioid.[128] Two other reports have shown endometrioid histology in 86–87% of LS-associated cases, as compared to >96% in both sporadic controls[129] and *MLH1* hypermethylated cases.[118,129] The nonendometrioid tumors were predominantly serous, clear cell, and carcinosarcoma in these reports.

It has been reported that the prevalence of LS is higher in patients with carcinoma of the lower uterine segment (29%) as compared to the general population with endometrial cancer.[130]

Molecular Features

EC can be associated with mutation in any of the MMR genes (*MSH2*, *MLH1*, *MSH6*, *PMS2*). However, the lifetime risk of EC appears to be highest in *MSH6* mutation, followed by *MSH2* and *MLH1*.[131] This is the inverse of the behavior seen for CRC in women, for which the lifetime risk is highest for *MLH1* mutants and lowest for *MSH6*. Indeed, while *MSH6* mutation has been considered something of a hypomorph from the viewpoint of CRC, it is potentially the most significant of the MMR proteins from the viewpoint of EC. Data on EC risk in *PMS2* mutants are relatively scarce, but in one series of 61 confirmed mutants, the cumulative risk of EC was 15% to age 70 years, showing the penetrance of *PMS2* mutation to probably be lower than the other three MMR genes.[132]

Ovarian Cancer

An estimated 5–10% of epithelial ovarian cancers (EOC) are hereditary, consisting mainly of those associated with *BRCA1* and *BRCA2* mutations.[110,133] LS patients make up most of the remaining 10–15% of hereditary epithelial ovarian cancer cases.[110,134] Although these figures suggest that approximately

1% of ovarian cancer is associated with LS, the MSI-H phenotype is present in approximately 12% of all EOC cases,[135] indicating that this defect probably arises de novo and plays a pathogenetic role in many sporadic tumors.

LS-associated ovarian cancers present at an earlier age than sporadic tumors (mean 49.5 versus 60.9 years).[134,136] These cases are also identified at earlier stages than sporadic tumors. In one study, the stage at diagnosis was FIGO I for LS-associated tumors, but FIGO III for sporadic ones.[136] Both age and stage differences, when they occur, probably reflect more active screening in the Lynch patients. However, a stage difference was not seen in a series of 37 hereditary ovarian cancers that included predominantly *BRCA* mutants, although these would presumably also have been heavily screened (in an era, however, predating the appreciation of the role of the fallopian tube in EOC carcinogenesis).[134]

Pathologic Features

EOCs in general exhibit several histologic patterns. In sporadic cases, the most common histology is serous (accounting for as many as 78% of all EOCs), followed by endometrioid, mucinous, clear cell, and malignant Brenner tumor in decreasing order of frequency.[137,138] Carcinomas of mixed or indeterminate (i.e., poorly differentiated) histology also occur. LS-associated and MMR-deficient EOCs appear to be enriched in nonserous histologies, which in one meta-analysis constituted 57% of LS-associated ovarian cancers (128 patients in 6 studies).[139] In this meta-analysis, 25% of LS-associated EOCs were endometrioid, 17% were clear cell, and 16% were mucinous. Similar proportions were found in MSI-H tumors occurring outside the context of Lynch syndrome, suggesting that the relative scarcity of serous tumors somehow reflects the biology of the MMR-deficient state.[86]

The prognosis of EOC in Lynch patients appears to be similar to that of non-Lynch controls. In one report, there was a small and statistically insignificant decrement in overall survival for Lynch patients,[136] conceivably attributable to these patients' risk of other malignancies. This situation contrasts with that for CRC, where survival is better in Lynch-associated tumors versus sporadic ones.[4]

Gastric Cancer

Gastric cancer was present, along with CRC and EC, in the original "family G of Warthin" in whom LS was initially described. A study of 60 families from a Brazilian registry found a history of gastric cancer in 12/1,040 = 1.1% of men and 12/1,055 = 1.1% of women meeting Amsterdam I or II criteria.[89] The prevalence of gastric cancer in a Dutch LS registry population was similar (21/948 = 2.2% of men, 11/1,066 = 1.0% of women); Kaplan-Meier analysis in this population gave an estimated incidence of 6.2% in men and 2.0% in women to age 70.[140] In the Dutch series, gastric cancer occurred only in *MSH2* and *MLH1* mutant kindreds. *MSH6* mutation was well represented in the sample, but was not associated with any gastric cancers. *PMS2* mutants had no gastric cancers, but represented only two of the 236 families.

The histology of Lynch-associated gastric cancers is predominantly intestinal type in the Lauren classification (at least two-thirds of patients), the remainder being of diffuse type.[140,141] This finding is somewhat unexpected, given that the diffuse type is statistically more likely to have a primary genetic etiology (e.g., in hereditary diffuse gastric carcinoma).[142,143] Intestinal-type tumors are numerically more common than diffuse type in the genetically normal background population (51% intestinal type, 37% diffuse type).[144] *H. pylori* was noted in only 20% of LS-associated gastric cancers,[141] a fraction that is lower relative to the general gastric cancer population and reflects the presence of an inherited cancer predisposition. The histologic pattern of LS-associated gastric cancer is not distinctive enough to be used to triage patients for further testing in the absence of contributory personal or family history.

Pancreatobiliary Carcinoma

The cumulative lifetime risk of pancreatobiliary carcinoma in confirmed and presumed MMR gene mutation carriers has been estimated at 2–4% to age 70,[87,96] compared with 0.2% in the general population. These tumors appear to be almost entirely cholangiocarcinomas arising at various sites along the biliary tract, including common bile duct (7/18 in a series of 315 Finnish subjects), ampulla of Vater (4/18), intrahepatic biliary tree (4/18), and pancreas (3/18).[145] A mucinous cholangiocarcinoma has been reported in a patient with Muir-Torre syndrome related to *MSH2* mutation.[146] LS does not seem to have an association with gallbladder cancer.

Small Intestinal Carcinoma

Carcinomas of the small bowel are approximately 100 times more common in LS than in the general population, with a cumulative lifetime risk of 4%.[147] This is roughly similar to the relative risk in Crohn disease or familial adenomatous polyposis.[148] The cancer risk is higher in *MSH2* and *MLH1* mutants, and lower in *MSH6* and *PMS2*.[149] Small bowel tumors in LS are adenocarcinomas, have up to 3:1 male:female bias,[147] have no particular site of predilection within the small bowel, and may occur synchronously at several sites.[148] The median age at diagnosis is 40–50, at least a decade younger than the general population with small bowel cancer.[147,148] As in the colon, the prognosis for patients with small bowel carcinoma in the setting of Lynch syndrome may be slightly better than for the general population.[148]

Transitional Cell Carcinoma

Lynch syndrome carries a 22-fold increased risk of transitional cell carcinoma (TCC) of the upper urinary tract (renal pelvis and ureter),[150] occurring in approximately 4% of the Lynch syndrome population.[87,111,151] There is no increase in TCC of the bladder in LS.[150,152] The tumors present around age 56, a decade earlier than in the background population.[150] They have an MSI phenotype,[153] confirming that they are part of the Lynch syndrome spectrum. Special histologic features of these tumors have not been described.

CNS Tumors in Turcot Syndrome

The eponym "Turcot syndrome" has been used to describe the association of colorectal and CNS tumors. It is now apparent that this association occurs in two distinct sets of patients with fundamentally different genetic lesions.[154] The larger group has APC mutations, with the characteristic florid pancolonic polyposis, and with medulloblastoma as the CNS manifestation. A smaller group of patients has MMR mutations, typical Lynch-type CRC, and glioblastoma as the CNS manifestation.[155] Intriguingly, much as CRC associated with Lynch syndrome has a favorable prognosis, the survival of Turcot patients with glioblastoma appears to be better than that of patients with sporadic glioblastoma, although the number of patients reported is small.[155]

Sebaceous Adenoma/Carcinoma in Muir-Torre Syndrome

The Torre syndrome,[156] simultaneously reported by Muir,[157] was initially believed to represent the co-occurrence of cutaneous lesions with visceral malignancies, without mention of any familial association. It was subsequently noted that several of these patients belonged to families with what was then known as the cancer family syndrome, now HNPCC/LS.[158] The cutaneous lesions are frequently sebaceous adenomas, sebaceous carcinomas, or keratoacanthomas, i.e., low-grade squamous cell carcinomas arising from the pilosebaceous unit.

Further study has confirmed Muir-Torre syndrome (MTS) to be a variant of Lynch syndrome[159] defined by the presence of sebaceous skin neoplasms. The skin lesions of MTS have MMR mutations, usually in *MSH2*,[160] and a MSI-H phenotype.[161,162] The presence of sebaceous neoplasms is variably penetrant, having been reported in 28% of families and 9.2% of individuals meeting criteria for LS. There were 42% of kindreds with *MSH2* mutations, and 44% of kindreds with *MLH1* mutations, that had at least one individual with MTS, while MTS was not found in kindreds with *MSH6* or *PMS2* mutation.

HNPCC/LS: Clinical Management

Colorectal Cancer

Carriers of DNA mismatch repair gene mutations seen in HNPCC/LS are recommended to have colonoscopic surveillance staring at early age.[61] Colonoscopy is recommended every 1–2 years starting at age 20–25 years (age 30 years for those with *MSH6* mutations). For individuals who will undergo surgical resection of colon cancer, subtotal colectomy may be favored.

Endometrial and Ovarian Cancer

Patients Without Known Lynch Syndrome

Although identification of a CRC meeting Amsterdam or Bethesda criteria has been suggested as a cue to screen for EC, it appears that EC is more common than CRC in these patients, indicating that EC with appropriate features may equally well be taken as a sentinel event to identify Lynch syndrome patients and families.[127] Examining the converse situation, in a prospective study of 100 women with endometrial cancer diagnosed before age 50, nine carried germline MMR mutations (seven *MSH2* mutants, one *MLH1* mutant, and one *MSH6* mutant).[116]

MMR testing by immunohistochemistry, MSI testing, or gene sequencing is commonly recommended when faced with a new diagnosis of colon cancer in an appropriate clinicopathologic setting. Similar reasoning dictates that EC patients of sufficiently low age be tested for MMR mutations (with age <50 years often suggested as a cutoff). As has been mentioned, the prevalence of such mutations is in the neighborhood of 9%.[116] As age rises, the relative number of Lynch-associated mutations would be expected to fall, as sporadic tumors begin to predominate, but in absolute terms, Lynch cases continue to accumulate. Furthermore, with rising age, sporadic hypermethylation begins to predominate as a cause of *MLH1* silencing, causing an apparent dMMR/MSI phenotype in a patient with no germline mutation and no increased tumor risk at other sites. Thus the relative diagnostic utility of immunohistochemistry as compared to other methods can be expected to change with age.

A consensus statement of the Society of Gynecologic Oncologists instructs practitioners to identify women who have a 20–25% chance of having an inherited predisposition to endometrial, colorectal, and related cancers, for whom genetic risk assessment is "recommended," and those with a 5–10% chance of the same, for whom genetic risk assessment "may be helpful".[163] The SGO statement does not specify the form that the risk assessment should take, but underlines the need for it to be integrated with genetic counseling and education. Since LS-associated malignancies are uncommon before age 21, it is suggested that the benefits of testing do not outweigh its potential adverse effects in this age group.

Strategies for risk assessment in the patient with EC and suspected Lynch syndrome resemble those available in CRC, with immunohistochemistry, MSI testing, and gene sequencing representing the state of the art in approximately increasing order of cost.[117] Application of the Amsterdam criteria to triage patients for testing increases specificity at the cost of decreased sensitivity. As in CRC, immunohistochemical staining of the endometrial tumor for MSH2, MLH1, MSH6, and PMS2 is a simple gatekeeper strategy that can serve as a useful initial screen. When sequencing is used, nonsense mutations are relatively simple to interpret, but missense mutations are heterogeneous and may or may not be of clinical significance.[82]

Several heuristics[116,163] or specific algorithms[4,105,117,124] have been proposed to combine clinicopathologic features with stepwise diagnostic testing in order to achieve sensitivity and specificity while minimizing cost.[117] While the relative merits of each specific testing strategy will depend on the cost–benefit tradeoffs one chooses to make, the lowest cost-effectiveness ratio appears to be achieved with four-protein immunohistochemistry, followed by confirmatory sequencing of any putatively affected gene.[117] When cost represents a major consideration, an initial panel consisting only of MSH6 and PMS2 IHC can provide clues regarding dMMR status at a reduced cost.[164]

Patients with Suspected Lynch Syndrome

Once a presumptive diagnosis of Lynch syndrome has been established, further management can involve a combination of surveillance and, potentially, prophylactic surgery. For women, in whom EC and EOC are the main malignancies to exclude, proposed surveillance models usually involve imaging, usually by ultrasound, and periodic endometrial sampling.[105,165–169]

Other HNPCC/LS Associated Carcinomas

Patients Without Known Lynch Syndrome

Endometrial and ovarian cancers are markedly more common than the other extracolonic Lynch-associated tumors and have been the focus of most of the research on screening. However, when other tumors associated with the syndrome present at a young age or with suspicious family history, tumor testing for features of Lynch syndrome is broadly recommended. As for endometrial cancer, IHC testing for loss of MMR proteins or molecular testing for MSI are both appropriate initial modalities, without clear consensus to favor one over the other.[152] DNA sequencing should be reserved for later steps of the investigation due to its expense and complexity.[170] For clinicians, it is important to emphasize the details of family history and to inform the pathologist of these details so that testing can be initiated or justified.

Patients with Suspected Lynch Syndrome

The heterogeneity in extracolonic tumors between Lynch kindreds and between patients within a given kindred,[111] combined with the relatively low frequency of any given extracolonic tumor, makes it difficult to recommend any specific screening protocol in patients with suspected or confirmed Lynch syndrome. For some tumors, such as glioblastoma, no specific screening method seems practical. In the case of the small bowel, screening by capsule endoscopy or double-balloon enteroscopy has been suggested; rough calculations with rather favorable assumptions suggest a reasonable cost per QALY if screening is performed once above age 40.[147] Urine cytology is a straightforward screening method for transitional cell carcinoma. None of these methods have been explicitly adopted or endorsed, and screening of the Lynch patient therefore seems to currently require an individualized approach.

Polyposis Syndromes of the Gastrointestinal Tract

Polyposis syndromes are characterized by the development of variable numbers of polypoid lesions throughout the colon, small intestine, and stomach and include developmental polypoid abnormalities or hamartomatous polyps, inflammatory-type polyps, and adenomas. The risk of adenocarcinoma is highest in the syndromes that develop adenomas, but increased risk of malignancy also characterizes the other polyposis syndromes. A summary of the gastrointestinal polyposis syndromes is depicted in Table 7.1.

Familial Adenomatous Polyposis

Clinical Features, Pathology, and Natural History

Familial adenomatous polyposis (FAP) is the most frequent gastrointestinal polyposis syndrome. Patients develop numerous adenomas preferentially involving the colorectum (Fig. 7.6), but also affecting the small intestine, in particular the duodenum and periampullary region.[171–173] The stomach typically develops numerous fundic gland polyps, although

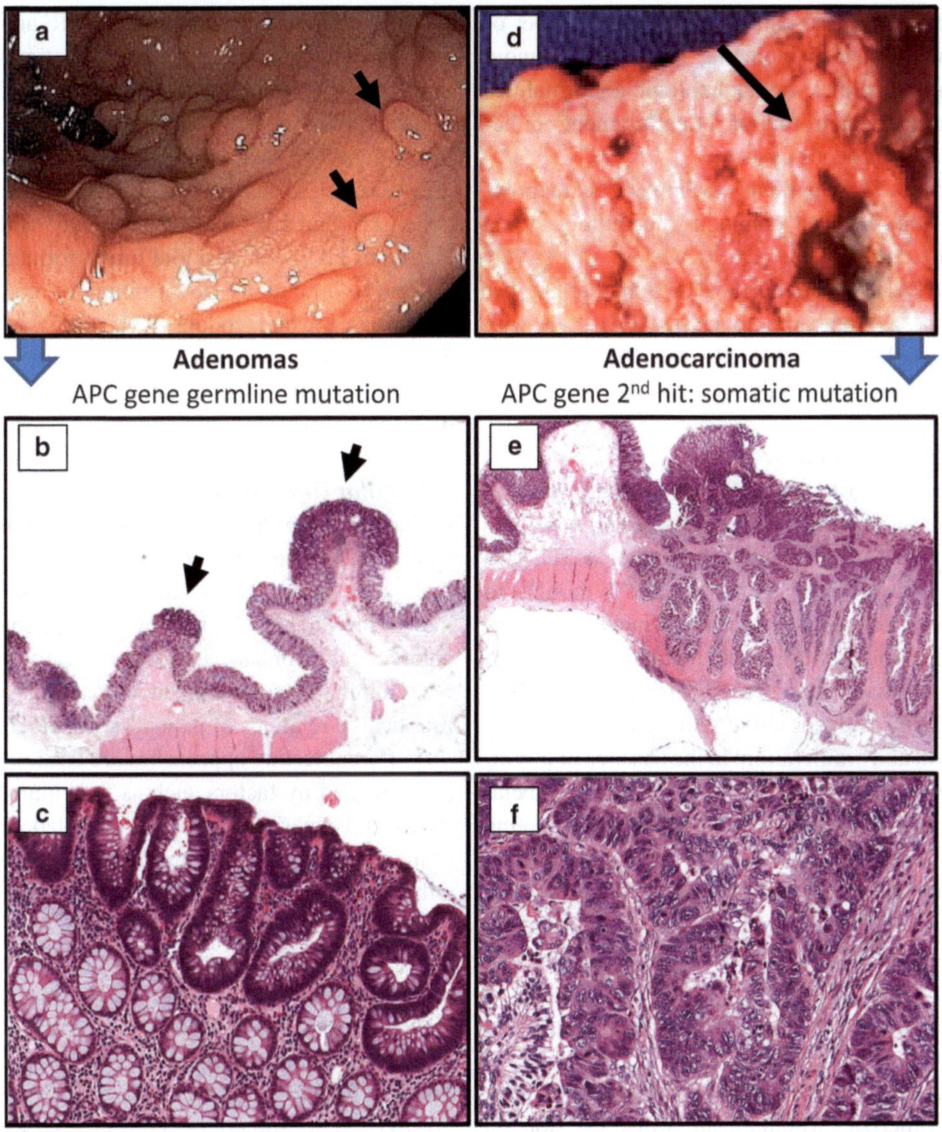

Fig. 7.6 Colonic adenomas and progression to adenocarcinoma in a patient with FAP. (**a**) Numerous polyps are identified at colonoscopy (image provided by courtesy of Dr. David Metz, University of Pennsylvania); (**b** and **c**) Histologic features of representative tubular adenomas. (**d**) Adenocarcinoma (*arrow*) arising in the background of numerous colonic polyps. (**e** and **f**) Histologically, the tumor is a moderately differentiated adenocarcinoma extending into the subserosal tissue

adenomas may also occur.[173–178] If the disease progresses through its natural history, 100% of affected individuals eventually develop colorectal cancer at early age[179] (Fig. 7.6). Overall, FAP patients represent less than 1% of all colorectal carcinoma cases in the United States, affecting 1 in 8,000–10,000 individuals.[180] FAP patients are also at higher risk of developing duodenal and ampullary carcinomas and have a slightly increased risk of gastric adenocarcinoma.[181]

The majority of FAP patients inherit germline mutations in the adenomatous polyposis coli (*APC*) gene on 5q21–22 chromosome locus,[182–184] but up to a third of FAP cases present as de novo germline mutations.[180,185]

In addition to the characteristic gastrointestinal polyposis, FAP patients manifest other lesions, including congenital hypertrophy of retinal pigmented epithelium (CHRPE) in 70–80% of FAP patients, desmoid tumors in 15% of cases, thyroid carcinoma (papillary and follicular types, including the characteristic cribriform-morular variant) in 1–2% of FAP patients,[174] and hepatoblastoma in young children.[174]

In addition to the classic FAP syndrome, inherited mutations in the *APC* gene are associated with several variants of FAP that include Gardner Syndrome, Turcot Syndrome, and Attenuated FAP (AFAP), summarized in Table 7.1.[173,180,181,186,187]

Gardner syndrome: These patients develop a number of extra-colonic manifestations including osteomas, desmoid tumors, dental abnormalities, ophthalmologic abnormalities including congenital hypertrophy of retinal pigment epithelium (CHRPE) and cutaneous cysts.

Turcot syndrome: These patients develop colorectal polyposis and brain tumors, most commonly medulloblastoma (see also above).

Attenuated FAP: These patients develop a smaller number of colonic polyps as compared to classic FAP, but with sufficient colonic polyposis (frequently over 15), suggesting an underlying polyposis syndrome.[181]

Genetic and Molecular Features

FAP provides the basis to understand the molecular pathways underlying the most common mechanisms of stepwise progression in colorectal cancer.[188] *APC* codes for a 312 kDa protein that is expressed in many tissues and is thought to participate in several cellular functions including Wnt-mediated signaling and transcriptional regulation, cell adhesion, cell migration, and chromosomal segregation. The *APC* gene product is a key mediator in the Wnt signaling pathway for cellular growth and proliferation. In the absence of a Wnt-mediated growth signal, APC occurs in a complex with beta-catenin, leading to beta-catenin phosphorylation and targeting it for destruction by the proteasome. When the Wnt pathway is activated by ligand binding, the APC–beta-catenin protein complex is disrupted, beta-catenin phosphorylation cannot occur, and this results in stability and nuclear localization of beta-catenin. Pathogenic mutations in the *APC* gene result in a disrupted APC–beta-catenin protein complex, leading to constitutive activation of the Wnt pathway.[188–190]

The APC protein contains multiple functional domains, including an oligomerization domain, an "armadillo" domain region which is thought to be involved in binding of APC to proteins related to cell morphology and motility, a beta-catenin-binding domain, an axin-binding domain, and a microtubule-binding domain.[174,191]

The majority of germline mutations associated with FAP are either frameshift or nonsense mutations that result in a truncated protein product, leading to disruption of interaction with beta-catenin, stabilization of beta-catenin with nuclear accumulation of the protein, and a phenotype of constitutive activation of the Wnt pathway.[191,192] The most common germline mutations occur at codons 1061 and 1309 and account for 17% and 11% of all germline APC mutations, respectively. The region between codons 1286 and 1513 is known as the "mutation cluster region" (MCR), and many of the identified *APC* mutations occur in this segment of the gene.[193] Some associations between the location of the germline APC mutation and the clinical phenotype have been found.[194] Mutations within the MCR are associated with extensive polyposis of typical FAP patients, whereas mutations in the 5′ end of the gene (exons 4 and 5), and mutations in the alternatively spliced form of exon 9 or the 3′ distal end of the gene, are seen in attenuated polyposis. An intermediate phenotype is observed in patients with mutations between codon 157 and 1249 and between 1465 and 1595. The association of FAP with desmoid tumor formation has been correlated to mutations downstream of codon 1400.[181,194,195] Mutations beyond codons 934, 1395, and within codons 564–1465 may be associated with upper gastrointestinal tumors. CHRPE is associated with mutations that occur between codons 311 and 1444.

Molecular Diagnosis

Molecular testing for germline mutations in the *APC* gene is recommended in specific settings as summarized by the American Gastroenterological Association.[171] The primary indications include high clinical suspicion for FAP (>100 colorectal adenomas), first-degree relatives of FAP patients, >20 cumulative colorectal adenomas (suspected AFAP), and first-degree relatives of patients with AFAP.[171,196]

Different testing approaches are used in various laboratories, dictated by factors such as the volume of testing, platforms, and experience available in the laboratory. Sequencing of the entire coding region is the gold standard for diagnosis. Other methods include protein truncation tests and mutation scanning.

As numerous pathogenic mutations have been described in *APC*, including large exonic or whole gene deletions, a comprehensive approach to molecular diagnosis is required.[197] If the patient has a phenotype suggestive of FAP but no mutations are found in the APC gene, underlying mutations in the *MUTYH* gene should be considered (see also below).[198] When a mutation is identified, targeted genetic testing can be offered to family members.

When germline mutations are not detected in patients clinically suspicious for FAP and related syndromes, other mechanisms of gene deficiency may be interrogated. These alternatives include alterations in epigenetic regulation of the *APC* gene, contribution of genes encoding other proteins involved in the beta-catenin pathway such as axin, alterations of allelic mRNA ratios, and somatic APC mosaicism.[199] Germline hypermethylation of the *APC* gene has been shown not to be a significant cause of FAP in *APC* mutation-negative cases.[200] In cases in which no other discrete mutation exists, unbalanced *APC* allelic mRNA expression, resulting in reduced "dosage" of *APC* and functional haploinsufficiency has been reported.[201]

Individuals who are carriers of an *APC* gene germline mutation are recommended to have regular surveillance starting early in life with annual sigmoidoscopy or colonoscopy, beginning at 10–12 years of age. Prophylactic colectomy is recommended, usually by the time the patient is in his or her early 20s. Regular esophagogastroduodenoscopy (EGD) is also recommended for identification of gastric, duodenal, and periampullary lesions. Additional recommendations are directed at extra-colonic manifestations and include annual palpation of the thyroid, serum alpha-fetoprotein (AFP) levels, and abdominal palpation every 6 months in young children of FAP families to detect hepatoblastoma.

MUTYH-Associated Polyposis (MAP)

MUTYH-associated polyposis is transmitted as an autosomal recessive colorectal cancer syndrome, occurring in patients with colorectal polyposis and underlying germline mutations in the DNA repair gene *MYH*[202–204] (Table 7.1). Patients with MAP usually present with fewer polyps, but they may show no polyps or even numerous polyps as seen in FAP.[204] Colorectal cancer arising in the background of MAP represents an estimated 0.5–1% of all colorectal cancers, with a lifetime risk of CRC reaching 80%, and as in FAP the risk of duodenal cancer is also increased.[204]

The *MUTYH* gene encodes a protein with glycosylase functions, involved in the base excision repair (BER) system critical to the repair of DNA damage caused by oxidative stress. The oxidized base 7,8-dihydroxy-8-oxoguanine (8-oxo-G) is often mistakenly paired with adenine (A), resulting in the appearance of guanine:cytosine>thymine:adenine (G:C>T:A) transversions at the next round of DNA replication, as the detection of stable 8-oxo-G:A base-pairs is missed by the replicative DNA polymerases.[205,206] The DNA damage-specific glycosylases OGG1, MUTYH, and MTH1 function by recognizing and facilitating the removal of 8-oxo-G adducts.[206] Consequently, deficient MUTYH function is associated with an increased frequency of G:C>T:A transversions,[207] which occur in regions of cancer-related genes such as *APC, KRAS,* and *BRCA1/2*. Mutations in two hotspots, Y165C and G382D, account for 70% of all *MUTYH* mutations in Caucasian patients. Germline mutational testing is indicated in individuals with greater than 10 adenomatous polyps (particularly with family history of colon cancer consistent with recessive inheritance) and significant polyposis similar to AFAP/FAP who test negative for mutations in *APC*.[204] Screening is recommended to begin at age 18–20 years with colonoscopies every 1–2 years. Colectomy can be considered in cases with larger numbers of polyps mimicking FAP. Guidelines for the screening of duodenal cancers in FAP/AFAP should be applied to MAP patients as well.[204]

References

1. Boland CR. Evolution of the nomenclature for the hereditary colorectal cancer syndromes. *Fam Cancer*. 2005;4:211–8.
2. Llor X, Pons E, Xicola RM, et al. Differential features of colorectal cancers fulfilling Amsterdam criteria without involvement of the mutator pathway. *Clin Cancer Res*. 2005;11:7304–10.
3. Boland CR, Shike M. Report from the Jerusalem workshop on Lynch syndrome-hereditary nonpolyposis colorectal cancer. *Gastroenterology*. 2010;138(2197):e1–7.
4. Lynch HT, Lynch PM, Lanspa SJ, Snyder CL, Lynch JF, Boland CR. Review of the Lynch syndrome: history, molecular genetics, screening, differential diagnosis, and medicolegal ramifications. *Clin Genet*. 2009;76:1–18.
5. Umar A. Lynch syndrome (HNPCC) and microsatellite instability. *Dis Markers*. 2004;20:179–80.
6. Peltomaki P. Deficient DNA, mismatch repair: a common etiologic factor for colon cancer. *Hum Mol Genet*. 2001;10:735–40.
7. Lynch HT, Lanspa SJ, Boman BM, et al. Hereditary nonpolyposis colorectal cancer–Lynch syndromes I and II. *Gastroenterol Clin North Am*. 1988;17:679–712.
8. Terdiman JP. HNPCC: an uncommon but important diagnosis. *Gastroenterology*. 2001;121:1005–8.
9. Lin KM, Shashidharan M, Thorson AG, et al. Cumulative incidence of colorectal and extracolonic cancers in MLH1 and MSH2 mutation carriers of hereditary nonpolyposis colorectal cancer. *J Gastrointest Surg*. 1998;2:67–71.
10. Vasen HF, Watson P, Mecklin JP, Lynch HT. New clinical criteria for hereditary nonpolyposis colorectal cancer (HNPCC, Lynch syndrome) proposed by the International Collaborative group on HNPCC. *Gastroenterology*. 1999;116:1453–6.
11. Young J, Simms LA, Biden KG, et al. Features of colorectal cancers with high-level microsatellite instability occurring in familial and sporadic settings: parallel pathways of tumorigenesis. *Am J Pathol*. 2001;159:2107–16.
12. Gologan A, Sepulveda AR. Microsatellite instability and DNA mismatch repair deficiency testing in hereditary and sporadic gastrointestinal cancers. *Clin Lab Med*. 2005;25:179–96.
13. Kim H, Jen J, Vogelstein B, Hamilton SR. Clinical and pathological characteristics of sporadic colorectal carcinomas with DNA replication errors in microsatellite sequences. *Am J Pathol*. 1994;145:148–56.
14. Alexander J, Watanabe T, Wu TT, Rashid A, Li S, Hamilton SR. Histopathological identification of colon cancer with microsatellite instability. *Am J Pathol*. 2001;158:527–35.
15. Dolcetti R, Viel A, Doglioni C, et al. High prevalence of activated intraepithelial cytotoxic T lymphocytes and increased neoplastic cell apoptosis in colorectal carcinomas with microsatellite instability. *Am J Pathol*. 1999;154:1805–13.
16. Greenson JK, Bonner JD, Ben-Yzhak O, et al. Phenotype of microsatellite unstable colorectal carcinomas: Well-differentiated and focally mucinous tumors and the absence of dirty necrosis correlate with microsatellite instability. *Am J Surg Pathol*. 2003;27:563–70.
17. Jass JR. Pathology of hereditary nonpolyposis colorectal cancer. *Ann N Y Acad Sci*. 2000;910:62–73. discussion 73–4.
18. Gologan A, Krasinskas A, Hunt J, Thull DL, Farkas L, Sepulveda AR. Performance of the revised Bethesda guidelines for identification of colorectal carcinomas with a high level of microsatellite instability. *Arch Pathol Lab Med*. 2005;129:1390–7.
19. De Jong AE, Morreau H, Van Puijenbroek M, et al. The role of mismatch repair gene defects in the development of adenomas in patients with HNPCC. *Gastroenterology*. 2004;126:42–8.

20. Lindgren G, Liljegren A, Jaramillo E, Rubio C, Lindblom A. Adenoma prevalence and cancer risk in familial non-polyposis colorectal cancer. *Gut*. 2002;50:228–34.
21. Jarvinen HJ, Aarnio M, Mustonen H, et al. Controlled 15-year trial on screening for colorectal cancer in families with hereditary non-polyposis colorectal cancer. *Gastroenterology*. 2000;118:829–34.
22. Vasen HF, den Hartog Jager FC, Menko FH, Nagengast FM. Screening for hereditary non-polyposis colorectal cancer: a study of 22 kindreds in The Netherlands. *Am J Med*. 1989;86:278–81.
23. Rijcken FE, Hollema H, Kleibeuker JH. Proximal adenomas in hereditary non-polyposis colorectal cancer are prone to rapid malignant transformation. *Gut*. 2002;50:382–6.
24. Bettstetter M, Dechant S, Ruemmele P, et al. Distinction of hereditary nonpolyposis colorectal cancer and sporadic microsatellite-unstable colorectal cancer through quantification of MLH1 methylation by real-time PCR. *Clin Cancer Res*. 2007;13:3221–8.
25. Leach FS, Nicolaides NC, Papadopoulos N, et al. Mutations of a mutS homolog in hereditary nonpolyposis colorectal cancer. *Cell*. 1993;75:1215–1225.
26. Bronner CE, Baker SM, Morrison PT, et al. Mutation in the DNA mismatch repair gene homologue hMLH1 is associated with hereditary non-polyposis colon cancer. *Nature*. 1994;368:258–261.
27. Nicolaides NC, Papadopoulos N, Liu B, et al. Mutations of two PMS homologues in hereditary nonpolyposis colon cancer. *Nature*. 1994;371:75–80.
28. Berends MJ, Wu Y, Sijmons RH, et al. Molecular and clinical characteristics of MSH6 variants: an analysis of 25 index carriers of a germline variant. *Am J Hum Genet*. 2002;70:26–37.
29. Kariola R, Raevaara TE, Lonnqvist KE, Nystrom-Lahti M. Functional analysis of MSH6 mutations linked to kindreds with putative hereditary non-polyposis colorectal cancer syndrome. *Hum Mol Genet*. 2002;11:1303–10.
30. Buttin BM, Powell MA, Mutch DG, et al. Penetrance and expressivity of MSH6 germline mutations in seven kindreds not ascertained by family history. *Am J Hum Genet*. 2004;74:1262–9.
31. Liu B, Parsons R, Papadopoulos N, et al. Analysis of mismatch repair genes in hereditary non-polyposis colorectal cancer patients. *Nat Med*. 1996;2:169–174.
32. Peltomaki P. DNA mismatch repair and cancer. *Mutat Res*. 2001;488:77–85.
33. Peltomaki P. Role of DNA mismatch repair defects in the pathogenesis of human cancer. *J Clin Oncol*. 2003;21:1174–9.
34. Liu B, Nicolaides C, Markowitz S, et al. Mismatch repair defects in sporadic colorectal cancers with microsatellite instability. *Nat Genet*. 1995;9:48–55.
35. Umar A, Boland CR, Terdiman JP, et al. Revised Bethesda Guidelines for hereditary nonpolyposis colorectal cancer (Lynch syndrome) and microsatellite instability. *J Natl Cancer Inst*. 2004;96:261–8.
36. Lynch HT, Lynch JF. Lynch syndrome: history and current status. *Dis Markers*. 2004;20:181–98.
37. Goel A, Nguyen TP, Leung HC, et al. De novo constitutional MLH1 epimutations confer early-onset colorectal cancer in two new sporadic Lynch syndrome cases, with derivation of the epimutation on the paternal allele in one. *Int J Cancer*. 2010;128:869–78.
38. Kolodner RD, Marsischky GT. Eukaryotic DNA mismatch repair. *Curr Opin Genet Dev*. 1999;9:89–96.
39. Lipkin SM, Wang V, Jacoby R, et al. MLH3: a DNA mismatch repair gene associated with mammalian microsatellite instability. *Nat Genet*. 2000;24:27–35.
40. Kolodner R. Biochemistry and genetics of eukaryotic mismatch repair. *Genes Dev*. 1996;10:1433–42.
41. Genschel J, Littman SJ, Drummond JT, Modrich P. Isolation of MutSbeta from human cells and comparison of the mismatch repair specificities of MutSbeta and MutSalpha. *J Biol Chem*. 1998;273:19895–901.
42. Umar A, Risinger JI, Glaab WE, Tindall KR, Barrett JC, Kunkel TA. Functional overlap in mismatch repair by human MSH3 and MSH6. *Genetics*. 1998;148:1637–46.
43. Palombo F, Gallinari P, Iaccarino I, et al. GTBP, a 160-kilodalton protein essential for mismatch-binding activity in human cells. *Science*. 1995;268:1912–4.
44. Marsischky GT, Filosi N, Kane MF, Kolodner R. Redundancy of Saccharomyces cerevisiae MSH3 and MSH6 in MSH2-dependent mismatch repair. *Genes Dev*. 1996;10:407–20.
45. Sia EA, Kokoska RJ, Dominska M, Greenwell P, Petes TD. Microsatellite instability in yeast: dependence on repeat unit size and DNA mismatch repair genes. *Mol Cell Biol*. 1997;17:2851–8.
46. Lu A-L. Biochemistry of mammalian DNA mismatch repair. Humana Press, 1998
47. Leung WK, Kim JJ, Wu L, Sepulveda JL, Sepulveda AR. Identification of a second MutL DNA mismatch repair complex (hPMS1 and hMLH1) in human epithelial cells. *J Biol Chem*. 2000;275:15728–15732.
48. Raschle M, Marra G, Nystrom-Lahti M, Schar P, Jiricny J. Identification of hMutLbeta, a heterodimer of hMLH1 and hPMS1. *J Biol Chem*. 1999;274:32368–75.
49. Lynch HT, Boman B, Fitzgibbons RJ Jr, Lanspa SJ, Smyrk TC. Hereditary nonpolyposis colon cancer: (Lynch syndrome I and II). A challenge for the clinician. *Nebr Med J*. 1989;74:2–7.
50. Lynch HT, Drouhard T, Lanspa S, et al. Mutation of an mutL homologue in a Navajo family with hereditary nonpolyposis colorectal cancer. *J Natl Cancer Inst*. 1994;86:1417–9.
51. Lynch HT, Lynch JF. 25 years of HNPCC. *Anticancer Res*. 1994;14:1617–24.
52. Lynch HT, Lynch JF. Hereditary cancer: family history, diagnosis, molecular genetics, ecogenetics, and management strategies. *Biochimie*. 2002;84:3–17.
53. Bessa X, Balleste B, Andreu M, et al. A prospective, multicenter, population-based study of BRAF mutational analysis for Lynch syndrome screening. *Clin Gastroenterol Hepatol*. 2008;6:206–14.
54. De Roock W, Claes B, Bernasconi D, et al. Effects of KRAS, BRAF, NRAS, and PIK3CA mutations on the efficacy of cetuximab plus chemotherapy in chemotherapy-refractory metastatic colorectal cancer: a retrospective consortium analysis. *Lancet Oncol*. 2010;11:753–62.
55. Deng G, Bell I, Crawley S, et al. BRAF mutation is frequently present in sporadic colorectal cancer with methylated hMLH1, but not in hereditary nonpolyposis colorectal cancer. *Clin Cancer Res*. 2004;10:191–5.
56. Palomaki GE, McClain MR, Melillo S, Hampel HL, Thibodeau SN. EGAPP supplementary evidence review: DNA testing strategies aimed at reducing morbidity and mortality from Lynch syndrome. *Genet Med*. 2009;11:42–65.
57. Vasen HF, Mecklin JP, Khan PM, Lynch HT. The International Collaborative Group on Hereditary Non-Polyposis Colorectal Cancer (ICG-HNPCC). *Dis Colon Rectum*. 1991;34:424–5.
58. Boland CR, Thibodeau SN, Hamilton SR, et al. A National Cancer Institute Workshop on Microsatellite Instability for cancer detection and familial predisposition: development of international criteria for the determination of microsatellite instability in colorectal cancer. *Cancer Res*. 1998;58:5248–57.
59. Syngal S, Fox EA, Eng C, Kolodner RD, Garber JE. Sensitivity and specificity of clinical criteria for hereditary non-polyposis colorectal cancer associated mutations in MSH2 and MLH1. *J Med Genet*. 2000;37:641–5.
60. Umar A, Risinger JI, Hawk ET, Barrett JC. Testing guidelines for hereditary non-polyposis colorectal cancer. *Nat Rev Cancer*. 2004;4:153–8.
61. Lindor NM, Petersen GM, Hadley DW, et al. Recommendations for the care of individuals with an inherited predisposition to Lynch syndrome: a systematic review. *JAMA*. 2006;296:1507–17.

62. Hampel H, Frankel WL, Martin E, et al. Screening for the Lynch syndrome (hereditary nonpolyposis colorectal cancer). *N Engl J Med.* 2005;352:1851–60.
63. Recommendations from the EGAPP Working Group: genetic testing strategies in newly diagnosed individuals with colorectal cancer aimed at reducing morbidity and mortality from Lynch syndrome in relatives. Genet Med 2009;11:35–41.
64. Hampel H, de la Chapelle A. The search for unaffected individuals with Lynch syndrome: do the ends justify the means? *Cancer Prev Res (Phila).* 2011;4:1–5.
65. Suraweera N, Duval A, Reperant M, et al. Evaluation of tumor microsatellite instability using five quasimonomorphic mononucleotide repeats and pentaplex PCR. *Gastroenterology.* 2002;123: 1804–11.
66. Goel A, Xicola RM, Nguyen TP, et al. Aberrant DNA methylation in hereditary nonpolyposis colorectal cancer without mismatch repair deficiency. *Gastroenterology.* 2010;138:1854–62.
67. Bacher JW, Flanagan LA, Smalley RL, et al. Development of a fluorescent multiplex assay for detection of MSI-High tumors. *Dis Markers.* 2004;20:237–50.
68. Murphy KM, Zhang S, Geiger T, et al. Comparison of the microsatellite instability analysis system and the Bethesda panel for the determination of microsatellite instability in colorectal cancers. *J Mol Diagn.* 2006;8:305–11.
69. Baudhuin LM, Burgart LJ, Leontovich O, Thibodeau SN. Use of microsatellite instability and immunohistochemistry testing for the identification of individuals at risk for Lynch syndrome. *Fam Cancer.* 2005;4:255–65.
70. Watson N, Grieu F, Morris M, et al. Heterogeneous staining for mismatch repair proteins during population-based prescreening for hereditary nonpolyposis colorectal cancer. *J Mol Diagn.* 2007;9:472–8.
71. Peltomaki P. Lynch syndrome genes. *Fam Cancer.* 2005;4:227–32.
72. Salahshor S, Koelble K, Rubio C, Lindblom A. Microsatellite Instability and hMLH1 and hMSH2 expression analysis in familial and sporadic colorectal cancer. *Lab Invest.* 2001;81:535–41.
73. Funkhouser WK Jr, Lubin IM, Monzon FA, et al. Relevance, pathogenesis, and testing algorithm for mismatch repair-defective colorectal carcinomas: a report of the association for molecular pathology. *J Mol Diagn.* 2012;14:91–103.
74. Grady WM. Genetic testing for high-risk colon cancer patients. *Gastroenterology.* 2003;124:1574–94.
75. Mutations MaM. http://www.insight-group.org/ Accessed September 2004.
76. Akiyama Y, Sato H, Yamada T, et al. Germ-line mutation of the hMSH6/GTBP gene in an atypical hereditary nonpolyposis colorectal cancer kindred. *Cancer Res.* 1997;57:3920–3.
77. Iino H, Simms L, Young J, et al. DNA microsatellite instability and mismatch repair protein loss in adenomas presenting in hereditary non-polyposis colorectal cancer. *Gut.* 2000;47:37–42.
78. Hampel H, Stephens JA, Pukkala E, et al. Cancer risk in hereditary nonpolyposis colorectal cancer syndrome: later age of onset. *Gastroenterology.* 2005;129:415–21.
79. Lindor NM, Rabe K, Petersen GM, et al. Lower cancer incidence in Amsterdam-I criteria families without mismatch repair deficiency: familial colorectal cancer type X. *JAMA.* 2005;293:1979–85.
80. Guillem JG, Wood WC, Moley JF, et al. ASCO/SSO review of current role of risk-reducing surgery in common hereditary cancer syndromes. *J Clin Oncol.* 2006;24:4642–60.
81. Hampel H, Frankel WL, Martin E, et al. Feasibility of screening for Lynch syndrome among patients with colorectal cancer. *J Clin Oncol.* 2008;26:5783–8.
82. Hampel H, Frankel W, Panescu J, et al. Screening for Lynch syndrome (hereditary nonpolyposis colorectal cancer) among endometrial cancer patients. *Cancer Res.* 2006;66:7810–7.
83. Hampel H, Panescu J, Lockman J, et al. Comment on: screening for lynch syndrome (hereditary nonpolyposis colorectal cancer) among endometrial cancer patients. *Cancer Res.* 2007;67:9603.
84. Mvundura M, Grosse SD, Hampel H, Palomaki GE. The cost-effectiveness of genetic testing strategies for Lynch syndrome among newly diagnosed patients with colorectal cancer. *Genet Med.* 2010;12:93–104.
85. Dunlop MG, Farrington SM, Carothers AD, et al. Cancer risk associated with germline DNA mismatch repair gene mutations. *Hum Mol Genet.* 1997;6:105–10.
86. Watson P, Butzow R, Lynch HT, et al. The clinical features of ovarian cancer in hereditary nonpolyposis colorectal cancer. *Gynecol Oncol.* 2001;82:223–8.
87. Aarnio M, Sankila R, Pukkala E, et al. Cancer risk in mutation carriers of DNA-mismatch-repair genes. *Int J Cancer.* 1999;81: 214–8.
88. Lynch HT, Boland CR, Gong G, et al. Phenotypic and genotypic heterogeneity in the Lynch syndrome: diagnostic, surveillance and management implications. *Eur J Hum Genet.* 2006;14: 390–402.
89. da Silva FC, de Oliveira LP, Santos EM, et al. Frequency of extracolonic tumors in Brazilian families with Lynch syndrome: analysis of a hereditary colorectal cancer institutional registry. *Fam Cancer.* 2010;9:563–70.
90. Vasen HF, Morreau H, Nortier JW. Is breast cancer part of the tumor spectrum of hereditary nonpolyposis colorectal cancer? *Am J Hum Genet.* 2001;68:1533–5.
91. Westenend PJ, Schutte R, Hoogmans MM, Wagner A, Dinjens WN. Breast cancer in an MSH2 gene mutation carrier. *Hum Pathol.* 2005;36:1322–6.
92. Risinger JI, Barrett JC, Watson P, Lynch HT, Boyd J. Molecular genetic evidence of the occurrence of breast cancer as an integral tumor in patients with the hereditary nonpolyposis colorectal carcinoma syndrome. *Cancer.* 1996;77:1836–43.
93. Nelson CL, Sellers TA, Rich SS, Potter JD, McGovern PG, Kushi LH. Familial clustering of colon, breast, uterine, and ovarian cancers as assessed by family history. *Genet Epidemiol.* 1993;10:235–44.
94. de Leeuw WJ, van Puijenbroek M, Tollenaar RA, et al. Exclusion of breast cancer as an integral tumor of hereditary nonpolyposis colorectal cancer. *Cancer Res.* 2003;62:1014–1019. Cancer Res 2003;63:1148–9.
95. Boyd J, Rhei E, Federici MG, et al. Male breast cancer in the hereditary nonpolyposis colorectal cancer syndrome. *Breast Cancer Res Treat.* 1999;53:87–91.
96. Watson P, Vasen HF, Mecklin JP, et al. The risk of extra-colonic, extra-endometrial cancer in the Lynch syndrome. *Int J Cancer.* 2008;123:444–9.
97. Jemal A, Murray T, Samuels A, Ghafoor A, Ward E, Thun MJ. Cancer statistics, 2003. *CA Cancer J Clin.* 2003;53:5–26.
98. Broaddus RR, Lynch PM, Lu KH, Luthra R, Michelson SJ. Unusual tumors associated with the hereditary nonpolyposis colorectal cancer syndrome. *Mod Pathol.* 2004;17:981–9.
99. Sijmons R, Hofstra R, Hollema H, et al. Inclusion of malignant fibrous histiocytoma in the tumour spectrum associated with hereditary non-polyposis colorectal cancer. *Genes Chromosomes Cancer.* 2000;29:353–5.
100. den Bakker MA, Seynaeve C, Kliffen M, Dinjens WN. Microsatellite instability in a pleomorphic rhabdomyosarcoma in a patient with hereditary non-polyposis colorectal cancer. *Histopathology.* 2003;43:297–9.
101. Kawaguchi K, Oda Y, Takahira T, et al. Microsatellite instability and hMLH1 and hMSH2 expression analysis in soft tissue sarcomas. *Oncol Rep.* 2005;13:241–6.
102. Suwa K, Ohmori M, Miki H. Microsatellite alterations in various sarcomas in Japanese patients. *J Orthop Sci.* 1999;4:223–30.

103. Soravia C, van der Klift H, Brundler MA, et al. Prostate cancer is part of the hereditary non-polyposis colorectal cancer (HNPCC) tumor spectrum. *Am J Med Genet.* 2003;121A:159–62.
104. Gallinger S, Aronson M, Shayan K, et al. Gastrointestinal cancers and neurofibromatosis type 1 features in children with a germline homozygous MLH1 mutation. *Gastroenterology.* 2004;126: 576–85.
105. Meyer LA, Broaddus RR, Lu KH. Endometrial cancer and Lynch syndrome: clinical and pathologic considerations. *Cancer Control.* 2009;16:14–22.
106. Garg K, Soslow RA. Lynch syndrome (hereditary non-polyposis colorectal cancer) and endometrial carcinoma. *J Clin Pathol.* 2009;62:679–84.
107. Manchanda R, Menon U, Michaelson-Cohen R, Beller U, Jacobs I. Hereditary non-polyposis colorectal cancer or Lynch syndrome: the gynaecological perspective. *Curr Opin Obstet Gynecol.* 2009;21:31–8.
108. Resnick KE, Hampel H, Fishel R, Cohn DE. Current and emerging trends in Lynch syndrome identification in women with endometrial cancer. *Gynecol Oncol.* 2009;114:128–34.
109. Taylor N, Mutch DG. Gynecologic manifestations of hereditary nonpolyposis colorectal cancer. From inherited to sporadic disease. *Oncology (Williston Park).* 2006;20:85–94.
110. Prat J, Ribe A, Gallardo A. Hereditary ovarian cancer. *Hum Pathol.* 2005;36:861–70.
111. Watson P, Lynch HT. Cancer risk in mismatch repair gene mutation carriers. *Fam Cancer.* 2001;1:57–60.
112. Lu KH, Dinh M, Kohlmann W, et al. Gynecologic cancer as a "sentinel cancer" for women with hereditary nonpolyposis colorectal cancer syndrome. *Obstet Gynecol.* 2005;105:569–74.
113. Obermair A, Youlden DR, Young JP, et al. Risk of endometrial cancer for women diagnosed with HNPCC-related colorectal carcinoma. *Int J Cancer.* 2010;127:2678–84.
114. Chadwick RB, Pyatt RE, Niemann TH, et al. Hereditary and somatic DNA mismatch repair gene mutations in sporadic endometrial carcinoma. *J Med Genet.* 2001;38:461–6.
115. Banno K, Susumu N, Yanokura M, et al. Association of HNPCC and endometrial cancers. *Int J Clin Oncol.* 2004;9:262–9.
116. Lu KH, Schorge JO, Rodabaugh KJ, et al. Prospective determination of prevalence of lynch syndrome in young women with endometrial cancer. *J Clin Oncol.* 2007;25:5158–64.
117. Resnick K, Straughn JM Jr, Backes F, Hampel H, Matthews KS, Cohn DE. Lynch syndrome screening strategies among newly diagnosed endometrial cancer patients. *Obstet Gynecol.* 2009;114:530–6.
118. Goodfellow PJ, Buttin BM, Herzog TJ, et al. Prevalence of defective DNA mismatch repair and MSH6 mutation in an unselected series of endometrial cancers. *Proc Natl Acad Sci USA.* 2003;100:5908–13.
119. Boks DE, Trujillo AP, Voogd AC, Morreau H, Kenter GG, Vasen HF. Survival analysis of endometrial carcinoma associated with hereditary nonpolyposis colorectal cancer. *Int J Cancer.* 2002;102:198–200.
120. MacDonald ND, Salvesen HB, Ryan A, Iversen OE, Akslen LA, Jacobs IJ. Frequency and prognostic impact of microsatellite instability in a large population-based study of endometrial carcinomas. *Cancer Res.* 2000;60:1750–2.
121. Basil JB, Goodfellow PJ, Rader JS, Mutch DG, Herzog TJ. Clinical significance of microsatellite instability in endometrial carcinoma. *Cancer.* 2000;89:1758–64.
122. Caduff RF, Johnston CM, Svoboda-Newman SM, Poy EL, Merajver SD, Frank TS. Clinical and pathological significance of microsatellite instability in sporadic endometrial carcinoma. *Am J Pathol.* 1996;148:1671–8.
123. Maxwell GL, Risinger JI, Alvarez AA, Barrett JC, Berchuck A. Favorable survival associated with microsatellite instability in endometrioid endometrial cancers. *Obstet Gynecol.* 2001;97:417–22.
124. Garg K, Leitao MM Jr, Kauff ND, et al. Selection of endometrial carcinomas for DNA mismatch repair protein immunohistochemistry using patient age and tumor morphology enhances detection of mismatch repair abnormalities. *Am J Surg Pathol.* 2009;33:925–33.
125. Shia J, Black D, Hummer AJ, Boyd J, Soslow RA. Routinely assessed morphological features correlate with microsatellite instability status in endometrial cancer. *Hum Pathol.* 2008;39: 116–25.
126. van den Bos M, van den Hoven M, Jongejan E, et al. More differences between HNPCC-related and sporadic carcinomas from the endometrium as compared to the colon. *Am J Surg Pathol.* 2004;28:706–11.
127. Walsh MD, Cummings MC, Buchanan DD, et al. Molecular, pathologic, and clinical features of early-onset endometrial cancer: identifying presumptive Lynch syndrome patients. *Clin Cancer Res.* 2008;14:1692–700.
128. Carcangiu ML, Radice P, Casalini P, Bertario L, Merola M, Sala P. Lynch syndrome–related endometrial carcinomas show a high frequency of nonendometrioid types and of high FIGO grade endometrioid types. *Int J Surg Pathol.* 2010;18:21–6.
129. Broaddus RR, Lynch HT, Chen LM, et al. Pathologic features of endometrial carcinoma associated with HNPCC: a comparison with sporadic endometrial carcinoma. *Cancer.* 2006;106:87–94.
130. Westin SN, Lacour RA, Urbauer DL, et al. Carcinoma of the lower uterine segment: a newly described association with Lynch syndrome. *J Clin Oncol.* 2008;26:5965–71.
131. Ramsoekh D, Wagner A, van Leerdam ME, et al. Cancer risk in MLH1, MSH2 and MSH6 mutation carriers; different risk profiles may influence clinical management. *Hered Cancer Clin Pract.* 2009;7:17.
132. Senter L, Clendenning M, Sotamaa K, et al. The clinical phenotype of Lynch syndrome due to germ-line PMS2 mutations. *Gastroenterology.* 2008;135:419–28.
133. Greggi S, Genuardi M, Benedetti-Panici P, et al. Analysis of 138 consecutive ovarian cancer patients: incidence and characteristics of familial cases. *Gynecol Oncol.* 1990;39:300–4.
134. Bewtra C, Watson P, Conway T, Read-Hippee C, Lynch HT. Hereditary ovarian cancer: a clinicopathological study. *Int J Gynecol Pathol.* 1992;11:180–7.
135. Pal T, Permuth-Wey J, Sellers TA. A review of the clinical relevance of mismatch-repair deficiency in ovarian cancer. *Cancer.* 2008;113:733–42.
136. Crijnen TE, Janssen-Heijnen ML, Gelderblom H, et al. Survival of patients with ovarian cancer due to a mismatch repair defect. *Fam Cancer.* 2005;4:301–5.
137. Seidman JD, Horkayne-Szakaly I, Haiba M, Boice CR, Kurman RJ, Ronnett BM. The histologic type and stage distribution of ovarian carcinomas of surface epithelial origin. *Int J Gynecol Pathol.* 2004;23:41–4.
138. Quirk JT, Natarajan N. Ovarian cancer incidence in the United States, 1992–1999. *Gynecol Oncol.* 2005;97:519–23.
139. Pal T, Permuth-Wey J, Kumar A, Sellers TA. Systematic review and meta-analysis of ovarian cancers: estimation of microsatellite-high frequency and characterization of mismatch repair deficient tumor histology. *Clin Cancer Res.* 2008;14:6847–54.
140. Capelle LG, Van Grieken NC, Lingsma HF, et al. Risk and epidemiological time trends of gastric cancer in Lynch syndrome carriers in the Netherlands. *Gastroenterology.* 2010;138:487–92.
141. Aarnio M, Salovaara R, Aaltonen LA, Mecklin JP, Jarvinen HJ. Features of gastric cancer in hereditary non-polyposis colorectal cancer syndrome. *Int J Cancer.* 1997;74:551–5.
142. Lehtola J. Family study of gastric carcinoma; with special reference to histological types. *Scand J Gastroenterol Suppl.* 1978;50: 3–54.
143. Lynch HT, Grady W, Suriano G, Huntsman D. Gastric cancer: new genetic developments. *J Surg Oncol.* 2005;90:114–33. discussion 133.

144. Lauren PA, Nevalainen TJ. Epidemiology of intestinal and diffuse types of gastric carcinoma. A time-trend study in Finland with comparison between studies from high- and low-risk areas. *Cancer*. 1993;71:2926–33.
145. Mecklin JP, Jarvinen HJ, Virolainen M. The association between cholangiocarcinoma and hereditary nonpolyposis colorectal carcinoma. *Cancer*. 1992;69:1112–4.
146. Vernez M, Hutter P, Monnerat C, Halkic N, Gugerli O, Bouzourene H. A case of Muir-Torre syndrome associated with mucinous hepatic cholangiocarcinoma and a novel germline mutation of the MSH2 gene. *Fam Cancer*. 2007;6:141–5.
147. Koornstra JJ, Kleibeuker JH, Vasen HF. Small-bowel cancer in Lynch syndrome: is it time for surveillance? *Lancet Oncol*. 2008;9:901–5.
148. Rodriguez-Bigas MA, Vasen HF, Lynch HT, et al. Characteristics of small bowel carcinoma in hereditary nonpolyposis colorectal carcinoma. International Collaborative Group on HNPCC. *Cancer*. 1998;83:240–4.
149. Schulmann K, Brasch FE, Kunstmann E, et al. HNPCC-associated small bowel cancer: clinical and molecular characteristics. *Gastroenterology*. 2005;128:590–9.
150. Watson P, Lynch HT. The tumor spectrum in HNPCC. *Anticancer Res*. 1994;14:1635–9.
151. Maul JS, Warner NR, Kuwada SK, Burt RW, Cannon-Albright LA. Extracolonic cancers associated with hereditary nonpolyposis colorectal cancer in the Utah Population Database. *Am J Gastroenterol*. 2006;101:1591–6.
152. Roupret M, Yates DR, Comperat E, Cussenot O. Upper urinary tract urothelial cell carcinomas and other urological malignancies involved in the hereditary nonpolyposis colorectal cancer (lynch syndrome) tumor spectrum. *Eur Urol*. 2008;54:1226–36.
153. Catto JW, Azzouzi AR, Amira N, et al. Distinct patterns of microsatellite instability are seen in tumours of the urinary tract. *Oncogene*. 2003;22:8699–706.
154. Sarin S, Bernath A. Turcot syndrome (glioma polyposis): a case report. *South Med J*. 2008;101:1273–4.
155. Hamilton SR, Liu B, Parsons RE, et al. The molecular basis of Turcot's syndrome. *N Engl J Med*. 1995;332:839–47.
156. Torre D. Multiple sebaceous tumors. *Arch Dermatol*. 1968;98: 549–51.
157. Muir EG, Bell AJ, Barlow KA. Multiple primary carcinomata of the colon, duodenum, and larynx associated with kerato-acanthomata of the face. *Br J Surg*. 1967;54:191–5.
158. Lynch HT, Lynch PM, Pester J, Fusaro RM. The cancer family syndrome. Rare cutaneous phenotypic linkage of Torre's syndrome. *Arch Intern Med*. 1981;141:607–11.
159. South CD, Hampel H, Comeras I, Westman JA, Frankel WL, de la Chapelle A. The frequency of Muir-Torre syndrome among Lynch syndrome families. *J Natl Cancer Inst*. 2008;100: 277–81.
160. Mangold E, Pagenstecher C, Leister M, et al. A genotype-phenotype correlation in HNPCC: strong predominance of msh2 mutations in 41 patients with Muir-Torre syndrome. *J Med Genet*. 2004;41:567–72.
161. Entius MM, Keller JJ, Drillenburg P, Kuypers KC, Giardiello FM, Offerhaus GJ. Microsatellite instability and expression of hMLH-1 and hMSH-2 in sebaceous gland carcinomas as markers for Muir-Torre syndrome. *Clin Cancer Res*. 2000;6:1784–9.
162. Mathiak M, Rutten A, Mangold E, et al. Loss of DNA mismatch repair proteins in skin tumors from patients with Muir-Torre syndrome and MSH2 or MLH1 germline mutations: establishment of immunohistochemical analysis as a screening test. *Am J Surg Pathol*. 2002;26:338–43.
163. Lancaster JM, Powell CB, Kauff ND, et al. Society of Gynecologic Oncologists Education Committee statement on risk assessment for inherited gynecologic cancer predispositions. *Gynecol Oncol*. 2007;107:159–62.
164. Mojtahed A, Schrijver I, Ford JM, Longacre TA, Pai RK. A two-antibody mismatch repair protein immunohistochemistry screening approach for colorectal carcinomas, skin sebaceous tumors, and gynecologic tract carcinomas. *Mod Pathol*. 2011;24: 1004–14.
165. Dove-Edwin I, Boks D, Goff S, et al. The outcome of endometrial carcinoma surveillance by ultrasound scan in women at risk of hereditary nonpolyposis colorectal carcinoma and familial colorectal carcinoma. *Cancer*. 2002;94:1708–12.
166. Rijcken FE, Mourits MJ, Kleibeuker JH, Hollema H, van der Zee AG. Gynecologic screening in hereditary nonpolyposis colorectal cancer. *Gynecol Oncol*. 2003;91:74–80.
167. Renkonen-Sinisalo L, Butzow R, Leminen A, Lehtovirta P, Mecklin JP, Jarvinen HJ. Surveillance for endometrial cancer in hereditary nonpolyposis colorectal cancer syndrome. *Int J Cancer*. 2007;120:821–4.
168. Lecuru F, Metzger U, Scarabin C, Le Frere Belda MA, Olschwang S, Laurent Puig P. Hysteroscopic findings in women at risk of HNPCC. Results of a prospective observational study. *Fam Cancer*. 2007;6:295–9.
169. Lecuru F, Le Frere Belda MA, Bats AS, et al. Performance of office hysteroscopy and endometrial biopsy for detecting endometrial disease in women at risk of human non-polyposis colon cancer: a prospective study. *Int J Gynecol Cancer*. 2008;18: 1326–31.
170. Lynch HT, Boland CR, Rodriguez-Bigas MA, Amos C, Lynch JF, Lynch PM. Who should be sent for genetic testing in hereditary colorectal cancer syndromes? *J Clin Oncol*. 2007;25:3534–42.
171. Bonis PA, Ahnen DJ, Axell L. Screening strategies in patients and families with familial colon cancer syndromes. In: Basow DE (Ed) UpToDate. Waltham, MA. 2008.
172. Doxey BW, Kuwada SK, Burt RW. Inherited polyposis syndromes: molecular mechanisms, clinicopathology, and genetic testing. *Clin Gastroenterol Hepatol*. 2005;3:633–41.
173. Lynch HT, Lynch JF, Shaw TG. Hereditary gastrointestinal cancer syndromes. *Gastrointest Cancer Res*. 2011;4:S9-S17.
174. Galiatsatos P, Foulkes WD. Familial adenomatous polyposis. *Am J Gastroenterol*. 2006;101:385–98.
175. Hofgartner WT, Thorp M, Ramus MW, et al. Gastric adenocarcinoma associated with fundic gland polyps in a patient with attenuated familial adenomatous polyposis. *Am J Gastroenterol*. 1999;94:2275–81.
176. Ahnen DJ, Axell L. Clinical features and diagnosis of familial adenomatous polyposis. UpToDate, Basow DS (Ed), Waltham, MA. 2008.
177. Abraham SC, Park SJ, Mugartegui L, Hamilton SR, Wu TT. Sporadic fundic gland polyps with epithelial dysplasia: evidence for preferential targeting for mutations in the adenomatous polyposis coli gene. *Am J Pathol*. 2002;161:1735–42.
178. Lam-Himlin D, Park JY, Cornish TC, Shi C, Montgomery E. Morphologic characterization of syndromic gastric polyps. *Am J Surg Pathol*. 2010;34:1656–62.
179. Lynch PM. Prevention of colorectal cancer in high-risk populations: the increasing role for endoscopy and chemoprevention in FAP and HNPCC. *Digestion*. 2007;76:68–76.
180. Lipton L, Tomlinson I. The genetics of FAP and FAP-like syndromes. *Fam Cancer*. 2006;5:221–6.
181. Rustgi AK. The genetics of hereditary colon cancer. *Genes Dev*. 2007;21:2525–38.
182. Bodmer WF, Bailey CJ, Bodmer J, et al. Localization of the gene for familial adenomatous polyposis on chromosome 5. *Nature*. 1987;328:614–6.
183. Kinzler KW, Nilbert MC, Su LK, et al. Identification of FAP locus genes from chromosome 5q21. *Science*. 1991;253:661–5.
184. Groden J, Thliveris A, Samowitz W, et al. Identification and characterization of the familial adenomatous polyposis coli gene. *Cell*. 1991;66:589–600.

185. Schulmann K, Pox C, Tannapfel A, Schmiegel W. The patient with multiple intestinal polyps. *Best Pract Res Clin Gastroenterol.* 2007;21:409–26.
186. Ahnen DJ. The genetic basis of colorectal cancer risk. *Adv Intern Med.* 1996;41:531–52.
187. Half E, Bercovich D, Rozen P. Familial adenomatous polyposis. *Orphanet J Rare Dis.* 2009;4:22.
188. Polakis P. The many ways of Wnt in cancer. *Curr Opin Genet Dev.* 2007;17:45–51.
189. Aoki K, Aoki M, Sugai M, et al. Chromosomal instability by beta-catenin/TCF transcription in APC or beta-catenin mutant cells. *Oncogene.* 2007;26:3511–20.
190. Schneikert J, Behrens J. The canonical Wnt signalling pathway and its APC partner in colon cancer development. *Gut.* 2007;56:417–25.
191. Senda T, Iizuka-Kogo A, Onouchi T, Shimomura A. Adenomatous polyposis coli (APC) plays multiple roles in the intestinal and colorectal epithelia. *Med Mol Morphol.* 2007;40:68–81.
192. Abdel-Rahman WM, Peltomaki P. Molecular basis and diagnostics of hereditary colorectal cancers. *Ann Med.* 2004;36:379–88.
193. Segditsas S, Tomlinson I. Colorectal cancer and genetic alterations in the Wnt pathway. *Oncogene.* 2006;25:7531–7.
194. Nieuwenhuis MH, Vasen HF. Correlations between mutation site in APC and phenotype of familial adenomatous polyposis (FAP): a review of the literature. *Crit Rev Oncol Hematol.* 2007;61:153–61.
195. Rozen P, Macrae F. Familial adenomatous polyposis: the practical applications of clinical and molecular screening. *Fam Cancer.* 2006;5:227–35.
196. Hegde MR, Roa BB (2006) Detecting mutations in the APC gene in familial adenomatous polyposis (FAP). Curr Protoc Hum Genet 2006; Chapter 10: Unit 10 8.
197. Michils G, Tejpar S, Thoelen R, et al. Large deletions of the APC gene in 15% of mutation-negative patients with classical polyposis (FAP): a Belgian study. *Hum Mutat.* 2005;25:125–34.
198. Nielsen M, Hes FJ, Nagengast FM, et al. Germline mutations in APC and MUTYH are responsible for the majority of families with attenuated familial adenomatous polyposis. *Clin Genet.* 2007;71:427–33.
199. Hes FJ, Nielsen M, Bik EC, et al. Somatic APC mosaicism: an underestimated cause of polyposis coli. *Gut.* 2008;57:71–6.
200. Romero-Gimenez J, Dopeso H, Blanco I, et al. Germline hypermethylation of the APC promoter is not a frequent cause of familial adenomatous polyposis in APC/MUTYH mutation negative families. *Int J Cancer.* 2008;122:1422–5.
201. Renkonen ET, Nieminen P, Abdel-Rahman WM, et al. Adenomatous polyposis families that screen APC mutation-negative by conventional methods are genetically heterogeneous. *J Clin Oncol.* 2005;23:5651–9.
202. Al-Tassan N, Chmiel NH, Maynard J, et al. Inherited variants of MYH associated with somatic G:C–>T:A mutations in colorectal tumors. *Nat Genet.* 2002;30:227–32.
203. Poulsen ML, Bisgaard ML. MUTYH Associated Polyposis (MAP). *Curr Genomics.* 2008;9:420–35.
204. Gala M, Chung DC. Hereditary colon cancer syndromes. *Semin Oncol.* 2011;38:490–9.
205. Cheadle JP, Sampson JR. MUTYH-associated polyposis–from defect in base excision repair to clinical genetic testing. *DNA Repair (Amst).* 2007;6:274–9.
206. Lu AL, Bai H, Shi G, Chang DY. MutY and MutY homologs (MYH) in genome maintenance. *Front Biosci.* 2006;11:3062–80.
207. Parker AR, Eshleman JR. Human MutY: gene structure, protein functions and interactions, and role in carcinogenesis. *Cell Mol Life Sci.* 2003;60:2064–83.

Molecular Pathology of Colon and Small Bowel Cancers: Sporadic Type

8

Asif Rashid

Introduction

Colorectal cancer (CRC) is the third most commonly diagnosed cancer and the third most common cause of cancer death in men and women in the USA and accounts for 9% of all new cancer cases and of all cancer deaths.[1] In contrast, the incidence of small bowel cancer is low and accounts for 0.4% of all new cases and 0.2% of all cancer deaths.[1] It is currently believed that most sporadic colorectal cancers arise from preexisting precursor lesions, including adenoma, dysplasia and recently serrated polyps, but a small percentage of colorectal cancers can arise de novo without identifiable precursor lesions. The majority of colorectal cancers develop through an "adenoma–carcinoma sequence" beginning from transformation of normal colorectal epithelium to an adenomatous intermediate and then to adenocarcinoma,[2] illustrated in Fig. 1.1. The molecular pathogenesis of colorectal cancer including genetic and epigenetic alterations has been extensively studied in the past two decades and is among one of the best understood among human neoplasms. Although the inherited forms of colorectal cancers contribute to a minority of all colorectal cancers, described in Chap. 7, the identification of specific underlying genetic defects in each inherited syndrome has laid a formidable groundwork for understanding the sporadic colorectal cancer pathogenesis.

Sporadic Colorectal Cancers

There are three major molecular pathways that have been well characterized in the sporadic colorectal cancers. The conventional chromosomal instability pathway characterized by wide spread imbalances in chromosome numbers and alterations of multiple tumor suppressor genes, including *adenomatous polyposis coli* (*APC*), *deleted in colorectal cancer* (*DCC*), *deleted in pancreatic cancer 4* (*DPC4*, *SMAD4*), and *TP53*, and oncogenes, including *KRAS* and *CTNNB1* (*β-catenin*) in the adenoma–carcinoma sequence accounts for a majority (60–70%) of sporadic colorectal cancers.[3] The "DNA methylator pathway" is a novel pathway characterized by methylation of multiple CpG islands in colorectal carcinomas, including genes known to be important in tumorigenesis such as the *CDKN2A* (*p16*) tumor suppressor gene and other loci and genes.[4–6] Approximately 15% of sporadic colorectal cancers arise through defects in a third distinct pathway, the "DNA mismatch repair pathway" due to CpG methylation of *human Mut long homologue-1* (*MLH1*) DNA mismatch repair gene promoter. Loss of *MLH1* expression underlies deficient DNA mismatch repair of mutations that occur during DNA replication, resulting in the accumulation of insertions or deletions of nucleotides in unstable repeated sequence such as microsatellites.[7–9] *MLH1* methylation is predominantly seen in tumors of the methylator pathway, but these tumors have extensive methylation involving many other genes and gene loci. Some of the clinic pathologic features, genetic alterations, prognosis, and response to chemotherapy are distinct among these three subgroups of colorectal carcinomas.

Chromosomal Instability Pathway

The molecular model following adenoma–carcinoma sequence involves multiple stepwise accumulations of genetic alterations in tumor suppressor genes and oncogenes and was first characterized by Fearon and Vogestein.[3] In this model, an ordered combination of multiple genetic alterations is required for the ultimate development of colorectal cancer and the presence of single genetic alteration is not sufficient for malignant transformation. Genome-wide sequencing of

A. Rashid, M.D., Ph.D. (✉)
Department of Pathology, The University of Texas M. D. Anderson Cancer Center, 1515 Holcombe, Houston, TX, USA
e-mail: arashid@mdanderson.org

A.R. Sepulveda and J.P. Lynch (eds.), *Molecular Pathology of Neoplastic Gastrointestinal Diseases*, Molecular Pathology Library 7, DOI 10.1007/978-1-4614-6015-2_8, © Springer Science+Business Media New York 2013

colorectal cancers have found ~80 mutations in an individual tumor but less than 15 mutations that were responsible for initiation, progression, or maintenance of the tumor.[10,11] In addition, a few genes are mutated in a large number of tumors but most genes are mutated in less than 5% of tumors, and single-base substitutions, especially missense mutations, are the most prevalent. Inactivation of *adenomatous polyposis coli* (*APC*) is the initiating event for adenomatous transformation in this model,[12,13] followed by activating mutations of *KRAS* gene,[14–16] followed by *TP53* (*p53*) inactivation,[17,18] and loss of chromosome 18q, chromosomal location of *deleted in colorectal cancer* (*DCC*) and *deleted in pancreatic cancer* (*DPC, SMAD4*) genes,[19,20] for malignant transformation to carcinoma. These tumors are aneuploid with imbalance in chromosome numbers, and allelic loss [loss of heterozygosity (LOH)], and genomic amplification due to mitotic disjunction, chromosomal deletion, translocation, and recombination between homologous chromosomes. Multiple tumor suppressor genes are involved in the development of colorectal cancers as evidenced by frequent chromosomal allelic loss of 1p, 5q (*APC* gene), 8p, 17p (*p53* gene), 18q (*SMAD2*, *SMAD4*, and *DCC* genes), and 22q.[12,20,21]

APC/B-catenin Alterations

The earliest genetic change in sporadic-type colorectal cancer occurs in the *APC* gene.[12] *APC* is a tumor suppressor gene located on chromosome 5q21, and first identified in familial adenomatous polyposis (FAP) syndrome.[13,22] *APC* gene has been regarded as a "gatekeeper" gene and plays a critical role in colorectal carcinogenesis. The inactivation of *APC* gene in colorectal neoplasm follows the Knudson's two-hit hypothesis. Allelic loss of chromosome 5q is present in 40–50% of sporadic colorectal adenomas and carcinomas and somatic mutation of *APC* gene can be identified in up to 70% of sporadic colorectal cancer.[23,24] The identification of *APC* mutation in dysplastic aberrant crypt foci, the earliest morphologic colorectal precursor lesion further supports the critical function of APC gene in colorectal pathogenesis.[25] The germline mutations of *APC* gene are clustered throughout the entire gene and contributes to phenotypic diversity in familial adenomatous polyposis but the somatic mutations are more frequent in a mutation cluster region between codons 1286 and 1513.[24] Methylation of the *APC* promoter is an alternative mechanism of *APC* gene inactivation in colorectal adenomas and carcinomas.[26]

The function of *APC* gene has been recently elucidated. The *APC* gene product is an integral component of the cytoskeletal framework through its interaction with cadherins and regulates adhesion, migration, polarity, differentiation, and chromosomal segregation. It also mediates Wnt/Wingless pathway by interacting with glycogen synthase kinase-3β, axin, and β-catenin[27] (Fig. 8.1). Phosphorylation of β-catenin by glycogen synthase kinase-3β leads to proteasome-dependent degradation. Mutant APC disrupts this complex and β-catenin can translocate to the nucleus, where it is a transcription factor in association with T-cell factor/lymphoid enhancer factor.[28] Mutations of other components of this complex, including serine or threonine phosphorylation sites in exon 3 of *β-catenin* gene and *axin* gene, are present in colorectal tumors without *APC* mutations.[29,30]

p53 Gene Alterations

Mutations of *p53* gene and allelic loss of chromosome 17p, and chromosomal location of *p53* gene, occur in up to 75% of colorectal cancers, but are infrequent in adenomas suggesting that p53 plays an important role in progression of adenoma to carcinoma, in sporadic CRC.[17,18,31] The p53 protein is a transcription factor that is involved in the cell cycle regulation and programmed cell death in response to DNA damage, aberrant proliferative signals, and cellular injury.[32,33] Under physiological conditions, p53 is negatively regulated by MDM2 and is degraded by ubiquitination. TP53 is upregulated in response to cellular injury and regulates multiple gene products, including p21 (CIP1/WAF1), the cell cycle inhibitor, and BAX, FAS, and DR5, which mediate apoptosis.[34] Most *p53* mutations are missense mutations.[35] The p53 protein with these missense point mutations can still be expressed with an abnormal half-life that can be detectable by immunohistochemistry.

Chromosome 18q Loss

Allelic loss of chromosomal 18q occurs in 70% of sporadic colorectal cancers and approximately in 50% of large adenomas.[19,20] A candidate tumor suppressor gene designated *DCC* (*deleted in colorectal cancer*) that belongs to the neural cell adhesion molecule (N-CAM) family has been identified.[36] Only a minority of colorectal cancers demonstrates somatic mutations in *DCC* in mutation analysis of the whole gene, but the protein expression is frequently reduced or absent in colorectal cancers. Other tumor suppressor genes, *SMAD4* (*DPC4*, *deleted in pancreatic cancer*) and *SMAD2*, are also located in chromosome 18q.[37,38] SMAD2 and SMAD4 are downstream intracellular mediators of the transforming growth factor-β (TGFβ) signaling pathway that is involved in cell growth, differentiation, and apoptosis. Mutations of *SMAD4* and *SMAD2* genes have been identified in 16% and 10% of colorectal cancers.[37,38] *Cables* is another candidate tumor suppressor gene on chromosome 18q that increases tyrosine phosphorylation of cyclin-dependent kinases.[39] Loss of *Cables*

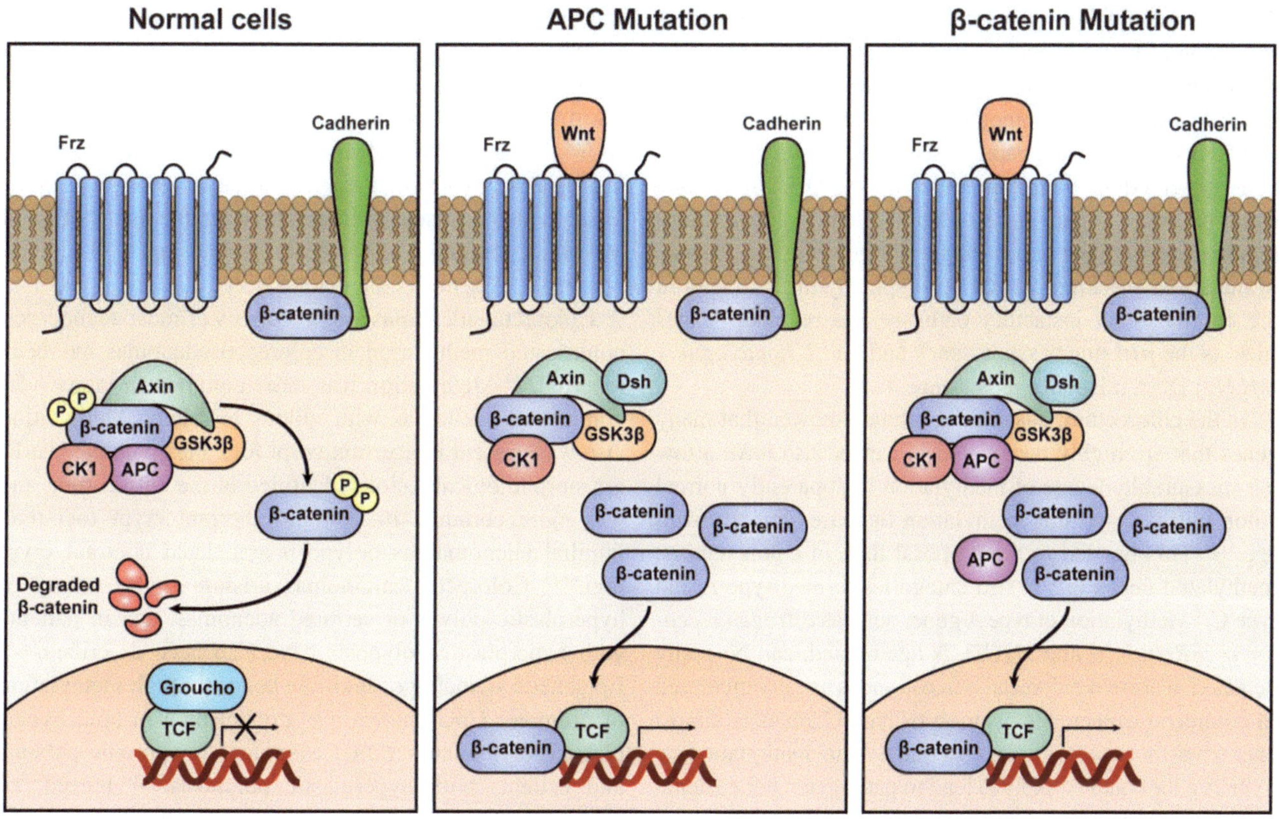

Fig. 8.1 The WNT signaling pathway. In the absence of WNT signal in normal cells, β-catenin is phosphorylated in the complex containing APC, axin, glycogen synthase kinase 3β, and casein kinase 1α/ε and degraded. In cancer cells with either APC alterations or β-catenin mutations, WNT signaling results in increased β-catenin in the cytoplasm and nuclear localization. In the nucleus, β-catenin displaces Groucho and interacts with TCF/lymphoid enhancer factor resulting in increased transcription of multiple genes

occur in 60–70% of colorectal cancers by loss of heterozygosity and CpG island methylation of the promoter region.[40]

KRAS, *BRAF*, and *Phosphatidylinositol 3 Kinase* Mutations

Among the oncogenes, *KRAS* gene is the most frequently mutated in colorectal adenomas and cancer. Activating mutation of *KRAS* oncogene has been detected in 40% of colorectal cancers and adenomas.[16] The majority of *KRAS* mutations are present at codons 12 and 13, and less frequently at codon 61, and lead to constitutive activation of guanosine triphosphate-bound enzyme that regulates multiple cellular functions. One of these is the Raf-mitogen-activated protein kinase kinase (MEK)-extracellular signal-regulated kinase (ERK) pathway. This pathway includes serine/threonine kinase BRAF that activates ERK1 and ERK2 and phosphorylates MEK1 and MEK2. *BRAF* mutations are present in 10% of colorectal cancers.[41] Ras-guanosine triphosphate also binds to the type I phosphatidylinositol 3 kinase (PIK3CA).[42,43] PIK3CA activates through AKT a number of pathways that influence cell growth, proliferation, and survival. *PIK3CA* mutations in exons 9 and 20 are present in 20% of colorectal cancers.

DNA Methylator Pathway

Methylation of cytosine is the only known modification of DNA in human cells, and methylated cytosines have been referred to as the elusive fifth base.[44] This epigenetic effect is particularly striking when DNA methylation affects promoter CpG islands.[45] CpG islands are 0.5–2 kb regions rich in the cytosine–guanine dinucleotides and are present in the 5′ region of about half of all human genes. Methylation of cytosines within CpG islands is associated with loss of protein expression by repression of transcription and is observed in physiological conditions such as X chromosome inactivation and imprinting.[44,45] Similar to other neoplastic cells, colorectal cancers have two paradoxical epigenetic changes involving methylated cytosines[46],global hypomethylation due to demethylation of cytosines,[47] and de novo hypermethylation of tumor-specific genes and other genes resulting in silencing of transcription.[48] Inactivation of gene function by methylation of the promoter region in the colorectal DNA methylator pathway overlaps closely with the genetic alterations observed in both conventional and DNA mismatch repair pathways. Methylation of CpG islands in the promoter region can inactivate tumor suppressor genes in the absence of mutations or chromosomal loss typically that are seen in the chromosomal instability pathway and regulates genes such as the *p16* tumor suppressor[49] and *mut L homologue* 1 (*MLH1*) DNA mismatch repair gene.[50]

In the colorectum, quantitative studies showed that many genes that are highly methylated in cancer also have a low but measurable degree of methylation in apparently normal colon mucosa, and this methylation increases linearly with age.[51,52] This has led to the proposal that, in colon tumors, methylated genes fall in two categories termed type A and type C.[4] Methylation of type A genes such as *estrogen receptor α* (*ERα*), *N33* and *MYOD*, is age related, can be easily detected in normal colorectal mucosa and is usually increased in colorectal cancer. Methylation of type C genes is almost exclusive to cancers, is less frequent than methylation of Type A genes, and is likely to lead to pathogenic gene silencing associated with a selective advantage.[4] Using either methylation-based screening techniques such as Methylated CpG island Amplification[4] or gene expression-reactivation-based techniques[53] have identified several genes that are methylated in colorectal cancers but a simple listing of these genes belittles the complexity of the process. It is clear that, of the hundreds of genes likely hypermethylated in a given tumor,[54] only a few play a significant functional role and are selected for the process. Many genes are likely hypermethylated in cancer simply as an extension of a process that begins in normal aging tissues, and paradoxically some genes whose expression should favor the neoplastic process such as *COX2* or *TERT* are downregulated in association with promoter methylation in some tumors.[55,56] Thus, DNA hypermethylation should be viewed as a global process analogous to microsatellite instability, whereby many loci are affected but only a few are functionally significant for the process of tumorigenesis.

The CpG island methylator phenotype (CIMP) was uncovered through a series of observations that included an association between microsatellite instability and hypermethylation of multiple genes in colorectal,[57] concordance between the methylation status of different genes in colorectal cancer[5] that was unrelated to gene function or chromosomal location, and a bimodal distribution of methylation when a selected subset of genes was studied quantitatively.[5,6] CIMP+ colorectal cancers have distinct clinical, pathological, and molecular genetic features. These cancers tend to occur proximally and are slightly more common in women and older patients.[6,58–60] They also have distinct pathologic features (mucinous, poorly differentiated), distinct genetic lesions (high frequencies of *KRAS* and *BRAF* mutations and low frequency of *p53* mutations) and a distinct prognosis.[6,58–61] About half of CIMP+ cancers also show microsatellite instability (MSI) via epigenetic inactivation of *MLH1*.[6] There is also a close association between the methylation of MGMT, a ubiquitous DNA repair enzyme, and G to A mutation in *KRAS* gene in colorectal cancer.[62]

Colorectal adenomas are precursors of most adenocarcinomas, and methylation in colorectal adenomas has been reported.[4,63] Methylation was more common in larger adenomas and adenomas with villous histology. Methylation also was present in aberrant crypt foci, the "putative" earliest morphological lesions identified in the colorectum, and was more common in sporadic aberrant crypt foci than familial adenomatous polyposis-associated aberrant crypt foci.[64,65] Colorectal carcinomas arising in the setting of hyperplastic polyps or serrated adenomas, and in patients with hyperplastic polyposis have also been described.[66–68] Epigenetic silencing of multiple genes through methylation of promoter CpG islands was documented in both hyperplastic polyps and serrated adenomas in sporadic patients and patients with hyperplastic polyposis.[69,70] Indeed, an alternative "serrated pathway" of colorectal carcinogenesis with a hyperplastic polyp-serrated adenoma–adenocarcinoma sequence has been proposed[71,72] (Fig. 8.2). The serrated pathway appears to be essentially driven by hypermethylation of multiple CpG islands. Not surprisingly, the proximal, mismatch repair-deficient colorectal cancers that have been proposed to arise primarily from this serrated adenoma pathway are also characterized by intense hypermethylation.[4,73]

DNA Mismatch Repair Pathway

MSI is due to mutations in microsatellites because of defective mismatch repair genes and has been observed in tumors arising in patients with hereditary nonpolyposis colorectal cancer (HNPCC) and in a subset (~15%) of sporadic colorectal cancers.[7–9] Microsatellites are tandem repeats of simple nucleotides sequence and are ubiquitously present throughout the human genome. The mismatch repair system detects and corrects replication errors by DNA polymerase in the newly synthesized DNA strand, including single base-pair mismatches and insertions or deletions of nucleotides. These errors are more prevalent in repetitive sequences, such as microsatellites. In HNPCC patients there are germline mutations of *MLH1*,[74,75] *MSH2*,[76,77] *MSH6*,[78,79] and *PMS2*[80] mismatch repair genes. In contrast, sporadic MSI colorectal cancers are due to silencing of *MLH1* by methylation of promoter region.[49,81,82]

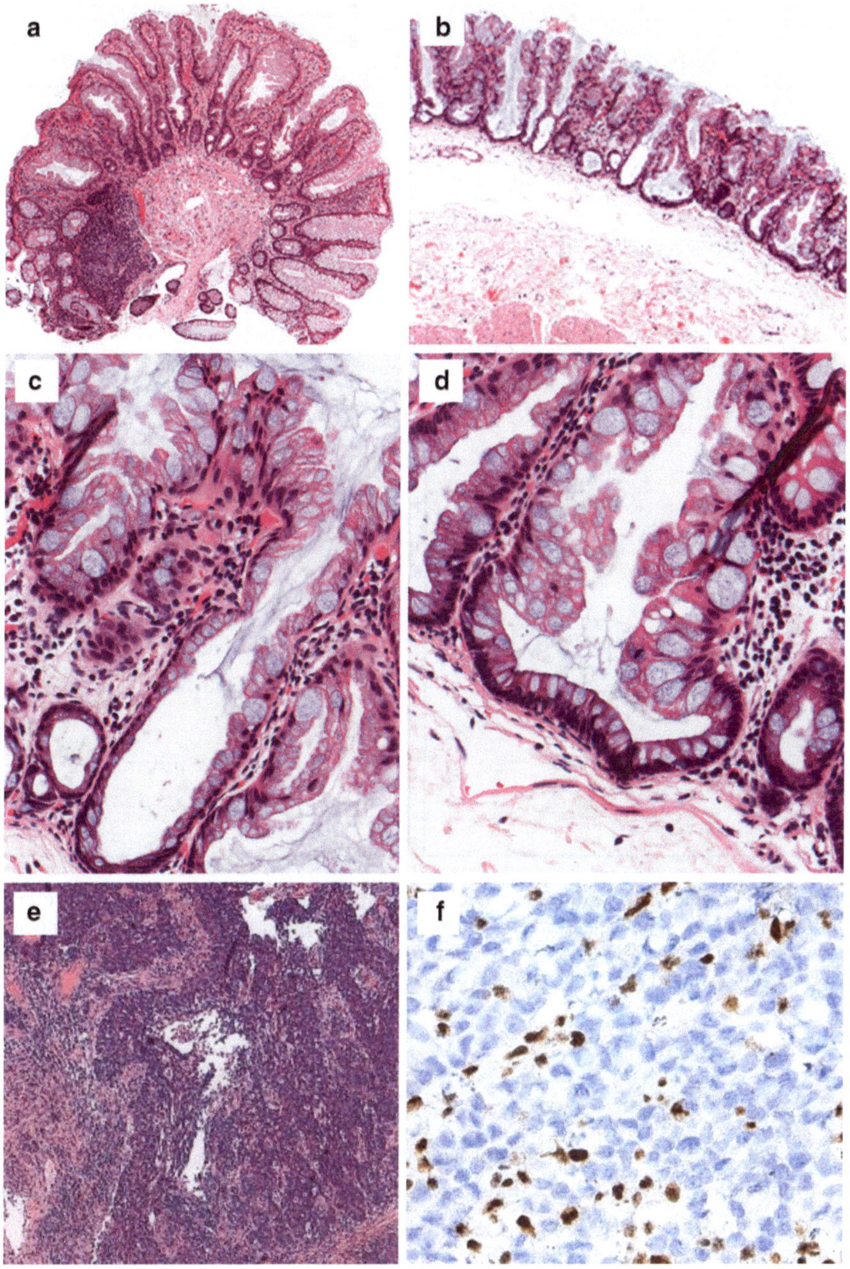

Fig. 8.2 Serrated pathway of colorectal carcinogenesis. (**a**) Hyperplastic polyp. (**b**) Sessile serrated adenoma/polyp. (**c**) and (**d**) High power illustrating the altered crypt architecture in a sessile serrated polyp with dilated and laterally expanded base of colonic crypts, but lacking evidence of epithelial cytologic dysplasia. (**e**) Low power view of poorly differentiated colonic adenocarcinoma showing loss of expression of MLH1 in tumor cell nuclei (**f**), while intratumoral lymphocytes show preserved expression of this DNA mismatch repair protein. Tumors of the serrated pathway often show loss of expression of MLH1 DNA mismatch repair protein associated with promoter hypermethylation and show microsatellite instability. (**a**)–(**e**) Hematoxylin & Eosin stains; (**f**) Immunohistochemistry for MLH1. Photomicrograph provided by Antonia R Sepulveda MD, PhD

MSI is tested by PCR amplification of microsatellite repeats. A consensus workshop recommended using two mononucleotide sequences (BAT25 and BAT26) and three dinucleotides sequences (D2S123, D5S346, and D17S250) to determine MSI.[83] Three MSI phenotypes have been defined in colorectal cancers: microsatellite stable (MSS), no allelic shift suggesting no change in microsatellite sequence; low frequency microsatellite instability (MSI-low), allelic shift of less than 40% of markers; and high frequency microsatellite instability (MSI-high), allelic shift of more than 40% of markers. MSI-high in colorectal cancers is due to either HNPCC with germline mutation of a mismatch repair gene and somatic inactivation of the other allele or due to biallelic methylation of *MLH1* gene in sporadic tumors.[7–9,49,81,82]

There are several distinct clinopathological features of sporadic MSI-high colorectal cancers as compared to microsatellite stable colorectal cancers. MSI-high cancers are more likely to present in older females, at a more advanced stage, proximally located and have better stage-specific survival after surgical and adjuvant therapies.[7,8,84,85] These tumors are more commonly bulky and exophytic, and about half of these cancers have a distinct histology with mucinous, solid, or variegated (multiple histologic components) components,

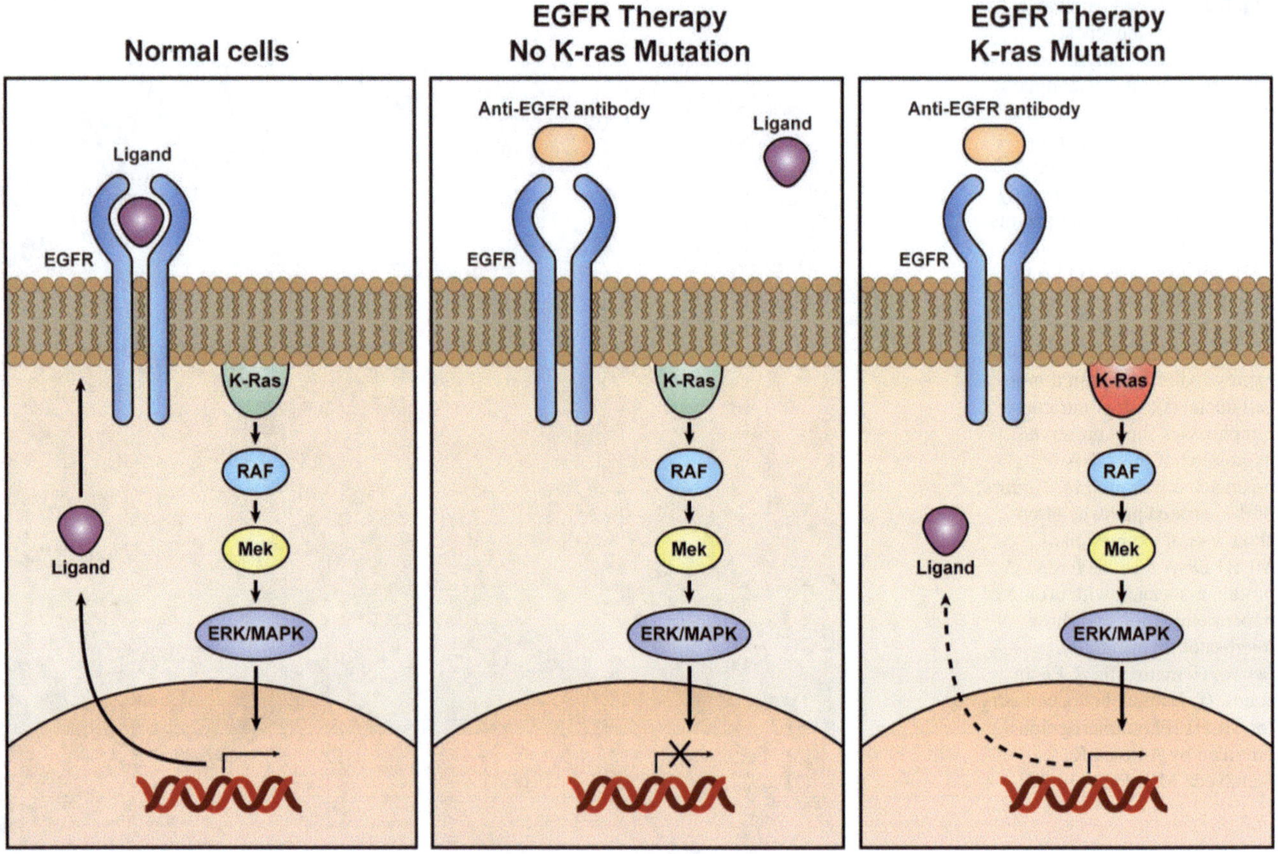

Fig. 8.3 Antiepidermal growth factor receptor (EGFR) therapy and *K-RAS* mutations in colorectal cancers. Binding of EGFR ligand activates signaling through K-RAS/MAPK pathway that in turn regulates ligand levels. Anti-EGFR antibody hinders ligand binding to EGFR by steric hindrance or immunomodulation and EGFR pathway is deactivated. *K-RAS* mutations activate MAPK pathway even in the absence of ligand binding of EGFR due to anti-EGFR antibody

and increased intratumoral lymphocytes and peritumoral lymphocytic infiltrate (Crohn-like reaction).[86–88] A frequent association with contiguous or noncontiguous hyperplastic or serrated polyps has been identified in sporadic MSI-high colorectal cancers, a characteristic shared with CIMP-high colorectal cancers.[71–73]

MSI-high colorectal carcinomas also have distinct genetic alterations. In contrast to the sporadic colorectal cancers with chromosomal instability pathway, tumors with MSI-high tend to have less frequent 18q allelic loss, *p53* and *KRAS* mutations[89,90] but more frequent *β-catenin* and *BRAF* mutations.[91,92] In addition, a distinct set of tumor suppressor genes containing short mononucleotide repeats in the encoding region such as *transforming growth factor β type II receptor* (*TGFβRII*), *insulin-like growth factor II receptor,* and *BAX* genes are frequently mutated in MSI-high colorectal cancers.[93–95] *TGFβRII* gene has a 10-base-pair long adenine tract that is mutated in more than 90% of MSI-high colorectal cancers.[96]

Prognostic and Therapeutic Implications of Molecular Markers in Colorectal Cancer

A variety of genetic and epigenetic alterations have been associated with prognosis, and respond to therapeutic agents in patients with colorectal carcinomas. Several chromosomal allelic losses have been associated with prognosis of patients with colorectal cancer (reviewed in[21]). Chromosomal allelic loss of 18q is frequently present in colorectal cancers and is associated with poor prognosis.[97,98] In contrast, MSI in sporadic colorectal carcinomas is associated with better prognosis[97–99], but CIMP+ is associated with poor prognosis.[100–102] Patients with colorectal cancers are treated with 5-fluorouracil-based therapy, but MSI or CIMP+ tumors may not benefit from such therapy.[100,102,103]

Epidermal growth factor receptor (EGFR) when activated by its ligand, epidermal growth factor, mediates signaling through KRAS/BRAF/MAPK is activated in a subset of colorectal carcinomas[104–109] (Fig. 8.3). A small subset of metastatic colorectal cancers respond to anti-EGFR antibody therapy by hindering ligand binding to EGFR by steric hindrance or immune modulation resulting in inactivation of the EGFR pathway. Cell lines or patients who have tumors with activating mutations of *KRAS*, *BRAF*, or *PIK3CA* do not respond to this treatment.[106–109]

Sporadic Small Intestinal Carcinomas

Compared to colorectal adenocarcinomas the genetic and epigenetic alterations in small intestinal adenocarcinomas have not been well characterized. Similar to the colorectum, an adenoma–carcinoma sequence has been reported, and similar to colorectal carcinomas chromosomal instability DNA methylator and DNA mismatch repair pathways have been reported for small intestinal carcinomas.[110] Sporadic small intestinal adenocarcinomas have chromosomal instability in 60% of tumors, CIMP-high in 30%, and MSI-high in 24% of tumors but with some overlap among the three pathways.[110]

Sporadic small intestinal carcinomas have gain of chromosomes 5p, 7, 8q, 9q, 13q, 16p, 19q, and 20 and loss of chromosomes 4p, 5q, 6q, 8p, 18q and 21 by comparative genomic hybridization.[110–113] Chromosomal loss of *APC* gene locus is infrequent[114] but *APC* gene missense and silent mutations are present in 42% of carcinomas and APC gene methylation in 48% of carcinomas.[111] Disruption of WNT signaling by either loss of *APC* or nuclear localization of B-catenin by immunohistochemistry is less frequent than in colorectal cancers.[115–117] Chromosome 18q loss is infrequent in some studies[111,112,114] but comparable to the frequency reported for colorectal carcinomas in another study,[110] and *DPC4* mutations have been reported.[112,114] *KRAS* mutations and infrequent *BRAF* mutations, similar to the frequencies observed in colorectal carcinomas, have been reported in small intestinal carcinomas,[110,114,116,118–120] and *BRAF* mutations are more common in MSI-high tumors.[110] Similarly, *p53* gene mutations have been reported in small intestinal carcinomas but are infrequent compared to colorectal cancers.[116,117,121]

MSI-high is present in 20% of small intestinal carcinomas[110–112,114] due to methylation of the promoter region of *MLH1* gene.[110,111,121] Duodenal cancers have a higher frequency of MSI-high.[122,123] Methylation of *p14*, *p16*, *MLH1*, *MGMT*, *retinoic acid receptor beta*, *immunoglobulin superfamily genes member 4*, *TIMP metallopeptidase inhibitor 3*, *APC*, *H-cadherin*, *paired box gene 6*, *estrogen receptor* genes, and MINT loci, that are methylated in colorectal carcinomas, have been reported in duodenal carcinomas, G-to-A *KRAS* mutations are associated with *MGMT* methylation in small intestinal carcinomas,[113,121] and CIMP+ has been reported.[110,121]

Conclusions

The molecular pathogenesis in sporadic colorectal and small bowel cancers are due to involvement of three major pathways: the conventional pathway involving accumulation of alterations of tumor suppressor genes and oncogenes, DNA mismatch repair pathway, and DNA methylator pathway. With the advance of molecular analysis, the precursor lesions for colorectal cancer have expanded from classic adenomas to the presumably non-neoplastic hyperplastic polyps and the earliest morphological precursor lesion, aberrant crypt foci. Although prognostic molecular makers and potential targets for therapies are still limited for colorectal cancers, with the advance of gene expression, microRNA and epigenetic profiling, through the application of novel high-throughput-based assays such as massively parallel sequencing, more prognostic molecular markers may be identified for both therapeutic and early detection purposes.

References

1. Jemal A, Siegel R, Xu J, et al. Cancer Statistics, 2010. *CA Cancer J Clin*. 2010;60:277–300.
2. Morson B. President's address: the polyp-cancer sequence in the large bowel. *Proc R Soc Med*. 1974;67:451–457.
3. Fearon E, Vogelstein B. A genetic model for colorectal tumorigenesis. *Cell*. 1990;61:759–767.
4. Toyota M, Ho C, Ahuja N, et al. Identification of differentially methylated sequences in colorectal cancer by methylated CpG island amplification. *Cancer Res*. 1999;59:2307–2312.
5. Toyota M, Ohe-Toyota M, Ahuja N, et al. Distinct genetic profiles in colorectal tumors with or without the CpG island methylator phenotype. *Proc Natl Acad Sci USA*. 2000;97:710–715.
6. Toyota M, Ahuja N, Ohe-Toyota M, et al. CpG Island methylator phenotype in colorectal cancer. *Proc Natl Acad Sci USA*. 1999;96:8681–8686.
7. Ionov Y, Peinado MA, Malkhosyan S, et al. Ubiquitous somatic mutations in simple repeated sequences reveal a new mechanism for colonic carcinogenesis. *Nature*. 1993;363:558–561.
8. Thibodeau SN, Berg G, Schaid D. Microsatellite instability in cancer of the proximal colon. *Science*. 1993;260:816–819.
9. Peltomaki P, Lothe RA, Aaltonen LA, et al. Microsatellite instability is associated with tumors that characterize the hereditary non-polyposis colorectal cancer syndrome. *Cancer Res*. 1993;53:5853–5855.
10. Wood LD, Parsons DW, Jones S, et al. The genomic landscapes of human breast and colorectal cancers. *Science*. 2007;318: 1108–1113.
11. Leary R, Lin J, Cummins J, et al. Integrated analysis of homozygous deletions, focal amplifications, and sequence alterations in breast and colorectal cancers. *Proc Natl Acad Sci USA*. 2008; 105:16226–16229.
12. Powell S, Zilz N, Beazer-Barclay Y, et al. APC mutations occur early during colorectal tumoriogenesis. *Nature*. 1992;359: 235–237.
13. Kinzler KW, Vogelstein B. Lessons from hereditary colorectal cancer. *Cell*. 1996;87:159–170.

14. Benhattar J, Losi L, Chaubert P, et al. Prognostic significance of K-ras mutations in colorectal carcinoma. *Gastroenterology.* 1993;104:1044–1048.
15. Moerkerk P, Arends JW, van Driel M, et al. Type and number of Ki-ras point mutations relate to stage of human colorectal cancer. *Cancer Res.* 1994;54:3376–3378.
16. Santini D, Loupakis F, Vincenzi B, et al. High concordance of KRAS status between primary colorectal tumors and related metastatic sites: implications for clinical practice. *Oncologist.* 2008;13:1270–1275.
17. Nigro JM, Baker SJ, Preisinger AC, et al. Mutations in the p53 gene occur in diverse tumor types. *Nature.* 1989;342:705–708.
18. Baker SJ, Preisinger AC, Jessup JM, et al. p53 gene mutations occur in combination with 17p allelic deletions as late event in colorectal tumorigenesis. *Cancer Res.* 1990;50:7717–7722.
19. Fearon ER, Cho KR, Nigro JM, et al. Identification of a chromosome 18q gene that is altered in colorectal cancers. *Science.* 1990;247:49–56.
20. Thiagalingam S, Lengauer C, Leach FS, et al. Evaluation of candidate tumor suppressor genes on chromosome 18 in colorectal cancers. *Nat Genet.* 1996;13:343–346.
21. Bacolod MD, Barany F. Gene dysregulation driven by somatic copy number aberrations-biological and clinical implications in colon tumors: a paper from the 2009 William Beaumont Hospital Symposium on Molecular Pathology. *J Mol Diag.* 2010;12:552–561.
22. Cottrell S, Bicknell D, Kaklamanis L, et al. Molecular analysis of APC mutations in familial adenomatous polyposis and sporadic colon carcinomas. *Lancet.* 1992;340:626–630.
23. Miyaki M, Konishi M, Kikuchi-Yanoshita R, et al. Characteristics of somatic mutation of the adenomatous polyposis coli gene in colorectal tumors. *Cancer Res.* 1994;54:3011–3020.
24. Miyoshi Y, Nagase H, Ando H, et al. Somatic mutations of the APC gene in colorectal tumors: mutation cluster region in the APC gene. *Hum Mol Genet.* 1992;1:229–233.
25. Otori K, Konishi M, Sugiyama K, et al. Infrequent somatic mutation of the adenomatous polyposis coli gene in aberrant crypt foci of human colon tissue. *Cancer.* 1998;83:896–900.
26. Esteller M, Sparks A, Toyota M, et al. Analysis of adenomatous polyposis coli promoter hypermethylation in human cancer. *Cancer Res.* 2000;60:4366–4371.
27. Rubinfeld B, Albert I, Porfiri E, et al. Binding of GSK3b to the APC-b-catenin complex and regulation of complex assembly. *Science.* 1996;272:1023–1026.
28. Mann B, Gelos M, Siedow A, et al. Target genes of beta-catenin-T-cell-factor/lymphoid-enhancer-factor signaling in human colorectal carcinomas. *Proc Natl Acad Sci USA.* 1999;96:1603–1608.
29. Sparks A, Morin P, Vogelstein B, et al. Mutational analysis of the APC/beta-catenin/Tcf pathway in colorectal cancer. *Cancer Res.* 1998;58:1130–1134.
30. Shimizu Y, Ikeda S, Fujimori M, et al. Frequent alterations in the Wnt signaling pathway in colorectal cancer with microsatellite instability. *Genes Chromosomes Cancer.* 2002;3:73–81.
31. Leslie A, Carey F, Pratt N, et al. The colorectal adenoma-carcinoma sequence. *Br J Surg.* 2002;89:845–860.
32. Vogelstein B, Lane D, Levine A. Surfing the p53 network. *Nature.* 2000;408:307–310.
33. Levine A. p53, the cellular gatekeeper for growth and division. *Cell.* 1997;88:323–331.
34. Menendez D, Inga A, Resnick MA. The expanding universe of p53 targets. *Nat Rev Cancer.* 2009;9:724–737.
35. Beroud C, Soussi T. The UMD-p53 database: new mutations and analysis tools. *Hum Mutat.* 2003;21:176–181.
36. Cho K, Oliner J, Simons J, et al. The DCC gene: structural analysis and mutations in colorectal carcinomas. *Genomics.* 1994;19:525–531.
37. Takagi Y, Kohmura H, Futamura M, et al. Somatic alterations of the DPC4 gene in human colorectal cancers in vivo. *Gastroenterology.* 1996;111:1369–1372.
38. Takagi Y, Koumura H, Futamura M, et al. Somatic alterations of the SMAD-2 gene in human colorectal cancers. *Br J Cancer.* 1995;78:1152–1155.
39. Wu C, Kirley S, Xiao H, et al. Cables enhances cdk2 tyrosine 152 phosphorylation by Wee1, inhibits cell growth, and is lost in many human colon and squamous cancers. *Cancer Res.* 2001;61:7325–7332.
40. Park do Y, Sakamoto H, Kirley S, et al. The Cables gene on chromosomes 18q is silences by promoter hypermethylation and allelic loss in human colorectal cancer. *Am J Pathol.* 2007;171:1509–1519.
41. Chan TL, Zhao W, Leung SY, et al. BRAF and KRAS mutations in colorectal hyperplastic polyps and serrated adenomas. *Cancer Res.* 2003;63:4878–4881.
42. Samuels Y, Wang Z, Bardelli A, et al. High frequency if mutations of the PIK3CA gene in human cancers. *Science.* 2004;304:554.
43. Samuels Y, Velculescu VE. Oncogenic mutations of PIK3CA in human cancers. *Cell Cycle.* 2004;3:1221–1224.
44. Jones PA, Takai D. The role of DNA methylation in mammalian epigenetics. *Science.* 2001;293:1068–1070.
45. Bird A. DNA methylation patterns and epigenetic memory. *Genes Dev.* 2002;16:6–21.
46. Baylin SB, Herman JG, Graff JR, et al. Alterations in DNA methylation—A fundamental aspect of neoplasia. *Adv Cancer Res.* 1998;72:141–196.
47. Feinberg AP, Vogelstein B. Hypomethylation distinguishes genes of some human cancers from their normal counterparts. *Nature.* 1983;301:89–92.
48. Jones PA, Laird PW. Cancer epigenetics comes of age. *Nat Genet.* 1999;21:163–167.
49. Kane MF, Loda M, Gaida GM, et al. Methylation of the hMLH1 promoter correlates with lack of expression of hMLH1 in sporadic colon tumors and mismatch repair-defective human tumor cell lines. *Cancer Res.* 1997;57:808–811.
50. Merlo A, Herman JG, Mao L, et al. 5′ CpG island methylation is associated with transcriptional silencing of the tumour suppressor p16/CDKN2/MTS1 in human cancers. *Nat Med.* 1995;1:686–692.
51. Ahuja N, Li Q, Mohan AL, et al. Aging and DNA methylation in colorectal mucosa and cancer. *Cancer Res.* 1998;58:5489–5494.
52. Issa JP, Ottaviano YL, Celano P, et al. Methylation of the oestrogen receptor CpG island links ageing and neoplasia in human colon. *Nat Genet.* 1994;7:536–540.
53. Suzuki H, Gabrielson E, Chen W, et al. A genomic screen for genes upregulated by demethylation and histone deacetylase inhibition in human colorectal cancer. *Nat Genet.* 2002;31:141–149.
54. Costello JF, Fruhwald MC, Smiraglia DJ, et al. Aberrant CpG-island methylation has non-random and tumour-type-specific patterns. *Nat Genet.* 2000;24:132–138.
55. Toyota M, Shen L, Ohe-Toyota M, et al. Aberrant methylation of the Cyclooxygenase 2 CpG island in colorectal tumors. *Cancer Res.* 2000;60:4044–4048.
56. Devereux TR, Horikawa I, Anna CH, et al. DNA methylation analysis of the promoter region of the human telomerase reverse transcriptase (hTERT) gene. *Cancer Res.* 1999;59:6087–6090.
57. Ahuja N, Mohan AL, Li Q, et al. Association between CpG island methylation and microsatellite instability in colorectal cancer. *Cancer Res.* 1997;57:3370–3374.
58. Hawkins N, Norrie M, Cheong K, et al. CpG island methylation in sporadic colorectal cancers and its relationship to microsatellite instability. *Gastroenterology.* 2002;122:1376–1387.
59. Whitehall VL, Wynter CV, Walsh MD, et al. Morphological and molecular heterogeneity within nonmicrosatellite instability-high colorectal cancer. *Cancer Res.* 2002;62:6011–6014.

60. Koinuma K, Shitoh K, Miyakura Y, et al. Mutations of BRAF are associated with extensive hMLH1 promoter methylation in sporadic colorectal carcinomas. *Int J Cancer*. 2004;108:237–242.
61. Wang L, Cunningham JM, Winters JL, et al. BRAF mutations in colon cancer are not likely attributable to defective DNA mismatch repair. *Cancer Res*. 2003;63:5209–5212.
62. Esteller M, Toyota M, Sanchez-Cespedes M, et al. Inactivation of the DNA repair gene O6-methylguanine-DNA methyltransferase by promoter hypermethylation is associated with G to A mutations in K-ras in colorectal tumorigenesis. *Cancer Res*. 2000;60:2368–2371.
63. Rashid A, Shen L, Morris JS, et al. CpG island methylation in colorectal adenomas. *Am J Pathol*. 2001;159:1129–1135.
64. Chan AO, Broaddus RR, Houlihan PS, et al. CpG island methylation in aberrant crypt foci of the colorectum. *Am J Pathol*. 2002;160:1823–1830.
65. Li H, Myeroff L, Smiraglia D, et al. SLC5A8, a sodium transporter, is a tumor suppressor gene silenced by methylation in human colon aberrant crypt foci and cancers. *Proc Natl Acad Sci USA*. 2003;100:8412–8417.
66. Torlakovic E, Snover DC. Serrated adenomatous polyposis in humans. *Gastroenterology*. 1996;110:748–755.
67. Rashid A, Houlihan PS, Booker S, et al. Phenotypic and molecular characteristics of hyperplastic polyposis. *Gastroenterology*. 2000;119:323–332.
68. Jeevaratnam P, Cottier DS, Browett PJ, et al. Familial giant hyperplastic polyposis predisposing to colorectal cancer: a new hereditary bowel cancer syndrome. *J Pathol*. 1996;179:20–25.
69. Park SJ, Rashid A, Lee JH, et al. Frequent CpG island methylation in serrated adenomas of the colorectum. *Am J Pathol*. 2003;162:815–822.
70. Chan AO, Issa JP, Morris JS, et al. Concordant CpG island methylation in hyperplastic polyposis. *Am J Pathol*. 2002;160:529–536.
71. Jass JR. Serrated route to colorectal cancer: back street or super highway? *J Pathol*. 2001;193:283–285.
72. Hawkins NJ, Bariol C, Ward RL. The serrated neoplasia pathway. *Pathology*. 2002;34:548–555.
73. Hawkins NJ, Ward RL. Sporadic colorectal cancers with microsatellite instability and their possible origin in hyperplastic polyps and serrated adenomas. *J Natl Cancer Inst*. 2001;93:1307–1313.
74. Bronner CE, Baker SM, Morrison PT, et al. Mutation in the DNA mismatch repair gene homologue hMLH1 is associated with hereditary non-polyposis colon cancer. *Nature*. 1994;368: 258–261.
75. Papadopoulos N, Nicolaides NC, Wei YF, et al. Mutation of a mutL homolog in hereditary colon cancer. *Science*. 1994;263: 1625–1629.
76. Leach FS, Nicolaides NC, Papadopoulos N, et al. Mutation of a Muts D homolog in hereditary nonpolyposis colorectal cancer. *Cell*. 1993;75:1215–1225.
77. Fishel R, Lescoe MK, Rao MR, et al. The human mutator gene homolog MSH2 and its association with hereditary nonpolyposis colon cancer. *Cell*. 1993;75:1027–1038 [Erratum, Cell 1994; 77:167].
78. Miyaki M, Konishi M, Tanaka K, et al. Germline mutation of MSH6 as the cause of hereditary nonpolyposis colorectal cancer. *Nat Genet*. 1997;17:271–272.
79. Koldner RD, Tytell JD, Schmeits JL, et al. Germ-line msh6 mutations in colorectal cancer families. *Cancer Res*. 1999;59: 5068–5074.
80. Nicolaides NC, Papadopoulos N, Liu B, et al. Mutations of two PMS homologues in hereditary nonpolyposis colon cancer. *Nature*. 1994;371:75–80.
81. Herman JG, Umar A, Polyak K, et al. Incidence and functional consequences of hMLH1 promoter hypermethylation in colorectal carcinoma. *Proc Natl Acad Sci USA*. 1998;95:6870–6875.
82. Veigel ML, Kasturi L, Olechnowicz J, et al. Biallelic inactivation of *hMLH1* by epigenetic gene silencing, a novel mechanism causing MSI cancers. *Proc Natl Acad Sci USA*. 1998;95: 8698–8702.
83. Boland CR, Thibodeau SN, Hamilton SR, et al. A National Cancer Institute Workshop on Microsatellite instability for cancer detection and familial predisposition: development of international criteria for the detection of microsatellite instability in colorectal cancer. *Cancer Res*. 1998;58:5248–5275.
84. Malkhosyan SR, Yamamoto H, Piao Z, et al. Late onset and high incidence of colon cancer of the mutator phenotype with hypermethylated *hMLH1* gene in women. *Gastroenterology*. 2000; 119:598.
85. Wright CM, Dent OF, Barker M, et al. The prognostic significance of extensive microsatellite instability in sporadic clinicopathologic stage C colorectal cancer. *Br J Surg*. 2000;87:1197–1202.
86. Alexander J, Watanabe T, Wu TT, et al. Histopathologic identification of colon cancer with microsatellite instability. *Am J Pathol*. 2001;98:527–735.
87. Kim H, Jen J, Vogelstein B, et al. Clinical and pathological characteristics of sporadic colorectal carcinomas with DNA replication errors in microsatellite sequences. *Am J Pathol*. 1994;145:148–156.
88. Rüschoff J, Dietmaier W, Lüttges J, et al. Poorly differentiated colonic adenocarcinoma, medullary type: clinical, phenotypic, and molecular characteristics. *Am J Pathol*. 1997;150: 1815–1825.
89. Fujiwara T, Stolker JM, Watanabe T, et al. Accumulated clonal genetic alterations in familial and sporadic colorectal carcinomas with widespread instability in microsatellite sequences. *Am J Pathol*. 1998;153:1063–1078.
90. Samowitz WS, Holden JA, Curtin K, et al. Inverse relationship between microsatellite instability and K-ras and p53 gene alteration in colon cancer. *Am J Pathol*. 2001;158:1517–1524.
91. Mirabelli-Primdahl L, Gryfe R, Kim H, et al. Beta-catenin mutations are specific for colorectal carcinomas with microsatellite instability but occur in endometrial carcinomas irrespective of mutator pathway. *Cancer Res*. 1999;59:3346–3351.
92. Deng G, Bell I, Crawley S, et al. BRAF mutation is frequently present in sporadic cancer with methylated hMLH1, but not in hereditary nonpolyposis colorectal cancer. *Clin Cancer Res*. 2004;10:191–195.
93. Markowitz S, Wang J, Myeroff L, et al. Inactivation of the type II TGF-β receptor in colon cancer cells with microsatellite instability. *Science*. 1995;268:1336–1338.
94. Souza RF, Appel R, Yin J, et al. The insulin-like growth factor II receptor gene is a target of microsatellite instability in human gastrointestinal tumors. *Nat Genet*. 1996;14:255–257.
95. Yamamoto H, Sawai H, Weber TK, et al. Somatic frameshift mutations in hereditary nonpolyposis colorectal cancer. *Cancer Res*. 1998;58:997–1003.
96. Parsons R, Myeroff L, Liu B, et al. Microsatellite instability and mutations of the transforming growth factor beta type II receptor gene in colorectal cancer. *Cancer Res*. 1995;55:5548–5550.
97. Jen J, Kim H, Piantadosi S, et al. Allelic loss of chromosome 18q and prognosis in colorectal cancer. *N Engl J Med*. 1994;331: 213–221.
98. Watanabe T, Wu T-T, Catalano PJ, et al. Molecular predictors of survival after chemotherapy for colon cancer. *N Engl J Med*. 2001;344:1196–1206.
99. Gryfe R, Kim H, Hsieh ET, et al. Tumor microsatellite instability and clinical outcome in young patients with colorectal cancer. *N Engl J Med*. 2000;342:69–77.
100. Shen L, Catalano PJ, Benson AB III, et al. Association between DNA methylation and shortened survival in patients with advanced colorectal cancer treated with 5-fluorouracil based chemotherapy. *Clin Cancer Res*. 2007;13:6093–6098.

101. Samowitz WS, Albertsen H, Herrick J, et al. Evaluation of a large, population-based sample supports a CpG island methylator phenotype in colon cancer. *Gastroenterology*. 2005;129:837–845.
102. Jover R, Nguyen T-P, Perez-Carbonell L, et al. 5-Fluorouracil adjuvant chemotherapy does not increase survival with CpG adjuvant chemotherapy does not increase survival in patients with CpG island methylator phenotype colorectal cancer. *Gastroenterology*. 2011;140:1174–1181.
103. Rubic CM, Sargent DJ, Moore MJ, et al. Tumor microsatellite-instability status as a predictor of benefit from fluorouracil-based adjuvant chemotherapy for colon cancer. *N Engl J Med*. 2003;349:247–257.
104. Liévre A, Bachet JB, Le Corre D, et al. KRAS mutation is predictive of response to cetuximab therapy in colorectal cancer. *Cancer Res*. 2006;66:3992–3995.
105. Liévre A, Bachet JB, Boige V, et al. KRAS mutation as an independent prognostic factor in patients with advanced colorectal cancer treated with cetuximab. *J Clin Oncol*. 2008;26:374–379.
106. Jhawer M, Goel S, Wilson AJ, et al. PIK3CA mutation/PTEN expression status predicts response of colon cancer cells to the epidermal growth factor receptor inhibitor cetuximab. *Cancer Res*. 2008;68:1953–1961 [Erratum, Cancer Res 2008;68:6859.].
107. Laurent-Puig P, Cayre A, Manceau G, et al. Analysis of PTEN, BRAF, and EGFR status in determining benefit from cetuximab therapy in wild-type KRAS metastatic colon cancer. *J Clin Oncol*. 2009;27:5924–5930.
108. van Cutsem E, Köhne C-H, Hitre E, et al. Cetuximab and chemotherapy as initial treatment for metastatic colorectal cancer. *N Eng J Med*. 2009;360:1408–1417.
109. De Roock W, Claes B, Bernasconi D, et al. Effects of KRAS, BRAF, NRAS, AND PIK3CA mutations on the efficacy of cetuximab plus chemotherapy in chemotherapy-refractory metastatic cancer: a retrospective consortium analysis. *Lancet Oncol*. 2010;11:753–762.
110. Warth A, Kloor M, Schirmacher P, et al. Genetics and epigenetics of small bowel adenocarcinoma: the interactions of CIN, MSI, and CIMP. *Mod Pathol*. 2011;24:564–570.
111. Diosdado B, Buffart TE, Watkins R, et al. High-resolution array comparative genomic hybridization in sporadic and celiac disease-related small bowel adenocarcinomas. *Clin Cancer Res*. 2010;16:1391–1401.
112. Blaker H, von Herbay A, Penzel R, et al. Genetics of adenocarcinomas of the small intestine: frequent deletions at chromosome 18q and mutations of the SMAD4 gene. *Oncogene*. 2002;21: 158–164.
113. Berkhout M, Nagtegaal ID, Cornelissen SJ, et al. Chromosomal and methylation alterations in sporadic and familial adenomatous polyposis-related duodenal carcinomas. *Mod Pathol*. 2007;20: 1253–1262.
114. Rashid A, Hamilton SR. Genetic alterations in sporadic and Crohn's-associated adenocarcinomas of the small intestine. *Gastroenterology*. 1997;113:127–135.
115. Wheeler JM, Warren BF, Mortensen NJ, et al. An insight into the genetic pathway of adenocarcinoma of the small intestine. *Gut*. 2002;50:218–223.
116. Arai M, Shimizu S, Imai Y, et al. Mutations of the Ki-ras, p53 and APC genes in adenocarcinomas of the human small intestine. *Int J Cancer*. 1997;70:390–395.
117. Zhang MQ, Chen ZM, Wang HL. Immunohistochemical investigation of tumorigenic pathways in small intestinal adenocarcinoma: a comparison with colorectal adenocarcinoma. *Mod Pathol*. 2006;19:573–580.
118. Younes N, Fulton N, Tanaka R, et al. The presence of K-12 ras mutations in duodenal adenocarcinomas and the absence of ras mutations in other small bowel adenocarcinomas and carcinoid tumors. *Cancer*. 1997;79:1804–1808.
119. Muneyuki T, Watanabe M, Yamanaka M, et al. Combination analysis of genetic alterations and cell proliferation in small intestinal carcinomas. *Dig Dis Sci*. 2000;45:2022–2028.
120. Schonleben F, Qiu W, Allendorf JD, et al. Molecular analysis of PIK3CA, BRAF, and RAS oncogenes in periampullary and ampullary adenomas and carcinomas. *J Gastrointest Surg*. 2009;13: 1510–1516.
121. Kim SG, Chan AOO, Wu TT, et al. Epigenetic and genetic alterations in duodenal carcinomas are distinct from biliary and ampullary carcinomas. *Gastroenterology*. 2003;124:1300–1310.
122. Overman MJ, Pozadzides J, Kopetz S, et al. Immunophenotype and molecular characterization of adenocarcinoma of the small intestine. *Br J Cancer*. 2010;102:144–150.
123. Lynch HT, Lynch JF, Lynch PM, et al. Hereditary colorectal cancer syndromes: molecular genetics, genetic counseling, diagnosis and management. *Fam Cancer*. 2008;7:27–39.

Cancers of the Rectum and Anal Canal

9

Jenia Jenab-Wolcott and Bruce Giantonio

Introduction

Colorectal cancer is the second leading cause of cancer in USA and remains a significant cause of mortality and morbidity throughout the world. In 2010 approximately 102,900 new cases of colon cancer and 39,670 rectal cancer were diagnosed with estimated 51,370 deaths in USA.[1,2] The profound impact of this disease on public health is underscored by the fact that 1 in 18 American men and 1 in 20 women are at risk of developing colorectal cancer in their lifetime.[3] While the overall incidence of colorectal cancer has decreased over the past three decades, since the 1980s there has been evidence for a left to right-sided shift in incidence of colorectal cancers.[4–7] The incidence of proximal (or right-sided) colorectal cancer rose from 20% to 30% whereas rectal cancer decreased from 22 to 11% between 1979 and 1994.[4,5] In a recent study of incidence of colorectal cancer in the USA between 1999 and 2004 the greatest burden of disease was in the proximal colon (21.8 per 100,000 population) vs. the distal colon (13 per 100,000 population) and the rectum (14.1 per 100,000 population).[6] Interestingly, an age-, gender-, and race-specific disparity in anatomic location of colorectal cancer (CRC) has been reported, where individuals aged ≥65 years, women, and blacks had the highest incidence rate of proximal lesions.[6,8,9] In the rectum, however, rates did not differ significantly by race and older whites had the highest incidence of rectal cancer.[6]

While the disparity change in the distribution of CRC lesions is unclear, some have argued that proximal and distal tumors arise from different pathogenetic pathways.[9–11] The right and left segments of the large intestine have distinct embryologic origin and biological behavior. The right side of the colon (cecum, proximal two-thirds of the transverse colon) arises from the midgut, and the left side of the colon (distal one-third of the transverse, descending and sigmoid colon, rectum) arises from the midgut. This difference in embryologic origin is further underscored by the dual blood supply of the colon. Moreover, tumors of the proximal and distal colon appear to have different, epidemiology, histology, genetics, and biological behavior. Differences in pathology of the right sided and left-sided colonic tumors have also been described.[12] Several studies have indicated distinct molecular biology in tumors arising from different segments of the large intestine. Distal tumors have been shown to have higher frequency of loss of p53 function, aneuploidy, and chromosomal instability, whereas proximal tumors are more mucinous, diploid, and of the microsatellite instability (MSI) phenotype.[13] Furthermore, clinical behavior is different where local recurrence is the major problem in rectal cancers and distant metastasis is a significant issue in the management of colon cancer. These observations have led to the hypothesis that the mechanisms of oncogenesis in colon and rectum are mediated via different cellular pathways.

Anatomy of Rectum and Anal Canal

The large intestine extends from the terminal ileum to the dentate line in the anal canal and it measures between 1.3 to 1.8 m.[14–16] It is divided into several sections: cecum, ascending colon, transverse colon, descending colon, sigmoid colon, and rectum. The right or proximal colon encompasses the region from cecum to the transverse colon, and the left or distal large intestine includes the segment from the splenic flexure to the rectum (Fig. 9.1). The rectum is approximately 12 cm and extends from the fusion of the taenia to the

J. Jenab-Wolcott, M.D., Ph.D. (✉)
Delaware County Memorial Hospital, 2100 Keystone Ave, Drexel Hill, PA, USA
e-mail: jenia.jenab.wolcott@gmail.com

B. Giantonio, M.D.
Department of Hematology/Oncology, University of Pennsylvania, Philadelphia, PA, USA

A.R. Sepulveda and J.P. Lynch (eds.), *Molecular Pathology of Neoplastic Gastrointestinal Diseases*, Molecular Pathology Library 7, DOI 10.1007/978-1-4614-6015-2_9,

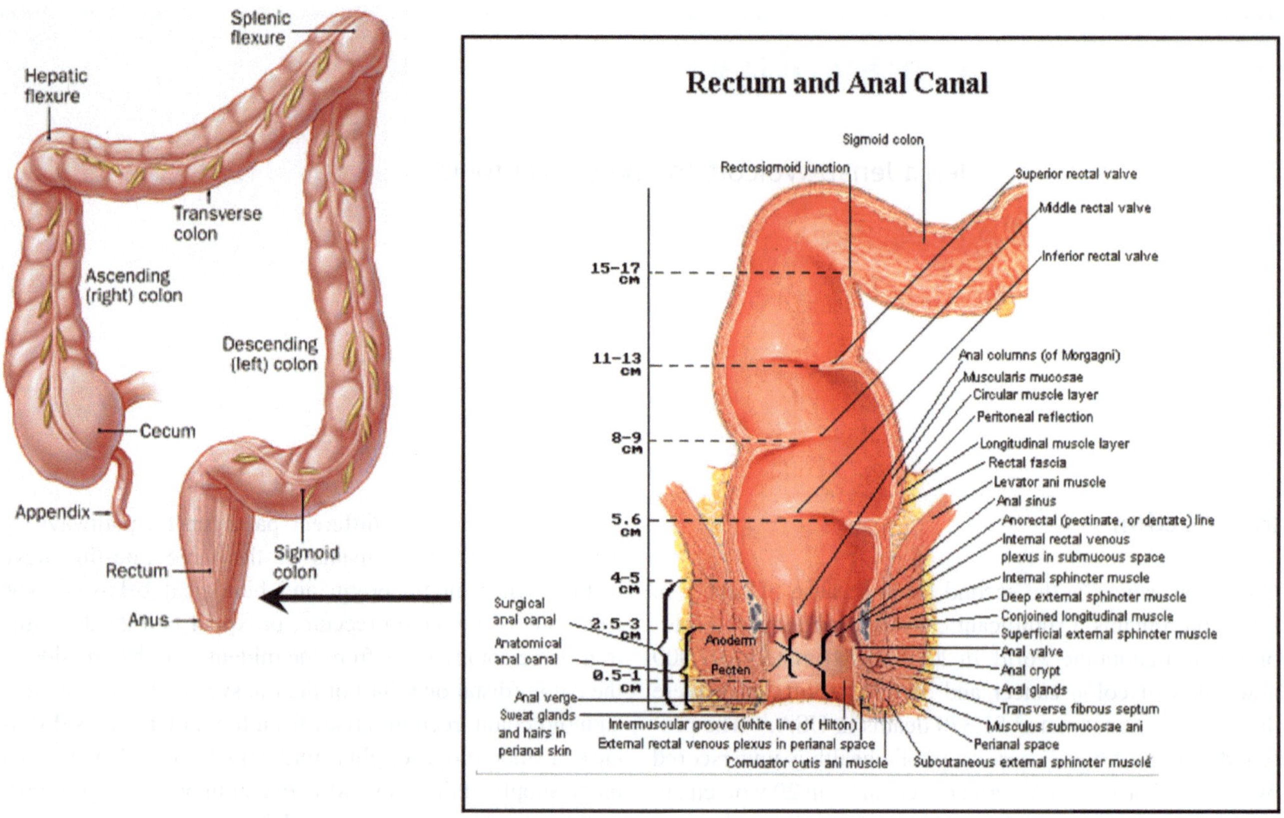

Fig. 9.1 Anatomy of the rectum and anus

puborectalis ring (palpable anorectal ring on digital rectal examination). It is divided into three segments, where the peritoneum covers the upper third on its anterior and lateral surfaces, the middle third on its anterior surface, and no covering of the lower third of the rectum which is known as the ampulla.

The location of the rectosigmoid junction is controversial, as there are different definitions of the relevant landmarks and the distance of the malignant lesion from the anal verge is important for cancer management. However the rectum is commonly defined as the region of the large intestine that is at least partially retroperitoneal. The location of rectal tumors is designated by the distance of the lower edge of the tumor from the anal verge, dentate (pectinate or mucocutaneous) line.

The anal canal measures 3–5 cm in length and extends from the rectal ampulla (level of pelvic floor) to the anal verge. The distal end of the anal canal, or the anal verge, is at the level of the squamous–mucocutaneous junction and the perianal skin. The pectinate line indicates the junction of the superior part of the anal canal, lined by columnar epithelium, and the inferior part, lined by non-keratinizing squamous epithelium. Distal to the dentate line, the squamous epithelium merges with the perianal skin or the true epidermis. Given the different types of epithelium found in the anal canal, two distinct categories of tumors can develop. Malignant lesions that arise from the mucosa (columnar, transitional, or squamous) are considered true anal canal cancers, whereas tumors arising from the epidermis or distal to the squamous–mucocutaneous junction are termed anal margin tumors.

Pathology

Gross Appearance

The macroscopic features of CRC depend on the extent of disease progression and the site of the lesion. Tumors in the proximal or right colon commonly appear as polypoid or fungating exophytic masses. Exophytic growth has been associated with lower stage,[17] lower risk of hematogenous spread,[18] and more favorable prognosis.[19,20] Tumors involving the distal or left colon however are more commonly annular producing an "apple core" appearance. These lesions often produce symptoms of bowel obstruction which is clinical maker of poor prognosis.[21–23]

Histological Subtypes and Molecular Biology

Adenocarcinoma

Although adenomas are the precursor lesions for all CRC, they evolve into different histological patterns with invasion and progression. Adenocarcinomas comprise the vast majority (85–90%) of cancers of the colon and rectum, which are further classified by histological grade.[24] These are gland-forming tumors, and the histological grade of differentiation takes into account the variability in gland size and shape (Fig. 9.2).

Mucinous and Signet Cell Tumors

Mucinous and signet cell tumors are related subtypes of colorectal adenocarcinomas with prominent mucin secretion (Fig. 9.2b). By convention a 50% or greater mucinous component is required for designation of mucinous carcinoma, and this morphology accounts for approximately 11–17% of colorectal cancers.[25,26] Mucinous carcinomas are more commonly found in the rectum and sigmoid and they tend to present as more advanced tumors.[27] Although older studies involving rectal cancers had suggested a more aggressive behavior for these tumors,[28,29] the College of American Pathology (CAP) consensus statement in 2000 indicated that the significance of mucinous histology is controversial and has not been proven to be a statistically significant independent prognostic indicator.[30] Signet cell carcinoma accounts for 1–2% of CRC. These are aggressive tumors with propensity for extensive intramural spread and peritoneal carcinomatosis.[31] The unique pathologic feature of these cells is the presence of intracytoplasmic mucin-containing vacuole that pushes the nucleus to the side. When ≥50% of the tumor is made up of this type of cell it is designated signet cell carcinoma.[24] Given the rarity of this morphologic subtype, a signet ring histology should prompt consideration of metastatic disease from other organs such as gastric carcinoma or lobular breast carcinoma.[24]

Signet ring cell carcinoma and mucinous cell carcinoma of colon and rectum are associated with distinct genetic features. Molecular studies demonstrate that tumors with minor signet ring or mucinous component (≤49%) have similar genetic features to those with abundant (≥50%) signet cell or mucinous component respectively.[32] Substantial mucin production is a feature of colorectal cancers with microsatellite instability (MSI) and both signet ring colorectal carcinoma and mucinous colorectal carcinoma are associated with high degree of MSI (MSI-H), as described in previous chapters.[33,34] Mucinous carcinomas have been shown to be twice likely as usual adenocarcinomas (30% vs. 15%) to exhibit MSI-H phenotype, and MSI-H mucinous carcinomas tend to have a better prognosis than their microsatellite stable (MSS) counterparts.[35] Approximately one-third of signet cell colorectal carcinomas are MSI-H and microsatellite instability status does not seem to be a predictor of survival for signet ring cell CRC.[33] Consistent with the MSI phenotype, loss of MLH1 expression by immunohistochemistry (IHC) is more common in both signet carcinomas (29–40%) and mucinous carcinomas

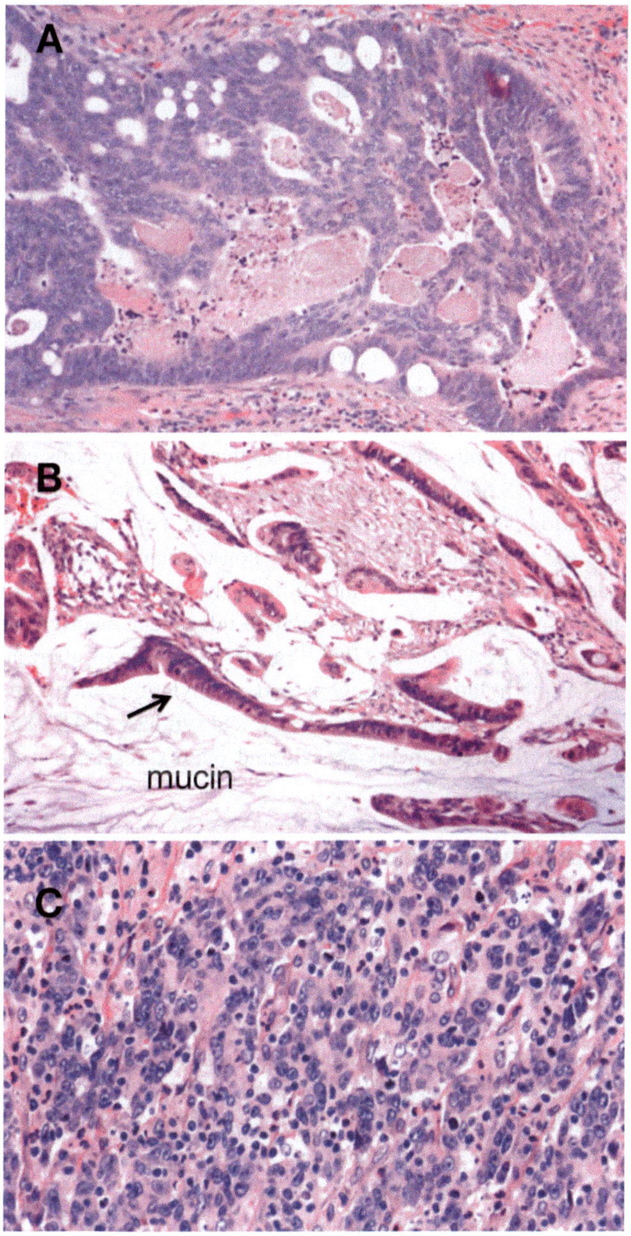

Fig. 9.2 Adenocarcinoma involving the sigmoid colon and rectum. (**a**) Moderately differentiated adenocarcinoma (original magnification ×100). (**b**) Mucinous adenocarcinoma. The *arrow* points to the strips of neoplastic epithelium in the background of mucin pools. (**c**) Poorly differentiated adenocarcinoma with associated intra-tumoral lymphocytes AKA medullary carcinoma (original magnification ×200). Hematoxylin and Eosin stains

(13–30%) than non-mucinous CRC (10%).[32] Since 30% of individuals with signet ring cell CRC have ulcerative colitis,[36] it has been suggested that differences in molecular basis and natural biology of signet cell carcinomas may confound the result of outcome studies.[24]

A number of other genes and cellular pathways have also been implicated in carcinogenesis of mucinous and signet cell tumors of colon and rectum. The RAS–RAF–MECK–ERK–MAP kinase pathway, involved in cellular response to growth signals, has been extensively studied in pathogenesis of colorectal cancers. Higher frequency of mutational activation of *BRAF* oncogene by Val600Glu (V600E) point mutation has been reported in both signet ring tumors (22–33%) and in mucinous cancers (15–27%) than non-mucinous carcinomas (8.6%).[32,34] In contrast lower frequency of *KRAS* mutations have been reported in signet cell carcinomas (36%), mucinous (38%) than in non-mucinous colorectal carcinomas (60%).[32,37] Other unique molecular features of mucinous colorectal tumors include infrequent inactivating mutations in *APC*,[34] or *TP53*,[32] but frequent rate of aberrant DNA methylation or CpG island methylation phenotype (CIMP),[34] and higher levels of fatty acid synthase (FASN) an enzyme involved in lipogenesis and overexpressed in colorectal cancers.[38,39]

Medullary Carcinoma

The term medullary carcinoma is applied to poorly differentiated non-gland forming large cell carcinomas with round nuclei, prominent nucleolus, that grow in solid sheets with heavy penetration of adjacent small lymphocytes (termed tumor infiltrating lymphocytes) (Fig. 9.2c).[40] This rare histological subtype appears to have a relatively indolent biology and improved survival.[41] Nearly all medullary carcinomas have MSI-H phenotype and have been described in both sporadic[42] and hereditary (Lynch syndrome) colorectal cancers.[43] The homeodomain intestinal transcription factor CDX2 is a useful immunohistochemical marker for identification of epithelial neoplasms of the gastrointestinal tract and loss of CDX2 expression has been strongly associated with medullary colorectal carcinoma.[44,45] Loss of CDX1 expression has been associated with mismatch repair defect and in both sporadic MSI-H CRC[44,46,47] and in 3.2% of Lynch syndrome CRC.[48] CDX2 negative colorectal cancers appear to have unique clinicopathological features including female gender, advanced stage, high tumor grade, aberrant methylation or CIMP-high phenotype, and poor prognosis in patients with a family history of CRC.[49]

Squamous Cell Carcinoma

Primary squamous cell carcinoma (SSC) of the rectum is a rare malignancy and only case reports and small case series have been published.[50–52] Review of colorectal cancers cases published in the English literature has estimated the incidence of the disease to be 0.1–0.25 per 1,000 CRC,[51,53] with the most frequent location in the rectum followed by the right colon.[54] Since the esophagus and the anus are the most common sites of SSC of the GI tract, the diagnostic criteria for rectal SSC include lack of continuity between the tumor and the anal canal, absence of evidence of metastatic SSC from another part of the body, lack of fistulous tract lined by squamous cells, in addition to squamous cell histology.[55] Immunohistochemical staining of biopsy specimen for cytokeratins can also aid in distinguishing SSC of rectum from that of the anus or other small poorly differentiated tumors. The cytokeratin CAM 5.2 characteristically stains rectal squamous cell and adenocarcinoma but not anal squamous cell tumors.[51,53] Cytokeratins AE1/AE3 stain positively for cells of squamous origin and can facilitate distinguishing this cell type from less well-differentiated lesions.[51] Furthermore, the squamous cell carcinoma antigen (SSC Ag) has been shown to be elevated in SSC of rectum with normalization of levels in response to therapy[56] and has been suggested as a potential useful tumor marker for monitoring disease response and progression.[51]

In light of the rarity of SSC of rectum, strong data regarding its epidemiology, natural history, and optimal therapy are limited. Risk factors implicated in the pathogenesis of this disease include inflammatory colorectal conditions[57] as well as infections such as Schistosomiasis,[58] Entamoeba histolytica,[55] and human papilloma virus (HPV).[59] While a clear association between HPV infection and SSC of anus has been established, studies relating HPV to SSC rectal cancer are sparse and varied in methodology and do not provide firm evidence for cause/effect relationship.[51] SSC of the rectum has been reported to be more common in women (66%) than in men (34%) and patients often present with advanced disease.[52] While early stage SSC of colon has been shown to have a similar outcome to node negative (stage I/II) adenocarcinoma of colon, node positive SSC have worse prognosis stage by stage.[60] Given the tendency for rectal cancer to have local lymph node involvement, the overall prognosis of SSC of rectum is poor.

Differential diagnosis of rectal carcinomas includes both rare primary rectal cancers as well as metastatic disease from other organs. Rare rectal cancers include carcinoid tumors, lymphoma, gastrointestinal stromal tumors, and Kaposi's sarcoma in individuals with acquired immunodeficiency syndrome. Also tumor invasion by direct extension (prostate, endometrium, and ovary) as well as metastatic disease from distant organs should be considered. The discussion of these malignancies is beyond the scope of this chapter.

Table 9.1 TNM staging for colorectal cancers adapted from AJCC cancer staging 7th edition

Primary tumor (T)	
Tx	Primary tumor cannot be assessed
T0	No evidence of primary tumor
Tis	Carcinoma in situ: intraepithelial or invasion of lamina propria[a]
T1	Tumor invades submucosa
T2	Tumor invades muscularis propria
T3	Tumor invades through the muscularis propria into pericolorectal tissues
T4a	Tumor penetrates to the surfaces of the visceral peritoneum[b]
T4b	Tumor directly invades or is adherent to other organs or structures[c]
Regional lymph nodes (N)[d,e]	
Nx	Regional lymph nodes cannot be assessed
N0	No regional lymph node metastasis
N1	Metastasis in 1–3 regional lymph nodes
N1a	Metastasis in one regional lymph node
N1b	Metastasis in 2–3 regional lymph node
N1c	Tumor deposit(s) in the subserosa, mesentery, or nonperitonealized pericolic, or perirectal tissues without regional nodal metastasis
N2	Metastasis in four or more regional lymph nodes
N2a	Metastasis in 4–6 regional lymph nodes
N2b	Metastasis in seven or more regional lymph nodes
Distant metastasis (M)	
M0	No distant metastasis
M1	Distant metastasis
M1a	Metastasis confined to one organ or site (e.g., liver, lung, ovary, nonregional node)
M1b	Metastases in more than one organ/site or the peritoneum

[a]Tis includes cancer cells confined within the glandular basement membrane (intraepithelial) or mucosal lamina propria (intramucosal) with no extension through the muscularis mucosae into the submucosa

[b]Direct invasion in T4 includes invasion of other organs or other segments of the colorectum as a result of direct extension through the serosa, as confirmed on microscopic examination (for example, invasion of the sigmoid colon by a carcinoma of the cecum) or for cancers in a retroperitoneal or subperitoneal location, direct invasion of other organs or structures by virtue of extension beyond the muscularis propria (i.e., respectively, a tumor on the posterior wall of the descending colon invading the left kidney or lateral abdominal wall; or a mid or distal rectal cancer with invasion of prostate, seminal vesicles, cervix, or vagina)

[c]Tumor that is adherent to other organs or structures, grossly, is classified cT4b. However, if no tumor is present in the adhesion, microscopically, the classification should be pT1-4a depending on the anatomical depth of wall invasion. The V and L classifications should be used to identify the presence or absence of vascular or lymphatic invasion whereas the PN site-specific factor should be used for perineural invasion

[d]A satellite peritumoral nodule in the pericolorectal adipose tissue of a primary carcinoma without histologic evidence of residual lymph node in the nodule may represent discontinuous spread, venous invasion with extravascular spread (V1/2), or a totally replaced lymph node (N1/2). Replaced nodes should be counted separately as positive nodes in the N category, whereas discontinuous spread or venous invasion should be classified and counted in the Site-Specific Factor category Tumor Deposits (TD)

[e]Expert panels recommend histological examination of at least 12 nodes for accurate determination of nodal status

Staging

The older Dukes' classification is rarely used in the modern literature, and the American Joint Committee on Cancer/International Union for Cancer Control (AJCC/UICC) has become the gold standard for staging CRC.[61] The most recent 7th edition 2010 tumor, node, metastasis (TNM) staging of AJCC is summarized in Tables 9.1 and 9.2.

Clinical stage (cT, cN, cM) is based on radiographic, endoscopic, and intraoperative findings, whereas pathologic stage (pT, pN, pM) requires gross and microscopic pathologic examination of the resected specimen. A modified pathologic staging is designated to surgical specimens post neoadjuvant therapy annotated by *y* prescript (ypT, ypN, ypM). Pathologic stage is the most powerful indicator of outcome after resection in CRC. Five-survival data adapted from the 2010 AJCC staging for rectal and colon cancer is shown in Tables 9.1 and 9.2.

While TNM staging incorporates anatomic elements of tumor extension, increasing number of independent prognostic indicators are being discovered for predicting outcome and response to therapy. In 1999 the College of American Pathologist (CAP) released a consensus document evaluating the prognostic role of a number of histopathologic factors in colorectal cancer.[30] Based on the strength of published evidence five categories of prognostic factors were defined. Category I represented definitively proven validated prognostic indicators generally used in patient management. Category IIA designated well-documented factors with sufficient importance to be included in the pathology report but that remain to be validated in statistically robust studies. Category IIB included prognostic factors promising in multiple studies, but with insufficient data for inclusion in category I or IIA. Category III referred to insufficiently studied factors with unproven prognostic value. Category IV included well studied markers that were shown to have no prognostic significance. These factors are discussed in the following section.

Molecular Pathways to Colorectal Tumorigenesis

Colorectal cancer (CRC) is a heterogeneous disease where accumulation of genetic and epigenetic alterations leads to progression from normal colonic epithelium to fully malignant invasive carcinoma. There is growing evidence that molecular defects and alteration in cellular signaling pathways determine tumor biology and clinical outcome in colorectal tumors. Classification of CRC into at least three distinct molecular pathways of genomic instability has been proposed[62] (Table 9.3). These pathways include chromosomal instability (CIN) pathway, DNA mismatch repair

Table 9.2 Staging and the observed survival rates for colon and rectal cancer

					3-year survival		5-year survival	
Stage	T	N	M	Dukes	Colon	Rectum	Colon	Rectum
0	Tis	N0	M0	–				
I	T1	N0	M0	A	82.6	83.4	74.0	74.1
	T2	N0	M0	A				
IIA	T3	N0	M0	B	77.8	76.6	66.5	64.5
IIB	T4a	N0	M0	B	69.1	65.9	58.6	51.6
IIC	T4b	N0	M0	B	45.3	45.4	37.3	32.3
IIIA	T1–2	N1/N1c	M0	C	83.6	85.8	79.1	74.0
	T1	N2a	M0	C				
IIIB	T3–T4a	N1/N1c	M0	C	59.3	63.6	46.3	45.0
	T2–T3	N2a	M0	C				
	T1–T2	N2b	M0	C				
IIIC	T4a	N2a	M0	C	39.0	48.8	32.9	33.4
	T3–T4a	N2b	M0	C				
	T4b	N1–N2	M0	C				
IVA	Any T	Any N	M1a	–	11.3[a]	13.7[a]	7.6[a]	6.0[a]
IVB	Any T	Any N	M1b	–				

Data based on 28,491 cases of colon cancer and 9,860 cases of rectal cancer from SEER registry 1973–2005 public use File diagnosed in years 1998–2000. The original source of this data is from the AJCC Cancer Staging Manual, 7th edition (2010) by Springer New York, Inc

[a]Rate for all stage IV disease

Table 9.3 Molecular pathways to colorectal carcinogenesis

	Chromosomal instability pathway	Mismatch repair pathway	Aberrant DNA methylation pathway			
Features	Hereditary or sporadic	Hereditary	Hereditary or sporadic			
BRAF	WT	WT	MT	MT	WT	WT
KRAS	WT	WT/MT	WT	WT	MT	MT
MSI	MSS	MSI-H	MSI-H	MSS	MSS/MSI-L	MSS/MSI-L
CIN	Present	Absent	Absent	Absent	Absent	Present/absent
CIMP	Negative	Negative	CIMP-H	CIMP-H	CIMP-H	CIMP-L
Anatomic location	Distal	Proximal	Proximal	Proximal	Proximal	Distal
Gender bias	Men	No gender bias	Women	Women	Women	Men
Prognosis	Intermediate	Good	Good	Poor	LD	Poor

Three distinct pathways have been implicated in pathogenesis of colorectal cancers. Each has unique molecular, histological, and clinical features

Table adapted from Leggett, B. and V. Whitehall, *Role of the serrated pathway in colorectal cancer pathogenesis.* Gastroenterology, 2009. 138(6): p. 2088–100; Noffsinger, A.E., *Serrated polyps and colorectal cancer: new pathway to malignancy.* Annu Rev Pathol, 2009. 4: p. 343–64

Abbreviations: CIMP CpG island methylator phenotype, *CIN* chromosomal instability, *MSI* microsatellite instability, *MSH-H* high level MSI, *MSI-L* low level MSI, *MSS* microsatellite stable, *LD* lack of strong data

pathway associated with epiphenomenon of microsatellite instability (MSI), and epigenomic instability or CpG island hypermethylation (CIMP) pathway.

Chromosomal Instability Pathway

Chromosomal instability (CIN) accounts for approximately 60–70% of sporadic CRC and is characterized by gain or loss of entire or large segments of chromosome and karyotypic abnormalities. The CIN phenotype was considered a hallmark feature of the classic model of multistep colorectal carcinogenesis originally proposed by Fearon and Vogelstein.[63] In this model, the initial mutational inactivation of the tumor suppressor gene, *adenomatous polyposis coli* (*APC*) was followed by activation of the *KRAS* proto-oncogene; subsequently, additional genetic defects involved mutations in the *transforming growth factor-β* (TGF-β), *PI3KCA*, *TP53*, and allelic loss of chromosome 18q (including putative genes including deleted in colorectal carcinoma, *DCC*, *SMAD4*, and *SMAD2*).[64] These tumors can be inherited, as typified by familial adenomatous polypsis (FAP) due to germline mutations in the *APC* gene, or they can occur sporadically.

The prognostic significance of aneuploidy in colorectal cancers was evaluated in a recent meta-analysis. Walther et al evaluated 63 studies that reported outcome on 10,126 patients with CRC.[65] They found that 60% of these tumors displayed CIN. A positive CIN status was associated with significantly worse outcome in all patients, including those with stage II and III CRC (overall HR 1.45, 95% CI 1.27–1.65, $P<0.001$). There was also inferior progression, free survival (PFS) (HR 1.71, 95% CI 1.51–1.94, $P<0.001$) in patients with CIN positive CRC. Given the clear demonstration of inferior outcome in CIN associated tumors, it has been suggested that chromosomal stability could be used as a molecular correlate in future clinical trial designs.

Microsatellite Instability Pathway

A subset of colorectal cancers is characterized by a defect in the cellular DNA mismatch repair (MMR) system. Deficient MMR leads to altered length of short nucleotide repeats in tumor DNA compared to normal DNA, a phenomenon termed microsatellite instability (MSI).[13] MSI is typically assessed by evaluation of five microsatellite markers (D2S123, D5S346, D17S250, BAT25, and BAT26) which are considered as the NCI consensus panel.[66] The term MSI, when otherwise not specified, denotes high frequency MSI (MSI-H) in which >30% of the markers are mutated as defined by Bethesda guidelines,[66] and these tumors are felt to represent a distinct clinicopathological entity. Colorectal tumors with 1 but <30% of microsatellite markers mutated are called low MSI (MSI-L) which have the same genotype and phenotype as microsatellite-stable tumors (MSS).

Defects in the DNA mismatch repair system can arise via inherited genetic mutations or through acquired epigenetic phenomenon that occur with aging. Germline mutations in any one of the MMR genes (predominantly MLH1, MSH2, MSH6, and PMS2) is the underlying genetic defect in the majority of hereditary non-polyposis colon cancer (HNPCC) also known a Lynch Syndrome.[67] Approximately 15% of sporadic CRC exhibit high frequency MSI (MSI-H) due to biallelic silencing of MLH1 gene expression by promoter hypermethylation.[68,69] It has been long appreciated that sporadic MSI CRC have distinct pathological and clinical features compared to tumors that arise through the classic CIN pathway. Histologically they are poorly differentiated, mucinous, and associated with peritumoral lymphocytic infiltration. These tumors are more commonly found in the proximal (right) colon, older individuals, and women.[13] The prognostic value of MSI in CRC has been extensively studied and is well accepted as an indicator of improved outcome. In fact, MSI is considered an important prognostic factor that is recommended for evaluation in the 2010 American Joint Committee on Cancer (AJCC) TNM staging criteria in CRC.[70]

Aberrant DNA Methylation Pathway

A third pathway, epigenomic instability, has gained recent recognition as an important pathway in colorectal carcinogenesis. Transcriptional silencing of tumor suppressor genes by cytosine methylation at the promoter CpG islands is commonly seen in human cancers..[71] Global promoter hypermethylation, known as CpG islands methylator phenotype, or CIMP, has been well described in a subset of CRC.[72] Promoter hypermethylation can occur in genes with no role in cancer development, denoted "methylated in tumor" or MINT. This mode of epigenetic silencing can also occur in known tumor suppressors such as p16, insulin-like growth factor 2 (IGF-2), and in DNA repair genes such a MLH1 and o-methylguanine methyltransferse (MGMT).[62,72] Although there is no consensus in the literature, a number of methylation markers and DNA methylation assays have been used to quantify the level of CpG island methylation in colorectal tumors. This has led to molecular subclassification of colorectal tumors as CIMP-high (or CIMP 1) vs. CIMP-low (CIMP 2) vs. CIMP-negative, the utility of which is not completely understood at this time.[73]

Promoter CpG methylation is associated with a serrated pathway of colorectal carcinogenesis,[74,75] distinct from the classic adenoma–carcinoma pathway described by Vogelstein.[63] These tumors are thought to represent a subset of CRC with unique biological and clinical features. CIMP tumors are associated with proximal location, female sex, mucinous histology, and poor tumor differentiation. These tumors often exhibit microsatellite instability, via somatic epigenetic silencing of MLH1 expression. While CIMP high tumors frequently carry *BRAF* V600E mutations, CIMP-low tumors have been proposed to be associated with more frequent k-ras mutation and male gender.[76] Additionally CIMP negative tumors appear to have chromosomal instability and to be distally located.

A complex prognostic relationship has been described between promoter CpG methylation status and other molecular markers in colorectal cancers. While most studies have indicated that high level CIMP is associated with poor prognosis,[77–79] contradictory results have been reported in the literature.[80] MSI-H/CIMP-negative colorectal cancers appear to have favorable prognosis.[77] Increasing level of CIMP confers worse prognosis in MSS CRC,[81] with CIMP-H cancers having worse prognosis than CIMP-negative tumors.

Prognostic Factors in Colorectal Cancers

The use of validated predictive (factors predicting response to therapy) and prognostic (factors associated with disease outcome) biomarkers has emerged as a critical component of individualized care of patients with colorectal cancers. Although the clinical management of colon and rectal cancers are different, these malignancies have been traditionally grouped with respect to epidemiology, staging, and molecular pathogenesis. At this time there is limited data on molecular biomarkers that are unique to malignancies of the rectum. This section will discuss the role of histological and genetic predictive and prognostic determinants in colorectal cancers with special focus on molecular markers relevant to rectal cancer.

In 1999 the College of American Pathologists (CAP) released a consensus statement on the biologic, genetic, and molecular prognostic factors in CRC.[30] The factors were grouped into categories based on the review of literature and strength of published evidence. The categories are as follows.

Category I Factors

Local tumor extent (pT category), regional lymph node involvement (pN), lymphovascular invasion, residual tumor post definitive surgery, and preoperative serum CEA were deemed strong predictors of outcome in CRC that merit inclusion in this category. Depth of tumor penetration was an independent predictor of survival[82,83] and number of involved regional lymph nodes was one of the strongest predictors of outcome in CRC.[84,85] In addition, venous and angiolymphatic invasion, residual tumor after definitive therapy, and lack of normalization of the CEA markers postsurgery was poor prognostic markers.[86]

Category IIA Factors

This category included tumor grade, circumferential resection (radial) margin (CRM), and tumor regression designated as ypTNM staging in resection specimen following neoadjuvant therapy. The radial margin corresponds to specimens with nonperitonealized surfaces such as mid and distal rectal cancers where the entire external surface of the specimen is considered a CRM. In rectal cancers, the CRM status (either negative or positive) was one of strongest predictors for local and distance recurrence as well for survival.[87–90] For patients who had not received preoperative radiation therapy, adjuvant radiation therapy to the positive radial margins was recommended if not administered preoperatively.

Category IIB Factors

This category included both histological (such as histological type, tumor border configuration, and morphologic features associated with MSI) and genetic (such as high degree MSI and loss of heterozygosity at 18q) prognostic factors. Although certain high grade subtypes (e.g., signet ring, poorly differentiated, or undifferentiated tumors) have more aggressive natural history, histological subtype in general has not been proven as an independent prognostic index in CRC.[91,92] Significance of the tumor border configuration as an independent predictor aside from tumor stage has been shown by several studies.[91,93] An infiltrating (irregular) pattern of growth in contrast to an expanding (pushing) border was associated with worse outcome, and in one study this was specifically significant for negative effect in rectal tumors in multivariate analysis. Perineural invasion alone and tumor "budding" (minute clusters of undifferentiated cancer cells ahead of the invasive front of the malignant lesion) at the tumor border have also been associated with more advanced disease and poor prognosis.[82,94]

Microstellite Instability

The predictive and prognostic significance of microsatellite instability in colorectal cancer has gained tremendous interest in the recent years.[95–97] MSI is a byproduct of defective DNA mismatch repair, and it has long been appreciated that MSI positive colorectal tumors have distinct clinicopathological features[98,99] and are associated with improved outcome.[100] In the seminal paper by Ribic et al the role of MSI was evaluated among 570 patients with stage II and III colon cancer prospectively enrolled to five randomized clinical trials of adjuvant chemotherapy or surgery alone.[101] Approximately 16.7% of the specimen in this study displayed high level MSI and were associated with improved rate of 5-year overall survival compared to MSS or low MSI tumors (hazard ratio [HR] 0.31, confidence interval [CI] 0.14–0.72, $P=0.004$). Furthermore, benefit of adjuvant chemotherapy in these cancers was limited to those with an intact MMR system. In a review of 32 studies with a total of 7,642 patients with CRC including 1,227 with MSI positive tumors, Popat et al showed that the combined HR estimate for overall survival associated with MSI was 0.65 (95% CI 0.59–0.71).[97] The analysis showed that patients whose tumors had MSI had 15% improvement in outcome compared to those without MSI. However tumors with MSI derived no benefit from adjuvant fluorouracil (FU)based chemotherapy (HR 1.24, 95% CI 0.72–2.14). In a recent study, Sargent et al updated their previous findings in a study involving an additional 457 patients with stage II and III colon cancer from five randomized trials of FU-based adjuvant chemotherapy.[102] Deficient MMR was prognostic of improved outcome with surgery alone and these patients derived no improvement in disease-free survival (DFS) with adjuvant FU chemotherapy (HR 1.1, 95% CI 0.42–2.91, $P=0.85$). Interestingly, systemic adjuvant chemotherapy in patients with MMR deficient stage II colon was associated with worse overall survival (HR = 2.95, 95% CI 1.02–8.5, $P=0.04$). As the use of adjuvant chemotherapy in stage II colon cancer[103–105] has yet to be determined, some authors have suggested determination of microsatellite stability status for decision-making for systemic therapy in stage II colon cancer.[102,106,107] In contrast to the above findings, a recent meta-analysis of seven studies including 810 patients with stage II and 2,444 patients with stage III CRC, showed similar relapse-free survival with or without adjuvant chemotherapy in MSI-H patients.[108] Therefore MSI status remains controversial as a predictive indicator of response to chemotherapy in colorectal cancer.

Microsatellite instability occurs rarely in the rectum and there is limited data regarding the predictive and prognostic value of this biomarker in distal colorectal tumors. MSI has been observed at a very low rate (<5%) in rectal cancers,[109–111] and it occurs 8.1 times more frequently in malignancies in the colon than in the rectum.[110] Patients with MSI positive rectal tumors often have clinical histories highly suggestive of hereditary nonpolyposis colorectal cancer (HNPCC)/ Lynch syndrome due to germline mutations in one of the MMR genes.[109] In fact, the presence of MSI in rectal cancers was shown to be independently related to fulfillment of the Bethesda Criteria for clinical diagnosis of patients with Lynch syndrome (odds ratio [OR] 7.0, $P=0.01$).[110] In an Italian study, statistically significant improvement in DFS and overall survival (OS) was reported for MSI positive rectal cancers compared with MSI negative ones, which was independent of administered therapy (radiotherapy, chemotherapy, or both).[112,113] Conversely, in a study of sporadic stage II and stage III rectal cancers from a Chinese Han population, MSI-H tumors did have a better clinical outcome and MSI status was non-prognostic.[112,113] Thus while this highly debated biomarker is promising, at this time there is insufficient data to support a definitive predictive or prognostic role in management of rectal cancer.

Chromosome 18q Deletion

Allelic loss of the long arm of chromosome 18 is the most common cytogenetic abnormality in CRC and has been associated with poor prognosis in.[114–116] Three putative genes are encoded in this region including DCC "deleted in colon cancer," SMAD4, and SMAD2. Point mutations in DCC have been reported in colorectal cancers and loss of DCC expression may have a negative prognostic value.[117–119] SMAD4 is a member of the transforming growth factor-beta (TGF-beta) signaling pathway, which is important in the biology of colorectal cancer.[120] Mutations in SMAD4 have been reported in a subset of CRC.[121,122] Decreased SMAD4 mRNA levels have been linked with worse outcome and inferior response to 5-FU-based chemotherapy.[123] SAMD2 is another candidate tumor suppressor gene implicated to play a role in CRC tumorigenesis.[121] However, the prognostic significance of these candidate genes has not been consistently shown across all studies,[124,125] and at this time there is no definitive link between loss of any locus on 18q and prognosis.

While the loss of heterozygosity (LOH) at 18q has been shown to be associated with inferior prognosis in CRC, the question remains if 18q loss is an independent predictor of outcome. Loss of 18q LOH is inversely associated with MSI, a favorable prognostic indicator, and there is conflicting evidence regarding prognostic value of 18 q LOH independent of MSI.[126–128] In fact, an expert panel by the American Society of Clinical Oncology (ASCO) convened in 2006 concluded that there was inadequate evidence for use of this maker in determining prognosis or to predict response to therapy.[129] We await the published result of the currently closed Eastern Cooperative Oncology Group (ECOG) 5202, which stratified stage II colon cancer patients to postoperative systemic therapy based on MSI status and LOH 18q, to shed further light on the pre-dictive value of these molecular markers.

Category III Factors

This category includes factors that have not been sufficiently studied to determine their prognostic significance. The factors grouped in this category included DNA content, perineural invasion, microvessel density, peritumoral fibrosis, peritumoral inflammatory response, focal neuroendocrine differentiation, nuclear organizing regions, and proliferation. The prognostic significance of aneuploidy, or aberrant DNA content in CRC has been debated, and contrasting results have been reported.[130,131] The 2006 ASCO guidelines for use of tumor markers in GI malignancies recommended against use of DNA ploidy to determine prognosis in CRC.[129] Perineural invasion (PNI) has long been appreciated as marker of more aggressive disease in a number of malignancies including rectal cancers.[132] PNI has been reported in 30% of rectal cancers and 19% of colon cancers. In the rectum, presence of PNI is associated with poor histopathologic variables including angiolymphatic invasion,[133,134] nodal involvement,[135] liver metastasis, and peritoneal dissemination.[134] In multivariate analysis extramural PNI has been shown to be a prognostic marker for local recurrence and long-term survival[134,136], independent of tumor depth or nodal status in rectal cancers.[135] In two recent studies, the prognostic significance of PNI as an independent predictor of outcome in both colon cancer and rectal carcinoma was demonstrated.[137,138] Microvessel density (MVD) in tumors is a measure of pathologic angiogenesis and can be immunohistochemically assessed, using monoclonal antibodies against endothelial markers (such as CD34, CD31, and von Willibrand factor). Although MVD has been associated with worse outcome in CRC in some studies,[139] standardization for evaluation and interpretation of MVD are lacking. The 2000 CAP consensus panel recommend this factor should be further validated in large studies using multivariate analysis.[30] There are inconsistent reports regarding the prognostic significance of peritumoral fibrosis[91,140,141] and the 2000 CAP consensus panel that this factor should be validated in large studies using multivariate analysis.[30] The few reports in the literature on the prognostic significance of peritumoral inflammatory response have indicated that this feature is associated with better outcome in CRC.[91,140] CAP recommended for separate evaluation of this feature to distinguish from host lymphoid response reaction.[30] Although significant neuroendocrine differentiation on H&E sections,[142,143] and high proliferative activity (assessed by analysis of argyrophilic nuclear organizing regions, mitotic index, or by IHC evaluation proliferation markers such as of Ki-67 nuclear antigen) are considered negative prognostic indicator in CRC,[144–146] data is conflicting and additional prospective studies are needed to demonstrate the true prognostic and predictive potential of these markers.

Additional factors included in category III of CAP prognostic factors in CRC included tumor cell-associated proteins or carbohydrates, and all other molecular markers (except with LOH18q and MSI-H). A wide variety of cell surface molecules (such as class I or II HLA molecules, CA19-9, E-cadherin to name a few) have been studied in colorectal cancer and full discussion is beyond the scope of this chapter. However none have been sufficiently studied in prospective clinical trials to meet criteria for specific recommendation.[30] The evaluation of predictive and prognostic biomarkers has become a critical component of correlative studies in colorectal clinical trials and a discussion of several key factors will be provided in the next section.

Category IV Factors

This section included factors that have been well studied and found to be of no prognostic significance. These include tumor size and gross tumor configuration.[30]

Molecular Markers in Cancers of Colon and Rectum

Adenomatous Polyposis Coli

The adenomatous polyposis coli (ACP) gene on chromosome 5q21 is perhaps the most critical gene in the pathogenesis of CRC. Inactivation of this tumor suppressor gene is regarded as the initiating event in the multistep genetic model of CRC tumorigenesis originally proposed by Fearon and Vogelstein in 1990. The main function of the *APC* gene product is to mediate proteolytic degradation of β-catenin, a glycogen synthase kinase essential to the Wnt signaling pathway of intestinal epithelial growth and differentiation. Germline mutations in *APC* are responsible for familial adenomatous polyposis (FAP), characterized by development of 100–1,000s of adenomatous polyps throughout the GI tract. In tumors obtained from FAP patients, somatic APC mutations, primarily involving the mutation cluster region (MCR), have been identified in 75% of the cases.[147,148] Mutations in the APC gene are emblematic of the common paradigm that genes involved in familial cancers are often mutated in sporadic forms of the same types of malignancies. Indeed APC mutations are frequently seen in sporadic colorectal cancers and are thought to be an early event in tumor progression. While 80% of these mutations are similar to APC germline mutations described in the FAP patients,[149,150] promoter hypermethylation is an alternate mechanism of APC gene inactivation that has been described in 18% of sporadic colorectal cancers.[151]

APC inactivation result in stabilization or nuclear localization of β-catenin and constitutive activation of the Wnt growth-promoting signaling pathway. Colorectal cancers with aberrant Wnt signaling pathway have been associated with unique molecular and pathological features. *APC* inactivation has been closely linked to tumors that exhibit chromosomal instability,[152] and significantly less associated with those that carry MSI-H phenotype.[153,154] *APC* mutations are more common in the rectum than the colon, with one report indicating significantly more nuclear β-catenin expression in the rectum than in the colon (65% vs. 400%, $P=0.04$).[154,155] While some studies have indicated that the presence of *APC* mutations in CRC is associated with worse prognosis,[156,157] others have reported no affect on survival.[158] Moreover in locally advanced rectal cancer, loss of heterozygosity at the APC gene was not prognostic of tumor regression after preoperative chemoradiation.[159] The *APC* gene mutation is a critical initiating event in CRC carcinogenesis and recent studies have provided indirect evidence for the role of Wnt pathway in the biology of rectal carcinomas. However, currently there are limited data regarding the prognostic and predictive value of changes in APC or β-catenin in CRC, and a clinical application of these biomarkers has not been established.

TP53

The *TP53* gene located on chromosome 17p is one of the most widely studied genes in CRC. It is mutated in 40–50% of colorectal cancers,[160] and it is thought to be a late event in colorectal tumorigenesis.[63,161] Inactivation of this gene occurs by mutation on one allele and loss of the remaining wildtype gene (LOH). The majority of TP53 mutations (approximately 80%) are point mutations,[162] that often lead to nuclear accumulation of an inactive protein that can be detected by immunohistochemical analysis (IHC). Two main techniques for detection of *TP53* mutations are either by DNA analysis for genetic alterations or by IHC detection of overexpressed p53 protein. The wildtype p53 protein is considered a tumor suppressor with multiple functions in control of cellular growth including cell cycle arrest, apoptosis, senescence, and differentiation. Given its central role in protecting the genome from DNA damage it is been coined the "guardian of the genome".[163,164]

The *TP53* gene has been extensively studied as a prognostic factor in colorectal cancers. A number of studies have demonstrated a higher frequency of *TP53* mutations in distal colon and rectal cancers (20–70%) compared to proximal adenocarcinomas (20–40%).[155,165–167] While most studies have demonstrated that defect in p53 is a negative prognostic marker of outcome and survival in CRC,[165] others have found no correlation between p53 expression and outcome measures.[158,168,169] Some have argued that anatomic tumor location, type of mutation, and adjuvant therapy may influence the prognostic significance of p53 alterations in CRC. Consistent with this hypothesis, abnormal p53 has been shown to be more important in the biology of rectal cancers than in colon malignancies and to be an independent predictor of worse DFS in rectal and not in colon tumors.[155,165] The "*TP53* Colorectal Cancer International Collaborative Study" is one of the largest pooled data that examined the prognostic and predictive significance of *TP53* mutations in CRC.[166] In this retrospective analysis of 3,583 patients, *TP53* mutations were significantly more common in the distal: and rectal cancers than proximal colon tumors (45%, 45%, and 34% respectively). In multivariate analysis, while *TP53* mutations causing loss of amino acids were associated with worse survival in distal tumors (relative risk [RR]=2.52, 95% CI, 1.28–4.93, $P=0.007$), mutations in exon 5 showed a trend toward statistically significant worse outcome in proximal colon tumors (RR=1.36, 95% CI 1.03–1.79; $P=0.03$). In the study, patients with Dukes' C cancers whose tumors harbored wildtype *TP53* and those with mutated *TP53* (proximal tumors) had significantly improved prognosis when treated with adjuvant chemotherapy.[166] Other lines of evidence have also argued that p53 tumor suppressor may play a stronger role in pathogenesis of distal colon/rectal cancers than in proximal colon tumors. For instance, rectal cancers have a higher frequency of aneuploidy, mutations in K-RAS and *TP53,* and MSS phenotype, whereas proximal colonic tumors have greater incidence of *BRAF* mutations, aberrant hypermethylation, diploidy, and MSI-H phenotype.[75,109,155,167,170] Moreover, an inverse relationship between high frequency MSI and genetic defects in *K-RAS* and *TP53* has been demonstrated in CRC.[171] These observations have led to the notion that rectal and colon cancers are molecularly distinct and evolve through different pathways.

The significance of *TP53* mutation as a predictive biomarker of response to chemo and radiation therapy in rectal cancer has been evaluated. Several recent reviews however have indicated contradictory evidence with respect to *TP53* status and response to chemotherapy or neoadjuvant chemoradiotherapy.[168,169,172] Therefore at this time determination of *TP53* status is not recommended for assessing either prognosis or response cytotoxic systemic therapy or radiation therapy.

Epidermal Growth Factor Receptor

Epidermal growth factor receptor (EGFR) is a member of the human epidermal growth factor receptor (HER-erbB) family of receptor tyrosine kinases. It is involved in activation of a number of oncogenic cellular pathways including the RAS–RAF–MAPK, phosphoinositide 3-kinase (PI3K)/Akt phospholipase C, and signal transducer and activator of transcription (STAT) and SRC/FAK pathways (Fig. 9.3). These pathways have been shown to play important role in tumor proliferation, angiogenesis, and cell survival. EGFR is an important therapeutic target in metastatic colorectal cancer (mCRC) and aberrant activation of signaling pathways downstream to EGFR play a critical role in CRC pathogenesis and mechanism of resistance to anti-EGFR monoclonal antibodies cetuximab and panitumumab.[173]

Deregulated EGFR activation can occur via mutational events or by gene amplification. While somatic EGFR mutations have been implicated in lung cancer,[174] these genetic defect are rare in CRC.[175] A number of techniques have been used for detection of EGFR expression including immunohistochemistry (IHC) determination of total protein expressed and fluorescence in situ hybridization (FISH) and PCR for detection of increased EGFR copy number. Overexpression of EGFR by amplification or increased copy number is seen in 10–15% of CRC[176,177] and EGFR expression by IHC has been reported in 25–75% of CRC.[178] Contrasting data has been reported in the literature with respect to the prognostic and predictive role of EGFR in CRC depending on the type of detection assay used. For instance, while FISH-positive CRC (high polysomy or amplification) have been shown to have improved outcome and higher response to anti-EGFR monoclonal antibody Cetuximab,[179] other investigators have observed tumor response without increased EGFR copy number by FISH[180] or by quantitative PCR.[181]

Several recent clinical trials have examined the predictive role of EGFR expression in locally advanced rectal cancers.[168,173] EGFR expression by IHC has been reported at the rate of 10–60% in rectal cancer. Overexpression of EGFR has been correlated with statistically significant increased risk of lymph node involvement, local recurrence, and worse disease-free survival, and overall survival.[182–186] Li et al showed in multivariate analysis, that EGFR expression in locally advanced rectal cancer was predictor of shorter DFS (relative risk [RR] 2.4, $P=0.041$) and distant metastasis-free survival (RR 2.6, $P=0.04$).[183] In contrast to these studies, Cunningham et al found no significant association between expression or coexpression of insulin-like growth factor type-I receptor (IGF-IR), HER2, or EGFR and clinicopathological features or overall survival in Dukes'C CRC.[187] Moreover, while a worse 3-year DFS has been shown for locally advanced rectal tumors expressing lower levels of vascular endothelial growth factor (VEGF) and EGFR[188] , other investigators have reported contrasting results with

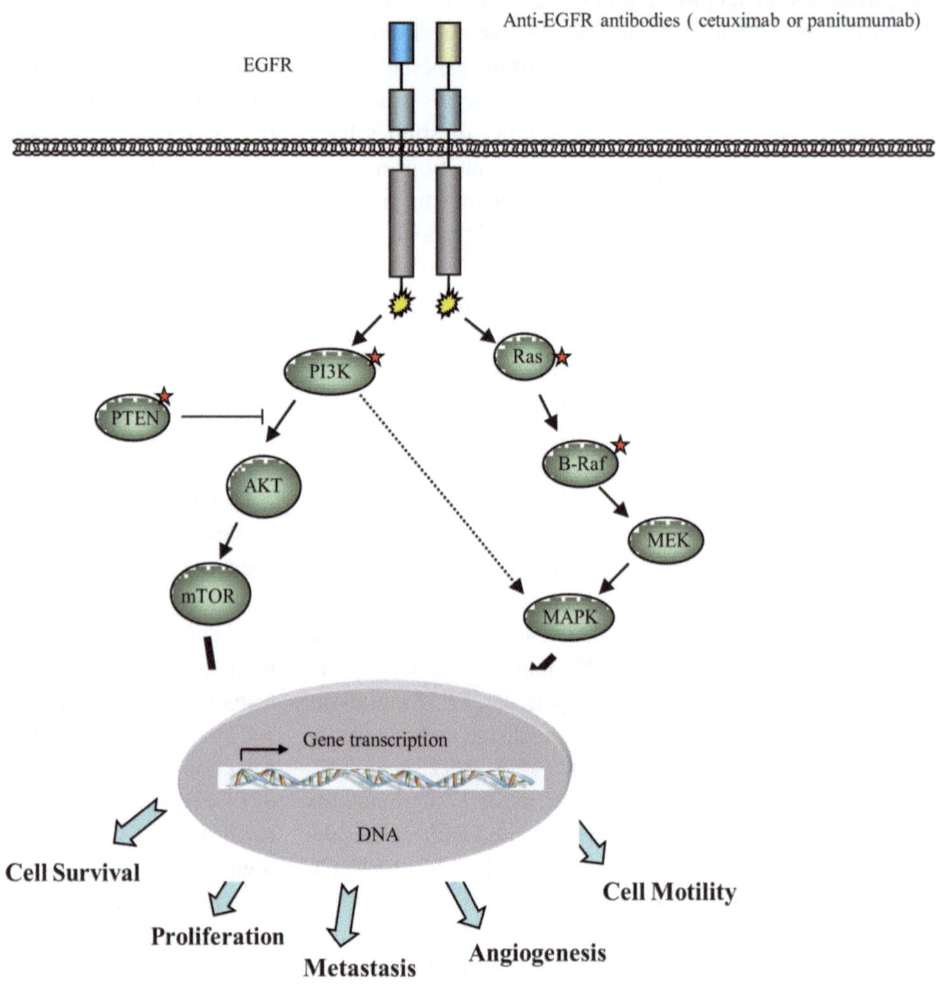

Fig. 9.3 The epidermal growth factor receptor (EFGR) signaling pathway. Molecules that are commonly affected by oncogenic alterations and are thought to serve as predictive biomarkers for the efficacy of EGFR antibodies are indicated with *red stars*

higher mRNA levels of VEGF, EGFR, and survivin (a molecule involved in apoptosis) in rectal tumors [189]

The prognostic significance of EGFR in rectal cancer has also been evaluated.[168,173] EGFR expression has been linked with lack of complete pathologic response (pCR) after preoperative radiotherapy and has been shown to be an independent predictor of poor tumor response to preoperative radiation and chemoradiation.[182–186] In contrast to these findings, others have reported EGFR overexpression to be a predictor of clinical response to fluoropyrimidines[190] in CRC.

Inconclusive results in the literature regarding the predictive and prognostic significance of EGFR expression in rectal cancer are likely due to a number of challenges in performing biomarker studies in modern clinical trials. These include study of nonhomogeneous patient populations with respect to grouping of colon and rectal cancers, use of different treatment protocols, numerous technical issues and non-standardization detection methods. At this time determination of EGFR expression is not ready for use as a predictive or prognostic tool in clinical decision-making.

KRAS

Due to the central role of KRAS in EGFR signaling pathway, there is currently intense interest in deciphering the predictive and prognostic significance of this biomarker in advanced CRC. *KRAS* mutations are common features of CRC with chromosomal instability (CIN) and follow the classic adenoma–carcinoma sequence carcinogenesis proposed by Vogelstein.[161] Mutations in the *KRAS* gene occur in 35–45% of tumors of colon and rectum, have been associated with more aggressive tumor biology, and thought to be an early step in the CRC tumorigenesis.[191,192] While some studies have suggested that *KRAS* mutations are more common in proximal colonic tumors than those in distal colon or rectum,[154,167] others have reported similar frequency in both locations.[193] A number of mutational events have been reported, with the most frequent mutations in exon 2 (codons 12 and 13) and to a lesser extent in exon 3 (codon 61). In a large, multicenter study (RASCAL) including 3,439 patients, codon 12 glycine-to-valine *KRAS* mutations was found to have highly statistically negative impact on DFS and OS in patients in stage III colon cancer.[194,195] In contrast data from CALGB 89803 (stage III colon cancer), PETACC-3 (stage II and III colon), and the National Cancer Institute of Canada CO.17 (stage IV CRC) suggest that *K-RAS* mutation status has no prognostic or predictive value for treatment with standard chemotherapy.[196–199]

Unlike the uncertain role of this proto-oncogene as a determinant of outcome in CRC, *KRAS* mutations have emerged as a major predictor of response to anti-EGFR monoclonal antibodies cetuximab and panitumumab.[200,201] Large randomized trials in treatment naïve and pretreated mCRC patients have demonstrated that patients with *KRAS* mutation tumors do not respond to EGFR inhibitors and derive neither survival nor quality of life benefit from this line of therapy.[199,202,203] Three large randomized phase III clinical trials have confirmed these findings. In first-line treatment of mCRC, the OPUS and CRYSTAL trials showed that the addition of cetuximab to oxaliplatin- or irinotecan-based chemotherapy conferred no benefit to patients with *KRAS* mutant tumors.[204–206] In fact the OPUS trial indicated a detrimental effect to addition of anti-EGFR therapy to these patients. Similarly in the National Cancer Institute of Canada Clinical Trials Group (NCIC-CTG) non-crossover design monotherapy study in relapsed/refractory patients, *KRAS* mutation was shown to be a negative predictor of outcome to cetuximab therapy in metastatic disease.[199,207] Given the results of these definitive clinical trials, anti-EGFR monoclonal therapy should not be used in treatment of patients with mCRC that harbor *KRAS* mutations. Indeed, the European health authorities have restricted the use EGFR monoclonal antibodies to *KRAS* wild type mCRC.[200] In 2009 American Cancer Society of Clinical Oncology released provisional recommendations for KRAS testing of patient with advanced CRC to predict response to this type of therapy.[208] Most recently, the US Food and Drug administration has provided similar guidelines indicating that anti-EGFR antibodies should not be given to patients with mCRC that have *KRAS* mutations in codon 12 or 13.[200]

BRAF

The *BRAF* oncogene is a downstream effector of KRAS in the EGFR-dependent signaling cascade (Fig. 9.3).[209] *BRAF* mutations have been reported in 5–10% of sporadic disease and have been linked to the serrated carcinoma pathway of colorectal tumorigenesis.[74,75] The most frequently reported *BRAF* mutation is the valine-to-glutamine amino acid (V600E) substitution. Mutations in the *BRAF* oncogene is exclusively seen in sporadic CRC, and the presence of these mutations suggests exclusion from criterion suspected of Lynch Syndrome-associated tumors.[210] These mutations are more commonly seen in the colon than the rectum, are associated epigenetic promoter silencing of one MLH1 (one of the mismatch repair family of molecules) resulting in MSI-H phenotype. Moreover these *BRAF* mutations are associated with CPG island hypermethylation phenotype, proximal tumors location, and reported to be more frequent in older women.[74,75]

Recent studies have indicated that *BRAF* mutations confer resistance to anti-EGFR monoclonal antibodies cetuximab and panitumumab.[179,211] In the original retrospectives analysis 132 patients with mCRC, none of the patients responding to EGFR-targeted therapy carried *BRAF* mutations, while 14% (11 of 79) of nonresponders had tumors with *BRAF* V600E mutations.[211] Thus *BRAF* mutations are an additional tool for selection of patients who may be resistant to anti-EGFR therapy. *BRAF* and *KRAS* mutations are known to be mutually exclusive in CRC. In fact it has been estimated that consideration of both *BRAF* and *KRAS* mutations together can potentially identify up to 55% (approximately 10% contribution from *BRAF* and 35–45% contribution from *KRAS*) of nonresponders to EGFR targeted therapy. Determination of mutational status in these two genes could avoid the expense and toxicities of an ineffective therapy in this subgroup of CRC patients.[200]

Oncogenic activation of BRAF has also been associated with poor prognosis in CRC. In a retrospective analysis of stage II and III colon cancer patient in the PETACC-3 study, *BRAF* mutations were prognostic of worse OS, particularly in patients with MSI-L and MSS tumors (HR 2.2, $P=0.0003$).[198] In metastatic colon cancer *BRAF* mutation was strongly associated with shorter DFS ($P<0.001$) and shorter OS ($P<0.001$).[179] Interestingly in some studies the positive prognosis conferred by an MSI-H phenotype was abrogated in the presence of simultaneous BRAF mutations.[80,212] In multivariate analysis, *BRAF* gene mutation has been shown to be an adverse prognostic marker in right-sided colon cancers independent of MSI status.[213] In the CAIRO-2 study, a randomized phase III trial of oxaliplatin, capecitabine, bevacizumab with or without cetuximab in mCRC, *BRAF* mutations was shown to be negative prognostic indicator, and in contrast to *KRAS* mutation, this effect was not restricted to anti-EGFR therapy.[214,215] In this study, both PFS and OS were significantly decreased in patients with *BRAF* mutation positive tumors compared to patients with *KRAS* mutation or those with *K-RAS/BRAF* wild type tumors in both arms of the study.[215]

BRAF mutations have emerged as a significant predictive and prognostic determinant in management of CRC. However, given the low frequency of these mutations and predilection for the proximal/right-sided colonic malignancies, the role of BRAF mutations in the pathogenesis of rectal cancer is unknown. At this time evaluation of BRAF mutational status has not recommended a predictive or prognostic marker of response to neoadjuvant therapy in locally advanced rectal cancer.

PI3KCA/PTEN

The EGFR-receptor also activates the PI3K/AKT pathway, and two well-characterized oncogenic events in colorectal cancers include *PI3KCA* mutations and loss of PTEN expression.[173,200] Activating mutations in PI3KCA p110 occur in 10–15% of CRC with hotspots in exons 1, 2, 9, and 20. Higher frequency of *PI3KCA* mutations have been reported in women and in tumors arising in the proximal colon.[216] The *PTEN* tumor-suppressor gene encodes a phosphatase and somatic mutations occur in 9% of CRC.[173] Inactivating mutations primarily involve epigenetic silencing of the promoter region. *PI3K3CA* and *PTEN* mutations are mutually exclusive although either mutation can coexist in a tumor with *K-RAS* or *BRAF* mutations.[217]

The predictive and prognostic significant of these biomarkers in CRC has gained a great deal of interest in the recent years. While conflicting results have been published regarding the impact of PI3KCA on response to anti-EGFR therapy in CRC patients,[218–220] most investigators agree that PTEN inactivation is a negative marker of response in CRC to this type of therapy.[217,221] The discrepant results on the value of PI3KCA as a predictive marker in part has been attributed to the lack of standardization of detection techniques in the literature and potentially different oncogenic potential of the various *PI3KCA* mutations.

Nevertheless, *PI3KCA* mutations and/or PTEN loss have been shown to be negative predictors of outcome in CRC.[179,222,223] He Y. et al evaluated the frequency and biological impact of *PI3KCA*, *K-RAS*, and *BRAF* mutations in 240 stage I–III rectal tumors from nonirradiated patients.[222] The frequency of *PI3KCA, K-RAS,* and *BRAF* mutations were seen in 19 (7.9%), 81 (33.9%), and 5 (2.1%) of the rectal specimens from total mesorectal excision (TME). The presence of *PI3KCA* mutations was associated with higher frequency of local recurrence (5-year risk, 27.8% vs. 9.4%, $P=0.006$) and a trend toward more rapid development of recurrence postsurgery (median local recurrence-free interval after surgery: 7.9 m vs. 19.6 m, $P=0.07$) that without this mutation. In multivariate analysis *PI3KCA* mutations was an independent predictor of local recurrence (HR 3.4, 95% CI 1.2–9.2, $P=0.017$).

At the current time, the frequency of *KRAS, BRAF, PI3KCA,* and *PTEN* mutational events and their oncogenic impact on the pathology of rectal cancer is not well understood. Although defining biomarkers and targeted therapies directed at the EGFR pathway has gained tremendous momentum in the treatment of advanced colorectal cancers, their role in clinical management of rectal cancer awaits further studies.

Vascular Endothelial Growth Factor

Angiogenesis plays a critical role in tumor formation and progression and vascular endothelial growth factor (VEGF) is considered a potent mediator of new blood vessel formation.[224–227] This process can be assessed by analysis of microvessel density (MVD) and by examining expression of angiogenic-promoting molecules, such as the VEGF ligands and their receptors. High microvessel count and elevated VEGF expression have been associated with aggressive biology, increased risk of metastatic disease, and poor prognosis in colorectal cancers.[139,228,229]

Study of VEGF family of molecules as predictive and prognostic markers and as therapeutic targets is an intense area of investigation in CRC. Positive VEGF expression evaluated by IHC, was reported in 57% of rectal cancers in one study and was found to be an indicator of poor DFS and distant metastasis following preoperative radiotherapy.[230] VEGF overexpression in postradiation-treated rectal specimens has also been associated with increased risk of distant metastasis.[231] In multivariate analysis, VEGF-C protein expression (a specific promoter of lymphangiogenesis) was found to be an independent predictor of local recurrence in rectal cancer and patients with positive VEGF-C tumors had worse prognosis compared to those with lack of expression of this factor.[232]

Microvessel density (MVD) and VEGF have also been evaluated as predictive markers of response to preoperative chemoradiotherapy in rectal cancer. Lower MVD in postirradiated rectal cancer tissue has been linked with statistically significant increased survival in rectal cancer patients.[233] Zlobec et al found a statistically significant association between mean VEGF expression and response to neoadjuvant radiotherapy, where the nonresponders had greater expression of VEGF protein.[234] The same investigators showed that loss of VEGF expression and positive EGFR expression were independent predictors of pCR post preoperative radiotherapy in rectal cancer.[235] In contrast to these results, other investigators have found that VEGF expression is not a significant predictor of response to radiotherapy or chemoradiation in rectal cancer.[236,237]

Treatment with the anti-VEGF monoclonal antibody, bevacizumab, has been extensively studied in solid tumors and has been shown to add 4.7 months to overall survival when added to standard chemotherapy in advanced CRC.[238] Bevacizumab has been shown to have radiosensitizing properties in rectal cancer.[172] Several early phase clinical trials have demonstrated safety and efficacy of preoperative bevacizumab combined with standard chemoradiotherapy in patients with locally advanced rectal cancers.[239,240] In these studies bevacizumab therapy was associated with improved tumor interstitial fluid and blood flow, decreased MVD, and baseline VEGF levels significantly correlated with outcome.

At this juncture, while angiogenesis plays an important role in pathogenesis of rectal cancer the role of angiogenic biomarkers and VEGF-targeted therapy in rectal tumors is not clear. Further prospective studies are needed to better define the role of MVD and VEGF as prognostic and predictive markers in rectal cancer, and the use of these factors outside of clinical trial studies cannot be recommended.

Thymidylate Synthase

Thymidylate synthase (TS) catalyzes a critical step in DNA synthesis and is the main molecular target for 5-fluorouracil (5-FU), which is the primary backbone of systemic chemotherapy in CRC. TS has been extensively studied in cancers of the lower digestive system as a prognostic and therapeutic predictive marker. High TS expression is associated with resistance to 5-FU chemotherapy and poor prognosis in colorectal cancers.[241,242] In a systemic review and a meta-analysis consisting of 3,497 CRC cases, TS overexpression was prognostic of worse OS in both advanced (HR 1.74, 95% CI 1.34–2.26) and adjuvant (HR 1.35, 95% CI 1.07–1.80) settings.[243] In contrast, other reports have indicated no prognostic implications with respect to TS expression level and DFS or OS in CRC patients treated with oral 5-FU-based chemotherapy.[244]

The role of TS as a predictive and prognostic biomarker has also been evaluated in rectal cancer. Elevated TS expression has been shown to be a poor prognostic marker in rectal cancers and indicator of increased risk of recurrence post-neoadjuvant chemoradiotherapy.[245,246] Elevated TS levels in preoperative rectal biopsy specimens were shown to be predictive of higher response to chemoradiation but not to radiation alone.[236] Conversely, other investigators have shown no significant correlation between TS expression level and inferior prognosis or treatment failure in rectal cancer.[247]

The discrepancy in the reported literature regarding the role of TS molecular marker in CRC once again points to the different TS detection assays, lack of standardization of techniques, and retrospective and small size of these biomarker studies. At this time no definitive conclusions can be drawn from the existing data and further prospectively validated studies of the predictive and prognostic role of TS expression in rectal cancer is warranted.

Other Molecular Markers and Microarray Assays

A number of genetic targets and cellular pathways have been investigated in rectal carcinomas as potential markers of outcome and/or response to neoadjuvant therapy. In addition to biomarkers discussed above, these have included markers of proliferation (Ki-67), cell cycle regulators (p21), apoptosis regulators (Bcl-2 and survivin), and global transcription factors (NF-kB).[168,169,172] However the value of these candidate genes is controversial; none has been unequivocally validated as a predictive or prognostic marker in rectal cancer.

Gene expression profiling based on microarray technology has shown promise in predicting recurrence in Dukes B colon cancer,[248] and in predicting response to drug therapy in colorectal cancer cell lines.[249] Several recent studies have used microarrays to evaluate differential gene expression patterns as surrogate of response to preoperative therapy in rectal tumors.[250–252] In all three studies, pretherapeutic prediction of response to neoadjuvant chemoradiotherapy was feasible. However there was no concordance among the genes differentially expressed in any of these studies (54 genes by Ghadimi et al,[250] 261 genes by Kim et al,[251] 42 genes by Rimkus et al[252]). Although microarray technology can result in interesting data and lead to discovery of novel candidate genes, at this time there is inadequate evidence in support of this technology for response prediction in rectal cancer.

Anal Neoplasms

Anal cancer accounts for approximately 4% of anorectal tumors and 1.5% of gastrointestinal malignancies. It is estimated to affect 5,260 patients (2,000 men and 3,260 women) and lead to approximately 720 deaths in 2010.[1] While considered an uncommon cancer of the digestive tract, the incidence of anal cancer has been increasing in both sexes worldwide over the past 25 years.[253–256] Well-described risk factors include human immunodeficiency virus (HIV) seropositivity, low CD4 count, persistent high-risk human papilloma virus (HPV) infection, receptive anal intercourse, increased number of sexual partners, anogenital warts, cervical dysplasia, or cancer.[257] Indeed, the key causative factors for anal tumorigenesis have been closely linked to sexually transmitted infections,[258–261] and some have described the biology of these cancers to be similar to malignancies of the genital tract.[262–264] The other risk factors implicated in pathogenesis of anal cancers include female gender, cigarette smoking, and chronic immunosuppression following solid organ transplant.[265–267]

Anatomy of the Anal Canal

The anal canal measures 3–5 cm in length and extends from the rectal ampulla (level of pelvic floor) to the anal verge (Fig. 9.1). The distal end of the anal canal, or the anal verge, is at the level of the squamous–mucocutaneous junction and the perianal skin. The pectinate line indicates the junction of the superior part of the anal canal, lined by columnar epithelium, and the inferior part, lined by nonkeratinizing squamous epithelium. Distal to the dentate line the squamous epithelium merges with the perianal skin or the true epidermis. The anatomic distribution is clinically significant, as it relates to lymphatic drainage and different types of precursor epithelium. Anal canal proximal to the dentate line drains into the perirectal and paravertebral nodes, similar to rectum; while the region of the anal canal below the dentate line drains into the lymphatics of the superficial inguinal and femoral nodes. Proximal malignant lesions that arise from the mucosa (columnar, transitional, or squamous) are considered true anal canal cancers and are generally treated the same. Tumors arising from the epidermis or distal to the squamous–mucocutaneous junction (also called the "anal" verge) are referred to as anal margin tumors (also known as perianal skin cancers). With the exception of melanomas, tumors arising in the hair-bearing skin below the squamous–mucocutaneous junction are biologically similar and classified, staged (Tables 9.4 and 9.5), and treated like cutaneous skin tumors and not like anal canal cancers.[268]

Table 9.4 TNM staging for anal cancer

Primary tumor (T)	
Tx	Primary tumor cannot be assessed
T0	No evidence of primary tumor
Tis	Carcinoma in situ[a]
T1	Tumor 2 cm or less in greatest dimension
T2	Tumor >2 cm but ≤5 cm in greatest dimension
T3	Tumor >5 cm in greatest dimension
T4	Tumor of any size invades adjacent organs(s), e.g., vagina, urethra, bladder[b]
Regional lymph nodes (N)	
Nx	Regional lymph nodes cannot be assessed
N0	No regional lymph node metastasis
N1	Metastasis in perirectal lymph nodes(s)
N2	Metastasis in unilateral internal iliac and/or inguinal lymph nodes(s)
N3	Metastasis in perirectal and inguinal lymph nodes and/or bilateral internal iliac and/or inguinal lymph nodes(s)
Distant metastasis (M)	
M0	No distant metastasis
M1	Distant metastasis

Table adapted from AJCC Cancer Staging Manual, 7th edition (2010) by Springer New York, Inc

[a] Bowen's disease, high-grade squamous intraepithelial lesion (HSIL), anal intraepithelial neoplasia II–III (AIN II–III)

[b] Direct invasion of the rectal wall, perirectal skin, subcutaneous tissue, or the sphincter muscle(s) is not classified as T4

[c] Expert panels recommend histological examination of at least 12 nodes for accurate determination of nodal status

Histological Subtypes and Molecular Biology

A variety of lesions comprise cancers of the anal canal and their diagnosis and treatment depends on tumor histology and anatomic location. The vast majority of these (80%) are squamous cell carcinoma, which is 1/10 that of rectal cancers[269] (Fig. 9.4). Other rare anal neoplasms include adenocarcinoma, melanoma, sarcoma, gastrointestinal stromal tumors (GIST), neuroendocrine tumors, and Kaposi sarcoma.[270] These malignancies and their respective molecular biology will be discussed below.

Squamous Cell Carcinoma of the Anus

Anal intraepithelial neoplasia (AIN) is a precursor of SSC and shares many features with cervical intraepithelial neoplasia (CIN), a precursor lesion to cervical cancer. Infection with HPV plays an important causative role in development of both CIN and AIN. Similar to CIN, grading system for AIN is designated by AIN I, AIN II, and AIN III, which indicate low-, moderate-, and high-grade dysplasia, respectively.[270] Recently however, the terminology of low-grade intraepithelial lesion (LSIL) and high-grade intraepithelial lesion (HSIL) has become more commonly adopted. The treatment of these lesions is debated. LSIL is felt to have low malignant potential and observation is acceptable. However, HSIL carries a higher risk for malignant transformation and local therapies such as 5-fluorouracil cream and surgical excision have been employed.[270]

Human Papilloma virus

The pathogenesis of anogenital squamous cell carcinoma is closely linked with infection with common human viruses and

Table 9.5 Anal cancer staging and patient outcome based on tumor histology (squamous and non-squamous)

				5-year survival rate		
Stage	T	N	M	Squamous	Non-squamous	*P*-value
0	Tis	N0	M0	–	–	–
I	T1	N0	M0	71.4	59.1	0.003
II	T2–3	N0	M0	63.5	52.9	0.001
IIIA	T1–4	N0–N1	M0	48.1	37.7	0.085
IIIB	T4	N1	M0	43.2	24.4	0.003
	Any T	N2	M0			
	Any T	N3	M0			
IV	Any T	Any N	M1	20.9	7.4	0.002

Data based on 3,598 cases of anal cancer in the National Cancer Database from 1998 to 1999
Adapted from the AJCC Cancer Staging Manual, 7th edition (2010) by Springer New York, Inc

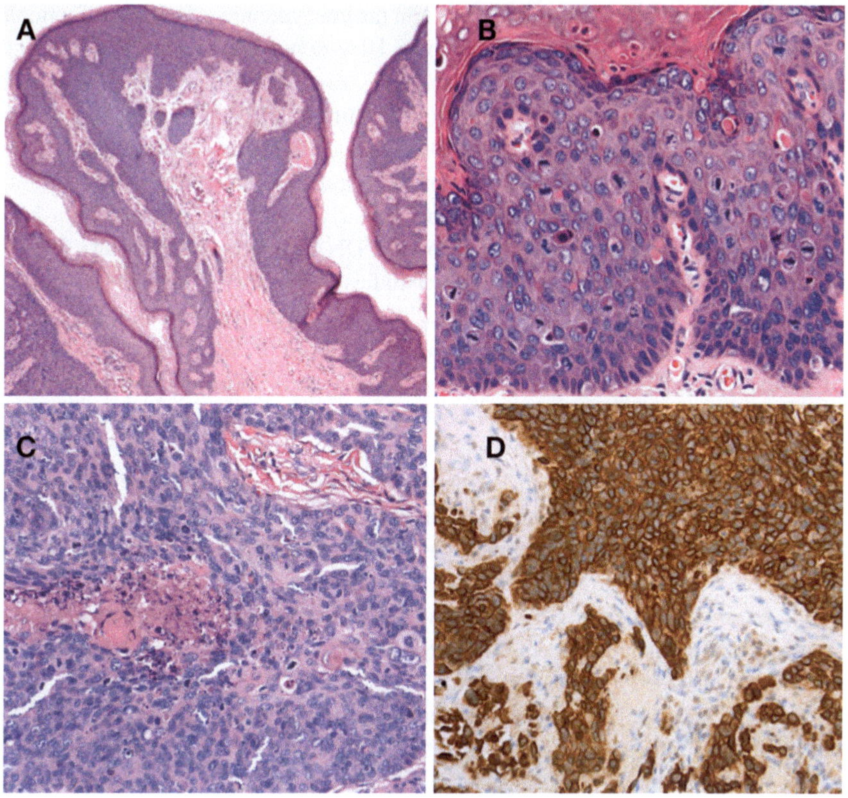

Fig. 9.4 (**a**) Condyloma accuminatum (original magnification ×10). (**b**) Squamous epithelium of Condyloma accuminatum with high-grade dysplasia/carcinoma in situ (original magnification ×200). (**c**) Squamous cell carcinoma of anus, high power view of the same tumor (original magnification ×200). (**d**) Immunohistochemistry for cytokeratin 5 and 6 (CK5/6) reveal strongly positive tumor cells (original magnification ×200). (**a**, **b,** and **c**: Hematoxylin and Eosin stain, **d**: Immunohistochemistry for CK5/6)

it has been used as a model of virus-induced carcinogenesis.[271–275] The human papilloma virus (HPV) is a common sexually transmitted disease and several studies have identified an association between HPV infections and anogenital cancers. Given the limited literature on the molecular biology of HPV infection in SSC of the anal canal, some of the data in this section is extrapolated from role of HPV in cervical squamous cell carcinoma.

HPV is a DNA tumor virus with over 100 different genotypes, of which some 23 have been associated with anogenital mucosal infection. Subtypes 6 and 11 are most commonly identified in lesion with low-grade dysplasia, while types 16, 18, 31, 33, and 35 are considered high-risk genotypes and more often identified in lesions with high-grade dysplasia and invasive carcinoma.[264] HPV-16 has been closely linked to anal cancers and is detected in approximately 70% of the cases in population-based studies.[258,276] HPV encodes for two transforming proteins, E6 and E7, which are thought to play a critical role in stimulating cellular growth and progression to invasive cancer. Both viral products (encoded by the high-risk HPV genotypes 16 and 18) are expressed in anal carcinomas.[277] The E6 oncoprotein is known to bind to cellular *TP53* and promote degradation of this tumor suppressor.[278,279] The observation that *TP53* gene is frequently wild type in cervical cancers,[280] has suggested that E6-mediated *TP53* degradation maybe functionally equivalent to inactivating *TP53* gene mutations.[281] The HPV-E7 protein complexes with the retinoblastoma tumor suppressor and targets it for degradation[282,283]; the efficacy with which E7 binds to RB correlates with the transforming capability of this oncoprotein.[284] Therefore E6/*TP53* and E7/RB1 interactions is thought to result in abrogation of cell cycle check points leading to aberrant DNA replication, DNA repair, apoptosis, and genomic instability.[285]

Several lines of evidence suggest that HPV infection, and subsequent E6 and E7 expression, is necessary but not sufficient for malignant progression in anogenital cancers. It is thought that additional oncogenic insults such as genomic instability are necessary for malignant transformation by the virus.[285] While in benign anogenital lesions the HPV viral genome replicates as an extra chromosomal episome, in malignant tumors the viral DNA integrates into the host chromosome.[286] In cervical cancer cell lines, HPV DNA integration was significantly associated with genomic rearrangements ($P < 10^{-10}$), resulting in increased amplification of both viral and cellular DNA sequences adjacent to the integration site.[287] The most common sites of HPV genomic integration in cervical cancers has been observed at 8q24[288] and 3p14,[289] two chromosomal regions that flank the *c-myc* oncogene and *fragile histidine triad* (*FHIT*) tumor suppressor genes respectively.[290] Overexpression of MYC mRNA and protein have been reported in genital tumor cell lines harboring HPV DNA insertion close to the MYC locus and no overexpression of MYC in lines where HPV insertion occurred at other sites.[291] Thus integration of the HPV DNA in the host genome can perturb genomic stability and promote HPV-dependent carcinogenesis.

Chromosomal instability is a hallmark feature of HPV-associated malignancies.[281,285] Genetic defects such as gains or loss of whole chromosomes (aneuploidy) and chromosomal rearrangements are thought to be an early event in HPV-induced cancers occurring prior to viral DNA integration into the host genome.[292] Cytogenetic studies of anal carcinomas have indicated recurrent loss of heterozygosity (LOH) at a number of loci including chromosome 3p (62% of cases), 5q (33% of cases), 11q (39–87% of cases), 17p (43% of cases), and at 18q (35–41% of cases).[293–295] These studies have indicated that tumor suppressors such as *TP53* (17p), APC (5q) and DCC (18q) maybe involved in the pathogenesis of anal squamous cell carcinomas. The frequent LOH at 11q23 in invasive cervical (40–62% of cases)[296,297] and anal SSC carcinomas has suggested the presence of a putative tumor suppressor gene that is important in progression of HPV-mediated cancers. However no specific functional gene has been identified to date.

The HPV-E6 and HPV-E7 oncoproteins appear to induce genomic instability by a number of different mechanisms. These viral-encoded products abrogate mitotic spindle checkpoints,[298,299] thereby inducing numerous defects including multipolar mitoses, centrosome duplication, anaphase bridges, and aneuploidy.[285] In high-risk HPV associated anal cancers, centrosome over-duplication has been observed which correlated with the presence of aberrant cell division.[300] E6 and E7 viral proteins also allow cells with mitotic defects to escape cell death by relaxing the *TP53*-regulated G2-M checkpoint[301] and by inhibition of apoptotic signals.[302] Moreover, E6 and E7 proteins can induce genomic instability by independently mediating numerical and structural chromosomal instability and by interrupting the ATM–ATR DNA damage response pathway.[285]

HIV

Prior to the HIV epidemic, older Caucasian women had the highest incidence of anal SSC. However after the emergence of HIV infection and introduction of highly active antiretroviral therapy (HAART), the demographics of this disease changed. Currently HIV-positive men who have sex with men (MSM) are at the highest risk for SSC of anal canal. History of receptive anal intercourse is associated with increased risk of anal cancer, (relative risk [RR] 33.1)[258] and this risk is even higher in HIV-infected homosexual men (RR 84.1).[303] In contrast to decrease in incidence of AIDS-defining illness in the era of HARRT, the incidence of anal cancers in HIV-infected homosexual men continues to increase.[304,305]

HIV infection does not appear to be the causative agent in anal SCC, yet infection with this retrovirus is a marker for coinfection with HPV, a major causative agent in anal SCC. In fact, approximately 95% of HIV-positive homosexual men are coinfected with HPV.[306,307] In general HIV infection is associated with a higher frequency of HPV-related preinvasive and invasive malignancies and these lesions occur at an earlier age.[273,308,309] In a series of 346 HIV-positive and HIV-negative homosexual men, the risk of AIN and HSIL was greater in setting of HIV infection (RR 5.7 and 3.7 respectively),[306] and the lower the CD4 count the higher the risk.[310,311] Anal cancer also occurs earlier in HIV-infected individuals by approximately two decades (mean age in HIV-positive individuals 37 years, HIV-negative men 58 years, and HIV-negative women 65 years).[312,313]

The independent impact of HIV infection on the biology of anal cancer is not fully understood, however most experts agree that HIV infection alters the natural history of HPV-related cancers by favoring persistent HPV infection. While HPV infection is cleared overtime in most immunocompetent individuals, HPV infection tends to persist and to be associated with higher prevalence of preinvasive lesions in immunocompromised individuals. In a study of 243 HIV-infected men and 231 controls, the overall HPV prevalence in urine samples of HIV-infected male was significantly higher than in the control group (27.5% vs. 12.6% respectively, $P<0.01$).[314] In HIV-infected men, there was a trend toward higher HPV prevalence and lower CD4 cell counts, however HAART therapy was associated with decreased HPV prevalence ($P=0.03$). There is also evidence that the natural history of AIN maybe different in HIV-positive than HIV-negative patients. Palefsky et al showed that the rate of progression from lower grade (AIN-1–2) to higher grade (AIN-3) anal intraepithelial neoplasia is accelerated in HIVpositive men (RR 2.4 95% CI 1.8–3.2) compared to HIV-negative men and the risk is increased with CD4 count lower than 200 cell/mm^3 (RR 3.1, 95% CI 2.3–4.1).[315]

Further data suggesting that HIV may alter the biology of anal cancer is reflected by a different type of genomic instability in HIV-associated neoplasia. High frequency of microsatellite instability (MSI) has been described in cancers obtained from HIV infected individuals including lung cancer, cervical intraepithelial tumors, Kaposi's sarcoma, immune deficiency-related lymphomas.[316–319] In contrast there was no evidence of such instability in lesions from HIV-negative patients. Moreover, while chromosomal instability, as reflected by LOH, is a key feature of HPV-related tumors, LOH is uncommon in anal cancers of HIV-positive patients. In a cohort of 18 HIV-negative and 10 HIV-positive patients with SCC of the anus, Gervaz et al showed that tumors from HIV-negative patients were more likely to present with LOH than tumors form HIV-positive individuals (24.1% vs. 6.6%, $P=0.0004$).[295] Allelic loss at specific loci,

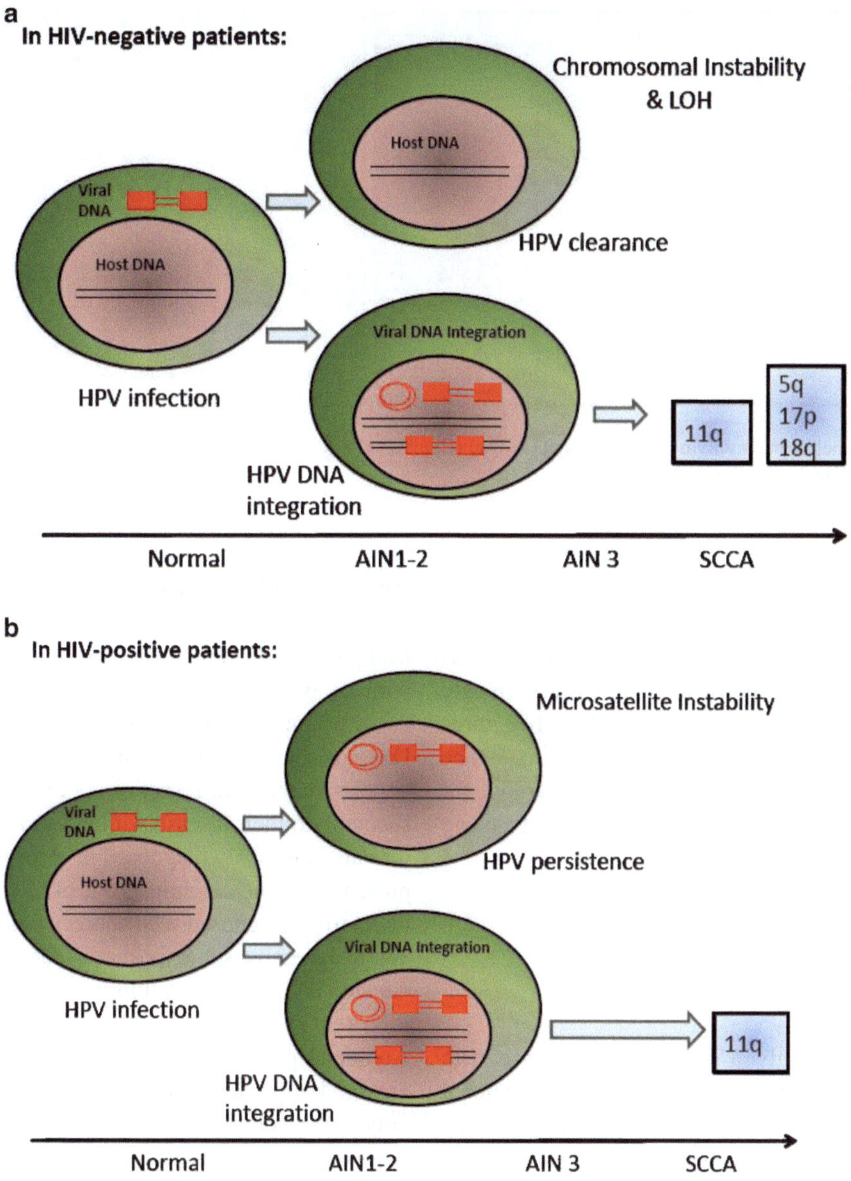

Fig. 9.5 Model of tumorigenesis in anal squamous cell carcinoma (SSCA) with respect to infection with the human immunodeficiency virus (HIV). (**a**) Following infection and integration of the human papillomavirus (HPV), progression of the neoplastic process requires loss of heterozygosity (LOH) at key loci including 17p (p53), 5q(APC), and 18q (DCC). Chromosome 11 is thought to harbor a putative tumor suppressor important in anal SSCA tumor progression, and LOH at 11q23 is thought to be an early event independent of HIV infection. This process takes an average time of 30–40 years, with the median age at the time of diagnosis being 60–70 years in this population. *AIN* anal intraepithelial neoplasia. (**b**) Progression of cancer is accelerated in the setting of HIV infection, with the median age at diagnosis being 37 years. The persistence of HPV infection and absence of LOH at 17p, 5q, 18q suggest an alternate molecular pathway perhaps via microsatellite instability in this population. *AIN* anal intraepithelial neoplasia (Adopted from Gervaz, British Journal of Surgery 2006)

such as 18q (DCC), 17p (*TP53*), and 5q (APC) were significantly lower in tumors of HIV-positive patients. Thus these data suggest that the molecular mechanisms involved in the pathogenesis of SCC of the anus may be dependent on HIV status. While chromosomal instability is the dominant feature in HIV-negative anal cancers, an alternate pathway of microsatellite instability may contribute to progression to invasive anal cancer in presence of HIV infection (see Fig. 9.5).[281,295]

EGFR

The epidermal growth factor receptor is expressed in a majority of squamous cell cancers of the anal canal. An analysis of 21 such cancers found that all overexpressed EGFR, but did not express HER2Neu.[320] More recently of 29 primary squamous carcinomas of the anal canal, 27 (93%) were found to express EGFR by IHC, while none of the specimen were found to carry a *K-RAS* mutation.[321] A report of seven patients

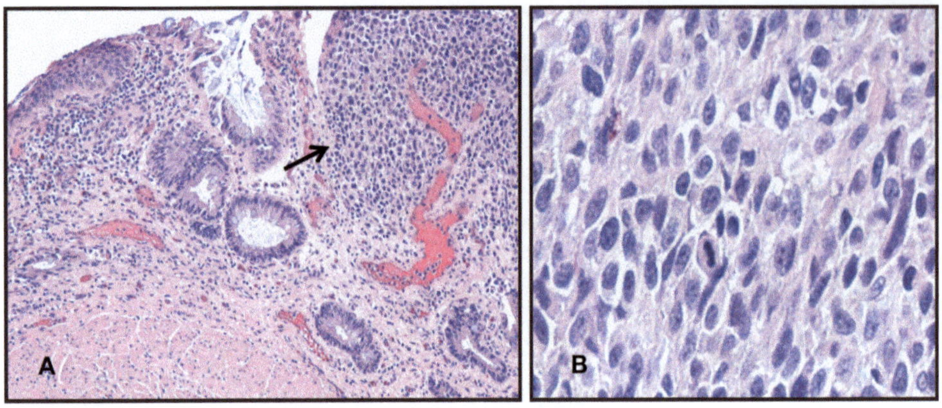

Fig. 9.6 (**a**) Malignant melanoma involving the anal canal (*arrow*) (Hematoxylin and Eosin stain, original magnification ×100). (**b**) High power view the same tumor (original magnification ×20)

with metastatic anal cancer treated with cetuximab, a recombinant chimeric monoclonal antibody to EGFR, found that two patients had *KRAS* mutations (EGFR determination was not done in this analysis). Response to therapy was seen only in those individuals with wild type *KRAS*: of those five, three had a partial response, and one had a minor response. [322] The addition of anti-EGFR agents to first-line therapy for squamous cell cancer of the anal canal is currently being investigated.

Molecular Markers of Response to Chemoradiation

Anal SCC is predominantly a locoregional disease with direct extension to the surrounding tissue and the regional lymphatics. Treatment involves combined modality therapy with upfront concurrent chemoradiation and surgery is often reserved for salvage therapy. There is paucity of data regarding predictive or prognostic biomarkers in anal cancer in the current literature. A recent study from M.D. Anderson Cancer Center evaluated the role of 10 biomarkers in predicting response to conventional chemoradiation in 30 patients with anal canal squamous cell carcinoma.[323] In multivariate analysis, tumor diameter ($P=0.002$), proliferation index Ki-67 ($P=0.005$), transcription factor NF-kB ($P=0.002$), and molecules involved in the Hedgehog signaling pathway including hedgehog ligand SHH ($P=0.002$) and the transcription factor Gli-1 ($P=0.02$) were associated with disease-free survival in 30 patients with anal canal SSC post conventional chemoradiation. Although these results are preliminary, if validated, this data can provide the basis for biomarker-driven understanding of the heterogeneous natural history of anal carcinomas.

Anorectal Melanoma

Malignant melanoma of the anorectum is a rare malignancy with an extremely poor prognosis (Fig. 9.6). It accounts for 0.3–1.6% of all melanomas and 2–4% of all anorectal. [324–326] Diagnosis is often made at an advanced stage, and even with aggressive surgical resection more than 80% of the patient succumb to their disease within 5 years.[327] Mucosal melanomas are commonly diagnosed in older individuals, with 50% presenting in their eighth decade of life. Women are also more likely to be diagnosed with anorectal melanomas than men.[328] While excessive sun exposure is considered a risk factor for cutaneous melanomas, ultraviolet (UV) radiation is not involved in development of these mucosal malignancies. Anorectal melanoma is more common in individuals with darker skin pigmentation, and rate of mucosal melanoma is only twice as high in Caucasians than in African Americans (whereas the risk of cutaneous and ocular melanoma is 5–20 times higher in Caucasians).[327] HIV infection has also been proposed as another risk factor for anal melanoma.[329]

Although the molecular pathogenesis of anal melanoma is poorly understood, there is recent evidence that c-KIT signaling may be the driving oncogenic event in this subset of melanomas.[330] The c-KIT receptor tyrosine kinase is critical in melanocyte development and its expression is lost in most melanomas. Recent studies have described an increased frequency of c-KIT aberrations in melanomas with no or little UV light exposure, namely mucosal melanomas and acral melanomas.[331,332] These c-KIT gene abnormalities, consisting of mutations or increase in copy number, have been reported in 16% of mucosal melanomas and acral melanomas[332] and in only approximately 2% of cutaneous melanomas.[333,334] Other evidence for distinct molecular pathogenesis of anal melanoma is the observation that *BRAF* and *NRAS* mutations, which are common in cutaneous melanomas,[335] are rarely found in anal melanomas.[336] Moreover there have been case reports of clinical efficacy of targeted therapies with c-KIT blockers in mucosal melanomas. Although the initial clinical trials with imatinib mesylate were disappointing,[337,338] several recent case reports have indicated clinical response with various c-KIT inhibitors (imatinib, sunitinib, dasatinib, or sorafenib) in patients with metastatic melanoma, includ-ing anal melanoma harboring c-KIT activating mutations.[339–344] Although the etiology of the observed differences is not fully understood, it has been hypothesized that c-KIT mutation or amplification, rather than protein expression, is relevant for susceptibility to c-KIT blockade therapy.[339]

Rare Anorectal Neoplasms

Uncommon tumors of the anal canal include gastrointestinal stromal tumors (GIST), Kaposi's sarcoma, neuroendocrine tumors, sarcomas, and lymphomas. According to the most recent data from the Epidemiology and End Results Program (SEER), the nonepidermoid/nonmelanoma cancers account for 2.3% of all cases of anal malignancies.[345] The non-squamous cancers of the anal canal have poor prognosis (Table 9.5) and have been traditionally managed by abdominoperineal resection as their definitive treatment. This section will discuss the molecular and clinical features of these rare anorectal tumors.

GIST

GISTs are the most common mesenchymal neoplasms of the digestive tract. They are most frequently found in the stomach (60%) and the small intestine (30%) and rarely found in the rectum or anus (5–10%).[346,347] While uncommon, GISTs arising in the small bowel, colon, rectum, or mesentery are more aggressive and associated with worse outcome than those arising in the stomach.[348] These tumors universally express CD117 antigen, which is part of the c-KIT receptor, a membrane tyrosine kinase.[349] Over 80% of these tumors harbor activating mutations in the c-KIT proto-oncogene; and approximately 5–7% KIT negative GIST cancers of others have mutations in a related tyrosine kinase PDGFα (platelet-derived growth factor α).[350]

Given the high sequence homology between KIT, PDGFα, and the BCR–ABL translocation in chronic myelogenous leukemia (CML), the small molecule tyrosine kinase inhibitor, imatinib mesylate has gained a great deal of interest for treatment of GIST. A number of studies have demonstrated the clinical efficacy of imatinib in advanced GIST,[351–353] with improvement in median survival from 20 to 60 months in these patients.[354] The type of mutation in KIT and PDGRA appears to influence clinical response to imatinib. In patients with KIT mutations, those with exon 11 mutant isoform appear to derive a higher objective response, longer time to progression, and improved median overall survival compared to those with exon 9 mutant isoform.[350,355] Several studies including a meta-analysis demonstrated that higher doses of imatinib (800 mg/day rather than the standard 400 mg/day) preferentially improved PFS in patients with exon 9 mutations without corresponding benefit in the overall survival.[355–357] GISTs that harbor PDGFRA mutations are more heterogeneous and only a subset of PDGFRA mutants are imatinib sensitive.[358,359] At this time PDGFRA mutational analysis is not routinely performed in clinical practice for management of GIST cancers.

The success of imatinib in advanced disease has spurred enthusiasm for use of this agent in the perioperative setting. While the gold standard for patients with primary resectable GIST is surgery, only one-half of the cases remain disease free at 5 years and adjuvant therapy is favored for patients at high risk for recurrence based on tumor size, mitotic index, and site of tumor origin. Several studies have demonstrated the benefit of imatinib in the adjuvant setting in these high risk patients. In the double-blinded multicenter ACOSOG Z9001 phase III trial, 713 patients with primary GIST of the intestinal tract at least 3 cm in size with IHC-proven positive KIT protein were randomized to 1 year of adjuvant imatinib (40 mg daily) or placebo.[360] The primary endpoint of the study was recurrence-free survival (RFS). The study was stopped early when the interim analysis disclosed significantly fewer recurrences in the treatment arm than the placebo arm. At median follow-up of 1 year, RFS rate was 98% vs. 83% favoring the imatinib arm (HR 0.35, 95% CI 0.22–0.53). Based on these results US FDA approved imatinib for adjuvant treatment of fully resected GIST ≥3 cm in size without providing guidance for optimal duration of therapy or the optimal patient selection.

Imatinib therapy has also been studied in neoadjuvant setting for primary unresectable or borderline respectable GIST tumors. Although data from randomized trials for use of imatinib in preoperative setting is not available, data from retrospective series[361,362] and a phase II trial[363] support the benefit of initial imatinib therapy. Moreover, several recent case reports have demonstrated that preoperative imatinib therapy in rectal GIST tumors can reduce tumor bulk and allow for subsequent resection of initially unresectable tumors.[364,365]

Carcinoid and Neuroendocrine Tumors

Anorectal carcinoid tumors are rare and account for 1.3% of all rectal cancers.[366] Nonetheless, the rectum is the second most common site of origin of neuroendocrine tumors of the digestive tract.[367] Most carcinoid tumors in the rectum are small (median diameter 0.6 cm) with over 90% located within 4–13 cm above the dentate line.[349,367] These tumors are

Table 9.6 TNM staging for carcinoid tumors of the colon and rectum

Primary tumor (T)	
Tx	Primary tumor cannot be assessed
T0	No evidence of primary tumor
T1	Tumor invades lamina propria or submucosa and size 2 cm or less
T1a	Tumor less than 1 cm in greatest dimension
T1b	Tumor size 1–2 cm in greatest dimension
T2	Tumor invades muscularis propria or size more than 2 cm with invasion of lamina propria or submucosa
T3	Tumor invades through the muscularis propria into the submucosa, or into the non-peritonealized pericolic or perirectal tissues
T4	Tumor invades peritoneum or other organs
	For any T add (m) for multiple tumors
Regional lymph nodes (N)	
Nx	Regional lymph nodes cannot be assessed
N0	No regional lymph node metastasis
N1	Regional lymph node metastasis
Distant metastasis (M)	
M0	No distant metastasis
M1	Distant metastasis

Table adapted from AJCC Cancer Staging Manual, 7th edition (2010) by Springer New York, Inc

Table 9.7 TNM staging for carcinoid tumors of colon and rectum

Stage	T	N	M
0	Tis	N0	M0
I	T1	N0	M0
IIA	T2	N0	M0
IIB	T3	N0	M0
IIIA	T4	N0	
IIIB	Any T	N1	
IV	Any T	Any N	M1

Adapted from the AJCC Cancer Staging Manual, 7th edition (2010) by Springer New York, Inc

hormonally inactive and unlike carcinoid tumors of the midgut, those arising in the rectum do not manifest carcinoid syndrome even in the setting of liver metastasis.[349,368]

Prognosis and optimal treatment of anorectal carcinoids depends on size of the primary tumor.[369] The risk of distant metastasis is minimal for small tumors that are <1 cm in size and can be treated with local excision.[370–372] Tumors >2 cm have 70% chance of distant metastasis and have been traditionally treated with extensive surgical resection similar to rectal adenocarcinomas.[370,371,373] However this practice has been questioned since improved survival has not been consistently shown compared to endoscopic removal.[374] Carcinoid tumors ranging 1–2 cm have intermediate risk of metastasis (4–30%) and treatment is more controversial.[370,371] While local excision may suffice for most of these tumors, more aggressive surgical resection has been proposed for tumors with unfavorable prognostic features such as invasion of the muscularis propria, ≥2 mitoses per high power field, and lymphovascular invasion.[375] In a proposed staging system based on SEER database, the 5-year survival rates for stages I through IV were 97%, 84%, 27%, and 20% respectively (Tables 9.6 and 9.7).[376]

Lymphoma

Primary anorectal lymphoma is a rare entity, representing 0.2% of rectal neoplasms and 9% of non-Hodgkins lymphomas (NHL).[377] Two risk factors associated with primary anorectal lymphoma include inflammatory bowel disease and immunosuppression (from HIV infection, post-transplant, or other immune disorders).[378–380] AIDS-related lymphomas are more aggressive with mean age of diagnosis 34 years (in contrast to 64 years of age in non-AIDS related cases) and they often present with disseminated disease at the time of diagnosis.[349,381] Treatment of primary anorectal lymphomas is controversial. However the current, National Comprehensive Cancer Network (NCCN) guidelines recommend observation if negative margins are obtained postexcision and locoregional radiation if the margins are positive. Advanced disease or systemic recurrence is treated similar to follicular lymphoma.

References

1. Jemal A, Siegel R, Xu J, Ward E. Cancer statistics, 2010. *CA Cancer J Clin.* 2010;60:277-300.
2. American Cancer Society. *Cancer facts & figures 2010.* Atlanta: American Cancer Society; 2010.
3. Jemal A, et al. Cancer statistics, 2009. *CA Cancer J Clin.* 2009;59(4):225-49.
4. Cucino C, Buchner AM, Sonnenberg A. Continued rightward shift of colorectal cancer. *Dis Colon Rectum.* 2002;45(8):1035-40.
5. Meza R, et al. Colorectal cancer incidence trends in the United States and United Kingdom: evidence of right- to left-sided biological gradients with implications for screening. *Cancer Res.* 2010;70(13):5419-29.
6. Rim SH, et al. Colorectal cancer incidence in the United States, 1999–2004: an updated analysis of data from the National Program of Cancer Registries and the Surveillance, Epidemiology, and End Results Program. *Cancer.* 2009;115(9):1967-76.
7. Levi F, Randimbison L, La Vecchia C. Trends in subsite distribution of colorectal cancers and polyps from the Vaud Cancer Registry. *Cancer.* 1993;72(1):46-50.
8. Cooper GS, et al. A national population-based study of incidence of colorectal cancer and age. Implications for screening in older Americans. *Cancer.* 1995;75(3):775-81.
9. Benedix F, et al. Comparison of 17,641 patients with right- and left-sided colon cancer: differences in epidemiology, perioperative course, histology, and survival. *Dis Colon Rectum.* 2010;53(1): 57-64.
10. Distler P, Holt PR. Are right- and left-sided colon neoplasms distinct tumors? *Dig Dis.* 1997;15(4–5):302-11.
11. Meguid R, et al. Is there a difference in survival between right- versus left-sided colon cancers? *Ann Surg Oncol.* 2008;15(9):2388-94.

12. Papagiorgis P, et al. The impact of tumor location on the histopathologic expression of colorectal cancer. *J BUON*. 2006;11(3): 317-21.
13. Boland CR, Goel A. Microsatellite instability in colorectal cancer. *Gastroenterology*. 2010;138(6):2073-2087. e3.
14. Abeloff M, et al. *Abeloff's clinical oncology*. 4th ed. Oxford, UK: Churchill Livingstone, An Imprint of Elsevier; 2008.
15. Agur AM, Dalley AF, Moore KL. *Clinically oriented anatomy*. 6th ed. Baltimore: Lippincott Williams and Wilkins; 2009.
16. DeVita VT, Hellman S, Rosenberg SA. *Cancer: principles and practice of oncology*. 7th ed. Philadelphia, PA: Lippincott Williams & Wilkins; 2005.
17. Cohen AM, et al. Pathological studies in rectal cancer. *Cancer*. 1980;45(12):2965-8.
18. Sontag SJ, et al. Fecal occult blood screening for colorectal cancer in a Veterans Administration Hospital. *Am J Surg*. 1983;145(1):89-94.
19. George SM, et al. Classification of advanced colorectal carcinomas by tumor edge morphology: evidence for different pathogenesis and significance of polypoid and nonpolypoid tumors. *Cancer*. 2000;89(9):1901-9.
20. Steinberg SM, et al. Prognostic indicators of colon tumors. The Gastrointestinal Tumor Study Group experience. *Cancer*. 1986;57(9):1866-70.
21. Carraro PG, et al. Obstructing colonic cancer: failure and survival patterns over a ten-year follow-up after one-stage curative surgery. *Dis Colon Rectum*. 2001;44(2):243-50.
22. Griffin MR, et al. Predictors of survival after curative resection of carcinoma of the colon and rectum. *Cancer*. 1987;60(9): 2318-24.
23. Wolmark N, et al. The prognostic significance of tumor location and bowel obstruction in Dukes B and C colorectal cancer. Findings from the NSABP clinical trials. *Ann Surg*. 1983;198(6):743-52.
24. Kelsen DP, et al. *Principles and practice of gastrointestinal oncology*. Philadelphia, PA: Lippincott Williams & Wilkins, Wolter Kluwer Health; 2008.
25. Green JB, et al. Mucinous carcinoma–just another colon cancer? *Dis Colon Rectum*. 1993;36(1):49-54.
26. Secco GB, et al. Primary mucinous adenocarcinomas and signet-ring cell carcinomas of colon and rectum. *Oncology*. 1994;51(1): 30-4.
27. Consorti F, et al. Prognostic significance of mucinous carcinoma of colon and rectum: a prospective case–control study. *J Surg Oncol*. 2000;73(2):70-4.
28. Sasaki O, Atkin WS, Jass JR. Mucinous carcinoma of the rectum. *Histopathology*. 1987;11(3):259-72.
29. Symonds DA, Vickery AL. Mucinous carcinoma of the colon and rectum. *Cancer*. 1976;37(4):1891-1900.
30. Compton CC, et al. Prognostic factors in colorectal cancer. College of American Pathologists Consensus Statement 1999. *Arch Pathol Lab Med*. 2000;124(7):979-94.
31. Nissan A, et al. Signet-ring cell carcinoma of the colon and rectum: a matched control study. *Dis Colon Rectum*. 1999;42(9):1176-80.
32. Ogino S, et al. Distinct molecular features of colorectal carcinoma with signet ring cell component and colorectal carcinoma with mucinous component. *Mod Pathol*. 2006;19(1):59-68.
33. Kakar S, Smyrk TC. Signet ring cell carcinoma of the colorectum: correlations between microsatellite instability, clinicopathologic features and survival. *Mod Pathol*. 2005;18(2):244-9.
34. Song GA, et al. Mucinous carcinomas of the colorectum have distinct molecular genetic characteristics. *Int J Oncol*. 2005;26(3):745-50.
35. Kakar S, et al. Mucinous carcinoma of the colon: correlation of loss of mismatch repair enzymes with clinicopathologic features and survival. *Mod Pathol*. 2004;17(6):696-700.
36. Ojeda VJ, et al. Primary colo-rectal linitis plastica type of carcinoma: report of two cases and review of the literature. *Pathology*. 1982;14(2):181-9.
37. Sasaki S, et al. Characteristics in primary signet-ring cell carcinoma of the colorectum, from clinicopathological observations. *Jpn J Clin Oncol*. 1998;28(3):202-6.
38. Rashid A, et al. Elevated expression of fatty acid synthase and fatty acid synthetic activity in colorectal neoplasia. *Am J Pathol*. 1997;150(1):201-8.
39. Visca P, et al. Immunohistochemical expression of fatty acid synthase, apoptotic-regulating genes, proliferating factors, and ras protein product in colorectal adenomas, carcinomas, and adjacent nonneoplastic mucosa. *Clin Cancer Res*. 1999;5(12):4111-8.
40. Jessurun J, Romero-Guadarrama M, Manivel JC. Medullary adenocarcinoma of the colon: clinicopathologic study of 11 cases. *Hum Pathol*. 1999;30(7):843-8.
41. Lanza G, et al. Medullary-type poorly differentiated adenocarcinoma of the large bowel: a distinct clinicopathologic entity characterized by microsatellite instability and improved survival. *J Clin Oncol*. 1999;17(8):2429-38.
42. Jass JR, et al. Morphology of sporadic colorectal cancer with DNA replication errors. *Gut*. 1998;42(5):673-9.
43. Jass JR, et al. Pathology of hereditary non-polyposis colorectal cancer. *Anticancer Res*. 1994;14(4B):1631-4.
44. Hinoi T, et al. Loss of CDX2 expression and microsatellite instability are prominent features of large cell minimally differentiated carcinomas of the colon. *Am J Pathol*. 2001;159(6): 2239-48.
45. Winn B, et al. Differentiating the undifferentiated: immunohistochemical profile of medullary carcinoma of the colon with an emphasis on intestinal differentiation. *Hum Pathol*. 2009;40(3): 398-404.
46. Wicking C, et al. CDX2, a human homologue of Drosophila caudal, is mutated in both alleles in a replication error positive colorectal cancer. *Oncogene*. 1998;17(5):657-9.
47. Lugli A, et al. Differential diagnostic and functional role of the multi-marker phenotype CDX2/CK20/CK7 in colorectal cancer stratified by mismatch repair status. *Mod Pathol*. 2008;21(11): 1403-12.
48. Yamaguchi T, et al. Accumulation profile of frameshift mutations during development and progression of colorectal cancer from patients with hereditary nonpolyposis colorectal cancer. *Dis Colon Rectum*. 2006;49(3):399-406.
49. Baba Y, et al. Relationship of CDX2 loss with molecular features and prognosis in colorectal cancer. *Clin Cancer Res*. 2009;15(14):4665-73.
50. Cabrera A, Pickren JW. Squamous metaplasia and squamous-cell carcinoma of the rectosigmoid. *Dis Colon Rectum*. 1967;10(4): 288-97.
51. Dyson T, Draganov PV. Squamous cell cancer of the rectum. *World J Gastroenterol*. 2009;15(35):4380-6.
52. Lafreniere R, Ketcham AS. Primary squamous carcinoma of the rectum. Report of a case and review of the literature. *Dis Colon Rectum*. 1985;28(12):967-72.
53. Nahas CS, et al. Squamous-cell carcinoma of the rectum: a rare but curable tumor. *Dis Colon Rectum*. 2007;50(9):1393-400.
54. Juturi JV, et al. Squamous-cell carcinoma of the colon responsive to combination chemotherapy: report of two cases and review of the literature. *Dis Colon Rectum*. 1999;42(1):102-9.
55. Williams GT, Blackshaw AJ, Morson BC. Squamous carcinoma of the colorectum and its genesis. *J Pathol*. 1979;129(3):139-47.
56. Rasheed S, et al. Chemo-radiotherapy: an alternative to surgery for squamous cell carcinoma of the rectum–report of six patients and literature review. *Colorectal Dis*. 2009;11(2):191-7.
57. Comer TP, Beahrs OH, Dockerty MB. Primary squamous cell carcinoma and adenocanthoma of the colon. *Cancer*. 1971;28(5): 1111-7.
58. Wiener MF, Polayes SH, Yidi R. Squamous carcinoma with schistosomiasis of the colon. *Am J Gastroenterol*. 1962;37:48-54.

59. Kong CS, Welton ML, Longacre TA. Role of human papillomavirus in squamous cell metaplasia-dysplasia-carcinoma of the rectum. *Am J Surg Pathol*. 2007;31(6):919-25.
60. Frizelle FA, et al. Adenosquamous and squamous carcinoma of the colon and upper rectum: a clinical and histopathologic study. *Dis Colon Rectum*. 2001;44(3):341-6.
61. The American Joint Committee on Cancer. *AJCC Cancer staging manual*. 7th ed. Chicago: Springer; 2010.
62. Ogino S, Goel A. Molecular classification and correlates in colorectal cancer. *J Mol Diagn*. 2008;10(1):13-27.
63. Fearon ER, Vogelstein B. A genetic model for colorectal tumorigenesis. *Cell*. 1990;61(5):759-67.
64. Pino MS, Chung DC. The chromosomal instability pathway in colon cancer. *Gastroenterology*. 2010;138(6):2059-72.
65. Walther A, Houlston R, Tomlinson I. Association between chromosomal instability and prognosis in colorectal cancer: a meta-analysis. *Gut*. 2008;57(7):941-50.
66. Boland CR, et al. A National Cancer Institute Workshop on Microsatellite Instability for cancer detection and familial predisposition: development of international criteria for the determination of microsatellite instability in colorectal cancer. *Cancer Res*. 1998;58(22):5248-57.
67. Lynch HT, et al. Genetics, natural history, tumor spectrum, and pathology of hereditary nonpolyposis colorectal cancer: an updated review. *Gastroenterology*. 1993;104(5):1535-49.
68. Ward R, et al. Microsatellite instability and the clinicopathological features of sporadic colorectal cancer. *Gut*. 2001;48(6):821-9.
69. Veigl ML, et al. Biallelic inactivation of hMLH1 by epigenetic gene silencing, a novel mechanism causing human MSI cancers. *Proc Natl Acad Sci USA*. 1998;95(15):8698-702.
70. Edge SB, et al. *AJCC (American Joint Committee on Cancer) Cancer Staging Manual Seventh Edition*. Chicago: Springer; 2010.
71. Laird PW. Cancer epigenetics. *Hum Mol Genet*. 2005;14(Spec No 1):R65-76.
72. Kim MS, Lee J, Sidransky D. DNA methylation markers in colorectal cancer. *Cancer Metastasis Rev*. 2010;29(1):181-206.
73. Shen L, et al. Integrated genetic and epigenetic analysis identifies three different subclasses of colon cancer. *Proc Natl Acad Sci USA*. 2007;104(47):18654-9.
74. Leggett B, Whitehall V. Role of the serrated pathway in colorectal cancer pathogenesis. *Gastroenterology*. 2009;138(6):2088-100.
75. Noffsinger AE. Serrated polyps and colorectal cancer: new pathway to malignancy. *Annu Rev Pathol*. 2009;4:343-64.
76. Ogino S, et al. CpG island methylator phenotype-low (CIMP-low) in colorectal cancer: possible associations with male sex and KRAS mutations. *J Mol Diagn*. 2006;8(5):582-8.
77. Sanchez JA, et al. Genetic and epigenetic classifications define clinical phenotypes and determine patient outcomes in colorectal cancer. *Br J Surg*. 2009;96(10):1196-204.
78. Ogino S, et al. CpG island methylation, response to combination chemotherapy, and patient survival in advanced microsatellite stable colorectal carcinoma. *Virchows Arch*. 2007;450(5):529-37.
79. Dahlin AM, et al. The role of the CpG island methylator phenotype in colorectal cancer prognosis depends on microsatellite instability screening status. *Clin Cancer Res*. 2010;16(6):1845-55.
80. Ogino S, et al. CpG island methylator phenotype, microsatellite instability, BRAF mutation and clinical outcome in colon cancer. *Gut*. 2009;58(1):90-6.
81. Barault L, et al. Hypermethylator phenotype in sporadic colon cancer: study on a population-based series of 582 cases. *Cancer Res*. 2008;68(20):8541-6.
82. Chapuis PH, et al. A multivariate analysis of clinical and pathological variables in prognosis after resection of large bowel cancer. *Br J Surg*. 1985;72(9):698-702.
83. Wiggers T, Arends JW, Volovics A. Regression analysis of prognostic factors in colorectal cancer after curative resections. *Dis Colon Rectum*. 1988;31(1):33-41.
84. Chang GJ, et al. Lymph node evaluation and survival after curative resection of colon cancer: systematic review. *J Natl Cancer Inst*. 2007;99(6):433-41.
85. Johnson PM, et al. Increasing negative lymph node count is independently associated with improved long-term survival in stage IIIB and IIIC colon cancer. *J Clin Oncol*. 2006;24(22):3570-5.
86. Compton C, et al. American Joint Committee on Cancer Prognostic Factors Consensus Conference: Colorectal Working Group. *Cancer*. 2000;88(7):1739-57.
87. Bozzetti F. Prognostic significance of radial margins of clearance in rectal cancer. *Br J Surg*. 1996;83(12):1798.
88. de Haas-Kock DF, et al. Prognostic significance of radial margins of clearance in rectal cancer. *Br J Surg*. 1996;83(6):781-5.
89. Nagtegaal ID, Quirke P. What is the role for the circumferential margin in the modern treatment of rectal cancer? *J Clin Oncol*. 2008;26(2):303-12.
90. Quirke P, et al. Local recurrence of rectal adenocarcinoma due to inadequate surgical resection. Histopathological study of lateral tumour spread and surgical excision. *Lancet*. 1986;2(8514):996-9.
91. Halvorsen TB, Seim E. Association between invasiveness, inflammatory reaction, desmoplasia and survival in colorectal cancer. *J Clin Pathol*. 1989;42(2):162-6.
92. Newland RC, et al. Pathologic determinants of survival associated with colorectal cancer with lymph node metastases. A multivariate analysis of 579 patients. *Cancer*. 1994;73(8):2076-82.
93. Roncucci L, et al. Survival for colon and rectal cancer in a population-based cancer registry. *Eur J Cancer*. 1996;32A(2):295-302.
94. Hase K, et al. Prognostic value of tumor "budding" in patients with colorectal cancer. *Dis Colon Rectum*. 1993;36(7):627-35.
95. Gryfe R, et al. Tumor microsatellite instability and clinical outcome in young patients with colorectal cancer. *N Engl J Med*. 2000;342(2):69-77.
96. Lothe RA, et al. Genomic instability in colorectal cancer: relationship to clinicopathological variables and family history. *Cancer Res*. 1993;53(24):5849-52.
97. Popat S, Hubner R, Houlston RS. Systematic review of microsatellite instability and colorectal cancer prognosis. *J Clin Oncol*. 2005;23(3):609-18.
98. Kim H, et al. Clinical and pathological characteristics of sporadic colorectal carcinomas with DNA replication errors in microsatellite sequences. *Am J Pathol*. 1994;145(1):148-56.
99. Smyrk TC, et al. Tumor-infiltrating lymphocytes are a marker for microsatellite instability in colorectal carcinoma. *Cancer*. 2001;91(12):2417-22.
100. Lanza G, et al. Immunohistochemical test for MLH1 and MSH2 expression predicts clinical outcome in stage II and III colorectal cancer patients. *J Clin Oncol*. 2006;24(15):2359-67.
101. Ribic CM, et al. Tumor microsatellite-instability status as a predictor of benefit from fluorouracil-based adjuvant chemotherapy for colon cancer. *N Engl J Med*. 2003;349(3):247-57.
102. Sargent DJ, et al. Defective mismatch repair as a predictive marker for lack of efficacy of fluorouracil-based adjuvant therapy in colon cancer. *J Clin Oncol*. 2010;28(20):3219-26.
103. Andre T, et al. Oxaliplatin, fluorouracil, and leucovorin as adjuvant treatment for colon cancer. *N Engl J Med*. 2004;350(23):2343-51.
104. Andre T, et al. Improved overall survival with oxaliplatin, fluorouracil, and leucovorin as adjuvant treatment in stage II or III colon cancer in the MOSAIC trial. *J Clin Oncol*. 2009;27(19):3109-16.

105. Benson AB 3rd, et al. American Society of Clinical Oncology recommendations on adjuvant chemotherapy for stage II colon cancer. *J Clin Oncol.* 2004;22(16):3408-19.
106. Kerr DJ, Midgley R. Defective mismatch repair in colon cancer: a prognostic or predictive biomarker? *J Clin Oncol.* 2010;28(20):3210-2.
107. Ng K, Schrag D. Microsatellite instability and adjuvant fluorouracil chemotherapy: a mismatch? *J Clin Oncol.* 2010;28(20):3207-10.
108. Des Guetz G, et al. Does microsatellite instability predict the efficacy of adjuvant chemotherapy in colorectal cancer? A systematic review with meta-analysis. *Eur J Cancer.* 2009;45(10):1890-6.
109. Fernebro E, et al. Predominance of CIN versus MSI in the development of rectal cancer at young age. *BMC Cancer.* 2002;2:25.
110. Hoogerbrugge N, et al. Very low incidence of microsatellite instability in rectal cancers from families at risk for HNPCC. *Clin Genet.* 2003;63(1):64-70.
111. Ishikubo T, et al. The clinical features of rectal cancers with high-frequency microsatellite instability (MSI-H) in Japanese males. *Cancer Lett.* 2004;216(1):55-62.
112. Colombino M, et al. Prevalence and prognostic role of microsatellite instability in patients with rectal carcinoma. *Ann Oncol.* 2002;13(9):1447-53.
113. Meng WJ, et al. Microsatellite instability did not predict individual survival in sporadic stage II and III rectal cancer patients. *Oncology.* 2007;72(1–2):82-8.
114. Jen J, et al. Allelic loss of chromosome 18q and prognosis in colorectal cancer. *N Engl J Med.* 1994;331(4):213-21.
115. Lanza G, et al. Chromosome 18q allelic loss and prognosis in stage II and III colon cancer. *Int J Cancer.* 1998;79(4):390-5.
116. Popat S, Houlston RS. A systematic review and meta-analysis of the relationship between chromosome 18q genotype, DCC status and colorectal cancer prognosis. *Eur J Cancer.* 2005;41(14):2060-70.
117. Kato M, et al. Detection of DCC and Ki-ras gene alterations in colorectal carcinoma tissue as prognostic markers for liver metastatic recurrence. *Cancer.* 1996;77(8 Suppl):1729-35.
118. Shibata D, et al. The DCC protein and prognosis in colorectal cancer. *N Engl J Med.* 1996;335(23):1727-32.
119. Itoh F, et al. Decreased expression of DCC mRNA in human colorectal cancers. *Int J Cancer.* 1993;53(2):260-3.
120. Hong S, Lee HJ, Kim SJ, Hahm KB. Connection between inflammation and carcinogenesis in gastrointestinal tract: focus on TGF-beta signaling. *World J Gastroenterol.* 2010;16(17):2080-93.
121. Eppert K, et al. MADR2 maps to 18q21 and encodes a TGFbeta-regulated MAD-related protein that is functionally mutated in colorectal carcinoma. *Cell.* 1996;86(4):543-52.
122. Xie W, et al. Loss of Smad signaling in human colorectal cancer is associated with advanced disease and poor prognosis. *Cancer J.* 2003;9(4):302-12.
123. Alhopuro P, et al. SMAD4 levels and response to 5-fluorouracil in colorectal cancer. *Clin Cancer Res.* 2005;11(17):6311-6.
124. Alazzouzi H, et al. SMAD4 as a prognostic marker in colorectal cancer. *Clin Cancer Res.* 2005;11(7):2606-11.
125. Carethers JM, et al. Prognostic significance of allelic lost at chromosome 18q21 for stage II colorectal cancer. *Gastroenterology.* 1998;114(6):1188-95.
126. Cohn KH, et al. The significance of allelic deletions and aneuploidy in colorectal carcinoma. Results of a 5-year follow-up study. *Cancer.* 1997;79(2):233-44.
127. Laurent-Puig P, et al. Survival and acquired genetic alterations in colorectal cancer. *Gastroenterology.* 1992;102(4 Pt 1):1136-41.
128. Zauber NP, et al. Ki-ras gene mutations, LOH of the APC and DCC genes, and microsatellite instability in primary colorectal carcinoma are not associated with micrometastases in pericolonic lymph nodes or with patients' survival. *J Clin Pathol.* 2004;57(9):938-42.
129. Locker GY, et al. ASCO 2006 update of recommendations for the use of tumor markers in gastrointestinal cancer. *J Clin Oncol.* 2006;24(33):5313-27.
130. Bazan V, et al. DNA ploidy and S-phase fraction, but not p53 or NM23-H1 expression, predict outcome in colorectal cancer patients. Result of a 5-year prospective study. *J Cancer Res Clin Oncol.* 2002;128(12):650-8.
131. Bottger TC, et al. Prognostic value of DNA analysis in colorectal carcinoma. *Cancer.* 1993;72(12):3579-87.
132. Liebig C, et al. Perineural invasion in cancer: a review of the literature. *Cancer.* 2009;115(15):3379-91.
133. Knudsen JB, et al. Venous and nerve invasion as prognostic factors in postoperative survival of patients with resectable cancer of the rectum. *Dis Colon Rectum.* 1983;26(9):613-7.
134. Shirouzu K, et al. Clinicopathologic study of perineural invasion in rectal cancer. *Kurume Med J.* 1992;39(1):41-9.
135. Ueno H, Hase K, Mochizuki H. Criteria for extramural perineural invasion as a prognostic factor in rectal cancer. *Br J Surg.* 2001;88(7):994-1000.
136. Shirouzu K, Isomoto H, Kakegawa T. Prognostic evaluation of perineural invasion in rectal cancer. *Am J Surg.* 1993;165(2):233-7.
137. Liebig C, et al. Perineural invasion is an independent predictor of outcome in colorectal cancer. *J Clin Oncol.* 2009;27(31):5131-7.
138. Poeschl EM, et al. Perineural invasion: correlation with aggressive phenotype and independent prognostic variable in both colon and rectum cancer. *J Clin Oncol.* 2010;28(21):e358-60. author reply e361-2.
139. Des Guetz G, et al. Microvessel density and VEGF expression are prognostic factors in colorectal cancer. Meta-analysis of the literature. *Br J Cancer.* 2006;94(12):1823-32.
140. Klintrup K, et al. Inflammation and prognosis in colorectal cancer. *Eur J Cancer.* 2005;41(17):2645-54.
141. Deans GT, et al. Jass' classification revisited. *J Am Coll Surg.* 1994;179(1):11-7.
142. de Bruine AP, et al. Endocrine cells in colorectal adenocarcinomas: incidence, hormone profile and prognostic relevance. *Int J Cancer.* 1993;54(5):765-71.
143. Grabowski P, et al. Neuroendocrine differentiation is a relevant prognostic factor in stage III-IV colorectal cancer. *Eur J Gastroenterol Hepatol.* 2001;13(4):405-11.
144. Ruschoff J, et al. Prognostic significance of nucleolar organizing regions (NORs) in carcinomas of the sigmoid colon and rectum. *Pathol Res Pract.* 1990;186(1):85-91.
145. Garrity MM, et al. Prognostic value of proliferation, apoptosis, defective DNA mismatch repair, and p53 overexpression in patients with resected Dukes' B2 or C colon cancer: a North Central Cancer Treatment Group Study. *J Clin Oncol.* 2004;22(9):1572-82.
146. Brown DC, Gatter KC. Ki67 protein: the immaculate deception? *Histopathology.* 2002;40(1):2-11.
147. Miyaki M, et al. Characteristics of somatic mutation of the adenomatous polyposis coli gene in colorectal tumors. *Cancer Res.* 1994;54(11):3011-20.
148. Levy DB, et al. Inactivation of both APC alleles in human and mouse tumors. *Cancer Res.* 1994;54(22):5953-8.
149. Powell SM, et al. APC mutations occur early during colorectal tumorigenesis. *Nature.* 1992;359(6392):235-7.
150. Miyoshi Y, et al. Somatic mutations of the APC gene in colorectal tumors: mutation cluster region in the APC gene. *Hum Mol Genet.* 1992;1(4):229-33.
151. Esteller M, et al. Analysis of adenomatous polyposis coli promoter hypermethylation in human cancer. *Cancer Res.* 2000;60(16):4366-71.
152. Rusan NM, Peifer M. Original CIN: reviewing roles for APC in chromosome instability. *J Cell Biol.* 2008;181(5):719-26.

153. Lovig T, et al. APC and CTNNB1 mutations in a large series of sporadic colorectal carcinomas stratified by the microsatellite instability status. *Scand J Gastroenterol*. 2002;37(10):1184-93.
154. Frattini M, et al. Different genetic features associated with colon and rectal carcinogenesis. *Clin Cancer Res*. 2004;10(12 Pt 1): 4015-21.
155. Kapiteijn E, et al. Mechanisms of oncogenesis in colon versus rectal cancer. *J Pathol*. 2001;195(2):171-8.
156. Jass JR, et al. APC mutation and tumour budding in colorectal cancer. *J Clin Pathol*. 2003;56(1):69-73.
157. Bondi J, et al. Expression of non-membranous beta-catenin and gamma-catenin, c-Myc and cyclin D1 in relation to patient outcome in human colon adenocarcinomas. *APMIS*. 2004;112(1):49-56.
158. Conlin A, et al. The prognostic significance of K-ras, p53, and APC mutations in colorectal carcinoma. *Gut*. 2005;54(9):1283-6.
159. Zauber NP, et al. Molecular genetic changes associated with colorectal carcinogenesis are not prognostic for tumor regression following preoperative chemoradiation of rectal carcinoma. *Int J Radiat Oncol Biol Phys*. 2009;74(2):472-6.
160. Iacopetta B. TP53 mutation in colorectal cancer. *Hum Mutat*. 2003;21(3):271-6.
161. Vogelstein B, et al. Genetic alterations during colorectal-tumor development. *N Engl J Med*. 1988;319(9):525-32.
162. Beroud C, Soussi T. The UMD-p53 database: new mutations and analysis tools. *Hum Mutat*. 2003;21(3):176-81.
163. Carson DA, Lois A. Cancer progression and p53. *Lancet*. 1995;346(8981):1009-11.
164. Efeyan A, Serrano M. p53: guardian of the genome and policeman of the oncogenes. *Cell Cycle*. 2007;6(9):1006-10.
165. Gervaz P, et al. Dukes B colorectal cancer: distinct genetic categories and clinical outcome based on proximal or distal tumor location. *Dis Colon Rectum*. 2001;44(3):364-72. discussion 372–3.
166. Russo A, et al. The TP53 colorectal cancer international collaborative study on the prognostic and predictive significance of p53 mutation: influence of tumor site, type of mutation, and adjuvant treatment. *J Clin Oncol*. 2005;23(30):7518-28.
167. Slattery ML, et al. A comparison of colon and rectal somatic DNA alterations. *Dis Colon Rectum*. 2009;52(7):1304-11.
168. Berardi R, et al. Locally advanced rectal cancer: from molecular profiling to clinical practice. A literature review: Part 2. *Expert Opin Pharmacother*. 2009;10(15):2467-78.
169. Kuremsky JG, Tepper JE, McLeod HL. Biomarkers for response to neoadjuvant chemoradiation for rectal cancer. *Int J Radiat Oncol Biol Phys*. 2009;74(3):673-88.
170. Makinen MJ. Colorectal serrated adenocarcinoma. *Histopathology*. 2007;50(1):131-50.
171. Samowitz WS, et al. Inverse relationship between microsatellite instability and K-ras and p53 gene alterations in colon cancer. *Am J Pathol*. 2001;158(4):1517-24.
172. Huerta S, Gao X, Saha D. Mechanisms of resistance to ionizing radiation in rectal cancer. *Expert Rev Mol Diagn*. 2009;9(5): 469-80.
173. Lievre A, Blons H, Laurent-Puig P. Oncogenic mutations as predictive factors in colorectal cancer. *Oncogene*. 2010;29(21): 3033-43.
174. Paez JG, et al. EGFR mutations in lung cancer: correlation with clinical response to gefitinib therapy. *Science*. 2004; 304(5676):1497-500.
175. Barber TD, et al. Somatic mutations of EGFR in colorectal cancers and glioblastomas. *N Engl J Med*. 2004;351(27):2883.
176. Sauer T, et al. Demonstration of EGFR gene copy loss in colorectal carcinomas by fluorescence in situ hybridization (FISH): a surrogate marker for sensitivity to specific anti-EGFR therapy? *Histopathology*. 2005;47(6):560-4.
177. Shia J, et al. Epidermal growth factor receptor expression and gene amplification in colorectal carcinoma: an immunohistochemical and chromogenic in situ hybridization study. *Mod Pathol*. 2005;18(10):1350-6.
178. Goldstein NS, Armin M. Epidermal growth factor receptor immunohistochemical reactivity in patients with American Joint Committee on Cancer Stage IV colon adenocarcinoma: implications for a standardized scoring system. *Cancer*. 2001;92(5): 1331-46.
179. Laurent-Puig P, et al. Analysis of PTEN, BRAF, and EGFR status in determining benefit from cetuximab therapy in wild-type KRAS metastatic colon cancer. *J Clin Oncol*. 2009;27(35):5924-30.
180. Italiano A, et al. Cetuximab shows activity in colorectal cancer patients with tumors for which FISH analysis does not detect an increase in EGFR gene copy number. *Ann Surg Oncol*. 2008;15(2):649-54.
181. Vallbohmer D, et al. Molecular determinants of cetuximab efficacy. *J Clin Oncol*. 2005;23(15):3536-44.
182. Kim JS, et al. Epidermal growth factor receptor as a predictor of tumor downstaging in locally advanced rectal cancer patients treated with preoperative chemoradiotherapy. *Int J Radiat Oncol Biol Phys*. 2006;66(1):195-200.
183. Li S, et al. Epidermal growth factor receptor as a prognostic factor in locally advanced rectal-cancer patients treated with preoperative chemoradiation. *Int J Radiat Oncol Biol Phys*. 2006;65(3): 705-12.
184. Giralt J, et al. The expression of epidermal growth factor receptor results in a worse prognosis for patients with rectal cancer treated with preoperative radiotherapy: a multicenter, retrospective analysis. *Radiother Oncol*. 2005;74(2):101-8.
185. Giralt J, et al. Epidermal growth factor receptor is a predictor of tumor response in locally advanced rectal cancer patients treated with preoperative radiotherapy. *Int J Radiat Oncol Biol Phys*. 2002;54(5):1460-5.
186. Azria D, et al. Prognostic impact of epidermal growth factor receptor (EGFR) expression on loco-regional recurrence after preoperative radiotherapy in rectal cancer. *BMC Cancer*. 2005;5:62.
187. Cunningham MP, et al. Coexpression of the IGF-IR, EGFR and HER-2 is common in colorectal cancer patients. *Int J Oncol*. 2006;28(2):329-35.
188. Toiyama Y, et al. Gene expression profiles of epidermal growth factor receptor, vascular endothelial growth factor and hypoxia-inducible factor-1 with special reference to local responsiveness to neoadjuvant chemoradiotherapy and disease recurrence after rectal cancer surgery. *Clin Oncol (R Coll Radiol)*. 2010;22(4): 272-80.
189. Yang D, et al. Gene expression levels of epidermal growth factor receptor, survivin, and vascular endothelial growth factor as molecular markers of lymph node involvement in patients with locally advanced rectal cancer. *Clin Colorectal Cancer*. 2006;6(4):305-11.
190. Takahari D, et al. Relationships of insulin-like growth factor-1 receptor and epidermal growth factor receptor expression to clinical outcomes in patients with colorectal cancer. *Oncology*. 2009;76(1):42-8.
191. Walther A, et al. Genetic prognostic and predictive markers in colorectal cancer. *Nat Rev Cancer*. 2009;9(7):489-99.
192. Worthley DL, et al. Colorectal carcinogenesis: road maps to cancer. *World J Gastroenterol*. 2007;13(28):3784-91.
193. Kalady MF, et al. Divergent oncogenic changes influence survival differences between colon and rectal adenocarcinomas. *Dis Colon Rectum*. 2009;52(6):1039-45.
194. Andreyev HJ, et al. Kirsten ras mutations in patients with colorectal cancer: the 'RASCAL II' study. *Br J Cancer*. 2001;85(5): 692-6.
195. Andreyev HJ, et al. Kirsten ras mutations in patients with colorectal cancer: the multicenter "RASCAL" study. *J Natl Cancer Inst*. 1998;90(9):675-84.

196. Fuchs C, et al. KRAS mutation, cancer recurrence, and patient survival in stage III colon cancer: Findings from CALGB 89803. In: 2009 ASCO Annual Meeting 2009. Orlando.
197. Ogino S, et al. KRAS mutation in stage III colon cancer and clinical outcome following intergroup trial CALGB 89803. *Clin Cancer Res*. 2009;15(23):7322-9.
198. Roth AD, et al. Prognostic role of KRAS and BRAF in stage II and III resected colon cancer: results of the translational study on the PETACC-3, EORTC 40993, SAKK 60–00 trial. *J Clin Oncol*. 2010;28(3):466-74.
199. Karapetis CS, et al. K-ras mutations and benefit from cetuximab in advanced colorectal cancer. *N Engl J Med*. 2008;359(17):1757-65.
200. Bardelli A, Siena S. Molecular mechanisms of resistance to cetuximab and panitumumab in colorectal cancer. *J Clin Oncol*. 2010;28(7):1254-61.
201. Sartore-Bianchi A, et al. Integrated molecular dissection of the epidermal growth factor receptor (EFGR) oncogenic pathway to predict response to EGFR-targeted monoclonal antibodies in metastatic colorectal cancer. *Target Oncol*. 2010;5(1):19-28.
202. Amado RG, et al. Wild-type KRAS is required for panitumumab efficacy in patients with metastatic colorectal cancer. *J Clin Oncol*. 2008;26(10):1626-34.
203. Lievre A, et al. KRAS mutations as an independent prognostic factor in patients with advanced colorectal cancer treated with cetuximab. *J Clin Oncol*. 2008;26(3):374-9.
204. Van Cutsem E, et al. Cetuximab and chemotherapy as initial treatment for metastatic colorectal cancer. *N Engl J Med*. 2009;360(14):1408-17.
205. Van Cutsem E, et al. (2008) KRAS status and efficacy in the first-line treatment of patients with metastatic colorectal cancer (mCRC) treated with FOLFIRI with or without cetuximab: The CRYSTAL experience. in: ASCO 2008 Annual Meeting,2009: J Clin Oncol 26: 2008 (May 20 suppl; abstr 2).
206. Bokemeyer C, et al. Fluorouracil, leucovorin, and oxaliplatin with and without cetuximab in the first-line treatment of metastatic colorectal cancer. *J Clin Oncol*. 2009;27(5):663-71.
207. Jonker DJ, et al. Cetuximab for the treatment of colorectal cancer. *N Engl J Med*. 2007;357(20):2040-8.
208. Allegra CJ, et al. American Society of Clinical Oncology provisional clinical opinion: testing for KRAS gene mutations in patients with metastatic colorectal carcinoma to predict response to anti-epidermal growth factor receptor monoclonal antibody therapy. *J Clin Oncol*. 2009;27(12):2091-6.
209. Rajagopalan H, et al. Tumorigenesis: RAF/RAS oncogenes and mismatch-repair status. *Nature*. 2002;418(6901):934.
210. Domingo E, et al. BRAF-V600E is not involved in the colorectal tumorigenesis of HNPCC in patients with functional MLH1 and MSH2 genes. *Oncogene*. 2005;24(24):3995-8.
211. Di Nicolantonio F, et al. Wild-type BRAF is required for response to panitumumab or cetuximab in metastatic colorectal cancer. *J Clin Oncol*. 2008;26(35):5705-12.
212. French AJ, et al. Prognostic significance of defective mismatch repair and BRAF V600E in patients with colon cancer. *Clin Cancer Res*. 2008;14(11):3408-15.
213. Zlobec I, et al. Clinicopathological and protein characterization of BRAF- and K-RAS-mutated colorectal cancer and implications for prognosis. *Int J Cancer*. 2010;127(2):367-80.
214. Tol J, et al. Chemotherapy, bevacizumab, and cetuximab in metastatic colorectal cancer. *N Engl J Med*. 2009;360(6):563-72.
215. Tol J, Nagtegaal ID, Punt CJ. BRAF mutation in metastatic colorectal cancer. *N Engl J Med*. 2009;361(1):98-9.
216. Benvenuti S, et al. PIK3CA cancer mutations display gender and tissue specificity patterns. *Hum Mutat*. 2008;29(2):284-8.
217. Frattini M, et al. PTEN loss of expression predicts cetuximab efficacy in metastatic colorectal cancer patients. *Br J Cancer*. 2007;97(8):1139-45.
218. Jhawer M, et al. PIK3CA mutation/PTEN expression status predicts response of colon cancer cells to the epidermal growth factor receptor inhibitor cetuximab. *Cancer Res*. 2008;68(6):1953-61.
219. Prenen H, et al. PIK3CA mutations are not a major determinant of resistance to the epidermal growth factor receptor inhibitor cetuximab in metastatic colorectal cancer. *Clin Cancer Res*. 2009;15(9):3184-8.
220. Sartore-Bianchi A, et al. PIK3CA mutations in colorectal cancer are associated with clinical resistance to EGFR-targeted monoclonal antibodies. *Cancer Res*. 2009;69(5):1851-7.
221. Perrone F, et al. PI3KCA/PTEN deregulation contributes to impaired responses to cetuximab in metastatic colorectal cancer patients. *Ann Oncol*. 2009;20(1):84-90.
222. He Y, et al. PIK3CA mutations predict local recurrences in rectal cancer patients. *Clin Cancer Res*. 2009;15(22):6956-62.
223. Ogino S, et al. PIK3CA mutation is associated with poor prognosis among patients with curatively resected colon cancer. *J Clin Oncol*. 2009;27(9):1477-84.
224. Carmeliet P, Collen D. Molecular basis of angiogenesis. Role of VEGF and VE-cadherin. *Ann N Y Acad Sci*. 2000;902:249-62. discussion 262–4.
225. Carmeliet P, Jain RK. Angiogenesis in cancer and other diseases. *Nature*. 2000;407(6801):249-57.
226. Folkman J. Tumor angiogenesis: therapeutic implications. *N Engl J Med*. 1971;285(21):1182-6.
227. Folkman J. What is the evidence that tumors are angiogenesis dependent? *J Natl Cancer Inst*. 1990;82(1):4-6.
228. Li C, et al. Both high intratumoral microvessel density determined using CD105 antibody and elevated plasma levels of CD105 in colorectal cancer patients correlate with poor prognosis. *Br J Cancer*. 2003;88(9):1424-31.
229. Winder T, Lenz HJ. Vascular endothelial growth factor and epidermal growth factor signaling pathways as therapeutic targets for colorectal cancer. *Gastroenterology*. 2010;138(6):2163-76.
230. Giralt J, et al. Prognostic significance of vascular endothelial growth factor and cyclooxygenase-2 in patients with rectal cancer treated with preoperative radiotherapy. *Oncology*. 2006;71 (5–6):312-9.
231. Nozue M, Isaka N, Fukao K. Over-expression of vascular endothelial growth factor after preoperative radiation therapy for rectal cancer. *Oncol Rep*. 2001;8(6):1247-9.
232. Noda E, et al. Predictive value of vascular endothelial growth factor-C expression for local recurrence of rectal carcinoma. *Oncol Rep*. 2007;17(6):1327-31.
233. Svagzdys S, et al. Microvessel density as new prognostic marker after radiotherapy in rectal cancer. *BMC Cancer*. 2009;9:95.
234. Zlobec I, Steele R, Compton CC. VEGF as a predictive marker of rectal tumor response to preoperative radiotherapy. *Cancer*. 2005;104(11):2517-21.
235. Zlobec I, et al. Combined analysis of VEGF and EGFR predicts complete tumour response in rectal cancer treated with preoperative radiotherapy. *Br J Cancer*. 2008;98(2):450-6.
236. Negri FV, et al. Biological predictive factors in rectal cancer treated with preoperative radiotherapy or radiochemotherapy. *Br J Cancer*. 2008;98(1):143-7.
237. Qiu H, et al. Molecular prognostic factors in rectal cancer treated by radiation and surgery. *Dis Colon Rectum*. 2000;43(4):451-9.
238. Hurwitz H, et al. Bevacizumab plus irinotecan, fluorouracil, and leucovorin for metastatic colorectal cancer. *N Engl J Med*. 2004;350(23):2335-42.
239. Czito BG, et al. Bevacizumab, oxaliplatin, and capecitabine with radiation therapy in rectal cancer: Phase I trial results. *Int J Radiat Oncol Biol Phys*. 2007;68(2):472-8.
240. Willett CG, et al. Efficacy, safety, and biomarkers of neoadjuvant bevacizumab, radiation therapy, and fluorouracil in rectal cancer: a multidisciplinary phase II study. *J Clin Oncol*. 2009;27(18): 3020-6.

241. Lenz HJ, et al. p53 and thymidylate synthase expression in untreated stage II colon cancer: associations with recurrence, survival, and site. *Clin Cancer Res.* 1998;4(5):1227-34.
242. Salonga D, et al. Colorectal tumors responding to 5-fluorouracil have low gene expression levels of dihydropyrimidine dehydrogenase, thymidylate synthase, and thymidine phosphorylase. *Clin Cancer Res.* 2000;6(4):1322-7.
243. Popat S, Matakidou A, Houlston RS. Thymidylate synthase expression and prognosis in colorectal cancer: a systematic review and meta-analysis. *J Clin Oncol.* 2004;22(3):529-36.
244. Yamada H, Iinuma H, Watanabe T. Prognostic value of 5-fluorouracil metabolic enzyme genes in Dukes' stage B and C colorectal cancer patients treated with oral 5-fluorouracil-based adjuvant chemotherapy. *Oncol Rep.* 2008;19(3):729-35.
245. Liersch T, et al. Lymph node status and TS gene expression are prognostic markers in stage II/III rectal cancer after neoadjuvant fluorouracil-based chemoradiotherapy. *J Clin Oncol.* 2006;24(25):4062-8.
246. Jakob C, et al. Prognostic value of histologic tumor regression, thymidylate synthase, thymidine phosphorylase, and dihydropyrimidine dehydrogenase in rectal cancer UICC Stage II/III after neoadjuvant chemoradiotherapy. *Am J Surg Pathol.* 2006;30(9):1169-74.
247. Bertolini F, et al. Prognostic and predictive value of baseline and posttreatment molecular marker expression in locally advanced rectal cancer treated with neoadjuvant chemoradiotherapy. *Int J Radiat Oncol Biol Phys.* 2007;68(5):1455-61.
248. Wang Y, et al. Gene expression profiles and molecular markers to predict recurrence of Dukes' B colon cancer. *J Clin Oncol.* 2004;22(9):1564-71.
249. Mariadason JM, et al. Gene expression profiling-based prediction of response of colon carcinoma cells to 5-fluorouracil and camptothecin. *Cancer Res.* 2003;63(24):8791-812.
250. Ghadimi BM, et al. Effectiveness of gene expression profiling for response prediction of rectal adenocarcinomas to preoperative chemoradiotherapy. *J Clin Oncol.* 2005;23(9):1826-38.
251. Kim IJ, et al. Microarray gene expression profiling for predicting complete response to preoperative chemoradiotherapy in patients with advanced rectal cancer. *Dis Colon Rectum.* 2007;50(9):1342-53.
252. Rimkus C, et al. Microarray-based prediction of tumor response to neoadjuvant radiochemotherapy of patients with locally advanced rectal cancer. *Clin Gastroenterol Hepatol.* 2008;6(1):53-61.
253. Johnson LG, et al. Anal cancer incidence and survival: the surveillance, epidemiology, and end results experience, 1973–2000. *Cancer.* 2004;101(2):281-8.
254. Chiao EY, et al. A population-based analysis of temporal trends in the incidence of squamous anal canal cancer in relation to the HIV epidemic. *J Acquir Immune Defic Syndr.* 2005;40(4):451-5.
255. Frisch M, Melbye M, Moller H. Trends in incidence of anal cancer in Denmark. *BMJ.* 1993;306(6875):419-22.
256. Brewster DH, Bhatti LA. Increasing incidence of squamous cell carcinoma of the anus in Scotland, 1975–2002. *Br J Cancer.* 2006;95(1):87-90.
257. Welton ML, Sharkey FE, Kahlenberg MS. The etiology and epidemiology of anal cancer. *Surg Oncol Clin N Am.* 2004;13(2):263-75.
258. Frisch M, et al. Sexually transmitted infection as a cause of anal cancer. *N Engl J Med.* 1997;337(19):1350-8.
259. Daling JR, et al. Sexual practices, sexually transmitted diseases, and the incidence of anal cancer. *N Engl J Med.* 1987;317(16):973-7.
260. Palefsky JM. Anal human papillomavirus infection and anal cancer in HIV-positive individuals: an emerging problem. *AIDS.* 1994;8(3):283-95.
261. Palefsky JM, Shiboski S, Moss A. Risk factors for anal human papillomavirus infection and anal cytologic abnormalities in HIV-positive and HIV-negative homosexual men. *J Acquir Immune Defic Syndr.* 1994;7(6):599-606.
262. Williams AB, et al. Anal and cervical human papillomavirus infection and risk of anal and cervical epithelial abnormalities in human immunodeficiency virus-infected women. *Obstet Gynecol.* 1994;83(2):205-11.
263. Melbye M, Sprogel P. Aetiological parallel between anal cancer and cervical cancer. *Lancet.* 1991;338(8768):657-9.
264. Zbar AP, et al. The pathology and molecular biology of anal intraepithelial neoplasia: comparisons with cervical and vulvar intraepithelial carcinoma. *Int J Colorectal Dis.* 2002;17(4):203-15.
265. Arends MJ, et al. Renal allograft recipients with high susceptibility to cutaneous malignancy have an increased prevalence of human papillomavirus DNA in skin tumours and a greater risk of anogenital malignancy. *Br J Cancer.* 1997;75(5):722-8.
266. Holmes F, et al. Anal cancer in women. *Gastroenterology.* 1988;95(1):107-11.
267. Penn I. Cancers of the anogenital region in renal transplant recipients. Analysis of 65 cases. *Cancer.* 1986;58(3):611-6.
268. Edge S, et al. AJCC Cancer Staging Manual, 7th Edition. 2010.
269. Martin FT, Kavanagh D, Waldron R. Squamous cell carcinoma of the anal canal. *Surgeon.* 2009;7(4):232-7.
270. Garrett K, Kalady MF. Anal neoplasms. *Surg Clin North Am.* 2010;90(1):147-61. Table of Contents.
271. Insinga RP, Dasbach EJ, Elbasha EH. Epidemiologic natural history and clinical management of Human Papillomavirus (HPV) Disease: a critical and systematic review of the literature in the development of an HPV dynamic transmission model. *BMC Infect Dis.* 2009;9:119.
272. Chin-Hong PV, et al. Anal human papillomavirus infection is associated with HIV acquisition in men who have sex with men. *AIDS.* 2009;23(9):1135-42.
273. Palefsky J. Human papillomavirus-related disease in people with HIV. *Curr Opin HIV AIDS.* 2009;4(1):52-6.
274. Grinsztejn B, et al. Factors associated with increased prevalence of human papillomavirus infection in a cohort of HIV-infected Brazilian women. *Int J Infect Dis.* 2009;13(1):72-80.
275. Palefsky J. Human papillomavirus and anal neoplasia. *Curr HIV/AIDS Rep.* 2008;5(2):78-85.
276. Daling JR, et al. Human papillomavirus, smoking, and sexual practices in the etiology of anal cancer. *Cancer.* 2004;101(2):270-80.
277. Da Costa MM, et al. Increased risk of high-grade anal neoplasia associated with a human papillomavirus type 16 E6 sequence variant. *J Infect Dis.* 2002;185(9):1229-37.
278. Scheffner M, et al. The E6 oncoprotein encoded by human papillomavirus types 16 and 18 promotes the degradation of p53. *Cell.* 1990;63(6):1129-36.
279. Werness BA, Levine AJ, Howley PM. Association of human papillomavirus types 16 and 18 E6 proteins with p53. *Science.* 1990;248(4951):76-9.
280. Lee JH, et al. p53 gene mutation is rare in human cervical carcinomas with positive HPV sequences. *Int J Gynecol Cancer.* 1994;4(6):371-378.
281. Gervaz P, Hirschel B, Morel P. Molecular biology of squamous cell carcinoma of the anus. *Br J Surg.* 2006;93(5):531-8.
282. Munger K, et al. Complex formation of human papillomavirus E7 proteins with the retinoblastoma tumor suppressor gene product. *EMBO J.* 1989;8(13):4099-105.
283. Dyson N, et al. The human papilloma virus-16 E7 oncoprotein is able to bind to the retinoblastoma gene product. *Science.* 1989;243(4893):934-7.
284. Heck DV, et al. Efficiency of binding the retinoblastoma protein correlates with the transforming capacity of the E7 oncoproteins of the human papillomaviruses. *Proc Natl Acad Sci USA.* 1992;89(10):4442-6.

285. Moody CA, Laimins LA. Human papillomavirus oncoproteins: pathways to transformation. *Nat Rev Cancer*. 2010;10(8):550-60.
286. Durst M, et al. The physical state of human papillomavirus type 16 DNA in benign and malignant genital tumours. *J Gen Virol*. 1985;66(Pt 7):1515-22.
287. Peter M, et al. Frequent genomic structural alterations at HPV insertion sites in cervical carcinoma. *J Pathol*. 2010;221(3): 320-30.
288. Wentzensen N, Vinokurova S, von Knebel Doeberitz M. Systematic review of genomic integration sites of human papillomavirus genomes in epithelial dysplasia and invasive cancer of the female lower genital tract. *Cancer Res*. 2004;64(11):3878-84.
289. Wilke CM, et al. FRA3B extends over a broad region and contains a spontaneous HPV16 integration site: direct evidence for the coincidence of viral integration sites and fragile sites. *Hum Mol Genet*. 1996;5(2):187-95.
290. Muller CY, et al. Abnormalities of fragile histidine triad genomic and complementary DNAs in cervical cancer: association with human papillomavirus type. *J Natl Cancer Inst*. 1998;90(6):433-9.
291. Peter M, et al. MYC activation associated with the integration of HPV DNA at the MYC locus in genital tumors. *Oncogene*. 2006;25(44):5985-93.
292. Duensing S, et al. Human papillomavirus type 16 E7 oncoprotein-induced abnormal centrosome synthesis is an early event in the evolving malignant phenotype. *Cancer Res*. 2001;61(6):2356-60.
293. Muleris M, et al. Recurrent deletions of chromosomes 11q and 3p in anal canal carcinoma. *Int J Cancer*. 1987;39(5):595-8.
294. Heselmeyer K, et al. A recurrent pattern of chromosomal aberrations and immunophenotypic appearance defines anal squamous cell carcinomas. *Br J Cancer*. 1997;76(10):1271-8.
295. Gervaz P, et al. Molecular biology of squamous cell carcinoma of the anus: a comparison of HIV-positive and HIV-negative patients. *J Gastrointest Surg*. 2004;8(8):1024-30. discussion 1031.
296. Bethwaite PB, et al. Loss of heterozygosity occurs at the D11S29 locus on chromosome 11q23 in invasive cervical carcinoma. *Br J Cancer*. 1995;71(4):814-8.
297. Hampton GM, et al. Loss of heterozygosity in cervical carcinoma: subchromosomal localization of a putative tumor-suppressor gene to chromosome 11q22-q24. *Proc Natl Acad Sci USA*. 1994;91(15):6953-7.
298. Thompson DA, et al. The human papillomavirus-16 E6 oncoprotein decreases the vigilance of mitotic checkpoints. *Oncogene*. 1997;15(25):3025-35.
299. Thomas JT, Laimins LA. Human papillomavirus oncoproteins E6 and E7 independently abrogate the mitotic spindle checkpoint. *J Virol*. 1998;72(2):1131-7.
300. Duensing A, et al. Analysis of centrosome overduplication in correlation to cell division errors in high-risk human papillomavirus (HPV)-associated anal neoplasms. *Virology*. 2008;372(1):157-64.
301. Patel D, et al. Human papillomavirus type 16 E6 and E7 cause polyploidy in human keratinocytes and up-regulation of G2-M-phase proteins. *Cancer Res*. 2004;64(4):1299-306.
302. Finzer P, Aguilar-Lemarroy A, Rosl F. The role of human papillomavirus oncoproteins E6 and E7 in apoptosis. *Cancer Lett*. 2002;188(1–2):15-24.
303. Melbye M, et al. High incidence of anal cancer among AIDS patients. The AIDS/Cancer Working Group. *Lancet*. 1994;343(8898):636-9.
304. Diamond C, et al. Increased incidence of squamous cell anal cancer among men with AIDS in the era of highly active antiretroviral therapy. *Sex Transm Dis*. 2005;32(5):314-20.
305. Piketty C, et al. Marked increase in the incidence of invasive anal cancer among HIV-infected patients despite treatment with combination antiretroviral therapy. *AIDS*. 2008;22(10):1203-11.
306. Palefsky JM, et al. High incidence of anal high-grade squamous intra-epithelial lesions among HIV-positive and HIV-negative homosexual and bisexual men. *AIDS*. 1998;12(5):495-503.
307. Critchlow CW, et al. Effect of HIV infection on the natural history of anal human papillomavirus infection. *AIDS*. 1998;12(10): 1177-84.
308. Nagle D. Anal squamous cell carcinoma in the HIV-positive patient. *Clin Colon Rectal Surg*. 2009;22(2):102-6.
309. Palefsky JM. Anal cancer prevention in HIV-positive men and women. *Curr Opin Oncol*. 2009;21(5):433-8.
310. Palefsky JM, et al. Anal squamous intraepithelial lesions in HIV-positive and HIV-negative homosexual and bisexual men: prevalence and risk factors. *J Acquir Immune Defic Syndr Hum Retrovirol*. 1998;17(4):320-6.
311. Palefsky JM, et al. Anal intraepithelial neoplasia and anal papillomavirus infection among homosexual males with group IV HIV disease. *JAMA*. 1990;263(21):2911-6.
312. Goedert JJ, et al. Spectrum of AIDS-associated malignant disorders. *Lancet*. 1998;351(9119):1833-9.
313. Maggard MA, Beanes SR, Ko CY. Anal canal cancer: a population-based reappraisal. *Dis Colon Rectum*. 2003;46(11):1517-23. discussion 1523–4; author reply 1524.
314. Jong E, et al. Effect of HIV viral load, CD4 cell count and antiretroviral therapy on human papillomavirus prevalence in urine samples of HIV-infected men. *Int J STD AIDS*. 2009;20(4):262-4.
315. Palefsky JM, et al. Virologic, immunologic, and clinical parameters in the incidence and progression of anal squamous intraepithelial lesions in HIV-positive and HIV-negative homosexual men. *J Acquir Immune Defic Syndr Hum Retrovirol*. 1998;17(4):314-9.
316. Wistuba II, et al. Comparison of molecular changes in lung cancers in HIV-positive and HIV-indeterminate subjects. *JAMA*. 1998;279(19):1554-9.
317. Wistuba II, et al. Comparison of molecular changes in cervical intraepithelial neoplasia in HIV-positive and HIV-indeterminate subjects. *Gynecol Oncol*. 1999;74(3):519-26.
318. Bedi GC, et al. Microsatellite instability in primary neoplasms from HIV + patients. *Nat Med*. 1995;1(1):65-8.
319. Duval A, et al. The mutator pathway is a feature of immunodeficiency-related lymphomas. *Proc Natl Acad Sci USA*. 2004;101(14):5002-7.
320. Le LH, Chetty R, Moore MJ. Epidermal growth factor receptor expression in anal canal carcinoma. *Am J Clin Pathol*. 2005;124(1):20-3.
321. Van Damme N, et al. EGFR and K-RAS gene status evaluation in anal canal squamous cell carcinoma, in 2008 ASCO Annual Meeting. 2008, J Clin Oncol 26: 2008 (May 20 suppl; abstr 15569).
322. Lukan N, et al. Cetuximab-based treatment of metastatic anal cancer: correlation of response with KRAS mutational status. *Oncology*. 2009;77(5):293-9.
323. Ajani JA, et al. Molecular biomarkers correlate with disease-free survival in patients with anal canal carcinoma treated with chemoradiation. *Dig Dis Sci*. 2010;55(4):1098-105.
324. Klas JV, et al. Malignant tumors of the anal canal: the spectrum of disease, treatment, and outcomes. *Cancer*. 1999;85(8):1686-93.
325. Wanebo HJ, et al. Anorectal melanoma. *Cancer*. 1981;47(7): 1891-900.
326. Iversen K, Robins RE. Mucosal malignant melanomas. *Am J Surg*. 1980;139(5):660-4.
327. Row D, Weiser MR. Anorectal melanoma. *Clin Colon Rectal Surg*. 2009;22(2):120-6.
328. McLaughlin CC, et al. Incidence of noncutaneous melanomas in the U.S. *Cancer*. 2005;103(5):1000-7.
329. Cagir B, et al. Changing epidemiology of anorectal melanoma. *Dis Colon Rectum*. 1999;42(9):1203-8.

330. Smalley KS, Sondak VK, Weber JS. c-KIT signaling as the driving oncogenic event in sub-groups of melanomas. *Histol Histopathol*. 2009;24(5):643-50.
331. Curtin JA, et al. Somatic activation of KIT in distinct subtypes of melanoma. *J Clin Oncol*. 2006;24(26):4340-6.
332. Satzger I, et al. Analysis of c-KIT expression and KIT gene mutation in human mucosal melanomas. *Br J Cancer*. 2008;99(12):2065-9.
333. Went PT, et al. Prevalence of KIT expression in human tumors. *J Clin Oncol*. 2004;22(22):4514-22.
334. Willmore-Payne C, et al. Human malignant melanoma: detection of BRAF- and c-kit-activating mutations by high-resolution amplicon melting analysis. *Hum Pathol*. 2005;36(5):486-93.
335. Omholt K, et al. NRAS and BRAF mutations arise early during melanoma pathogenesis and are preserved throughout tumor progression. *Clin Cancer Res*. 2003;9(17):6483-8.
336. Antonescu CR, et al. L576P KIT mutation in anal melanomas correlates with KIT protein expression and is sensitive to specific kinase inhibition. *Int J Cancer*. 2007;121(2):257-64.
337. Kim KB, et al. Phase II trial of imatinib mesylate in patients with metastatic melanoma. *Br J Cancer*. 2008;99(5):734-40.
338. Ugurel S, et al. Lack of clinical efficacy of imatinib in metastatic melanoma. *Br J Cancer*. 2005;92(8):1398-405.
339. Satzger I, et al. Anal mucosal melanoma with KIT-activating mutation and response to imatinib therapy–case report and review of the literature. *Dermatology*. 2010;220(1):77-81.
340. Alexis JB, Martinez AE, Lutzky J. An immunohistochemical evaluation of c-kit (CD-117) expression in malignant melanoma, and results of imatinib mesylate (Gleevec) therapy in three patients. *Melanoma Res*. 2005;15(4):283-5.
341. Carvajal RD, et al. A phase II study of flavopiridol (Alvocidib) in combination with docetaxel in refractory, metastatic pancreatic cancer. *Pancreatology*. 2009;9(4):404-9.
342. Su DM, et al. Two types of human malignant melanoma cell lines revealed by expression patterns of mitochondrial and survival-apoptosis genes: implications for malignant melanoma therapy. *Mol Cancer Ther*. 2009;8:1292-304.
343. Woodman SE, et al. Activity of dasatinib against L576P KIT mutant melanoma: molecular, cellular, and clinical correlates. *Mol Cancer Ther*. 2009;8(8):2079-85.
344. Quintas-Cardama A, et al. Complete response of stage IV anal mucosal melanoma expressing KIT Val560Asp to the multikinase inhibitor sorafenib. *Nat Clin Pract Oncol*. 2008;5(12):737-40.
345. Madeleine M, Newcomer LM. Cancers of the anus. In: Madeleine M, Newcomer LM, eds. *National Cancer Institute's Surveillance, Epidemiology, and End Results Program (SEER)*. Bethesda, MD: National Cancer Institute; 2007.
346. DeMatteo RP, et al. Two hundred gastrointestinal stromal tumors: recurrence patterns and prognostic factors for survival. *Ann Surg*. 2000;231(1):51-8.
347. Miettinen M, et al. Gastrointestinal stromal tumors, intramural leiomyomas, and leiomyosarcomas in the rectum and anus: a clinicopathologic, immunohistochemical, and molecular genetic study of 144 cases. *Am J Surg Pathol*. 2001;25(9):1121-33.
348. Miettinen M, Lasota J. Gastrointestinal stromal tumors: pathology and prognosis at different sites. *Semin Diagn Pathol*. 2006;23(2): 70-83.
349. Peralta EA. Rare anorectal neoplasms: gastrointestinal stromal tumor, carcinoid, and lymphoma. *Clin Colon Rectal Surg*. 2009;22(2):107-14.
350. Heinrich MC, et al. Kinase mutations and imatinib response in patients with metastatic gastrointestinal stromal tumor. *J Clin Oncol*. 2003;21(23):4342-9.
351. Joensuu H, et al. Effect of the tyrosine kinase inhibitor STI571 in a patient with a metastatic gastrointestinal stromal tumor. *N Engl J Med*. 2001;344(14):1052-6.
352. Demetri GD, et al. Efficacy and safety of imatinib mesylate in advanced gastrointestinal stromal tumors. *N Engl J Med*. 2002;347(7):472-80.
353. Blanke CD, et al. Phase III randomized, intergroup trial assessing imatinib mesylate at two dose levels in patients with unresectable or metastatic gastrointestinal stromal tumors expressing the kit receptor tyrosine kinase: S0033. *J Clin Oncol*. 2008;26(4): 626-32.
354. Blanke CD, et al. Long-term results from a randomized phase II trial of standard- versus higher-dose imatinib mesylate for patients with unresectable or metastatic gastrointestinal stromal tumors expressing KIT. *J Clin Oncol*. 2008;26(4):620-5.
355. Heinrich MC, et al. Correlation of kinase genotype and clinical outcome in the North American Intergroup Phase III Trial of imatinib mesylate for treatment of advanced gastrointestinal stromal tumor: CALGB 150105 Study by Cancer and Leukemia Group B and Southwest Oncology Group. *J Clin Oncol*. 2008;26(33):5360-7.
356. Van Glabbeke MM, et al. Comparison of two doses of imatinib for the treatment of unresectable or metastatic gastrointestinal stromal tumors (GIST): A meta-analyis based on 1,640 patients (pts), in 2007 ASCO Annual Meeting. 2007.
357. Debiec-Rychter M, et al. KIT mutations and dose selection for imatinib in patients with advanced gastrointestinal stromal tumours. *Eur J Cancer*. 2006;42(8):1093-103.
358. Corless CL, et al. PDGFRA mutations in gastrointestinal stromal tumors: frequency, spectrum and in vitro sensitivity to imatinib. *J Clin Oncol*. 2005;23(23):5357-64.
359. Medeiros F, et al. KIT-negative gastrointestinal stromal tumors: proof of concept and therapeutic implications. *Am J Surg Pathol*. 2004;28(7):889-94.
360. Dematteo RP, et al. Adjuvant imatinib mesylate after resection of localised, primary gastrointestinal stromal tumour: a randomised, double-blind, placebo-controlled trial. *Lancet*. 2009;373(9669): 1097-104.
361. Lang I, et al. Case 3. Resection of originally inoperable liver metastases of gastrointestinal stromal tumor after imatinib mesylate therapy. *J Clin Oncol*. 2003;21(18):3538-40.
362. Andtbacka RH, et al. Surgical resection of gastrointestinal stromal tumors after treatment with imatinib. *Ann Surg Oncol*. 2007;14(1):14-24.
363. Eisenberg BL, et al. Phase II trial of neoadjuvant/adjuvant imatinib mesylate (IM) for advanced primary and metastatic/recurrent operable gastrointestinal stromal tumor (GIST): early results of RTOG 0132/ACRIN 6665. *J Surg Oncol*. 2009;99(1):42-7.
364. Hou YY, et al. Imatinib mesylate neoadjuvant treatment for rectal malignant gastrointestinal stromal tumor. *World J Gastroenterol*. 2009;15(15):1910-3.
365. Lo SS, et al. Neoadjuvant imatinib in gastrointestinal stromal tumor of the rectum: report of a case. *Dis Colon Rectum*. 2005;48(6):1316-9.
366. Caldarola VT, et al. Carcinoid Tumors of the Rectum. *Am J Surg*. 1964;107:844-9.
367. Soga J. Early-stage carcinoids of the gastrointestinal tract: an analysis of 1914 reported cases. *Cancer*. 2005;103(8):1587-95.
368. Orloff MJ. Carcinoid tumors of the rectum. *Cancer*. 1971;28(1):175-80.
369. Koura AN, et al. Carcinoid tumors of the rectum: effect of size, histopathology, and surgical treatment on metastasis free survival. *Cancer*. 1997;79(7):1294-8.
370. Pinchot SN, et al. Carcinoid tumors. *Oncologist*. 2008;13(12): 1255-69.
371. Jetmore AB, et al. Rectal carcinoids: the most frequent carcinoid tumor. *Dis Colon Rectum*. 1992;35(8):717-25.
372. Mani S, et al. Carcinoids of the rectum. *J Am Coll Surg*. 1994;179(2):231-48.

373. Modlin IM, Lye KD, Kidd M. A 5-decade analysis of 13,715 carcinoid tumors. *Cancer*. 2003;97(4):934-59.
374. Sauven P, et al. Anorectal carcinoid tumors. Is aggressive surgery warranted? *Ann Surg*. 1990;211(1):67-71.
375. Naunheim KS, et al. Rectal carcinoid tumors–treatment and prognosis. *Surgery*. 1983;94(4):670-6.
376. Landry CS, et al. A proposed staging system for rectal carcinoid tumors based on an analysis of 4701 patients. *Surgery*. 2008; 144(3):460-6.
377. Shepherd NA, et al. Primary malignant lymphoma of the colon and rectum. A histopathological and immunohistochemical analysis of 45 cases with clinicopathological correlations. *Histopathology*. 1988;12(3):235-52.
378. Hatch KF, et al. Tumors of the rectum and anal canal. *World J Surg*. 2000;24(4):437-43.
379. Bartolo D, Goepel JR, Parsons MA. Rectal malignant lymphoma in chronic ulcerative colitis. *Gut*. 1982;23(2):164-8.
380. Fan CW, et al. Perforated rectal lymphoma in a renal transplant recipient: report of a case. *Dis Colon Rectum*. 1997;40(10):1258-60.
381. Bilsel Y, et al. Clinical and therapeutic considerations of rectal lymphoma: a case report and literature review. *World J Gastroenterol*. 2005;11(3):460-1.

Molecular Pathology of Inflammatory Bowel Disease-Associated Neoplasia

10

Takeshi Uehara, Deqin Ma, and Antonia R. Sepulveda

Introduction

Inflammatory bowel diseases (IBD) are chronic diseases presenting clinically as ulcerative colitis or Crohn's disease and affecting approximately 1.4 million US patients. While ulcerative colitis is limited to the colon, Crohn's disease often affects multiple segments of the gastrointestinal (GI) tract, including the small intestine (enteritis) and colon (colitis), and may involve the upper GI tract, primarily manifesting as chronic gastritis.

A major concern of these patients is their greatly enhanced risk of developing colorectal cancer (CRC) as compared to patients without colitis. CRC in IBD patients develops in the background colon affected by chronic injury to the epithelial lining in a stepwise cascade of alterations that include a large background field of colitis characterized by variable grades of mucosal inflammation and epithelial injury, development of dysplastic lesions that include flat or polypoid lesions, and finally cancer (adenocarcinoma). Patients with IBD sequentially develop foci of low-grade dysplasia (LGD), which may progress to high-grade dysplasia (HGD), and ultimately invasive adenocarcinoma (Fig. 10.1). The risk of colon cancer for patients with IBD was reported to increase by 0.5–1.0% every year after 8–10 years of diagnosis.[1] The incidence of CRC in IBD is 20-fold higher and is detected on average in patients 20 years younger than those with CRC in the non-IBD population.[2,3] Current guidelines recommend colonoscopic surveillance with random biopsies every 1–2 years after 8–10 years of pancolitis.[4,5] Most studies of neoplasia in IBD have been conducted in patients with ulcerative colitis (UC). Therefore, this chapter will primarily describe the molecular features of ulcerative colitis-associated neoplasia. It is likely that most of these alterations are similar in Crohn's disease-associated cancers, but the data are more limited in this patient population.

T. Uehara, M.D.
Department of Laboratory Medicine, Shinshu University School of Medicine, Matsumoto, Japan
e-mail: uehara@med.u-toyama.ac.jp

D. Ma, M.D., Ph.D.
Department of Pathology, University of Iowa Hospitals and Clinics, 200 Hawkins Drive BT6008GH, Iowa City, 52242 IA, USA

A.R. Sepulveda, M.D., Ph.D. (✉)
Department of Pathology & Cell Biology, Columbia University, 630 W 168th Street, VC-14 RM 212, New York, NY 10032, USA
e-mail: as4400@columbia.edu

Molecular Mechanisms Underlying Dysplasia and Cancer in IBD-Associated Colitis

Genomic Alterations and Mutagenesis

Numerous genetic and epigenetic abnormalities accumulate during colitis and are critical for progression to neoplasia (dysplasia and cancer) lesions in IBD. The molecular alterations of IBD-associated carcinogenesis are generally similar to those seen in sporadic colorectal carcinogenesis, but the timing of molecular events appears to be different, suggesting different cancer-driver pathways in IBD-associated neoplasia.

Activation of NF-KappaB occurs in the colonic epithelium with chronic colitis.[6] NF-KappaB can activate the expression of COX2, pro-inflammatory cytokines including IL-1, TNF-alpha, IL-12p40, and IL-23p19, anti-apoptotic factor inhibitor of apoptosis protein (IAP), and B-cell leukemia/lymphoma (Bcl-XL).[7] Prostaglandins and Cytokines such as IL-6 are released in the inflammatory environment and can activate intracellular serine-threonine kinase Akt signaling,[8,9] leading to inhibition of pro-apoptotic factors p53, BAD, and FoxO1 and increased cell survival.[10,11]

Similar to sporadic CRC, colitis-associated cancers show genetic instability manifested by chromosomal (CIN) and microsatellite instability (MSI), occurring in 85% and 15% of the cases, respectively.[12,13] Clonal chromosomal alterations were present in 85% of UC-associated cancers, 86% of

A.R. Sepulveda and J.P. Lynch (eds.), *Molecular Pathology of Neoplastic Gastrointestinal Diseases*, Molecular Pathology Library 7,
DOI 10.1007/978-1-4614-6015-2_10, © Springer Science+Business Media New York 2013

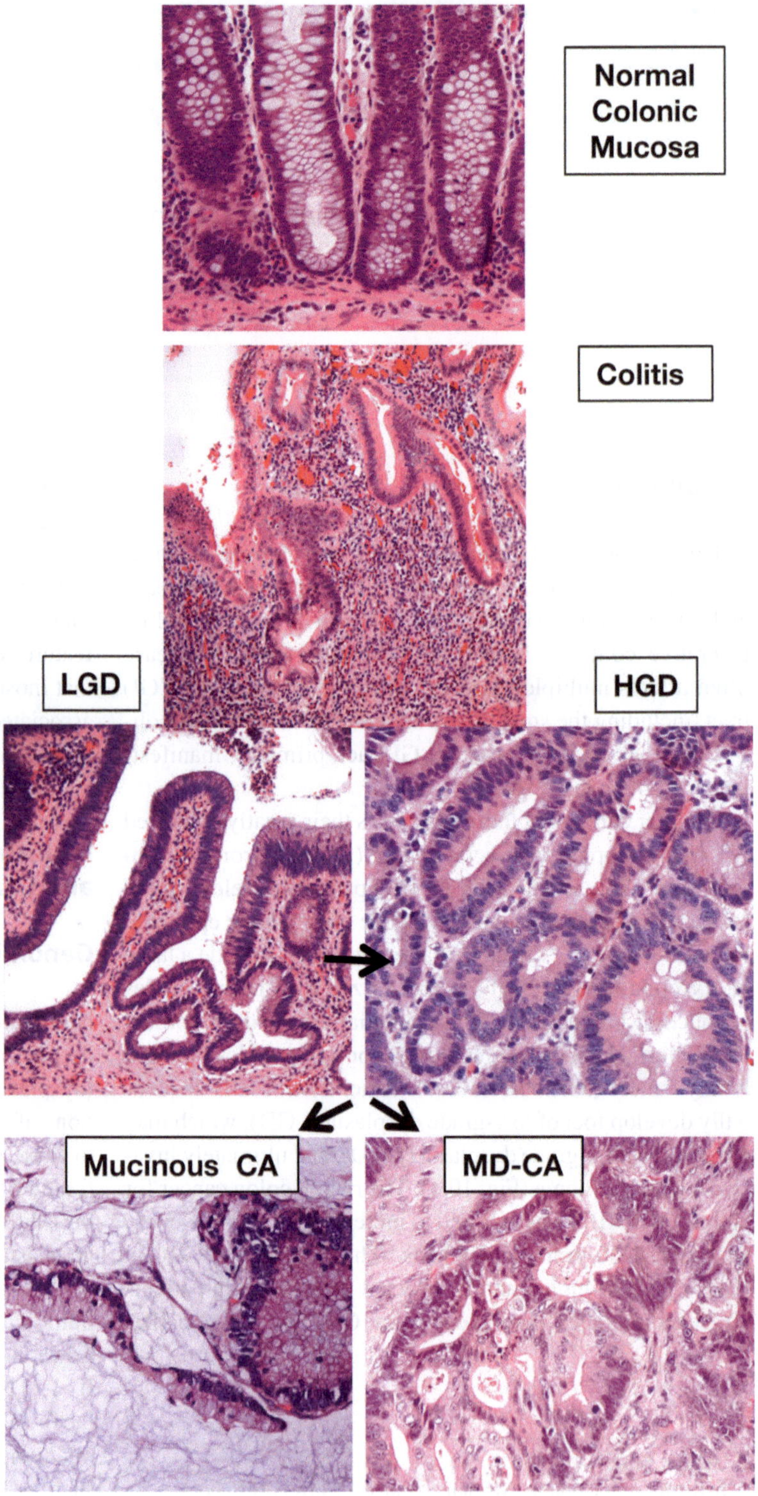

Fig. 10.1 Pathologic features of colitis-associated neoplasia. Colonic mucosa with chronic active colitis shows marked crypt architectural distortion in a background on increased inflammation in the mucosa. Chronic colitis may progress to the dysplastic lesions low-grade dysplasia (LGD), high-grade dysplasia (HGD), and invasive adenocarcinoma. Adenocarcinomas arising in the setting of IBD show morphologic features that are indistinguishable from sporadic CRC. The figure shows examples of moderately differentiated colonic adenocarcinoma and mucinous adenocarcinoma, in patients with ulcerative colitis. Other morphologic patterns similar to those seen in sporadic CRC may occur in IBD patients. The photomicrographs are from Hematoxylin and Eosin stains of routine formalin-fixed paraffin-embedded tissue sections

UC-associated dysplastic lesions, and 36% of non-dysplastic UC mucosa. Losses of chromosome 18 or 18q and chromosome 5 or 5q were common in UC-associated cancer and dysplasia and were occasionally detected in UC-associated non-dysplastic colonic mucosa.[14] By FISH, abnormalities in chromosomal arms (8, 11, 17, and 18), especially losses, were more common and discriminatory between UC-associated neoplasia (dysplasia or cancer) and non-dysplastic colitic mucosa.[15] In UC-associated CRC, *APC* mutations or LOH of the *APC* locus were reported in 14–33% of cancers.[16–19] Loss of chromosome 5 or 5q was detected in 36% UC-associated dysplasias and 54% UC-associated carcinomas.[14] Importantly, in UC-associated neoplasia, *APC* mutations occur late, in the transition from high-grade dysplasia to carcinoma.[12] This contrasts with sporadic colon carcinogenesis, where the *APC* gene is mutated in the majority (80%) of tumors and occurs early in the neoplastic process.[20] As compared to sporadic colon cancers, in UC, *APC* inactivation may not be necessary to drive the early steps of colitis-associated dysplasia, since other molecular mechanisms, such as activation of NF-KappaB in crypt epithelial cells by inflammatory cytokines, can promote cell proliferation and inhibit apoptosis.[6]

The tumor suppressor gene *TP53* is mutated at a high rate in both sporadic and UC colon cancers. However, in contrast to sporadic cancers, in UC, *TP53* mutations occur earlier in the colitis-associated neoplastic pathway.[21–25] In UC, *TP53* mutations were detected in 19% of colon biopsies without dysplasia, increasing in frequency with higher grades of dysplasia.[26] This contrasts with sporadic CRC in which *TP53* mutations and LOH happen during the progression from high-grade dysplasia to cancer.[20] It is possible that the early loss of *TP53* function in UC-associated neoplasia contributes to the rapid progression to CRC observed in these patients. In the normal epithelial cells, p53 induces p21 gene expression and delays cell cycle progression in S-phase to allow for repair of the damaged DNA. Reduced p53 function and increased DNA damage associated with inflammatory by-products in active colitis result in persistence of significant mutations in daughter cells, clonal selection, and ultimately cancer development.[27]

In UC, the frequent loss of 18q in dysplasia and occasionally in non-dysplastic mucosa suggests that these changes may be an important early event in IBD-associated neoplasia. In contrast, in sporadic colorectal cancer, allelic loss of 18q is thought to be a later event and is associated with metastatic disease.[28] Loss of chromosome 18 or 18q was present in 69% of UC-associated cancers, 43% of UC-associated dysplasias, and in 20% of UC non-dysplastic mucosa.[14] 18q21 is the location of three putative tumor suppressor genes, *DCC*, *SMAD4*, and *SMAD2*, suggesting that one or more of these genes may play an important role in UC-related carcinogenesis.

The long arm of chromosome 20 (20q) is frequently amplified in UC-associated neoplasms as well as other gastrointestinal cancers.[29] Overexpression of the anti-apoptotic protein Bcl-xl was detected in UC-associated dysplasias, suggesting a role in the pathogenesis of UC-associated carcinoma. The *BCLXL* gene is located adjacent to one of the amplified clones on chromosome 20q11, which may be a mechanism underlying the increased Bcl-xl protein expression in UC-associated carcinoma.[30]

Chromosome 6q abnormalities occur in a variety of human cancers and LOH involving 6q27 was detected in colitic mucosa. Deletions in 6q27 were frequently observed in the dysplastic and non-dysplastic tissue of UC patients who had progressed to neoplasia but not in control UC without neoplasia.[31] Losses in 2q14 were also reported in UC progressors but not in UC patients who were neoplasia free.[31]

Epigenetic Abnormalities

Alterations in epigenetic regulation, in particular CpG island hypermethylation, are also known to contribute to neoplastic development and progression in UC-associated CRC (Fig. 10.2). Methyl binding proteins recognize hypermethylated sites and recruit histone deacetylases, leading to histone deacetylation, chromatin condensation, and inactivation of genes. Several genes have been reported to be hypermethylated in dysplasia and/or cancer in UC, including genes that have been reported as targets of CpG island methylation in sporadic colorectal cancer,[32] such as the *MLH1* promoter,[33,34] and the *p16INK4a* promoter regions.[35,36] Extensive methylation characteristic of the CpG island methylator phenotype (CIMP) was observed in 17% of the UC-related cancers, and global DNA methylation measured with a LINE-1 assay was seen in 58% of UC-associated cancers.[37]

In microsatellite instability (MSI)-positive UC colon cancers, the underlying mechanism of high levels of MSI (MSI-H) is loss of MLH1 protein expression associated with *MLH1* by promoter hypermethylation.[33] Interestingly, MSI in the non-neoplastic mucosa is significantly more frequent in the colitic mucosa as compared to the background non-neoplastic mucosa of sporadic colon cancers.[6] This may be explained by reduced expression and function of DNA repair enzymes induced by oxidative stress.[38,39] A similar phenomenon is seen in gastric carcinogenesis in the setting of chronic inflammation associated with *H. pylori* gastritis.[40–42] Unlike sporadic colon cancers, in UC-associated colon cancers with MSI, *TGFBR2* mutations are much less common (17%)[12] and occur early in the neoplastic process.[43]

Issa et al. reported increased methylation levels in high-grade dysplasia (HGD) of patients with ulcerative colitis compared to controls without ulcerative colitis, for estrogen receptor (*ER*), *MYOD*, *CDKN2A* (*p16* exon 1), and *CSPG2*.[44] Hypermethylation of three of these genes was also detected in the colitic mucosa of patients with HGD.[44] The p16 methylation levels averaged 2% in the mucosa of controls, 3% in the mucosa of UC patients without dysplasia, 8% in the normal appearing epithelium of patients with HGD/CA, and 9% in the dysplastic epithelium (HGD/CA).[44] In addition, they found that CpG methylation was present in both the neoplastic and non-neoplastic-appearing epithelium from UC patients with HGD/cancer, suggesting that the increased levels of methylation are widespread in the inflammation affected colon and occur early in the process of carcinogenesis, preceding the histological appearance of dysplasia.[44]

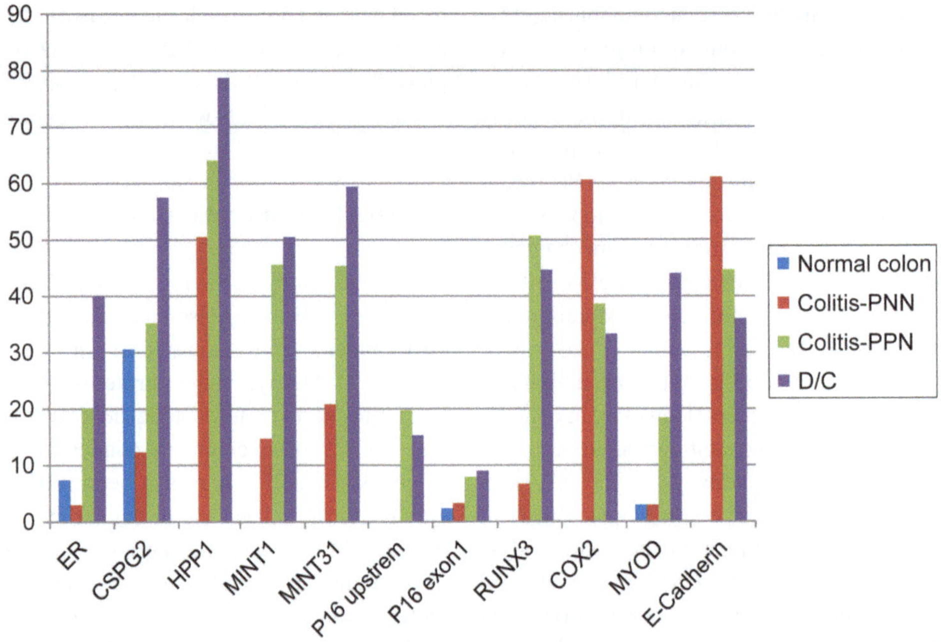

Fig. 10.2 Molecular events in the stepwise lesions of inflammatory bowel disease-associated neoplasia. Methylation levels are indicated in the *Y* axis. Summary of data from.[37,44,58] CpG methylation was determined in colonic mucosa with colitis in patients negative for neoplasia (Colitis-PNN); colonic mucosa with colitis in patients positive for neoplasia (Colitis-PPN); and dysplasia or cancer lesions (D/C)

Methylation of the hyperplastic polyposis gene 1 (*HPP1*) was observed in 50% of UC adenocarcinomas and in 40% of dysplasias but not in non-neoplastic UC mucosa.[45] Methylation of the E-cadherin (*CDH1*) promoter was detected in 93% of the patients with dysplastic biopsy samples, in contrast to only 6% of the patients without dysplasia and by immunohistochemistry areas of dysplasia displayed reduced E-cadherin expression levels.[46] The DNA repair protein O6-methylguanine-DNA methyltransferase gene (*MGMT*) was found to be more frequently methylated in sporadic adenomas and carcinomas than in IBD.[36,47,48] In IBD, promoter hypermethylation of *MGMT* was detected in 16.7% adenocarcinomas and in 3.7% mucosal samples with mild inflammation.[47] Mikami et al reported that the frequency of promoter methylation of *MGMT* and *MLH1* was lower in UC-associated tumors than in sporadic CRC.[36]

Methylation of the *WNT* signaling genes is an early event seen in patients with IBD colitis with a progressive increase in methylation of the *WNT* genes during development of IBD-associated neoplasia.[49] Seven CpG sites with differential methylation in intestinal tissues of IBD patients were identified by the Golden Gate assay.[50] Interestingly, different methylation patterns associated with CD and UC were reported, suggesting that IBD-associated changes in DNA methylation in intestinal tissue may be disease subtype specific.[50]

Hypomethylation in ulcerative colitis also occurs, but its relationship to carcinogenesis in UC is not clear.[51]CpG methylation testing in IBD has used a number of technical approaches. Methylation-dependent restriction enzyme-based approaches and bisulfite conversion followed by methylation-specific PCR (MSP) were most used in earlier studies of CpG methylation.[45–47,52] More recently, quantitative CpG methylation methods such as pyrosequencing, allowing the determination of ratios of methylated and unmethylated DNA within a population of molecules[37,52], and quantitative real-time PCR assays[42,52] have been employed in CpG methylation studies. High-throughput bisulfite-based approaches such as Golden Gate technology and bisulfite-modified DNA followed by genome-wide, massively parallel sequencing offer enormous potential to characterize epigenetic abnormalities in neoplasia.[50]

EGFR Pathway

Activation of the Raf/MEK/ERK (MAPK) kinase pathway through either *RAS* or *BRAF* mutation was detected in 27% of all UC-related cancers. Non-dysplastic UC mucosa of patients with UC cancer did not show *BRAF* mutations, indicating that *BRAF* mutations are not an initiating event in UC-related carcinogenesis but are associated with mismatch-repair deficiency through *MLH1* promoter hypermethylation in advanced lesions.[53] Conversely, *KRAS* mutations may occur not only in dysplasia, but also in villous regeneration in the mucosa and in active colitis.[54] *KRAS* mutations are inversely correlated with *BRAF* mutations in UC cancers, in that all tested UC cancers with *KRAS* mutations had an intact *BRAF* gene and the cancers with *BRAF* mutations had an intact *KRAS* gene, similar to sporadic CRC.[53]

MicroRNAs

Unique microRNA (miRNA) expression profiles have been reported in mucosal tissues of patients with ulcerative colitis, Crohn's ileitis, and colitis as well as in peripheral blood of IBD patients. MicroRNA expression profiles were also shown to change in the progression from normal colonic tissue to dysplastic lesions. Three miRNAs (miR-192, miR-375, and miR-422b) were reported to be significantly decreased in UC tissues, while eight miRNAs (miR-16, miR-21, miR-23a, miR-24, miR-29a, miR-126, miR-195, and let-7f) were significantly increased in active UC tissues.[55] Important targets of miRNAs in UC patients, identified by genome-wide mRNA microarray analyses, include the macrophage inflammatory peptide-2α (MIP-2α), a chemotactic cytokine, mediated by TNF-α (reviewed in[56]).

Olaru et al identified 32 miRNAs that were increased and 10 that were decreased in IBD dysplasia using miRNA microarray analyses.[57] MicroRNA-31 expression seemed to change in a stepwise fashion from normal to inflamed to neoplastic tissue in IBD. Increased expression of miR-31 was seen in mucosa of IBD patients compared to controls. No difference in miR-31 expression was found between the IBD dysplasia and IBD carcinomas. MicroR-31 expression was also significantly increased in sporadic CRC specimens compared to normal controls, although levels were lower in sporadic CRC when compared with IBD-associated neoplasia. Further, miR-31 expression levels were able to differentiate IBD-associated neoplasia from normal colonic, unaffected tissue from IBD patients and from inflamed tissue from IBD patients ([57], and reviewed in[56]). A hydroxylase called factor-inhibiting hypoxia inducible factor 1 (*FIH1*), which may be involved in tumor angiogenesis, was identified as a putative target of miR-31.

In summary, alterations of miRNA expression in colitis mucosa and progressive neoplastic lesions may serve as markers of disease progression in IBD and may become useful as biomarkers for the detection of dysplasia.

References

1. Munkholm P. Review article: the incidence and prevalence of colorectal cancer in inflammatory bowel disease. *Aliment Pharmacol Ther*. 2003;18(Suppl 2):1–5.
2. Harpaz N, Talbot IC. Colorectal cancer in idiopathic inflammatory bowel disease. *Semin Diagn Pathol*. 1996;13:339–57.
3. Itzkowitz SH, Harpaz N. Diagnosis and management of dysplasia in patients with inflammatory bowel diseases. *Gastroenterology*. 2004;126:1634–48.
4. Kornbluth A, Sachar DB. Ulcerative colitis practice guidelines in adults (update): American College of Gastroenterology, Practice Parameters Committee. *Am J Gastroenterol*. 2004;99:1371–85.
5. Kornbluth A, Sachar DB. Ulcerative colitis practice guidelines in adults: American College Of Gastroenterology, Practice Parameters Committee. *Am J Gastroenterol*. 2010;105:501–23. quiz 524.
6. Boland CR, Luciani MG, Gasche C, Goel A. Infection, inflammation, and gastrointestinal cancer. *Gut*. 2005;54:1321–31.
7. Karrasch T, Jobin C. NF-kappaB and the intestine: friend or foe? *Inflamm Bowel Dis*. 2008;14:114–24.
8. Rose-John S, Scheller J, Elson G, Jones SA. Interleukin-6 biology is coordinated by membrane-bound and soluble receptors: role in inflammation and cancer. *J Leukoc Biol*. 2006;80:227–36.
9. Chalaris A, Garbers C, Rabe B, Rose-John S, Scheller J. The soluble Interleukin 6 receptor: generation and role in inflammation and cancer. *Eur J Cell Biol*. 2011;90:484–94.
10. Vivanco I, Sawyers CL. The phosphatidylinositol 3-Kinase AKT pathway in human cancer. *Nat Rev Cancer*. 2002;2:489–501.
11. Stenson WF. Prostaglandins and epithelial response to injury. *Curr Opin Gastroenterol*. 2007;23:107–10.
12. Itzkowitz SH. Molecular biology of dysplasia and cancer in inflammatory bowel disease. *Gastroenterol Clin North Am*. 2006;35:553–71.
13. Maia L, Dinis J, Cravo M, et al. Who takes the lead in the development of ulcerative colitis-associated colorectal cancers: mutator, suppressor, or methylator pathway? *Cancer Genet Cytogenet*. 2005;162:68–73.
14. Willenbucher RF, Aust DE, Chang CG, et al. Genomic instability is an early event during the progression pathway of ulcerative-colitis-related neoplasia. *Am J Pathol*. 1999;154:1825–30.
15. Bronner MP, O'Sullivan JN, Rabinovitch PS, et al. Genomic biomarkers to improve ulcerative colitis neoplasia surveillance. *Am J Pathol*. 2008;173:1853–60.
16. Aust DE, Terdiman JP, Willenbucher RF, et al. The APC/beta-catenin pathway in ulcerative colitis-related colorectal carcinomas: a mutational analysis. *Cancer*. 2002;94:1421–7.
17. Redston MS, Papadopoulos N, Caldas C, Kinzler KW, Kern SE. Common occurrence of APC and K-ras gene mutations in the spectrum of colitis-associated neoplasias. *Gastroenterology*. 1995;108:383–92.
18. Tomlinson I, Ilyas M, Johnson V, et al. A comparison of the genetic pathways involved in the pathogenesis of three types of colorectal cancer. *J Pathol*. 1998;184:148–52.
19. Greenwald BD, Harpaz N, Yin J, et al. Loss of heterozygosity affecting the p53, Rb, and mcc/apc tumor suppressor gene loci in dysplastic and cancerous ulcerative colitis. *Cancer Res*. 1992;52: 741–5.
20. Lynch HT, Lynch JF. Hereditary cancer: family history, diagnosis, molecular genetics, ecogenetics, and management strategies. *Biochimie*. 2002;84:3–17.
21. Burmer GC, Rabinovitch PS, Haggitt RC, et al. Neoplastic progression in ulcerative colitis: histology, DNA content, and loss of a p53 allele. *Gastroenterology*. 1992;103:1602–10.
22. Yin J, Harpaz N, Tong Y, et al. p53 point mutations in dysplastic and cancerous ulcerative colitis lesions. *Gastroenterology*. 1993; 104:1633–9.
23. Brentnall TA, Crispin DA, Rabinovitch PS, et al. Mutations in the p53 gene: an early marker of neoplastic progression in ulcerative colitis. *Gastroenterology*. 1994;107:369–78.
24. Hussain SP, Amstad P, Raja K, et al. Increased p53 mutation load in noncancerous colon tissue from ulcerative colitis: a cancer-prone chronic inflammatory disease. *Cancer Res*. 2000;60:3333–7.
25. Yagishita H, Yoshida T, Ishiguro K, Numata Y, Okayasu I. Epithelial and stromal genetic instability linked to tumor suppressor genes in ulcerative colitis-associated tumorigenesis. *Scand J Gastroenterol*. 2008;43:559–66.
26. Holzmann K, Klump B, Borchard F, et al. Comparative analysis of histology, DNA content, p53 and Ki-ras mutations in colectomy specimens with long-standing ulcerative colitis. *Int J Cancer*. 1998;76:1–6.
27. Meek DW. The p53 response to DNA damage. *DNA Repair (Amst)*. 2004;3:1049–56.

28. Jen J, Kim H, Piantadosi S, et al. Allelic loss of chromosome 18q and prognosis in colorectal cancer. *N Engl J Med.* 1994;331: 213–21.
29. van Dieren JM, Wink JC, Vissers KJ, et al. Chromosomal and microsatellite instability of adenocarcinomas and dysplastic lesions (DALM) in ulcerative colitis. *Diagn Mol Pathol.* 2006;15:216–22.
30. van der Woude CJ, Moshage H, Homan M, Kleibeuker JH, Jansen PL, van Dekken H. Expression of apoptosis related proteins during malignant progression in chronic ulcerative colitis. *J Clin Pathol.* 2005;58:811–4.
31. Chen R, Bronner MP, Crispin DA, Rabinovitch PS, Brentnall TA. Characterization of genomic instability in ulcerative colitis neoplasia leads to discovery of putative tumor suppressor regions. *Cancer Genet Cytogenet.* 2005;162:99–106.
32. Takahashi T, Shigematsu H, Shivapurkar N, et al. Aberrant promoter methylation of multiple genes during multistep pathogenesis of colorectal cancers. *Int J Cancer.* 2005;118:924–31.
33. Fleisher AS, Esteller M, Harpaz N, et al. Microsatellite instability in inflammatory bowel disease-associated neoplastic lesions is associated with hypermethylation and diminished expression of the DNA mismatch repair gene, hMLH1. *Cancer Res.* 2000;60:4864–8.
34. Schulmann K, Mori Y, Croog V, et al. Molecular phenotype of inflammatory bowel disease-associated neoplasms with microsatellite instability. *Gastroenterology.* 2005;129:74–85.
35. Hsieh CJ, Klump B, Holzmann K, Borchard F, Gregor M, Porschen R. Hypermethylation of the p16INK4a promoter in colectomy specimens of patients with long-standing and extensive ulcerative colitis. *Cancer Res.* 1998;58:3942–5.
36. Mikami T, Yoshida T, Numata Y, et al. Low frequency of promoter methylation of O6-methylguanine DNA methyltransferase and hMLH1 in ulcerative colitis-associated tumors: comparison with sporadic colonic tumors. *Am J Clin Pathol.* 2007;127:366–73.
37. Konishi K, Shen L, Wang S, Meltzer SJ, Harpaz N, Issa JP. Rare CpG island methylator phenotype in ulcerative colitis-associated neoplasias. *Gastroenterology.* 2007;132:1254–60.
38. Chang DK, Goel A, Ricciardiello L, et al. Effect of H(2)O(2) on cell cycle and survival in DNA mismatch repair-deficient and -proficient cell lines. *Cancer Lett.* 2003;195:243–51.
39. Hofseth LJ, Saito S, Hussain SP, et al. Nitric oxide-induced cellular stress and p53 activation in chronic inflammation. *Proc Natl Acad Sci USA.* 2003;100:143–8.
40. Kim J, Leung W, Wu L, Graham D, Sepulveda A. *Helicobacter pylori* impairs DNA mismatch repair in gastric epithelial cells: a link with gastric carcinogenesis. *Gastroenterology.* 2000;118:A867.
41. Park DI, Park SH, Kim SH, et al. Effect of Helicobacter pylori infection on the expression of DNA mismatch repair protein. *Helicobacter.* 2005;10:179–84.
42. Sepulveda AR, Yao Y, Yan W, et al. CpG methylation and reduced expression of O6-methylguanine DNA methyltransferase is associated with Helicobacter pylori infection. *Gastroenterology.* 2010; 138:1836–44.
43. Souza RF, Lei J, Yin J, et al. A transforming growth factor beta 1 receptor type II mutation in ulcerative colitis-associated neoplasms [see comments]. *Gastroenterology.* 1997;112:40–5.
44. Issa JP, Ahuja N, Toyota M, Bronner MP, Brentnall TA. Accelerated age-related CpG island methylation in ulcerative colitis. *Cancer Res.* 2001;61:3573–7.
45. Sato F, Shibata D, Harpaz N, et al. Aberrant methylation of the HPP1 gene in ulcerative colitis-associated colorectal carcinoma. *Cancer Res.* 2002;62:6820–2.
46. Azarschab P, Porschen R, Gregor M, Blin N, Holzmann K. Epigenetic control of the E-cadherin gene (CDH1) by CpG methylation in colectomy samples of patients with ulcerative colitis. *Genes Chromosomes Cancer.* 2002;35:121–6.
47. Matsumura S, Oue N, Ito R, et al. The promoter methylation status of the DNA repair gene O6-methylguanine-DNA methyltransferase in ulcerative colitis. *Virchows Arch.* 2003;443:518–23.
48. Petko Z, Ghiassi M, Shuber A, et al. Aberrantly methylated CDKN2A, MGMT, and MLH1 in colon polyps and in fecal DNA from patients with colorectal polyps. *Clin Cancer Res.* 2005;11: 1203–9.
49. Dhir M, Montgomery EA, Glockner SC, et al. Epigenetic regulation of WNT signaling pathway genes in inflammatory bowel disease (IBD) associated neoplasia. *J Gastrointest Surg.* 2008;12:1745–53.
50. Lin Z, Hegarty JP, Cappel JA, et al. Identification of disease-associated DNA methylation in intestinal tissues from patients with inflammatory bowel disease. *Clin Genet.* 2011;80:59–67.
51. Gloria L, Cravo M, Pinto A, et al. DNA hypomethylation and proliferative activity are increased in the rectal mucosa of patients with long-standing ulcerative colitis. *Cancer.* 1996;78:2300–6.
52. Sepulveda AR, Jones D, Ogino S, et al. CpG methylation analysis–current status of clinical assays and potential applications in molecular diagnostics: a report of the Association for Molecular Pathology. *J Mol Diagn.* 2009;11:266–78.
53. Aust DE, Haase M, Dobryden L, et al. Mutations of the BRAF gene in ulcerative colitis-related colorectal carcinoma. *Int J Cancer.* 2005;115:673–7.
54. Benhattar J, Saraga E. Molecular genetics of dysplasia in ulcerative colitis. *Eur J Cancer.* 1995;31A:1171–3.
55. Wu F, Zhang S, Dassopoulos T, et al. Identification of microRNAs associated with ileal and colonic Crohn's disease. *Inflamm Bowel Dis.* 2010;16:1729–38.
56. Dalal SR, Kwon JH. The role of MicroRNA in inflammatory bowel disease. *Gastroenterol Hepatol (N Y).* 2010;6:714–22.
57. Olaru AV, Selaru FM, Mori Y. et al. Dynamic changes in the expression of MicroRNA-31 during inflammatory bowel disease-associated neoplastic transformation. *Inflamm Bowel Dis.* 2011;17:221–31.
58. Garrity-Park MM, Loftus EV Jr, Sandborn WJ, Bryant SC, Smyrk TC. Methylation status of genes in non-neoplastic mucosa from patients with ulcerative colitis-associated colorectal cancer. *Am J Gastroenterol.* 2010;105:1610–9.

Part III

Non-epithelial Neoplastic Tumors

Molecular Biology and Pathology of Gastrointestinal Stromal Tumors

11

Paul J. Zhang

Introduction

Gastrointestinal stromal tumors (GISTs) are mesenchymal tumors of the gastrointestinal (GI) tract with characteristic histologic and molecular features. These tumors are *KIT* or *PDFGRA* mutation-driven mesenchymal tumors of the gastrointestinal tract originating from the interstitial cells of Cajal (ICC) or their precursors,[1,2] and they generally express CKIT protein. GISTs are the most common malignant mesenchymal tumors of the gastrointestinal (GI) tract and about 5,000 new cases are diagnosed each year in the United States.[1,2]

GIST was first recognized in the stomach as a distinct clinicopathological entity by Mazur et al in 1983.[3] It was later recognized that it could arise in any part of the gastrointestinal tract with decreasing order of incidence as follows: in stomach (60–70%), small intestine (20–30%), large bowel (5%), and rarely esophagus and gallbladder.[4–9] In addition to the gastrointestinal sites, GISTs were also reported in omentum and other soft tissue sites outside the gastrointestinal tract.[10] Histologically, most GISTs show characteristic spindle cell morphology and increasing mitotic activity as tumors become more aggressive (Fig. 11.1). In addition to its distinct histologic features, GISTs were also found to be positive for CD34 and KIT immunoreactivity in 2000, which significantly facilitated the recognition and diagnosis of these tumors[11–14] (Fig. 11.1).

Because of its distinct phenotype and ultrastructural characteristics, the histogenesis of GIST was related to intestinal cells of Cajal (ICC), a special interstitial cell in the GI tract with pacemaker function.[15,16] Development and function of the ICC are critically dependent on the KIT-SCF axes.[17] However, the most important breakthrough in understanding the biology of GIST was the discovery of gain of function mutations of KIT in the oncogenesis of human GIST by Hirota et al,[18] which subsequently lead to the discovery of the use of tyrosine kinase inhibitors as a novel targeted therapy for GIST.[19,20]

The biologic behavior of GIST ranges from benign to frankly malignant. In routine practice, various pathological factors such as tumor site, size, cell type, necrosis, mitotic activity, and Ki67 index have been used to assess or predict the malignant risk of the tumor.[1,21,22] Tumor location in different portions of the GI tract as well as different KIT mutations is also known to have impact in tumor biologic behavior.[22–25] Approximately 20–25% of gastric and 40–50% of small bowel GISTs are expected to be malignant.[1]

When the tumors were treated by surgery alone, 5-year disease-specific survival after surgical removal of a primary tumor was approximately 20% for tumors larger than 10 cm and was approximately 60% for tumors less than 5 cm.[26] In patients whose disease was considered cured by surgery, the 5-year and 10-year survival rates were 81% and 67%.[27] As GISTs generally do not respond to conventional chemotherapy and radiation, the survival remained dismal until the early 2000s when imatinib became available. Imatinib mesylate (Gleevec, ST11571), an ATP-competitive inhibitor that inhibits BCR-ABL, KIT, and PDGFRA, has been used effectively for treating recurrent and unresectable GIST with *KIT* or *PDGFRA* mutations.[28–31] Response to imatinib treatment has been related to specific types of the *KIT* or *PDGFRA* mutations.[32–35] Secondary *KIT* or *PDGFRA* mutations are responsible for resistance to imatinib in about 40–60% of the tumors which originally respond to the treatment.[36–39]

P.J. Zhang, M.D. (✉)
Department of Pathology and Lab Medicine,
University of Pennsylvania Medical Center, 3400 Spruce Street – Six Founders, Philadelphia, PA 19104, USA
e-mail: pjz@mail.med.upenn.edu

A.R. Sepulveda and J.P. Lynch (eds.), *Molecular Pathology of Neoplastic Gastrointestinal Diseases*, Molecular Pathology Library 7,
DOI 10.1007/978-1-4614-6015-2_11, © Springer Science+Business Media New York 2013

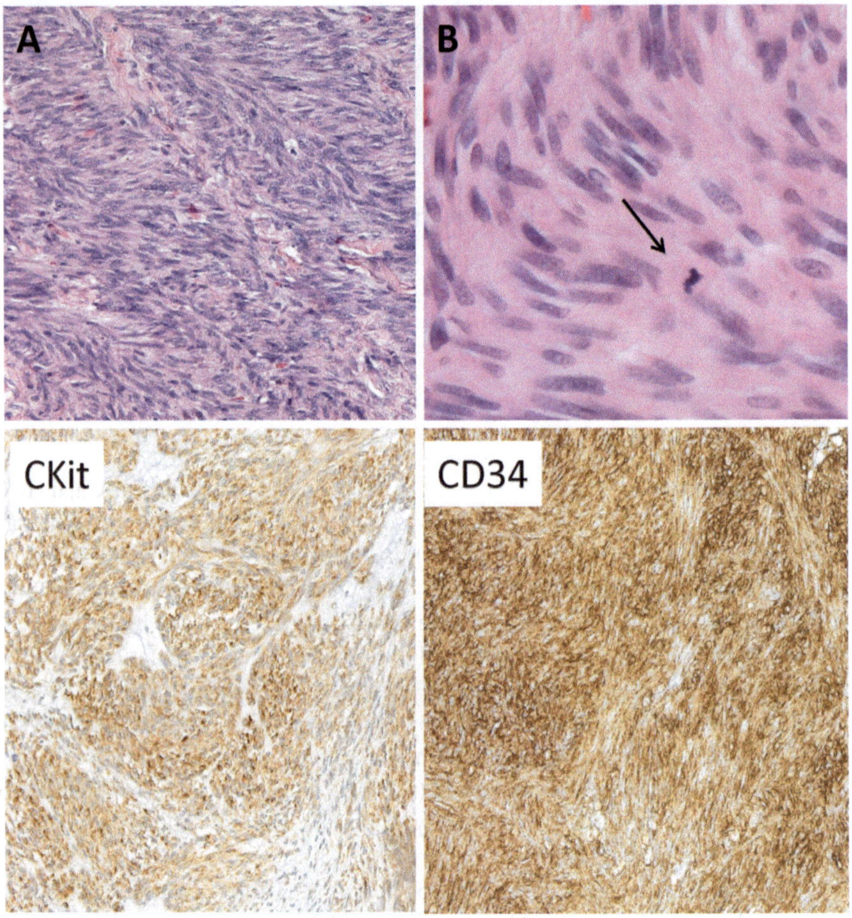

Fig. 11.1 Histopathology of a typical GIST shows relatively uniform spindle cell morphology (**a**). A rare mitotic figure is indicated by the *arrow* in a low-grade GIST (**b**). GISTs characteristically express KIT protein (**c**) and often CD34 (**d**), detected in tumor tissue sections by immunohistochemistry

Oncogenesis

Primary Mutations

About 90% of GISTs harbor activation mutations in *KIT* or *PDGFRA* genes. Both *KIT* and *PDGFRA* are located pericentromerically at 4q12 and have probably evolved as a duplication of an ancestral gene.[40] They both encode a protein that has structural characteristics of type III receptor tyrosine kinase family.[41] KIT is a 145-kd transmembrane glycoprotein that serves as the receptor for stem cell factor (SCF).[42–44] It is composed of an extracellular ligand-binding domain, a transmembrane sequence, a juxtamembrane domain, and two cytoplasmic kinase domains (TKI: ATP-binding pocket and TKII: kinase activation loop).[41,45] The KIT transmembrane protein is critical to the development of ICCs as well as to the development of hematopoietic progenitor cells, mast cells, germ cells, and melanocytes.[43,46–48] The binding of SCF to KIT results in receptor homodimerization and activation of the tyrosine kinase with phosphorylation of a number of effectors regulating various signal transduction pathways.[11,47] The KIT activity is normally inhibited by its juxtamembrane domain exon 11 which inhibits its receptor dimerization in the absence of SCF.[2,11]

The gain of function associated with mutation of *KIT* or *PDGFRA* in interstitial cells of Cajal (ICC) or their precursors is now believed to be the earliest event in the oncogenesis of GISTs.[1,2,11,18,49,50] Mutation in the *KIT* or *PDGFRA* gene could involve the receptor regulatory domains, extracellular and juxtamembrane domains, and the cytoplasmic enzymatic domains (TKI and TKII). Mutations of the juxtamembrane domain release the kinase from auto-inhibition and lead to constitutive activation of *KIT* or *PDFGRA*, activating either the extracellular or cytoplasmic domains of the receptor in absence of the ligand, and subsequent phosphorylation of all the downstream target proteins with activation of signal transduction cascades that regulate cell proliferation, survival, chemotaxis, and adhesion[47,51–54] (Table 11.1).

KIT Mutations

In GISTs, most *KIT* mutations (70%) occur in the juxtamembrane intracellular domain (exon 11) followed by mutations

Table 11.1 Genes Regulated by Mutations of *KIT* and *PDGFRA*

Gene	Target Genes	Downstream Signaling Factors		Signaling Consequences
KIT mutation	*MAPK*	JAK1/2	STAT	Induce progression through cell cycle; prevent apoptosis
		ERK1/2(P44/22)	P90RSK	Inhibit cell differentiation
			MSK	
			ELK-1, STAT	
		p38	PLA2, MNK1, PRAK, Hsp27, STAT1, ELK-1	Inhibit apoptosis
	GRB2	SOS, RAS, RAF, MEK, ERK	P90RSK, MSK, ELK-1, STAT	Inhibit apoptosis
	PI3K	p70S6K	RPS6, ELF-4	Regulate cell growth
		PKB(AKT)↓	mTOR signaling (p70S6K, RPS6, ELF4, STAT)	Regulate cell growth
			RAF, ERK, p70S6K↓	Inhibit apoptosis
			p21, p27	Regulate cell cycle and proliferation
			cyclinD1, p53	
			BAD, FXHR/AFX↓	Induce cell survival
			p53, NF-KB	Modulate cell death
		BAD↓	BCL-XL, BCL-2	Inhibit apoptosis
		NF-KB	IKB, IKK, et al	Inhibit cell differentiation
	SHP1/2	—	—	Negative regulation of KIT signaling pathway
	CBL	—	—	Unknown
	SHC	—	—	Unknown
	EPHA4	—	—	Unknown
	Paxillin	—	—	Unknown
PDGFRA mutation	*MAPK*	JAK1/2, ERK1/2, p38	STAT, P90RSK, MSK, ELK-1, PLA2, MNK1, PRAK, Hsp27	Inhibit apoptosis; inhibit cell differentiation; induce progression through cell cycle
	AKT (with controversy)	mTOR signaling (p70S6K, RPS6, ELF4, STAT)	—	Regulate cell growth
		RAF, ERK, p70S6K	—	Modulate cell growth
		p21, p27	—	Regulate cell cycle and proliferation
		cyclinD1	—	Modulate cell cycle (indirectly)
		BAD, FXHR/AFX	—	Induce cell survival
		p53, NF-KB	—	Modulate cell death (indirectly)
	STAT	—	—	Induce progression through cell cycle; prevent apoptosis

Adapted from Yang et al[51]

involving the extracellular domain (exon 9) and cytoplasmic domains in exons 13 and 17.[2,11,32,55] Point mutations, deletions, and duplications of 3' region and insertion have all been identified in *KIT*.[1,2,11,56] The most common type of KIT exon 11 mutations is isolated in-frame deletion.[35] Mutations commonly involve the 5'end of exon 11 (codons between 550 and 563).[18,57] Exon 9 encodes the end of the extracellular domain and is mutated in 3–21% of the cases.[18,58,59] Exon 9 mutations likely disrupt an antidimerization motif in the extracellular domain and insertion of six nucleotides in duplications Ala501 Tyr502 is common in exon 9 mutations.[32,58,60,61] Mutations in exons 13 (kinase I domain) and 17 (activation loop) are the least common and account for 1–2% of the cases. Mutation in exon 13 or 17 is usually a point mutation only (1945A-G Glu642Lys in exon 13 and Asn822His and Asn832Lys in exon 17).[32,62,63] Mutations in either exon 13 or 17 can cause constitutive activation of the kinase domain and ligand-independent activation of the receptor.[32] Most of the primary *KIT* mutations occur as single events, but rarely de novo double primary mutations in *KIT* exon 11 have been reported, usually as missense point mutations or deletions of different alleles in exon 11.[64,65] Figure 11.2 depicts the involved exons and common mutation types in *KIT* and *PDGFRA*.[1]

PDGFRA Mutations

PDGFRA mutations occur in about 8% of GISTs that are negative for *KIT* mutations (*KIT* wild type GIST).[66,67] The signal transduction profiles of *PDGFRA*-mutant tumor are indistinguishable from *KIT*-mutant tumors suggesting that PDGFRA can substitute for *KIT* in GIST oncogenesis.[66] Exon 18 (TK II: kinase activatin loop) and exon 14 (TK I: ATP-binding pocket are involved in 6–7% of the GISTs with exon 12 (juxtamembrane domain) involved in <1% of the

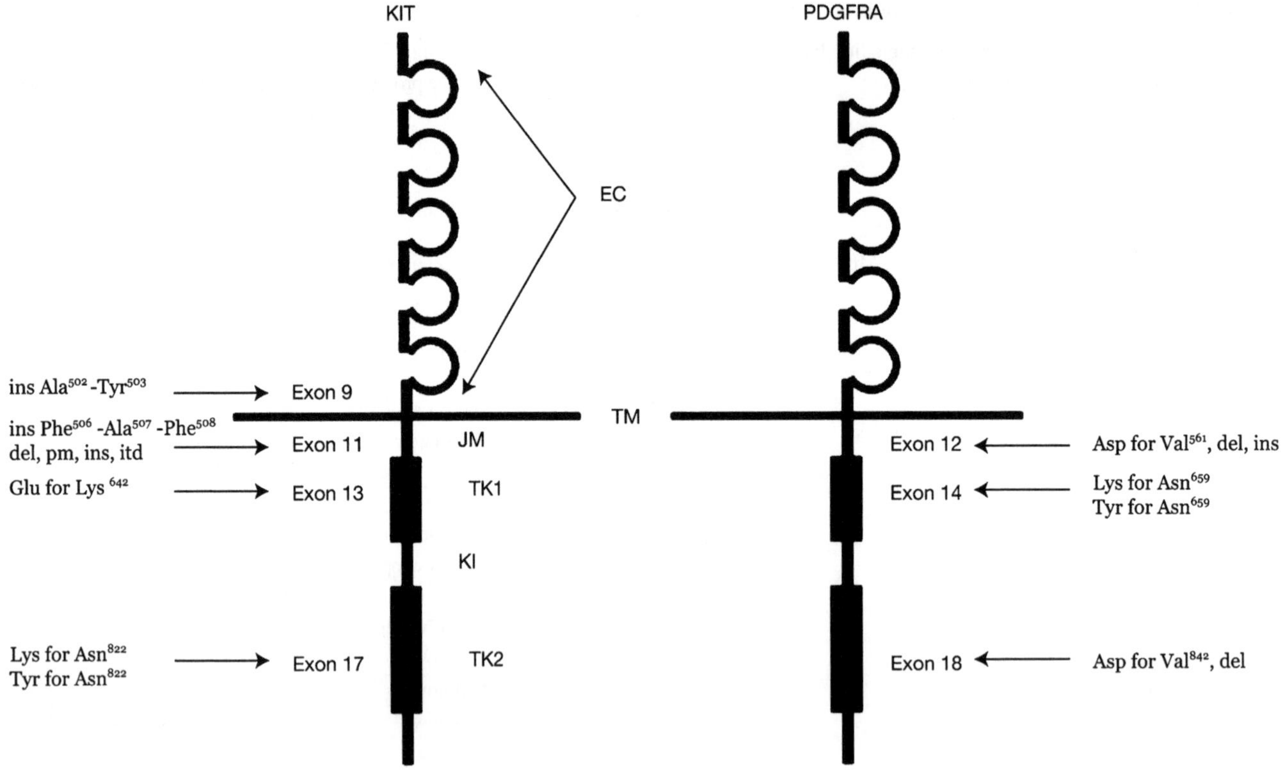

Fig. 11.2 Schematic representation of KIT and platelet-derived growth factor receptor alpha (PDGFRA) molecules and *KIT* and *PDGFRA* mutations in gastrointestinal stromal tumor (GIST), EC-extracellular domain; TM-transmembrane domain; JM-juxtamembrane domain; TK-tyrosine kinase domain. Adapted from Miettinen and Lasota[1]

cases. D842V point mutation (missense mutation) in exon 18 is the most common mutation type.[2,32,66,68]

Mutation or activation of *PDGFRA* or *KIT* is mutually exclusive in untreated GIST.[32,66] Roughly 10% of GISTs do not have a mutation in either *KIT* or *PDGFRA*. Figure 11.2 depicts the involved exons and common mutations in *KIT* and *PDGFRA*[1] that have been observed in GISTs. The non-gastrointestinal GISTs have similar patterns of *KIT* and *PDGFRA* mutations but at a lower frequency.[69]

Molecular and Genetic Aberrations Other than KIT or PDGFRA

The *KIT* and *PDGFRA* mutations are an early event in GIST development and important to its oncogenesis. However, these mutations seem to have little critical impact in malignant transformation.[2,70] Additional genetic hits are now known to have more significance in determining the tumor's clinical behavior. Either monosomy 14 or partial loss of 14q has been demonstrated in two-thirds of *KIT* or *PDGFRA* mutant GISTs.[71,72] In these cases, 14q11.1–14q22–24 has been identified to be hot spots for deletions and represent likely sites for important tumor-suppressor genes that play a role in preventing GIST formation.[73–76] Loss of the long arm of chromosome 22 is observed in 50% of GISTs and is associated with progression to a borderline or malignant lesion.[72,77] Other abnormalities less frequently observed are losses on chromosomes 1p, 9p, 11p, 13q, 17q, and 15q and gains on chromosomes 8q and 17q, which have been associated with malignant behavior.[71,75,78,79] One of the genes in 9p is *CDKN2A* (*p16 ink4A*), which is inactivated by several mechanisms in GISTs.[80]

According to these findings, a sequence of oncogenic events in GISTs has been suggested as follows: *KIT* or *PDGFRA* mutation –>14q deletion-22q deletion –> 1p deletion -8q gain-11p deletion- 9p deletion –> 17q gain.[49] A recent study using high-resolution CGH genomic analysis has proposed a tumor-progression genetic staging system (Genomic Instability Staging/GIS) in GISTs which were shown to progress from GIS 1 with deletion of distal 1p, 19, and 22q, to GIS 2 with deletion of 14q, then GIS 3 with deletions of proximal 1p and 15q and GIS 4 with loss of chromosome 10.[81]

In addition to *KIT* and *PDGFAR*, other genes known to have roles in proliferation and maintenance of the ICCs are also involved in GIST. ETV1 is a transcription factor that belongs to the ETS family. Structural alterations or amplification of *ETV1*, located at 7p21.3, have been implicated in EWS, prostate cancer, and melanoma.[82–84] Recently,

ETV1 has been shown to be selectively expressed in myenteric ICCs and intramuscular ICCs of the bowel and to be highly expressed in all GISTs.[85] Chi et al showed that ETV1 was selectively required for development of myenteric and intramuscular ICCs which give rise to GIST, and there was dual requirement of KIT and ETV1 in normal ICC development and GIST survival.[85] However, the oncologic role of *ETV1* in GIST is different from other ETV1 driven tumors as there are no abnormal aberrations in *ETV1* in GIST. Rather, the ETV1 expression in GIST is considered inherited from myenteric and intramuscular ICCs, for which ETV1 is also a survival factor. ETV1 therefore has been implicated as a lineage-specific survival factor for the ICC-GIST lineage and efforts to find ETV1 inhibitors for treating imatinib resistant GISTs are currently underway.[85] Hox11L1 gene, located on chromosome 2, has a role in proliferation of neuronal myenteric Cajal cells. Homozygous loss of the *Hox11L1* gene has been found in 10% of the GISTs and this is associated with more aggressive behavior.[86] Protein kinase C theta (PKC-theta) is a serine/threonine kinase which belongs to the PKC superfamily composed of at least 11 related protein kinases.[87] PKC-theta is selectively expressed in ICCs and is strongly activated in most of GISTs.[88–92] PKC-theta knockdown KIT+ GIST cell lines showed antiproliferative effects similar to that seen after direct KIT knockdown. Because of its role in regulating KIT expression and proliferation in GISTs, it likely functions as an oncogene in GIST and represents a new potential therapeutic target.

In addition to genes known to have role in regulating ICCs proliferation, a wide variety of proto-oncogenes and tumor suppressor genes have been found abnormal in GISTs. These include amplification or mutations of *C-MYC*, *MDM2*, *EFGR1*, *RB1*, *E2F1*, *KRAS BRAF*, and *CCND1*[73,93–95] and loss/down regulation or mutations of various tumor-suppressor genes such as *p16*, *p27*, *p53*, *RKIP*, *PARP2*, *APEX1*, *NF2*, and *NDRG2*.[71,73,96–98] Mutations in *BRAF*, an oncogene frequently mutated in many other tumors such as melanoma and papillary thyroid cancer, typically involve exon 15 (V600E) in 7% of the adult GISTs with wild-type *KIT* and *PDGFRA*.[94] The *BRAF* mutated, *KIT* wild-type tumors tend to locate in small bowel in female patients with high risk of malignancy. The abnormal expression of these proto-oncogenes and tumor suppressor genes has been shown to be associated with more aggressive behavior in GISTs.

KIT and *PDGFRA*-Targeted Therapy

Tumors with *KIT* exon 11 mutations are most frequent in low-risk group GISTs and show the highest (80%) imatinib response rate. Tumors with Exon 9 have the lower imatinib response (<50%) and D816V point mutations in exon 17 are also responsible for poor response to imatinib. *PDGFRA* exon 18 mutation (D842V) is less responsive to imatinib.[32,35,99]

As the effectiveness of imatinib depends on the specific type of *KIT* and *PDGRA* mutations, molecular testing to determine the mutation type can predict the therapeutic response of GISTs to imatinib treatment and has been used clinically to guide targeted therapy.[2]

Secondary Mutations and Development of Imatinib Resistance

Tumor progression within the first 6 months of imatinib treatment is referred to as primary resistance. Secondary resistance refers to tumor progression after 12–36 months in patients who initially show good response or stable disease after the treatment.[2,100] Secondary resistance is usually a result of secondary mutations in the *KIT* kinase domain and rarely *KIT*/*PDFGRA* genomic amplification and activation of alternative oncogenes.[100–102] Secondary mutations and overexpression or amplification of *KIT* or *PDGFRA* are generally referred as "target resistance" and resistance mechanisms resulting from other newly activated systems are generally referred to as "biological resistance" where *KIT* expression has disappeared and tumors show the morphological appearance of rhabdomyoblastic differentiation.[100,103] Secondary resistance mutations have been reported in 44–83% of GISTs progressing after imatinib therapy.[33,34, 36] In addition to the primary mutations, tumor cells gain second novel kinase mutations in the same or different alleles of *KIT* in exons 13, 14, 17, and 18. These second mutations are nonrandomly distributed and are associated with decreased sensitivity or binding to imatinib as compared to typical primary exon 11 mutations. These imatinib-resistant GIST cells remain dependent upon KIT kinase activity for activation of downstream signaling pathways. The most common secondary mutation in patients with primary KIT exon 11 mutant GISTs is 1982 T-C (V654A) point mutation in the ATP-binding pocket in kinase domain I (exon 13), which is novel and only seen in imatinib-treated tumors with aggressive behavior.[33,38,104] Sunitinib, a second-line tyrosinase kinase inhibitor after imatinib failure, has been shown to be effective against secondary mutations located in the ATP-binding pocket (exons 13 and 14) but not the kinase activation loop (exons 17 and 18).[61,105,106] Various other kinase inhibitors have also recently been evaluated to treat imatinib resistant GISTs.[107] As either imatinib-sensitive or imatinib-resistant GIST cells were recently shown to require ETV1 for survival, efforts to find ETV1 inhibitors are currently underway to identify novel therapeutic agents for imatinib-resistant GIST.

Secondary *PDGFRA* mutation is significantly less frequent than *KIT* mutation and has been reported in exons 14 and 18 (H687Y and D842Y).[37,101] Although primary *KIT* and *PDGFRA* mutations are known to be mutually exclusive in untreated GISTs, secondary *PDFGRA* mutations have been reported in GISTs with primary *KIT* mutation after imatinib treatment.[37] In addition to secondary mutations, "Kinase switch" from *KIT* to *AXL* which shows no binding to imatinib and amplification and activation of other *RTKS* with loss of KIT oncoprotein expression have been also implicated in tumors that developed imatinib resistance.[11,100] *BRAF* V600E mutation, in addition to occur as a primary mutation in some of the *KIT* wild type GISTs, was also found rarely as secondary mutation responsible for imatinib resistance.[94]

Correlation of *KIT/PDGFRA* Mutation Types and Clinicopathological Characteristics in Sporadic GISTs (Table 11.2)

In addition to their major role in GIST oncogenesis and as a target for tyrosine kinase inhibitors, various specific *KIT/PDFGRA* mutations are also associated with various specific clinicopathological features of these tumors.

KIT Mutations

GISTs with *KIT* mutations frequently show spindle morphology and have high levels of KIT expression. Some studies have shown that deletion mutations in and around exon 11 codon 557–558 were adverse prognostic factors compared to point mutation in exon 11[25] in gastric GISTs but showed no difference in progression-free survival or overall survival between patients with KIT exon 11 point mutations and deletions in other GISTs.[35] Tandem repeat mutations in the distal part of exon 11 were mainly seen in female gastric GISTs and associated with a quite indolent course.[108] Exon 9 mutations preferentially occur in small bowel GIST. In addition to a low imatinib response, tumors with exon 9 mutations are more aggressive than tumors with exon 11.[109] In gastric GIST, tumors with exon 13 mutations predict a more aggressive course.[62] Additionally, detection of more than one mutation in different alleles is associated with more aggressive features.[65]

PDGFRA mutations

PDGFRA mutations occur preferentially in GISTs located in gastric, omental, and peritoneal sites. Tumors with *PDGFRA* mutations tend to show epithelioid morphology (epithelioid GIST). On immunohistochemistry, tumors with *PDFGRA* mutations have lower or no KIT expression and show higher PDFGRA expression. Clinically, tumors with *PDGFRA* mutation have lower malignant behavior with more favorable clinical course. Tumors with a D842Vmutation in exon 18 are resistant to imatinib and sunitinib.[32,35,99]

Gene Expression Profiles

The status of *KIT/PDGFRA* mutations is known to affect the global gene expression profiles in GISTs, which is different from those of other mesenchymal tumors.[110] Microarray global gene expression analyses have shown that the gene expression profiles of *KIT*-mutated GISTs are homogeneous and tightly clustered with *KIT* as the prominent or highest ranked discriminator. Closely included in the GIST-associated expression cluster were the gene for protein kinase C theta (PKCTeta) and members of the superfamily of adenosine triphosphate-binding cassette transporters (ABCB1 and ABCC3), bcl-2, Sprouty 1, Sprouty 4, and G-coupled receptor (GPR20). Gene profiling has also been shown to be able to distinguish site and the grade of GISTs.[111]

FLJ10261, a gene highly expressed in GIST and encoding a novel protein with unknown function, was identified through

Table 11.2 *KIT* and *PDGFR* mutations and their significance in gastrointestinal stromal tumors

Gene	Specific aberrations	Potential clinical significance	Imatinib response
KIT	Exon 11 deletions	Independent adverse prognostic factor in patients with GISTs (preimatinib)	>80%
	Exon 11 mutations	Independent predictors for disease-free survival, mixed histologic pattern; more frequent liver metastasis; poor prognosis for gastric GISTs (preimatinib)	
	Exon 11 duplication	Gastric GISTs	
	Exon 9 mutations	Small intestinal GISTs	<50%
	Exon 13	More aggressive clinical course	Response in vitro, clinical response observed
	Exon 17		Response in vitro, clinical response observed
	LOH	Possible role in liver metastasis	
PDGFR	Exon 18 (D842V)		Imatinib resistance
Wild type			Poor

gene expression analyses in GIST. It was subsequently named as TMEM16A or DOG-1 (discovered on GIST 1).[112] Immunohistochemical detection of DOG1 has been used as a very sensitive and specific diagnostic marker for GIST.[113]

GIST Tumor Syndromes

It has been estimated that less than 5% of GIST are associated with 1 of 3 tumor syndromes: neurofibromatosis type 1, Carney Triad/Carney-Stratakis dyad, and familial GIST syndrome, in order of decreasing frequency[1].

Hereditary GIST Tumor syndromes

Familial GISTs due to heritable mutations in *KIT* and *PDGFRA* are very rare. Several kindreds have been reported to have heritable germline mutations in exon 11 (W557R, delv559, or V559A), rarely exon 13 (K642E) and exon 17 (D820Y).[114–116] Affected individuals had multiple GISTs usually in adulthood. In addition, patients with exon 11 mutations were also reported to show skin pigmentation, urticaria pigmentosa and mastocytosis, suggesting that the same mutations might also affect melanogenesis and mast cell proliferation.[114,117] Familial GISTs are likely low malignant risk tumors as < 20% of the patients with familial GIST die of the disease.[118]

A study showed that 6% of duodenal GIST patients had neurofibromatosis[119] and another study showed that 7% of NF1 patients had GISTs.[120] In these cases, GISTs are usually multiple in small bowel and occur in early adulthood. No *KIT or PDGFRA* mutations are identified in the majority of patients, with only rare exceptions.[121,122] The disease seems to involve a pathogenesis different from that of sporadic GISTs and tumors are usually of low risk for malignancy.[123]

Malignant GIST–paraganglioma syndrome (Carney–Stratakis dyad) is composed of multiple paragangliomas and gastric GISTs. The disease usually develops in young adults and affects males and females equally.[124] The disease is autosomal dominant with germline mutations found in three genes called *SDHB*, *SDHC*, and *SDHD*. No *KIT* or *PDGFRA* mutations are identified in the associated GIST tumors.

Nonhereditary GIST syndrome

Carney Triad (GIST–pulmonary chondroma–paraganglioma syndrome) is very rare and accounts for <1% of all GIST cases. It does not have *KIT*, *PDGFRA*, or *SDH* mutations and its genetic basis is not known currently. Likely it is sporadic rather than familial. It usually presents as multiple GISTs with frequent lymph node metastasis in younger age. Different from the hereditary Carney–Stratakis dyad, Carney triad affects younger age females more frequently (male:female=1:6).[125,126] The behavior of GISTs in Carney Triad is not predictable by usual GIST risk factors and these GISTs neither respond to chemotherapy and radiation nor have consistent response to imatinib.[125,126]

Pediatric GISTs

Approximately 1–2% of GISTs occur in pediatric patients. Pediatric GISTs have a marked female predominance with stomach as the preferential location and frequently show lymph node metastasis. Pediatric GISTs are nearly all wild type for either *KIT* or *PDGFRA* suggesting a different oncogenic event in these tumors. The possibility of Carney triad should be considered in these patients. In general, pediatric GISTs are resistant to imatinib but respond to sunitinib.[127,128]

Immunohistochemical Detection of KIT Expression in GIST

Overall 95% of the GISTs exhibit KIT immunostaining. The majority of *KIT*-mutated GISTs have detectable KIT expression by immunohistochemical methods on paraffin sections (Fig. 11.1), but *PDGFRA*-mutated GISTs tend to be KIT negative.[1,2,12] Immunohistochemical detection of KIT expression has been used routinely in the histologic diagnosis of GIST.[1,2,12,14] The extent and patterns of KIT immunoreactivity generally do not correlate with the type of *KIT* mutations and the likelihood of response to imatinib.[2] As GISTs with negative or poor KIT immunoreactivity are more likely *KIT* wild type, KIT immunostaining on routine surgical pathology specimen has also been used to guide kinase inhibitor therapy clinically when molecular tests are not available. Treatment responses have been associated with alterations in immunohistochemical staining patterns; KIT positive GISTs may lose KIT immunoreactivity after imatinib treatment and become imatinib resistant.[100,103]

However, a negative KIT immunostaining does not exclude a GIST diagnosis or indicate imatinib resistance as some immunohistochemically KIT negative GISTs would still have mutations in either *KIT* or the *PDGFRA* gene. Molecular screening for *KIT* and *PDGFRA* mutations should be used when available to determine tumor response to imatinib therapy. In addition to KIT, immunodetection of DOG1 has been recently used to diagnose GIST in routine clinical practice.[113] Immunodetection of other markers such as PKC-theta and ETV1 has also been shown to have potential value in diagnosing KIT negative GISTs.[85,88]

References

1. Miettinen M, Lasota J. Gastrointestinal stromal tumors: review on morphology, molecular pathology, prognosis, and differential diagnosis. *Arch Pathol Lab Med*. 2006;130:1466–78.
2. Liegl-Atzwanger B, Fletcher JA, Fletcher CD. Gastrointestinal stromal tumors. *Virchows Arch*. 2010;456:111–27.
3. Mazur MT, Clark HB. Gastric stromal tumors. Reappraisal of histogenesis. *Am J Surg Pathol*. 1983;7:507–19.
4. Tworek JA, Goldblum JR, Weiss SW, Greenson JK, Appelman HD. Stromal tumors of the anorectum: a clinicopathologic study of 22 cases. *Am J Surg Pathol*. 1999;23:946–54.
5. Miettinen M, Sarlomo-Rikala M, Sobin LH, Lasota J. Esophageal stromal tumors: a clinicopathologic, immunohistochemical, and molecular genetic study of 17 cases and comparison with esophageal leiomyomas and leiomyosarcomas. *Am J Surg Pathol*. 2000;24:211–22.
6. Tworek JA, Goldblum JR, Weiss SW, Greenson JK, Appelman HD. Stromal tumors of the abdominal colon: a clinicopathologic study of 20 cases. *Am J Surg Pathol*. 1999;23:937–45.
7. Brainard JA, Goldblum JR. Stromal tumors of the jejunum and ileum: a clinicopathologic study of 39 cases. *Am J Surg Pathol*. 1997;21:407–16.
8. Haque S, Dean PJ. Stromal neoplasms of the rectum and anal canal. *Hum Pathol*. 1992;23:762–7.
9. Ortiz-Hidalgo C, de Leon Bojorge B, Albores-Saavedra J. Stromal tumor of the gallbladder with phenotype of interstitial cells of Cajal: a previously unrecognized neoplasm. *Am J Surg Pathol*. 2000;24:1420–3.
10. Sakurai S, Hishima T, Takazawa Y, et al. Gastrointestinal stromal tumors and KIT-positive mesenchymal cells in the omentum. *Pathol Int*. 2001;51:524–31.
11. Corless CL, Fletcher JA, Heinrich MC. Biology of gastrointestinal stromal tumors. *J Clin Oncol*. 2004;22:3813–25.
12. Miettinen M, Sobin LH, Sarlomo-Rikala M. Immunohistochemical spectrum of GISTs at different sites and their differential diagnosis with a reference to CD117 (KIT). *Mod Pathol*. 2000;13:1134–42.
13. Miettinen M, Virolainen M. Maarit Sarlomo R. Gastrointestinal stromal tumors–value of CD34 antigen in their identification and separation from true leiomyomas and schwannomas. *Am J Surg Pathol*. 1995;19:207–16.
14. Hornick JL, Fletcher CD. Immunohistochemical staining for KIT (CD117) in soft tissue sarcomas is very limited in distribution. *Am J Clin Pathol*. 2002;117:188–93.
15. Perez-Atayde AR, Shamberger RC, Kozakewich HW. Neuroectodermal differentiation of the gastrointestinal tumors in the Carney triad. An ultrastructural and immunohistochemical study. *Am J Surg Pathol*. 1993;17:706–14.
16. Kindblom LG, Remotti HE, Aldenborg F, Meis-Kindblom JM. Gastrointestinal pacemaker cell tumor (GIPACT): gastrointestinal stromal tumors show phenotypic characteristics of the interstitial cells of Cajal. *Am J Pathol*. 1998;152:1259–69.
17. Huizinga JD, Thuneberg L, Kluppel M, Malysz J, Mikkelsen HB, Bernstein A. W/kit gene required for interstitial cells of Cajal and for intestinal pacemaker activity. *Nature*. 1995;373:347–9.
18. Hirota S, Isozaki K, Moriyama Y, et al. Gain-of-function mutations of c-kit in human gastrointestinal stromal tumors. *Science*. 1998;279:577–80.
19. Heinrich MC, Blanke CD, Druker BJ, Corless CL. Inhibition of KIT tyrosine kinase activity: a novel molecular approach to the treatment of KIT-positive malignancies. *J Clin Oncol*. 2002;20:1692–703.
20. Druker BJ, Tamura S, Buchdunger E, et al. Effects of a selective inhibitor of the Abl tyrosine kinase on the growth of Bcr-Abl positive cells. *Nat Med*. 1996;2:561–6.
21. Fletcher CD, Berman JJ, Corless C, et al. Diagnosis of gastrointestinal stromal tumors: a consensus approach. *Hum Pathol*. 2002;33:459–65.
22. Dematteo RP, Gold JS, Saran L, et al. Tumor mitotic rate, size, and location independently predict recurrence after resection of primary gastrointestinal stromal tumor (GIST). *Cancer*. 2008;112:608–15.
23. Miettinen M, Makhlouf H, Sobin LH, Lasota J. Gastrointestinal stromal tumors of the jejunum and ileum: a clinicopathologic, immunohistochemical, and molecular genetic study of 906 cases before imatinib with long-term follow-up. *Am J Surg Pathol*. 2006;30:477–89.
24. Emory TS, Sobin LH, Lukes L, Lee DH, O'Leary TJ. Prognosis of gastrointestinal smooth-muscle (stromal) tumors: dependence on anatomic site. *Am J Surg Pathol*. 1999;23:82–7.
25. Miettinen M, Sobin LH, Lasota J. Gastrointestinal stromal tumors of the stomach: a clinicopathologic, immunohistochemical, and molecular genetic study of 1765 cases with long-term follow-up. *Am J Surg Pathol*. 2005;29:52–68.
26. DeMatteo RP, Lewis JJ, Leung D, Mudan SS, Woodruff JM, Brennan MF. Two hundred gastrointestinal stromal tumors: recurrence patterns and prognostic factors for survival. *Ann Surg*. 2000;231:51–8.
27. Hasegawa T, Matsuno Y, Shimoda T, Hirohashi S. Gastrointestinal stromal tumor: consistent CD117 immunostaining for diagnosis, and prognostic classification based on tumor size and MIB-1 grade. *Hum Pathol*. 2002;33:669–76.
28. Judson I. Gastrointestinal stromal tumours (GIST): biology and treatment. *Ann Oncol*. 2002;13(Suppl 4):287–9.
29. Druker BJ, Lydon NB. Lessons learned from the development of an abl tyrosine kinase inhibitor for chronic myelogenous leukemia. *J Clin Invest*. 2000;105:3–7.
30. Joensuu H, Roberts PJ, Sarlomo-Rikala M, et al. Effect of the tyrosine kinase inhibitor STI571 in a patient with a metastatic gastrointestinal stromal tumor. *N Engl J Med*. 2001;344:1052–6.
31. Demetri GD, von Mehren M, Blanke CD, et al. Efficacy and safety of imatinib mesylate in advanced gastrointestinal stromal tumors. *N Engl J Med*. 2002;347:472–80.
32. Heinrich MC, Corless CL, Demetri GD, et al. Kinase mutations and imatinib response in patients with metastatic gastrointestinal stromal tumor. *J Clin Oncol*. 2003;21:4342–9.
33. Heinrich MC, Corless CL, Blanke CD, et al. Molecular correlates of imatinib resistance in gastrointestinal stromal tumors. *J Clin Oncol*. 2006;24:4764–74.
34. Agaram NP, Besmer P, Wong GC, et al. Pathologic and molecular heterogeneity in imatinib-stable or imatinib-responsive gastrointestinal stromal tumors. *Clin Cancer Res*. 2007;13:170–81.
35. Debiec-Rychter M, Sciot R, Le Cesne A, et al. KIT mutations and dose selection for imatinib in patients with advanced gastrointestinal stromal tumours. *Eur J Cancer*. 2006;42:1093–103.
36. Wardelmann E, Merkelbach-Bruse S, Pauls K, et al. Polyclonal evolution of multiple secondary KIT mutations in gastrointestinal stromal tumors under treatment with imatinib mesylate. *Clin Cancer Res*. 2006;12:1743–9.
37. Lim KH, Huang MJ, Chen LT, et al. Molecular analysis of secondary kinase mutations in imatinib-resistant gastrointestinal stromal tumors. *Med Oncol*. 2008;25:207–13.
38. Antonescu CR, Besmer P, Guo T, et al. Acquired resistance to imatinib in gastrointestinal stromal tumor occurs through secondary gene mutation. *Clin Cancer Res*. 2005;11:4182–90.
39. Prenen H, Cools J, Mentens N, et al. Efficacy of the kinase inhibitor SU11248 against gastrointestinal stromal tumor mutants refractory to imatinib mesylate. *Clin Cancer Res*. 2006;12:2622–7.
40. Stenman G, Eriksson A, Claesson-Welsh L. Human PDGFA receptor gene maps to the same region on chromosome 4 as the KIT oncogene. *Genes Chromosomes Cancer*. 1989;1:155–8.

41. Pawson T. Regulation and targets of receptor tyrosine kinases. *Eur J Cancer*. 2002;38(Suppl 5):S3–10.
42. Geissler EN, Liao M, Brook JD, et al. Stem cell factor (SCF), a novel hematopoietic growth factor and ligand for c-kit tyrosine kinase receptor, maps on human chromosome 12 between 12q14.3 and 12qter. *Somat Cell Mol Genet*. 1991;17:207–14.
43. Lev S, Blechman J, Nishikawa S, Givol D, Yarden Y. Interspecies molecular chimeras of kit help define the binding site of the stem cell factor. *Mol Cell Biol*. 1993;13:2224–34.
44. Sattler M, Salgia R, Shrikhande G, et al. Steel factor induces tyrosine phosphorylation of CRKL and binding of CRKL to a complex containing c-kit, phosphatidylinositol 3-kinase, and p120(CBL). *J Biol Chem*. 1997;272:10248–53.
45. Hubbard SR. Juxtamembrane autoinhibition in receptor tyrosine kinases. *Nat Rev Mol Cell Biol*. 2004;5:464–71.
46. Maeda H, Yamagata A, Nishikawa S, Yoshinaga K, Kobayashi S, Nishi K. Requirement of c-kit for development of intestinal pacemaker system. *Development*. 1992;116:369–75.
47. Blume-Jensen P, Claesson-Welsh L, Siegbahn A, Zsebo KM, Westermark B, Heldin CH. Activation of the human c-kit product by ligand-induced dimerization mediates circular actin reorganization and chemotaxis. *EMBO J*. 1991;10:4121–8.
48. Nocka K, Majumder S, Chabot B, et al. Expression of c-kit gene products in known cellular targets of W mutations in normal and W mutant mice–evidence for an impaired c-kit kinase in mutant mice. *Genes Dev*. 1989;3:816–26.
49. Heinrich MC, Rubin BP, Longley BJ, Fletcher JA. Biology and genetic aspects of gastrointestinal stromal tumors: KIT activation and cytogenetic alterations. *Hum Pathol*. 2002;33:484–95.
50. Ogasawara N, Tsukamoto T, Inada K, et al. Frequent c-Kit gene mutations not only in gastrointestinal stromal tumors but also in interstitial cells of Cajal in surrounding normal mucosa. *Cancer Lett*. 2005;230:199–210.
51. Yang J, Du X, Lazar AJ, et al. Genetic aberrations of gastrointestinal stromal tumors. *Cancer*. 2008;113:1532–43.
52. Longley BJ, Reguera MJ, Ma Y. Classes of c-KIT activating mutations: proposed mechanisms of action and implications for disease classification and therapy. *Leuk Res*. 2001;25:571–6.
53. Ma Y, Cunningham ME, Wang X, Ghosh I, Regan L, Longley BJ. Inhibition of spontaneous receptor phosphorylation by residues in a putative alpha-helix in the KIT intracellular juxtamembrane region. *J Biol Chem*. 1999;274:13399–402.
54. Chan PM, Ilangumaran S, La Rose J, Chakrabartty A, Rottapel R. Autoinhibition of the kit receptor tyrosine kinase by the cytosolic juxtamembrane region. *Mol Cell Biol*. 2003;23:3067–78.
55. Kitayama H, Kanakura Y, Furitsu T, et al. Constitutively activating mutations of c-kit receptor tyrosine kinase confer factor-independent growth and tumorigenicity of factor-dependent hematopoietic cell lines. *Blood*. 1995;85:790–8.
56. Duffaud F, Blay JY. Gastrointestinal stromal tumors: biology and treatment. *Oncology*. 2003;65:187–97.
57. Lasota J, Jasinski M, Sarlomo-Rikala M, Miettinen M. Mutations in exon 11 of c-Kit occur preferentially in malignant versus benign gastrointestinal stromal tumors and do not occur in leiomyomas or leiomyosarcomas. *Am J Pathol*. 1999;154:53–60.
58. Lux ML, Rubin BP, Biase TL, et al. KIT extracellular and kinase domain mutations in gastrointestinal stromal tumors. *Am J Pathol*. 2000;156:791–5.
59. Lasota J, Wozniak A, Sarlomo-Rikala M, et al. Mutations in exons 9 and 13 of KIT gene are rare events in gastrointestinal stromal tumors. A study of 200 cases. *Am J Pathol*. 2000;157:1091–5.
60. Lasota J, Miettinen M. Clinical significance of oncogenic KIT and PDGFRA mutations in gastrointestinal stromal tumours. *Histopathology*. 2008;53:245–66.
61. Heinrich MC, Owzar K, Corless CL, et al. Correlation of kinase genotype and clinical outcome in the North American Intergroup Phase III Trial of imatinib mesylate for treatment of advanced gastrointestinal stromal tumor: CALGB 150105 Study by Cancer and Leukemia Group B and Southwest Oncology Group. *J Clin Oncol*. 2008;26:5360–7.
62. Lasota J, Corless CL, Heinrich MC, et al. Clinicopathologic profile of gastrointestinal stromal tumors (GISTs) with primary KIT exon 13 or exon 17 mutations: a multicenter study on 54 cases. *Mod Pathol*. 2008;21:476–84.
63. Rubin BP, Singer S, Tsao C, et al. KIT activation is a ubiquitous feature of gastrointestinal stromal tumors. *Cancer Res*. 2001;61:8118–21.
64. Ichikawa Y, Miyagi Y, Fujii S, et al. Gastrointestinal stromal tumor with two genetic abnormalities on different alleles: report of a case. *Surg Today*. 2010;40:262–6.
65. Duensing A, Medeiros F, McConarty B, et al. Mechanisms of oncogenic KIT signal transduction in primary gastrointestinal stromal tumors (GISTs). *Oncogene*. 2004;23:3999–4006.
66. Heinrich MC, Corless CL, Duensing A, et al. PDGFRA activating mutations in gastrointestinal stromal tumors. *Science*. 2003;299:708–10.
67. Hirota S, Ohashi A, Nishida T, et al. Gain-of-function mutations of platelet-derived growth factor receptor alpha gene in gastrointestinal stromal tumors. *Gastroenterology*. 2003;125:660–7.
68. Wardelmann E, Hrychyk A, Merkelbach-Bruse S, et al. Association of platelet-derived growth factor receptor alpha mutations with gastric primary site and epithelioid or mixed cell morphology in gastrointestinal stromal tumors. *J Mol Diagn*. 2004;6:197–204.
69. Yamamoto H, Oda Y, Kawaguchi K, et al. C-kit and PDGFRA mutations in extragastrointestinal stromal tumor (gastrointestinal stromal tumor of the soft tissue). *Am J Surg Pathol*. 2004;28:479–88.
70. Corless CL, McGreevey L, Haley A, Town A, Heinrich MC. KIT mutations are common in incidental gastrointestinal stromal tumors one centimeter or less in size. *Am J Pathol*. 2002;160:1567–72.
71. Fukasawa T, Chong JM, Sakurai S, et al. Allelic loss of 14q and 22q, NF2 mutation, and genetic instability occur independently of c-kit mutation in gastrointestinal stromal tumor. *Jpn J Cancer Res*. 2000;91:1241–9.
72. Debiec-Rychter M, Lasota J, Sarlomo-Rikala M, Kordek R, Miettinen M. Chromosomal aberrations in malignant gastrointestinal stromal tumors: correlation with c-KIT gene mutation. *Cancer Genet Cytogenet*. 2001;128:24–30.
73. Astolfi A, Nannini M, Pantaleo MA, et al. A molecular portrait of gastrointestinal stromal tumors: an integrative analysis of gene expression profiling and high-resolution genomic copy number. *Lab Invest*. 2010;90:1285–94.
74. Wozniak A, Sciot R, Guillou L, et al. Array CGH analysis in primary gastrointestinal stromal tumors: cytogenetic profile correlates with anatomic site and tumor aggressiveness, irrespective of mutational status. *Genes Chromosomes Cancer*. 2007;46:261–76.
75. el-Rifai W, Sarlomo-Rikala M, Miettinen M, Knuutila S, Andersson LC. DNA copy number losses in chromosome 14: an early change in gastrointestinal stromal tumors. *Cancer Res*. 1996;56:3230–3.
76. El-Rifai W, Sarlomo-Rikala M, Andersson LC, Miettinen M, Knuutila S. High-resolution deletion mapping of chromosome 14 in stromal tumors of the gastrointestinal tract suggests two distinct tumor suppressor loci. *Genes Chromosomes Cancer*. 2000;27:387–91.
77. Kim NG, Kim JJ, Ahn JY, et al. Putative chromosomal deletions on 9P, 9Q and 22Q occur preferentially in malignant gastrointestinal stromal tumors. *Int J Cancer*. 2000;85:633–8.
78. Lasota J, Vel Dobosz AJ, Wasag B, et al. Presence of homozygous KIT exon 11 mutations is strongly associated with malignant clinical behavior in gastrointestinal stromal tumors. *Lab Invest*. 2007;87:1029–41.
79. Schurr P, Wolter S, Kaifi J, et al. Microsatellite DNA alterations of gastrointestinal stromal tumors are predictive for outcome. *Clin Cancer Res*. 2006;12:5151–7.

80. Zhang Y, Cao H, Wang M, et al. Loss of chromosome 9p21 and decreased p16 expression correlate with malignant gastrointestinal stromal tumor. *World J Gastroenterol*. 2010;16:4716–24.
81. Ylipaa A, Hunt KK, Yang J, et al. Integrative genomic characterization and a genomic staging system for gastrointestinal stromal tumors. *Cancer*. 2010;117:380–9.
82. Jane-Valbuena J, Widlund HR, Perner S, et al. An oncogenic role for ETV1 in melanoma. *Cancer Res*. 2010;70:2075–84.
83. Jeon IS, Davis JN, Braun BS, et al. A variant Ewing's sarcoma translocation (7;22) fuses the EWS gene to the ETS gene ETV1. *Oncogene*. 1995;10:1229–34.
84. Hermans KG, van Marion R, van Dekken H, Jenster G, van Weerden WM, Trapman J. TMPRSS2:ERG fusion by translocation or interstitial deletion is highly relevant in androgen-dependent prostate cancer, but is bypassed in late-stage androgen receptor-negative prostate cancer. *Cancer Res*. 2006;66:10658–63.
85. Chi P, Chen Y, Zhang L, et al. ETV1 is a lineage survival factor that cooperates with KIT in gastrointestinal stromal tumours. *Nature*. 2010;467:849–53.
86. Kaifi JT, Wagner M, Schurr PG, et al. Allelic loss of Hox11L1 gene locus predicts outcome of gastrointestinal stromal tumors. *Oncol Rep*. 2006;16:915–9.
87. Mellor H, Parker PJ. The extended protein kinase C superfamily. *Biochem J*. 1998;332(Pt 2):281–92.
88. Blay P, Astudillo A, Buesa JM, et al. Protein kinase C theta is highly expressed in gastrointestinal stromal tumors but not in other mesenchymal neoplasias. *Clin Cancer Res*. 2004;10:4089–95.
89. Ou WB, Zhu MJ, Demetri GD, Fletcher CD, Fletcher JA. Protein kinase C-theta regulates KIT expression and proliferation in gastrointestinal stromal tumors. *Oncogene*. 2008;27:5624–34.
90. Southwell BR. Localization of protein kinase C theta immunoreactivity to interstitial cells of Cajal in guinea-pig gastrointestinal tract. *Neurogastroenterol Motil*. 2003;15:139–47.
91. Poole DP, Van Nguyen T, Kawai M, Furness JB. Protein kinases expressed by interstitial cells of Cajal. *Histochem Cell Biol*. 2004;121:21–30.
92. Duensing A, Joseph NE, Medeiros F, et al. Protein Kinase C theta (PKCtheta) expression and constitutive activation in gastrointestinal stromal tumors (GISTs). *Cancer Res*. 2004;64:5127–31.
93. Tornillo L, Duchini G, Carafa V, et al. Patterns of gene amplification in gastrointestinal stromal tumors (GIST). *Lab Invest*. 2005;85:921–31.
94. Agaram NP, Wong GC, Guo T, et al. Novel V600E BRAF mutations in imatinib-naive and imatinib-resistant gastrointestinal stromal tumors. *Genes Chromosomes Cancer*. 2008;47:853–9.
95. Haller F, Gunawan B, von Heydebreck A, et al. Prognostic role of E2F1 and members of the CDKN2A network in gastrointestinal stromal tumors. *Clin Cancer Res*. 2005;11:6589–97.
96. Martinho O, Gouveia A, Silva P, Pimenta A, Reis RM, Lopes JM. Loss of RKIP expression is associated with poor survival in GISTs. *Virchows Arch*. 2009;455:277–84.
97. Ryu T, Lee H, Kim T, et al. p53 mutations as a determinant of prognosis in GIST patients treated imatinib mesylate. *J Clin Oncol*. 2005;23(16S):9018. ASCO Annual Meeting Proceedings.
98. Schmieder M, Wolf S, Danner B, et al. p16 expression differentiates high-risk gastrointestinal stromal tumor and predicts poor outcome. *Neoplasia*. 2008;10:1154–62.
99. Corless CL, Schroeder A, Griffith D, et al. PDGFRA mutations in gastrointestinal stromal tumors: frequency, spectrum and in vitro sensitivity to imatinib. *J Clin Oncol*. 2005;23:5357–64.
100. Nishida T, Takahashi T, Miyazaki Y. Gastrointestinal stromal tumor: a bridge between bench and bedside. *Gastric Cancer*. 2009;12:175–88.
101. Debiec-Rychter M, Cools J, Dumez H, et al. Mechanisms of resistance to imatinib mesylate in gastrointestinal stromal tumors and activity of the PKC412 inhibitor against imatinib-resistant mutants. *Gastroenterology*. 2005;128:270–9.
102. Liegl B, Kepten I, Le C, et al. Heterogeneity of kinase inhibitor resistance mechanisms in GIST. *J Pathol*. 2008;216:64–74.
103. Liegl B, Hornick JL, Antonescu CR, Corless CL, Fletcher CD. Rhabdomyosarcomatous differentiation in gastrointestinal stromal tumors after tyrosine kinase inhibitor therapy: a novel form of tumor progression. *Am J Surg Pathol*. 2009;33:218–26.
104. Chen LL, Trent JC, Wu EF, et al. A missense mutation in KIT kinase domain 1 correlates with imatinib resistance in gastrointestinal stromal tumors. *Cancer Res*. 2004;64:5913–9.
105. Heinrich MC, Maki RG, Corless CL, et al. Primary and secondary kinase genotypes correlate with the biological and clinical activity of sunitinib in imatinib-resistant gastrointestinal stromal tumor. *J Clin Oncol*. 2008;26:5352–9.
106. George S. Sunitinib, a multitargeted tyrosine kinase inhibitor, in the management of gastrointestinal stromal tumor. *Curr Oncol Rep*. 2007;9:323–7.
107. Guo T, Agaram NP, Wong GC, et al. Sorafenib inhibits the imatinib-resistant KITT670I gatekeeper mutation in gastrointestinal stromal tumor. *Clin Cancer Res*. 2007;13:4874–81.
108. Lasota J, Dansonka-Mieszkowska A, Stachura T, et al. Gastrointestinal stromal tumors with internal tandem duplications in 3' end of KIT juxtamembrane domain occur predominantly in stomach and generally seem to have a favorable course. *Mod Pathol*. 2003;16:1257–64.
109. Antonescu CR, Sommer G, Sarran L, et al. Association of KIT exon 9 mutations with nongastric primary site and aggressive behavior: KIT mutation analysis and clinical correlates of 120 gastrointestinal stromal tumors. *Clin Cancer Res*. 2003;9:3329–37.
110. Nielsen TO, West RB, Linn SC, et al. Molecular characterisation of soft tissue tumours: a gene expression study. *Lancet*. 2002;359:1301–7.
111. Yamaguchi U, Nakayama R, Honda K, et al. Distinct gene expression-defined classes of gastrointestinal stromal tumor. *J Clin Oncol*. 2008;26:4100–8.
112. West RB, Corless CL, Chen X, et al. The novel marker, DOG1, is expressed ubiquitously in gastrointestinal stromal tumors irrespective of KIT or PDGFRA mutation status. *Am J Pathol*. 2004;165:107–13.
113. Espinosa I, Lee CH, Kim MK, et al. A novel monoclonal antibody against DOG1 is a sensitive and specific marker for gastrointestinal stromal tumors. *Am J Surg Pathol*. 2008;32:210–8.
114. Beghini A, Tibiletti MG, Roversi G, et al. Germline mutation in the juxtamembrane domain of the kit gene in a family with gastrointestinal stromal tumors and urticaria pigmentosa. *Cancer*. 2001;92:657–62.
115. Isozaki K, Terris B, Belghiti J, Schiffmann S, Hirota S, Vanderwinden JM. Germline-activating mutation in the kinase domain of KIT gene in familial gastrointestinal stromal tumors. *Am J Pathol*. 2000;157:1581–5.
116. Nishida T, Hirota S, Taniguchi M, et al. Familial gastrointestinal stromal tumours with germline mutation of the KIT gene. *Nat Genet*. 1998;19:323–4.
117. Maeyama H, Hidaka E, Ota H, et al. Familial gastrointestinal stromal tumor with hyperpigmentation: association with a germline mutation of the c-kit gene. *Gastroenterology*. 2001;120:210–5.
118. Nishida T, Hirota S, Matsuda H, Kitamura Y. Familial gastrointestinal stromal tumors as a cancer syndrome. *Gann Monogr Cancer Res*. 2004;53:59–66.
119. Miettinen M, Kopczynski J, Makhlouf HR, et al. Gastrointestinal stromal tumors, intramural leiomyomas, and leiomyosarcomas in the duodenum: a clinicopathologic, immunohistochemical, and molecular genetic study of 167 cases. *Am J Surg Pathol*. 2003;27:625–41.

120. Zoller ME, Rembeck B, Oden A, Samuelsson M, Angervall L. Malignant and benign tumors in patients with neurofibromatosis type 1 in a defined Swedish population. *Cancer*. 1997;79:2125–31.
121. Takazawa Y, Sakurai S, Sakuma Y, et al. Gastrointestinal stromal tumors of neurofibromatosis type I (von Recklinghausen's disease). *Am J Surg Pathol*. 2005;29:755–63.
122. Cheng SP, Huang MJ, Yang TL, et al. Neurofibromatosis with gastrointestinal stromal tumors: insights into the association. *Dig Dis Sci*. 2004;49:1165–9.
123. Stewart DR, Corless CL, Rubin BP, et al. Mitotic recombination as evidence of alternative pathogenesis of gastrointestinal stromal tumours in neurofibromatosis type 1. *J Med Genet*. 2007;44:e61.
124. Pasini B, McWhinney SR, Bei T, et al. Clinical and molecular genetics of patients with the Carney-Stratakis syndrome and germline mutations of the genes coding for the succinate dehydrogenase subunits SDHB, SDHC, and SDHD. *Eur J Hum Genet*. 2008;16:79–88.
125. Zhang L, Smyrk TC, Young WF Jr, Stratakis CA, Carney JA. Gastric stromal tumors in Carney triad are different clinically, pathologically, and behaviorally from sporadic gastric gastrointestinal stromal tumors: findings in 104 cases. *Am J Surg Pathol*. 2010;34:53–64.
126. Carney JA. Gastric stromal sarcoma, pulmonary chondroma, and extra-adrenal paraganglioma (Carney Triad): natural history, adrenocortical component, and possible familial occurrence. *Mayo Clin Proc*. 1999;74:543–52.
127. Janeway KA, Albritton KH, Van Den Abbeele AD, et al. Sunitinib treatment in pediatric patients with advanced GIST following failure of imatinib. *Pediatr Blood Cancer*. 2009;52:767–71.
128. Prakash S, Sarran L, Socci N, et al. Gastrointestinal stromal tumors in children and young adults: a clinicopathologic, molecular, and genomic study of 15 cases and review of the literature. *J Pediatr Hematol Oncol*. 2005;27:179–87.

Neuroendocrine Tumors

12

Joseph R. Pisegna

Introduction

Neuroendocrine tumors of the digestive tract share many pathologic and molecular features as well as management approaches. This chapter will focus on neuroendocrine tumors of the pancreas.

Neuroendocrine tumors (NETs) of the pancreas, although previously thought to be relatively rare, are becoming increasingly recognized in clinical practice and continue to pose a significant challenge to both clinicians and pathologists. The diagnosis is facilitated when there is a high index of suspicion based on clinical symptoms, and confirmation can be made by biopsy or cytological sampling and pathological diagnosis. The utility of biochemical testing is a useful adjunct not only for the diagnosis but also for the prognosis and therapeutic follow-up. Over the past decade, there has been significant progress made in the identification of the biology and treatment of NETs. In this chapter, we will review the epidemiology, pathology, and clinical syndromes for the pancreatic neuroendocrine tumors, formerly referred to as pancreatic or islet cell tumors. The latter part of this chapter will focus on the more recent advances in localization modalities and treatment options, especially given the newly FDA-approved chemotherapy for their treatment.

Nomenclature of NETs

As a group, NETs arising in digestive organs can be broken down into two general groups: pancreatic and gastrointestinal neuroendocrine tumors, depending on the site of origin. Pancreatic NETs can be generally divided into two major groups: functional and nonfunctional. Each occurs in relatively equal frequency; however, the former tumors may come to clinical attention sooner and therefore may be detected earlier in the course of the disease. Nonfunctional NETs generally are diagnosed incidentally during abdominal imaging studies unrelated to a clinical syndrome. This distinction is based on the release of biologically active peptides and/or biogenic amines that result in the characteristic syndromes, which will be described in more detail later in this chapter. The functional pancreatic NETs include gastrinomas, insulinomas, glucagonomas, VIPomas, PPomas, somatostatinomas, and some which cannot be characterized biochemically and were previously thought to represent nonsecreting NETs. The latter probably release peptides or biogenic amines which have not been characterized as of yet using either ELISA or RIA and are therefore referred to as nonfunctional NETs. Functional and nonfunctional NETs secrete chromogranins (CGA), neuron-specific enolase (NSE), and ghrelin in varying amounts, which can be measured biochemically. In patients with gastrinoma (see Zollinger Ellison Syndrome), the tumors have been shown to arise in distant sites such as lung, heart, and ovary; however, the majority arise within the duodenum or pancreas. The second general group of NETs arises in the foregut, midgut, and hindgut. The foregut NETs (previously designated as carcinoids) include bronchial carcinoids and the larger group of gastric carcinoids. The midgut carcinoids include tumors arising from the small bowel or right side of the colon. The hindgut carcinoids arise from the distal large bowel and rectum (Fig. 12.1). In general, NETs exhibit biologic and pathologic heterogeneity and there has been previously confusion with regard to their diagnosis. More recently, the use of the term "neuroendocrine tumor" has supplanted the terms previously used such as carcinoids or carcinoid tumor. In approximately a third of patients with NETs, the recent identification of a mutation on the MENIN gene locus 11q13 (occurring in MEN I Syndrome) should be recognized since the natural history of the disease may be different than in patients without this gene mutation (sporadic NETs).

J.R. Pisegna, M.D. (✉)
Chief, Division of Gastroenterology and Hepatology, VA Greater Los Angeles Healthcare System, Bldg 115, Room 316, 11301 Wilshire Blvd, Los Angeles, CA 90073, USA
e-mail: jpisegna@ucla.edu

A.R. Sepulveda and J.P. Lynch (eds.), *Molecular Pathology of Neoplastic Gastrointestinal Diseases*, Molecular Pathology Library 7,
DOI 10.1007/978-1-4614-6015-2_12,

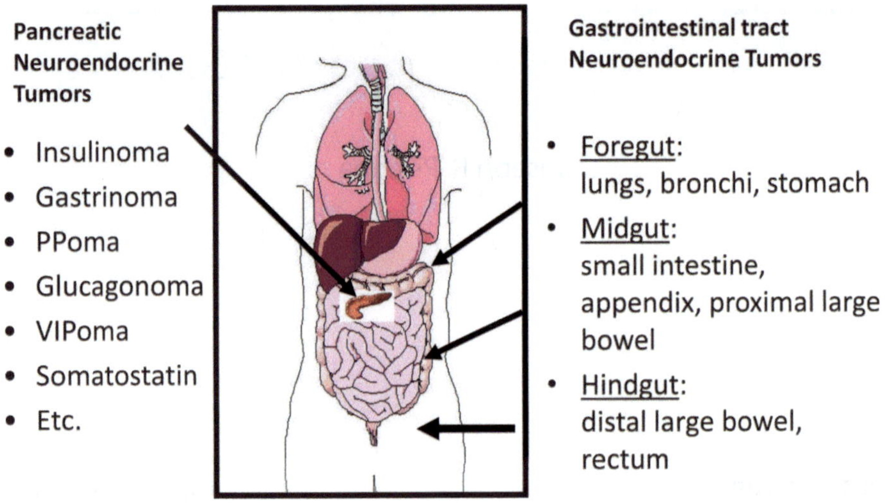

Fig. 12.1 Classification of NETs. On the *left panel*, pancreatic NETs are classified whereas the gastrointestinal neuroendocrine tumor family is shown in the *right panel*

Previously in the literature, there has been confusion regarding the definition of NETs owing in part to their localization (i.e., endocrine vs. islet cell vs. neuroendocrine) and differentiation (i.e., carcinoids vs. neuroendocrine). The term neuroendocrine has gained popularity in the field because it more accurately reflects that these tumor cells possess both neural and endocrine features. The World Health Organization (WHO) classification of tumors now uses the term neuroendocrine. Another area of confusion is whether NETs should be referred to as "tumors" or "neoplasms" with the former now in common use, although these terms should be considered synonymous given the natural history of these tumors.

Epidemiology

The annual incidence of NETs has increased to approximately 40–50 cases per million.[1] It is assumed that this increase in incidence is related to increased recognition within the clinical community and the increased use of diagnostic imaging studies in the population. However, NETs are relatively rare and account for less than 2% of gastrointestinal tumors.[1] Insulinomas are the most prevalent of the pancreatic NETs (pNETs) and account for about 90% of the cases with the majority being benign.[2] In contrast, gastrinomas accounting for the Zollinger Ellison Syndrome are the next most commonly diagnosed pNETs with the vast majority being malignant (~65%). The calculated annual incidence of pNETs is less than one per 100,000 population.[3] The majority of pNETs occur in middle age with an age range from 14 to 78 years old (mean 48 years) and a median age of 60 years. The majority of pNETs are present for many years prior to diagnosis, especially in patients with the MEN I Syndrome. In an autopsy series, the incidence was 0.11% with the majority being insulinomas (62%) and the remaining being gastrinomas (6%) and glucagonomas (4%).

Pathology

Neuroendocrine tumors (NET) are a heterogeneous group of tumors characterized by combinations of argentaffin cells possessing granules that stain positive for chromogranins, synaptophysins, neuron-specific enolase, or neurotensin.[1,4] Under light microscopy, these tumors range from well to poorly differentiated. Well-differentiated NETs consist of tumor cells that may be arranged in acinar or lobular patterns and separated by a fibrovascular stroma. The well-differentiated tumors give the appearance of an "organoid" arrangement with a distinct trabecular pattern (Fig. 12.2). In tumors that are less well differentiated, sheets of cells can be identified that are separated by septations, which demonstrate a fibrous component (Fig. 12.2). By electron microscopy, the cells contain electron dense granules that contain either biologically active amines or peptides.[1] In addition, these granules contain chromogranins (A and C), neuron-specific enolase, and synaptophysins in varying concentrations. Although neuroendocrine tumors can arise throughout the body, they all share common histopathological features and pathological grading. The most recent NET classification is based on the localization of the tumor, the degree of differentiation, and using markers for differentiation. Tumors are characterized as being well differentiated or poorly differentiated and markers include the use of Ki-67. The tumor differentiation refers to the resemblance of the tumor to normal cellular architecture. It should be noted here that poorly differentiated NETs (High Grade NETS, G3 category) behave clinically like small cell or large cell neuroendocrine carcinomas and are thus clinically more aggressive. These poorly differentiated or anaplastic tumors have a more diffuse architecture with irregularly arranged nuclei, possess less secretory granules, and may not stain by immunohistochemistry with

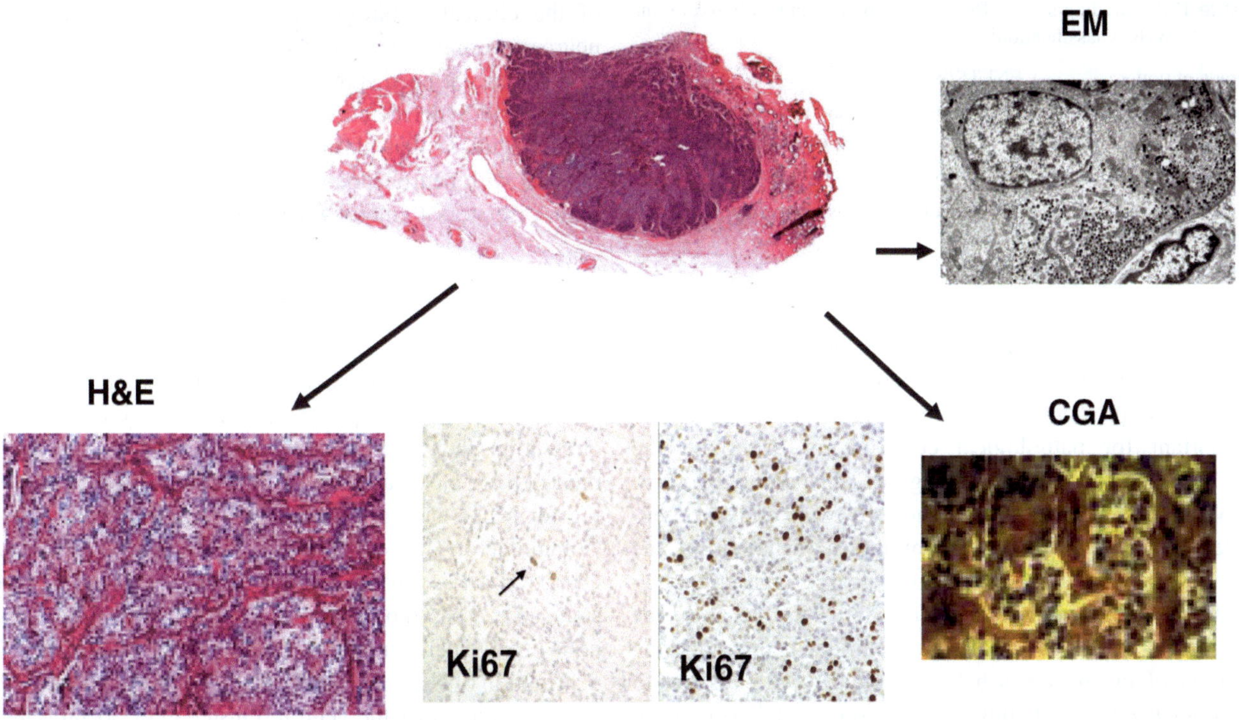

Fig. 12.2 Histopathology of NETs. A duodenal gastrinoma is shown in the *upper panel* under low magnification and at higher magnification in the *left bottom panel* (H&E stain); *middle panels* in the *bottom*: immunohistochemistry for Ki67; chromogranin A staining in the *bottom right*. A typical EM is shown in the *upper right*

Table 12.1 Comparison of nomenclature for Gastroentero-Pancreatic Neuroendocrine Tumors[4] GEP-NETs/ENETS

Grade	GEP-NETs/ENETS	GEP-NETs/WHO	Pancreatic NET
Low	NET Grade 1 (G1)	Neuroendocrine neoplasm, grade 1	Well-differentiated pancreatic endocrine neoplasm, low grade
Intermediate	NET, grade 2 (G2)	Neuroendocrine neoplasm, grade 2	Well-differentiated pancreatic endocrine neoplasm, intermediate grade
High	Neuroendocrine carcinoma grade 3, (G3) either small cell or large cell variant	Neuroendocrine carcinoma grade 3, small cell carcinoma or large cell carcinoma	Poorly differentiated pancreatic endocrine carcinoma, either small cell or large cell variant

neuroendocrine markers. Thus, a sharp difference with regard to biological behavior can be made between the well-differentiated (G1), intermediately differentiated (G2), and poorly differentiated (G3/neuroendocrine carcinoma) NETs. Tumor stage is used to determine the degree of biological aggressiveness and can be determined by the tumor size, the extent by which the NET invades tissue planes, organs, or lymph nodes. A number of pathological classification systems have been developed such as the World Health Organization (WHO) to be able to better categorize NETs and perhaps predict the biological aggression of these tumors. The most recent nomenclature has been developed by the North American Neuroendocrine Tumor Society and a Consensus Guideline is summarized in Table 12.1 (4). As demonstrated in Table 12.1, the various nomenclatures used are described, which includes both the specific tumor grade and grading system, which are necessary to properly characterize the tumor.

More recently, the description of the proliferative rate has proven to be important for both diagnosis and therapy and thus should be used to classify the tumor. The decision to undergo surgical resection, chemotherapy, or more conservative approaches to therapy will be based in part on an understanding of the tumor's proliferative rate. The proliferative rate can be determined by evaluating the number of mitoses per high-power field (scored in 10 high-power fields) or based on the staining pattern using Ki-67, or both (Table 12.2). The European Neuroendocrine Tumor Society (ENETS) system utilizing Ki-67 had been widely in use in Europe and is now becoming increasingly utilized in the USA whenever there is sufficient tissue to permit staining. A combination of utilizing Ki-67 and mitotic index probably has the most clinical utility.

Table 12.2 Grading system for neuroendocrine tumors based on the ENETS, WHO Classification[4]

Grade of tumor	ENETS/WHO
Low (Grade 1)	<2 mitoses/10 HPF and Ki67 index <3%
Intermediate (Grade 2)	2–10 mitoses/10 HPF or Ki67 index 3–20%
High (Grade 3)	>10 mitosis/10 HPF or Ki67 >10%

Grade 3 neuroendocrine tumors are diagnosed as neuroendocrine carcinomas (small or large cell type)

Since the majority of NETs secrete either one or a combination of neuroamines, neuropeptides, or other biologically active peptides, immunohistochemical analysis is also important for pathological confirmation. Although the NETs demonstrate varying degrees of staining of chromogranin A, neuron-specific enolase, synaptophysin, peptide, or biogenic amine, the biological behavior of the tumors may be similar. Thus, the degree of immunohistochemical staining does not provide an insight as to the biological course of disease. In addition, neuroendocrine tumors of the pancreas behave similarly with respect to their localization, capability for metastases, and histopathological characteristics. In one series, immunohistochemical stains showed evidence of multi-hormone production in 18% of cases with all tumors having staining for at least one of the six markers that included neuron-specific enolase (NSE), chromogranin (CG), synaptophysin (SYN), insulin (INS), glucagon (GLU), or somatostatin (SOM). Three markers, chromogranin, neuron-specific enolase, and synaptophysin led to the detection of 92% of the tumors.[1] It should be noted that many other tumors might also stain positive with these immunohistochemical stains, including colorectal adenomas and adenocarcinomas with areas of neuroendocrine differentiation, which may be predictive of more aggressive biology.[5] For example, adenocarcinomas of the colon and rectum may stain positive using chromogranin staining, suggesting a greater likelihood for malignant potential.[6,7] The majority of pancreatic islet cell tumors stain positive for multiple peptide hormones and the staining patterns are not necessarily predictive of the serum expression of these hormones.[8] It is also possible that some NETs may express granules and secrete the more recently identified neuropeptide, pituitary adenylate cyclase-activating polypeptide (PACAP), a close peptide related to vasoactive intestinal polypeptide (VIP) and glucagon or ghrelin, a peptide that stimulates appetite.[9]

In general, the biochemical levels of a particular peptide hormone have limited predictive value for assessing the malignant potential of pancreatic neuroendocrine tumors but may be useful for evaluating tumor recurrence in a patient either postoperatively or during chemotherapy. Similarly, the size or extent of a neuroendocrine tumor does not correlate with the level of peptide hormone production or the severity of the clinical syndrome. The best characterized of the neuroendocrine tumors are gastrinomas. The level of serum gastrin has not been shown to correlate with the degree of gastric acid hypersecretion. More recently, there is increasing recognition that plasma ghrelin levels are elevated in patients with neuroendocrine tumors. Plasma ghrelin levels may correlate with metastatic potential of NETs.[9]

Staging

Although the size of neuroendocrine tumors bears little relation to the levels of a particular hormone secreted into the circulation, their size may have important implications into their risk for metastatic spread. More recently, a TNM staging for NETs has been established by The American Joint Committee on Cancer (Table 12.3). Previously, NETs were characterized as having either localized, regional, or metastatic spread based on the presence of local invasion, lymph node involvement, or hepatic involvement, respectively. The distribution of NETs may be a result of embryological development from either the ventral (cluster 1) or dorsal (cluster 2) pancreatic buds with the ventral tumors (gastrinomas, pancreatic polypeptide (PP)-secreting tumors, and somatostatinomas) occurred in 75% of cases to the right of the superior mesenteric artery and dorsal tumors (insulinoma and glucagonoma) occurring in 75% of cases to the left of the superior mesenteric artery.[10] A special case can be made for the association of pancreatic neuroendocrine tumors arising in the setting of multiple endocrine neoplasia type 1 (MEN I) given the multipotentiality of the tumors arising at multiple sites.

Natural History and Clinical Presentation

Glucagonomas "Sweet's Syndrome" (Alpha Cell Tumors)

Glucagonomas are tumors involving functioning pancreatic alpha cells of the pancreas that result in the "Sweet Syndrome." Tumors of the alpha cells are rare and are characterized by a very distinctive rash, weight loss, stomatitis, glossitis, mild diabetes, hypoaminoacidemia, a normochromic, normocytic anemia, and a susceptibility to deep vein thrombosis and neuropsychiatric disturbances. Glucagonomas are more common in women than in men with a peak incidence in patients from 50 to 60 years of age. These tumors are usually larger than 5 cm in diameter, with the majority being malignant at the time of diagnosis. Although earlier reports suggested that these tumors were more commonly located in the body and tail of the pancreas, more recent reports indicate that location in the head of the pancreas was not uncommon.[10,11]

Table 12.3 The American Joint Committee on Cancer (AJCC) and European Neuroendocrine Tumors Society (ENETS) staging classifications for pancreatic neuroendocrine tumors with cross-tabulation of stage distributions (Strosberg JR, et al. JCO 2011;29:3044–3049)

AJCC staging classification				ENETS staging classification			
T1	Tumor limited to the pancreas, <2 cm			T1	Tumor limited to the pancreas, <2 cm		
T2	Tumor limited to the pancreas, >2 cm			T2	Tumor limited to the pancreas, 2–4 cm		
T3	Tumor extends beyond the pancreas, but not involving the celiac axis or SMA			T3	Tumor limited to the pancreas, > 4 cm, or invading duodenum or CBD		
T4	Tumor involves the celiac axis or SMA			T4	Tumor invades adjacent structures		
N0	No regional LN metastasis			N0	No regional LN metastasis		
N1	Regional LN metastasis			N1	Regional LN metastasis		
M0	No distant metastasis			M0	No distant metastasis		
M1	Distant metastasis			M1	Distant metastasis		
Stage	T	N	M	Stage	T	N	M
IA	T1	N0	M0	I	T1	N0	M0
IB	T2	N0	M0	IIA	T2	N0	M0
IIA	T3	N0	M0	IIB	T3	N0	M0
IIB	T1-3	N1	M0	IIIA	T4	N0	M0
III	T4	N0-1	M0	IIIB	Any T	N1	M0
IV	Any T	Any N	M1	IV	Any T	Any N	M1
		ENETS I		ENETS II	ENETS III		ENETS IV
AJCC I		25		59	0		0
AJCC II		0		4	37		0
AJCC III		0		0	18		0
AJCC IV		0		0	0		282

The characteristic skin rash in glucagonoma patients is the necrolytic migratory erythema, first described by Wilkinson.[12] The cardinal features of the rash are erosions and crusting, which tend to be seen in a truncal distribution affecting the buttocks, groin, central parts of the face, and distal aspects of the lower extremities. Fungal and bacterial superinfections as well as sparse scalp hair and thin, friable nails are also commonly noted. The factors associated with the development of this skin rash have not been determined, although it may be associated with the development of hypoaminoaciduria and elevated utilization of amino acids used for gluconeogenesis secondary to hypergluconemia.[13] Zinc treatment may improve the hypoaminoacidemia and rash.[14–18] The response to both local and oral zinc supplementation as well as omega-3-essential fatty acids suggests that zinc deficiency is important in the pathogenesis of the rash in patients with glucagonomas.[19] Treatment with the somatostatin analogue octreotide (400 μg/day) may also be a useful adjunct to therapy.[20]

This hyperglucagonemia is directly responsible for the mild diabetes through its stimulation of hepatic glucose production via enhanced glycogenolysis and gluconeogenesis; however, frank diabetes occurs in only a subset of patients and likely is related to the size of tumor. It is not uncommon for patients to be normoglycemic despite elevated plasma glucagon.[14,21–24] Pre-proglucagon has been identified as enteroglucagon, which may be produced in the cells in the intestine and is a putative growth factor for gut mucosa by acting at the GLP-2 receptor and may account for mucosal thickening and villous hypertrophy throughout the small intestine in patients with glucagonoma.[25–28] The weight loss associated with this syndrome may result from the direct actions of glucagon on catabolism and improvement has been reported with the use of octreotide.[29]

The diagnosis of glucagonoma should be considered in a patient presenting with the classic "4 D's": Dermatitis; DVT; Depression; and Diarrhea. Frequently, the diagnosis is first suspected by a dermatologist.[30,31] A definitive diagnosis is made by finding a high plasma glucagon concentration in the absence of any other cause, such as renal failure with plasma levels generally >500 pg/mL (normal glucagon levels being <50 pg/mL). A plasma level of glucagon greater than 1,000 pg/ml is virtually pathognomonic for the diagnosis of glucagonoma. There are no specific provocative studies to confirm an elevated glucagon level but there may be other peptides, which may be elevated such as gastrin, ACTH, pancreatic polypeptide, or PTH.

Insulinomas or Beta Cell Tumors

Insulinomas are tumors involving functioning pancreatic beta cells of the pancreas.[1] Insulinomas are generally benign tumors of the pancreas that secrete excessive amounts of insulin and clinically manifest with hypoglycemia as the predominant symptoms.[32] Insulinomas more commonly occur in women than in men and are usually diagnosed in patients in the fourth and fifth decades but may also occur in children.[33–39] The majority of patients with insulinomas have single benign adenomas with only 10% having malignant features, and about 10% occurring multifocal as benign tumors that are frequently associated with the MEN I Syndrome. Insulinomas differ from the other NETs in that they are more typically small, usually less than 2 cm in diameter, and are located with equal frequency in the head, body, and tail of the pancreas. A diagnosis of insulinomas should be considered in patients presenting with symptoms of hypoglycemia such as tachycardia, diaphoresis, and syncope occurring during fasting conditions. Chronic hyperinsulinemia and hypoglycemia lead to excessive caloric intake and lipogenesis leading to weight gain as noted in animal models.[40–44]

The diagnosis of insulinoma is generally made in the presence of high serum insulin levels for the resulting glucose concentration occurring during fasting conditions with the majority of patients developing symptomatic hypoglycemia within 72 h. Although glucose concentrations may drop as low as 30–35 mg/dl in the normal patient after a 72-h fast, insulin levels decrease in the normal state, whereas in insulinoma patients, the serum insulin levels remain elevated.[45] There are several ways to relate glucose and insulin concentrations during fasting[46] such as the simple insulin ((U/ml)-to-glucose (mg/dl)) ratio[47] and in normal state this will remain below 0.3 as fasting continues, whereas in patients with inappropriate insulin secretion, the ratio will almost always rise above 0.3.[48] Hypoglycemia associated with symptoms occurs within 24 h of the start of the fast in two-thirds of the patients with insulinomas and within 48 h in 95% with the remaining 5% of patients requiring the full 3 days of fasting. An elevated or high insulin concentration is not essential to make the diagnosis of insulinoma; the diagnosis can oftentimes only be made in the fasting state. For example, a value of 25–40 (U/ml) at a time when glucose concentration has fallen to less than 40 mg/dl would be considered positive. During this provocative test, should the patient develop symptoms of hypoglycemia or if the serum glucose drops below 40 mg/dL the test should be terminated.

The measurement of proinsulin and C peptide is also helpful in diagnosing insulinomas. Because the beta islet cells synthesize proinsulin, the percentage of proinsulin in the fasting plasma is less than 20% of the total immunoreactive insulin, whereas this is increased to 25–75% among patients with an insulinoma.[49–51] Aggressive insulinomas are more often associated with the highest levels of proinsulin, which may help to distinguish benign from malignant insulinomas.[50] Malignant insulinomas have metastatic potential and result in profound hypoglycemia, and the treatment strategies may include using diazoxide, octreotide, debulking surgery, and peripheral hyperalimentation to maintain stable glucose levels. Insulin and the C-peptide are secreted in similar amounts and patients with insulinoma have increased amounts of circulating proinsulin and either a normal or elevated level of C-peptide.[52] The major advantage of measuring C-peptide is the ability to distinguish endogenous insulin levels from exogenous insulin that may confound the diagnosis in cases of factitious hypoglycemia and given the small size of these tumors making surgical identification difficult.[53–58]

Delta Cell Tumors (Gastrinoma and Zollinger Ellison Syndrome)

Gastrinoma is the second most common pancreatic NET and the resulting Zollinger Ellison syndrome (ZES) is characterized by hypergastrinemia resulting in gastric acid hypersecretion.[59,60] In 1955, Zollinger and Ellison published their landmark article that characterized the gastrinoma syndrome and presented a hypothesis for the pancreatic endocrine origin of the gastric hypersecretion and ulcer disease.[1] Classically, duodenal post-bulbar ulcers result in gastrointestinal hemorrhage in patients with this syndrome, although the majority of patients present with symptoms of epigastric abdominal pain, diarrhea, or gastroesophageal reflux disease.[61] Gastrinomas are estimated to occur in 0.1–3 per million in the USA, but the actual numbers may be underreported because of the more prevalent use of potent gastric acid inhibitors.[62] Gastrinoma tumors occur with nearly equal frequency in both the duodenum and pancreas and are both equally malignant.[63] The duodenal gastrinomas are smaller and more difficult to localize than the tumors occurring in the pancreas requiring the use of operative endoscopic transillumination of the bowel wall for their localization.[63] Gastrinomas are associated with MEN I in approximately one-third of patients and about one-third of patients with MEN I syndrome will develop gastrinomas.[59,64,65] A family history of endocrinopathy and the presence of other tumors that are characteristic of MEN I, especially parathyroid and pituitary tumors, characterize the co-occurrence of ZES with the MEN I syndrome. Patients with sporadic gastrinomas usually have solitary tumors that are larger, whereas in patients with MEN I, the tumors can be multifocal and are typically smaller.[63,66,67]

Endoscopic examination of the stomach in patients with ZES demonstrates large gastric folds (Fig. 12.3 left panel). Microscopic examination of the gastric mucosa typically shows hypertrophic mucosa with parietal cell hyperplasia and ECL cell hyperplasia as a result of the trophic effects of hypergastrinemia (Fig. 12.3). The diagnosis of ZES is suspected in patients with severe gastroduodenal ulcer symptoms; however, diarrhea and abdominal pain occur due to the large volume of gastric juice that enters the duodenum, inactivating pancreatic lipase. The normal duodenal bicarbonate secretion is unable to neutralize this acid load resulting

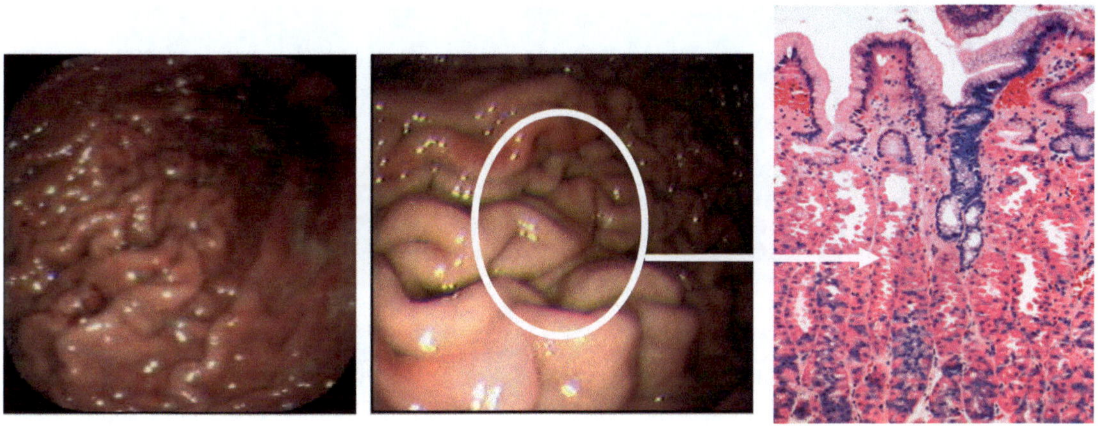

Fig. 12.3 Prominent gastric folds associated with hypertrophic mucosa and hyperplastic parietal cells in a typical patient with Zollinger Ellison Syndrome

in damage to the small bowel mucosa resulting in a malabsorption syndrome. Endoscopic examination of the duodenal bulb may demonstrate heterotropic, hypertrophic gastric mucosa.[68] The diagnosis of ZES is suggested when the fasting serum gastrin is greater than 100 pg/ml in the absence of achlorhydria (Fig. 12.4). Patients with gastrinoma usually have levels exceeding 500 pg/ml, and a level >1,000 pg/ml is diagnostic of ZES in the absence of other causes of hypergastrinemia, such as renal insufficiency, atrophic gastritis, gastric outlet obstruction, and retained antrum syndrome, or in the presence of high dose PPI therapy. In patients taking proton pump inhibitors, elevations in serum gastrin are common and occur in the setting of reduced acid secretion; however, their serum gastrin is generally <200 pg/ml. In addition, lipemic serum can also falsely elevate the gastrin levels.[69] Renal insufficiency can also result in an elevated serum gastrin from a reduction in the renal clearance of gastrin.[70] Intravenous administration of gastrin in humans[71] and rodents[72] is associated with an increase in renal excretion of sodium that is mediated, at least in part, by the gastrin receptor, CCKB (CCK2), that has been cloned in both species.[72,73]

In order to make a diagnosis with certainty, provocative testing with secretin can be used.[74,75] Gastrinoma tumors typically express receptors for secretin, and following secretin binding to the secretin receptor, there is activation of intracellular cAMP resulting in the release of gastrin. This is especially useful when the serum gastrin levels are borderline or if the clinical syndrome is not confirmed by gastric acid hypersecretion.[76] The secretin test is performed by the bolus administration of intravenous secretin (2 units/kg) and measuring plasma gastrin at baseline and several minutes following secretin administration. An increase in the gastrin level of >200 pg/ml within 15 min is diagnostic of gastrinoma in 87–93% of patients with ZES.[75] Alternatively, because gastrinoma tumors express the calcium sensing receptor (CaSR) intravenous Ca^{2+} provocative testing can be performed but is less sensitive and more prone to adverse events.[76]

Once the diagnosis of ZES is made, the inhibition of gastric acid secretion is the important clinical goal in patient management in order to prevent the development of peptic ulcerations, control the associated diarrhea, and prevent gastrointestinal hemorrhage.[77] Gastric analysis is therefore useful both in the diagnosis of ZES (Fig. 12.4) and also in the clinical management of gastric acid secretion. Gastric analysis is performed by measuring the volume and titratable acidity of gastric juice collected by either nasogastric tube or endoscopic measurement.[78] In ZES, the basal acid output (BAO) is >10 mEq/h. The maximal acid output (MAO), a direct measure of parietal cell mass, can be determined by the measurement of gastric acid secretion following administration of pentagastrin subcutaneously.[77–81] Following curative gastrinoma resection, the BAO may continue to be elevated due to the long-term effects of hypergastrinemia.[81] Another effect of the long-term effects of hypergastrinemia occurs in the gastric mucosa resulting in ECL cell hyperplasia and the development of Type I gastric carcinoids especially if there is coexistent MEN I Syndrome (see chapter on gastric carcinoids).

The pharmacologic control of gastric acid hypersecretion is readily accomplished with the use of potent proton pump inhibitors.[62,82–94] The goal of antisecretory therapy should be to control gastric acid secretion to <5 mEq/h. Acid secretion can be controlled acutely in patients unable to take oral medications with intravenous PPIs such as pantoprazole (Fig. 12.5) at a dose of 80 mg BID or TID.[95,96] PPIs have proved over the past 2 decades to be safe and efficacious with little to no change in the gastric ECL cell hyperplasia and without the development of gastric carcinoids in humans.[97–102] Once the gastric acid hypersecretion is controlled, the next objective is to determine whether the gastrinoma tumor is localized or metastatic (Fig. 12.6). The localization of NETs has improved with radiological imaging studies. If the disease is localized and not metastatic, surgical resection may be curative in over 60% of patients

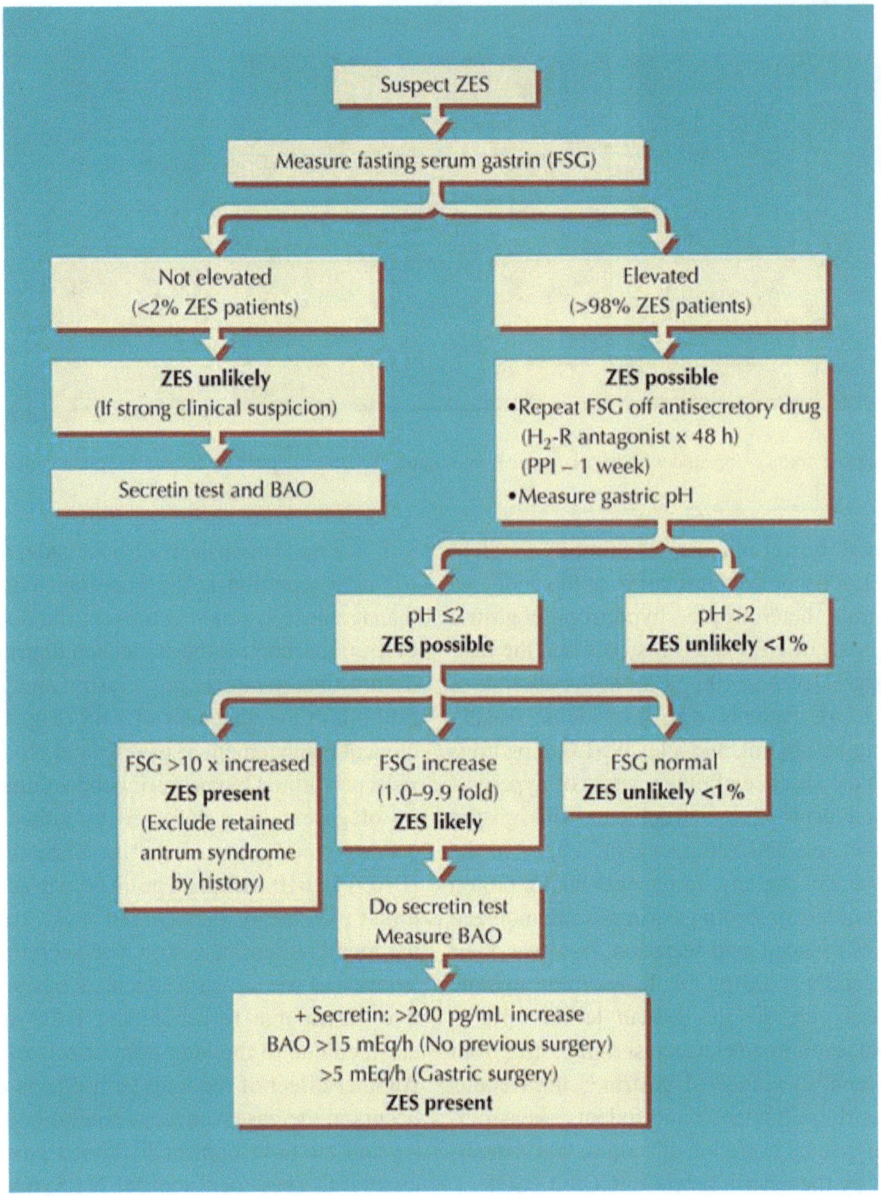

Fig. 12.4 Diagnostic algorithm for the diagnosis of ZES. This algorithm is based on the measurement of gastric acid secretion and the gastrin level

with sporadic gastrinomas. However, in patients with ZES and MEN I, the role of surgery is debatable.[103]

Verner–Morrison Syndrome (VIPomas)

The Verner–Morrison Syndrome, alternatively referred to as diarrheogenic tumor of the pancreas, pancreatic cholera or watery diarrhea, hypokalemia, and achlorhydria syndrome (WDHA), results when the pancreatic NET releases vasoactive intestinal polypeptide (VIP).[104] Although relatively rare, the syndrome is manifested by profuse watery diarrhea, massive gastrointestinal losses of potassium, a low serum potassium, and extreme weakness. VIPomas are typically single and large occurring in the pancreas and are generally advanced with metastases at the time of initial diagnosis. Achlorhydria develops even after stimulation with pentagastrin due to the inhibitory effects of VIP on gastric acid secretion.[105] The diagnosis of this syndrome is generally not subtle as patients are typically quite ill. The volume of diarrhea averages ~5 l per day during acute episodes and contains >300 mEq of potassium and there is severe bicarbonate wasting resulting in metabolic acidosis. Other laboratory abnormalities may result such as hypercalcemia probably from the release of PTH by the VIPoma and abnormal glucose tolerance presumably from decreased insulin secretion resulting

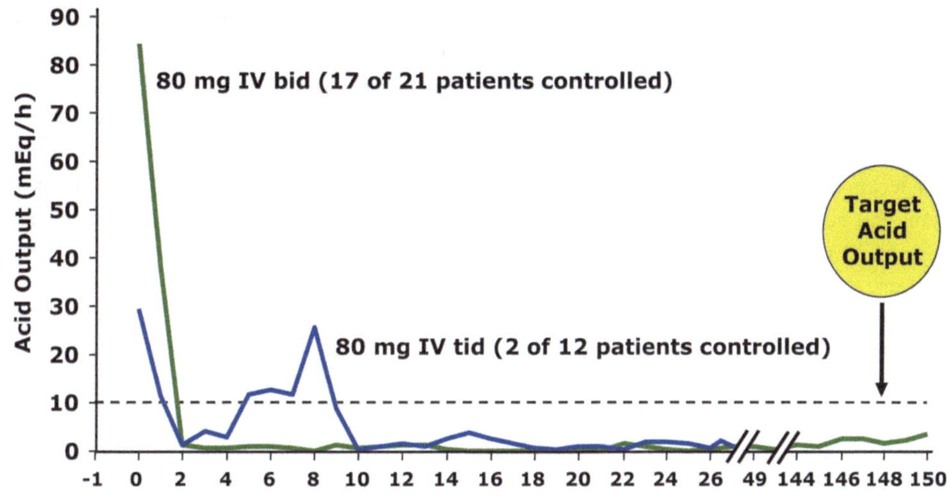

Lew EA, Pisegna JR et al. *Gastroenterology*. 2000;118:696–704.

Fig. 12.5 The effects of IV pantoprazole (80 mg BID) on gastric acid secretion

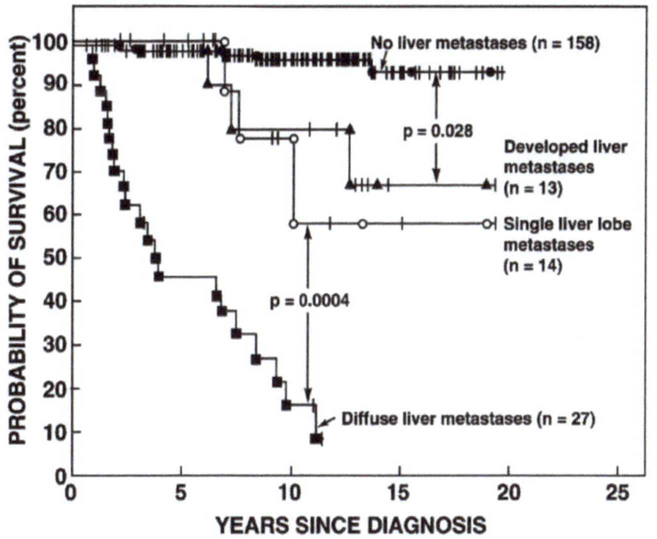

Norton, J and Jensen, R. Resolved and Unresolved Controversies in the Surgical Management of Patients With ZES. 2004. Annals of Surgery. Vol 240;5, p. 757-773.

Fig. 12.6 Kaplan–Meier results in patients with ZES. Note that there is a significant difference in survival that is dependent on the presence or absence of hepatic metastases

from the profound hypokalemia. The diagnosis of VIPoma should be considered in patients with a severe diarrhea associated with hypokalemia but should be distinguished from patients with psuedopancreatic cholera syndrome and laxative abuse, and a reliable VIP radioimmunoassay is generally needed.[106] Misdiagnosis may occur if the serum is not properly handled at the time of collection because VIP can be degraded in the serum. It is recommended that the laboratory determination be made on serum fractionated and snap frozen to avoid peptide degradation. In patients with confirmed VIPomas, serum VIP levels > 900 pg/ml are commonly observed[106,107] and prepro-VIP levels can be detected in the circulation.[108] Immunohistochemical staining of VIPomas typically stain positive with VIP stains. After the diagnosis of VIPoma is confirmed, radiological imaging, endoscopic ultrasonography, spiral CT, and/or angiogram should perform staging. Approximately 80% of VIPomas are solitary, and are located in the body or tail, and therefore amenable to surgical resection if not metastatic. About half of the lesions are malignant, and three-fourths of these have metastasized by the time of exploration. In children, however, most tumors secreting VIP are ganglioneuromas rather than islet cell lesions.[106] The symptoms can be controlled with the subcutaneous administration of somatostatin analogue, octreotide as either monotherapy or as adjunctive therapy as well as repletion of intravascular volume and potassium.

Somatostatinoma

Somatostatinomas are D-cell tumors that arise in the pancreas, although these tumors may also arise in the intestine.[109–114] The syndrome results from secretion of somatostatin, a tetradecapeptide. In most cases, somatostatinomas are malignant and accompanied by hepatic metastases. Since somatostatin has numerous effects on exocrine and endocrine functions, there are multiple facets in the clinical presentation. Activation of the somatostatin receptor results in activation of the intracellular G protein Gαi2 that inhibits intracellular Ca^{2+} release. Thus, the net result is that somatostatin is a potent inhibitor of secretion and motility. In the stomach, somatostatin, normally released by the gastric D cells, is a potent inhibitor of gastric acid secretion by inhibiting the release of histamine from the ECL cell.[105,115] Because there are receptors for somatostatin throughout the small bowel, somatostatin hypersecretion results in malabsorption. It should be noted that the majority of cases of pancreatic somatostatinomas are symptomatic, whereas the majority of intestinal somatostatinomas are silent and the tumor is identified unexpectedly at the time of surgery for other conditions.[114] In the majority of cases due to the excessive production of somatostatin, the presenting features include diabetes mellitus, cholelithiasis, diarrhea, and steatorrhea. Somatostatin inhibits pancreatic acinar function and reduces the release of pancreatic enzymes by cholecystokinin resulting in pancreatic steatorrhea and a reduction in the intestinal absorption of lipid and vitamins such as B12 and folate.[116] In addition, somatostatin is a potent inhibitor of intestinal and gallbladder smooth muscle contraction and increases the likelihood of gallstones. Despite this theoretical risk, in one series, 23 cases of pancreatic somatostatinoma were reviewed and there were no cases of cholelithiasis.[117] The protean effects of somatostatin on gastrointestinal hormone secretion are the primary reason that octreotide has utility in the management of NETs.[118–124] Although there is no specific provocative test to detect or diagnose somatostatinomas, tolbutamide and arginine may stimulate an increase in somatostatin levels of the serum.[89,125,126] However, in the majority of cases, the diagnosis is generally confirmed on pathological evaluation. There are only about 30 patients with this rare syndrome that have been reported in the literature.[116,127–130] More recently, duodenal somatostatinomas associated with carcinoids tumors,[131–133] Von Hippel-Lindau disease, and von Recklinghausen's disease/neurofibromatosis[131,132,134,135] have been described.

Pancreatic Polypeptide-Secreting Tumors of the Pancreas (PPoma)

NETs that secrete pancreatic peptide (PP) are broadly classified as either PPomas or nonfunctional NETs because there is a lack of clinical syndrome associated with PP release. The presentation is typically that of a patient being worked up for cachexia, weight loss, and hepatomegaly and the PPoma is identified by abdominal imaging. Thus, the majority of these patients are identified incidentally. The diagnosis of PPoma is confirmed by the histological identification of a pancreatic NET that may stain positive with anti-PP staining in addition to positive staining for chromogranins A, neuron-specific enolase, and synaptophysin with the biochemical presence of elevated serum levels of pancreatic polypeptide.[136–138] Patients with PPoma generally present later in life, generally at 5th and 6th decades of life and it is not unusual for patients up the eight decade of life to have these tumors diagnosed.[136–139] The majority of these patients will have widely metastatic disease at the time of diagnosis (70–90% of cases). The primary tumors are almost invariably situated in the pancreas and are large (7.5 cm) at the time of imaging. Once diagnosed, surgical extirpation is possible for solitary small lesions without metastatic spread. There is a paucity of data in the literature regarding the long-term cure rate following pancreatic resection in these cases.

Growth Hormone-Releasing Factor Tumor (GRFomas), Neurotensinomas, and ACTHomas

GRFomas, although rare, occur predominantly in the pancreas and secrete excessive amounts of GRF leading to a syndrome characterized by acromegaly or gigantism. The first case was identified in the literature in 1982.[140,141] The diagnosis is generally established on clinical grounds and by measuring the basal levels of growth hormone and IGF-1, which are elevated in a subset of patients. Confirmation of the diagnosis is made when the levels of GH are not suppressed to an oral glucose tolerance test, somatostatin inhibition test, or a bromocriptine suppression test. The tumors are generally large and the majority are benign. There is an association with patients with ZES and the MEN I syndrome. GRFomas should be considered in the differential diagnosis of acromegaly, especially when associated with ZES and MEN I.

Neurotensinomas remain rare and truly difficult to identify because the symptom complex produced results from excessive VIP secretion making the clinical diagnosis difficult to differentiate. These patients present with edema, hypotension, cyanosis, and flushing.[115]

The Cushing's syndrome has been observed in a subset of patients with NETs when the tumors secrete ACTH, producing the characteristic syndrome. The diagnosis is made in patients exhibiting the classical Cushing's Syndrome based on the elevated secretion of cortisone, adrenal androgen, and 11-deoxycortisone. Generally, the presence of Cushing's syndrome in a patient with a NET suggests more advanced disease.

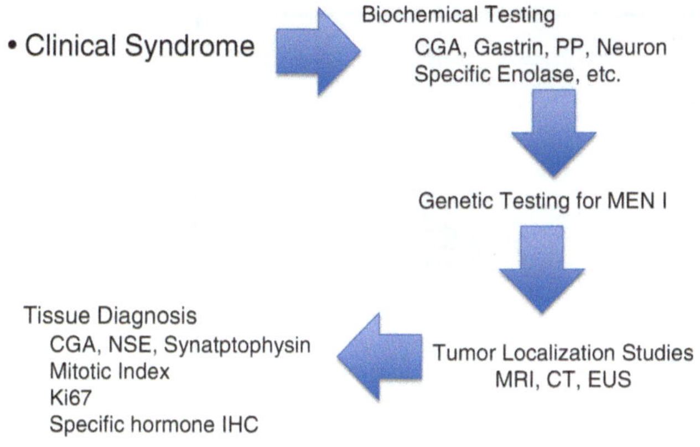

Fig. 12.7 Diagnostic algorithm for NETs

NET Localization and Diagnosis

Advances in gastrointestinal imaging studies have increased the yield for the detection of both primary and metastatic NETs.[142] Once there is a suspicion of a clinical syndrome and suggestion based on biochemical testing (Fig. 12.7), localization studies should be performed. Since the localization of the majority of pancreatic NETs is in the pancreas or peripancreatic area, imaging studies with a high sensitivity of visualizing these areas are important. Endoscopic ultrasound, computerized tomography, somatostatin receptor scintigraphy (Octreoscan), and magnetic resonance imaging have all been studied and shown to be sensitive and specific for the preoperative staging of disease (Fig. 12.8). Magnetic resonance imaging may be more sensitive for the detection of hepatic metastases and is useful for follow-up evaluations since there is no ionizing radiation.[143] Endoscopic ultrasonography (Fig. 12.9) is performed more routinely by gastroenterologists and has been shown to be very sensitive for the detection of primary pancreatic and duodenal NETs and allows the cytological evaluation of suspected tumors.[144,145]

Of the remaining islet cell tumors of the pancreas, gastrinoma have been the most studied of the tumors with respect to the diagnostic sensitivity and specificity of the localization studies. The ability to localize and resect gastrinoma has been greatly facilitated by the use of advanced imaging studies as with the long-acting somatostatin analogue, octreotide, which is frequently useful as a tracer to localize tumors.[146,147] In addition, ultrasonography, computerized tomography, magnetic resonance imaging, endoscopic ultrasonography, and intraoperative duodenal transillumination and sonography have greatly increased the yield for identification of the tumors.[143,148–150] With these improved imaging studies, duodenal wall gastrinomas have become more frequently detected and now account for nearly half of the total cases.[63] In some cases, the use of portal venous sampling (PVS) and angiography with stimulation can lead to a sensitivity for detecting tumors that approaches 70–80% in selected series.[151–153]

Surgical Management

Insulinoma

Surgery remains the mainstay of therapy for the management of insulinomas because the majority are benign and therefore surgery results in a cure in over 90% of cases. Because 10% of the tumors are small and not easily identified at surgery, every effort should be directed at preoperative localization of these tumors. The majority of insulinomas lesions are not identified by radiological and nuclear imaging studies because of their small size. Intraoperative imaging with ultrasonography may be required to identify the tumors.[154] Preoperatively, selective angiography demonstrates the tumor only in about 50% of cases and percutaneous transhepatic venous sampling may be required to identify an insulin gradient along the portal or splenic venous tributaries to assist in the localization of these tumors.[155] Endoscopic ultrasound appears to be the most sensitive technique (~85%) for localization (Fig. 12.9) of insulinomas.[154] At surgery, the standard approach may be to enucleate the tumor, especially if superficial; however, a partial pancreatectomy may be required especially if the tumor is deep and not readily removable. A Whipple procedure may be appropriate if the tumor is situated in the head of the pancreas. If the tumor cannot be found and the results of venous sampling studies suggest its location, that portion of the pancreas should be resected. The curative resection rate for insulinomas is high with >80% cured operatively.[156] The role of surgery for malignant or metastatic insulinomas is more controversial. Some feel that debulking of tumor may be useful for improved glycemic control; however, now with the approval of chemotherapy options, this will need to be further investigated.

Gastrinoma

Over 80% of these tumors are found in the "gastrinoma triangle," which includes the area of the common bile duct, the duodenum, and the head and neck of the pancreas, as described previously by Passaro et al.[157] The surgical approach to the management of gastrinoma (ZES) has been perhaps the best studied with several rigorous clinical trials reported with successful cure rates approaching 60%. Surgical treatment should be directed at complete tumor resection in order to effect cure of the syndrome, and to prevent the development of metastasis in all patients with the sporadic form of the disease.[158] However, in patients with

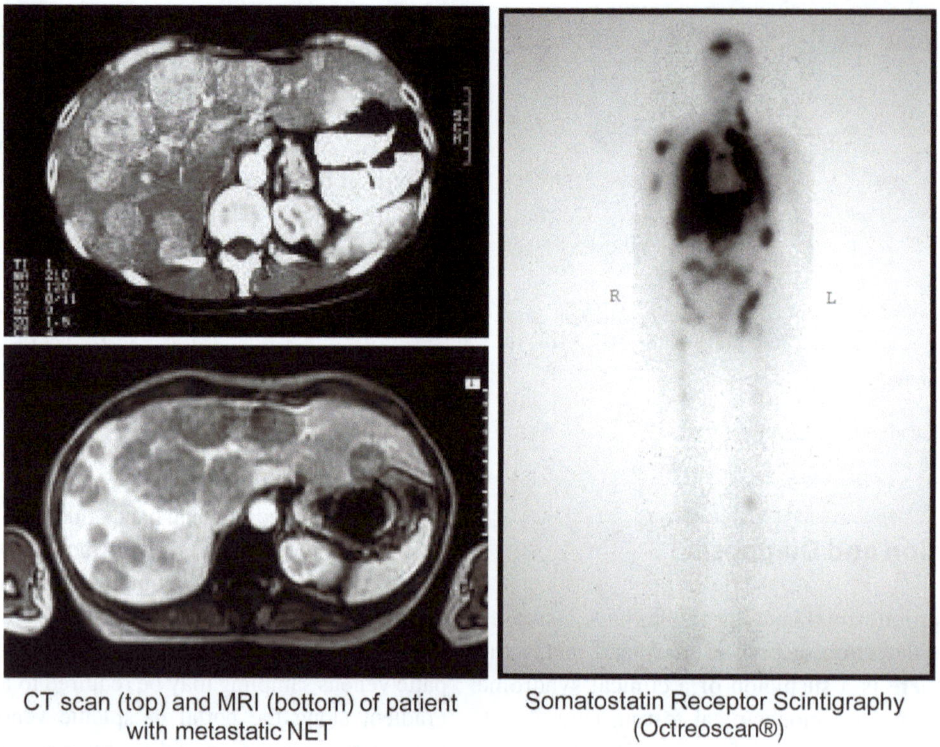

Fig. 12.8 Diagnosis: CT/MRI vs. SRS (somatostatin receptor scintigraphy)

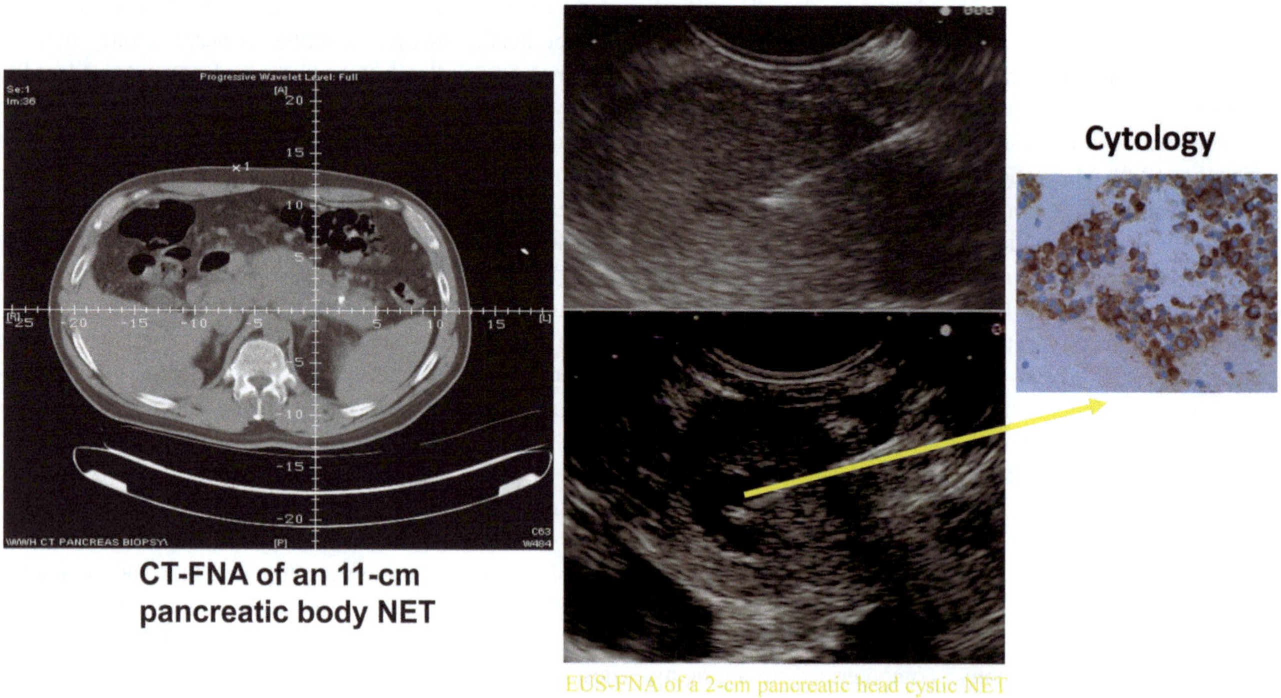

Fig. 12.9 EUS-guided fine needle aspiration (FNA) accurately diagnoses smaller pancreatic neuroendocrine tumors compared to CT-guided FNA

MEN I, the role of surgery is more controversial since the pancreatic NETs typically tend to be multifocal and the recurrence rate is high owing to the genetic mutation and dysfunction of the MENIN protein.[159–161] At surgery, the approach may be to enucleate the gastrinoma tumor when possible. Since about 50% of gastrinomas occur in the wall of the duodenum and are typically small, intraoperative endoscopy to transilluminate the duodenal wall may be required.[68] If the gastrinoma is present in the pancreatic tail, a distal pancreatectomy may be required.[162] Immediately postoperatively, successful removal of the gastrinoma tumor will result in normalization of the serum gastrin levels, measurements that are helpful in long-term follow-up to determine whether there is tumor recurrence.[163–165]

Glucagonomas, PPomas, and Somatostatinomas

Most of these lesions are malignant and have metastasized by the time of diagnosis; therefore the role of surgery may be more palliative or unnecessary. If surgery is being performed for palliation, the tumor should be resected, and if metastases are present, they should be debulked, and subtotal resection may result in considerable palliation. With widespread hepatic metastases, placement of a hepatic artery catheter is indicated for postoperative therapy. Interestingly, the characteristic rash of glucagonoma will usually improve within several days and clear rapidly, even with debulking, and improved glycemic control may occur. As stated earlier, the somatostatinomas of the intestine or pancreas are heterogenous; however, their occurrence is uncommon.[165]

Liver Transplantation

The role of liver transplantation is more controversial. In a recent retrospective study of patients undergoing liver transplantation for metastatic NETs using the UNOS database, 150 OLTs were performed (34% carcinoids; 4% insulinoma; 2%glucagonoma; 7% gastrinoma; 6% VIPoma; and 47% non-secreting). The study showed that the 1-, 3-, and 5-year survival rates for patients with NETs undergoing isolated LT were 81%, 65%, and 49%, respectively, which was similar to the survival observed for patients with hepatocellular carcinoma.[166]

Medical Approaches to Therapy

Until recently, chemotherapy resulted in only mixed results in a number of clinical studies. Dacarbazine had been used previously for the treatment of symptomatic glucagonoma.[167–172] In general, the use of stroptozotocin in combination with 5-fluorouracil (5-FU) is not effective for the management of glucagonomas.[173] The elevations in the serum glucagon levels may be responsive to hormonal therapy with octreotide.[174, 175] In patients with symptomatic insulinomas, the use of diazoxide (Hyperstat), an antihypertensive administered as a 100 mg oral dose three times a day, inhibits insulin levels by the pancreatic islets and blocks peripheral glucose utilization.[176–180] Additional options for treatment include using phenytoin, chlorpromazine, propranolol, verapamil, and octreotide to reduce the effects of hyperinsulinemia, especially in patients with the malignant forms of disease.[181–187] More recently, the use of the mTOR inhibitor, everolimus (Affinitor®), was investigated in three patients with metastatic, symptomatic insulinoma. All three patients demonstrated control of their hypoglycemia within 2 weeks of starting 10 mg of everolimus with a significant reduction (14–64%) of serum insulin levels following 1 month of treatment.[188]

Chemotherapy had been extensively studied in patients with metastatic gastrinoma who show evidence of active growth by serial imaging studies over a decade ago. A combination of streptozotocin, 5-FU, and adriamycin demonstrates short-lived responses in up to 40% of patients.[162, 189–192] However, given the short-lived response and excessive toxicities with these therapies, they were rarely used except for the recalcitrant tumors.[193,194] The more recent introduction of interferons in the 1990s demonstrated some activity against metastatic NETs.[193] This had largely been supplanted by the use of either radiofrequency ablation or transarterial embolization more recently.[195] The combination of consensus interferon when used along with long-acting octreotide has been studied and shown to have a static response against NET growth in the majority of patients.[196]

Recently, everolimus has been approved by the FDA for the treatment of metastatic NETs of pancreatic origin (Fig. 12.10). Affinitor is an active rapamycin derivative and therefore not a prodrug. It has oral bioavailability with a serum half-life of about 30 h and therefore is taken as a once a day medication. This drug has broad antitumor activity (Fig. 12.10) and was shown in preclinical studies to inhibit cell growth and slow the S-phase entry. This agent appears to also enhance the activity of other chemotherapeutic agents and radiation. As a class, rapamycin inhibits mTOR, which will reduce NETs by inhibiting cell growth and proliferation, angiogenesis, and glucose uptake. There is a rationale for combining octreotide with mTOR inhibition in NETs because octreotide has been shown to inhibit IGF-1R signaling and because the PI3-K/AKT/mTOR pathway has been thought to be activated by IGF-1 signaling in NET tumors. Thus, the use of Affinitor with octreotide may have a synergistic effect to arrest growth, inhibit angiogenesis, and reduce the release of secretory hormones. In an open-label, Phase II study of everolimus, there was a partial response observed in almost 10% of patients while two-thirds of the patients had stable disease and nearly a 2-month medial progression-free survival.[197] In Phase III clinical studies (RADIANT 3,[198]), everolimus extended progression-free survival (Fig. 12.11) compared to placebo. Furthermore, patients receiving Affinitor experienced decrease in size of their target lesions as compared to placebo. The side-effect profile was extensively studied in international trials with Affinitor with the most frequent adverse events including stomatitis, skin rash, diarrhea, and fatigue. In our case series of five patients, progressive disease was not seen in patients taking Affinitor (Fig. 12.12).

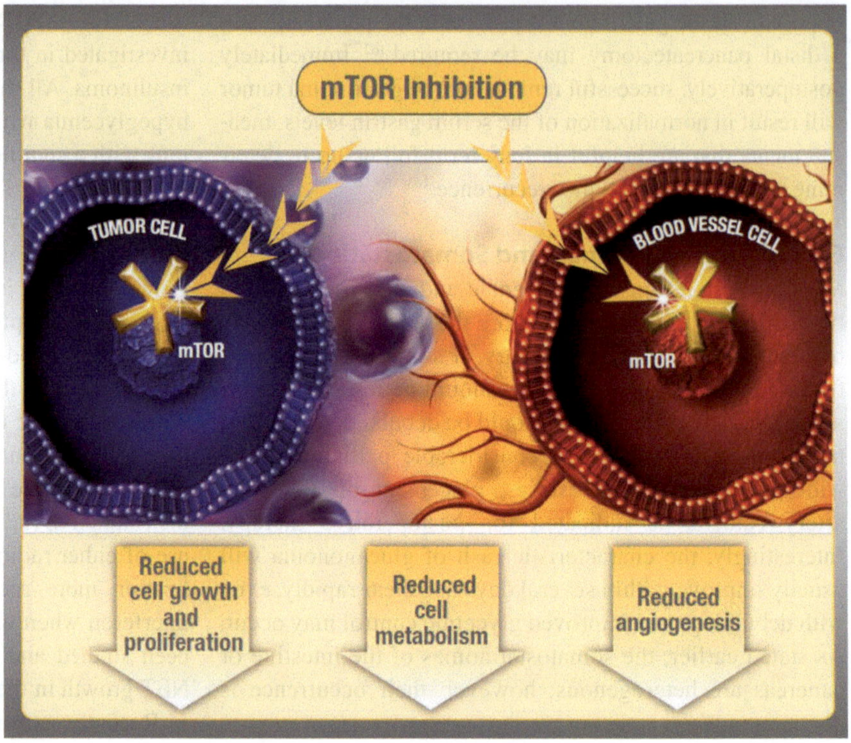

Fig. 12.10 Demonstration of the biological effects of mTOR inhibition on NET growth and angiogenesis

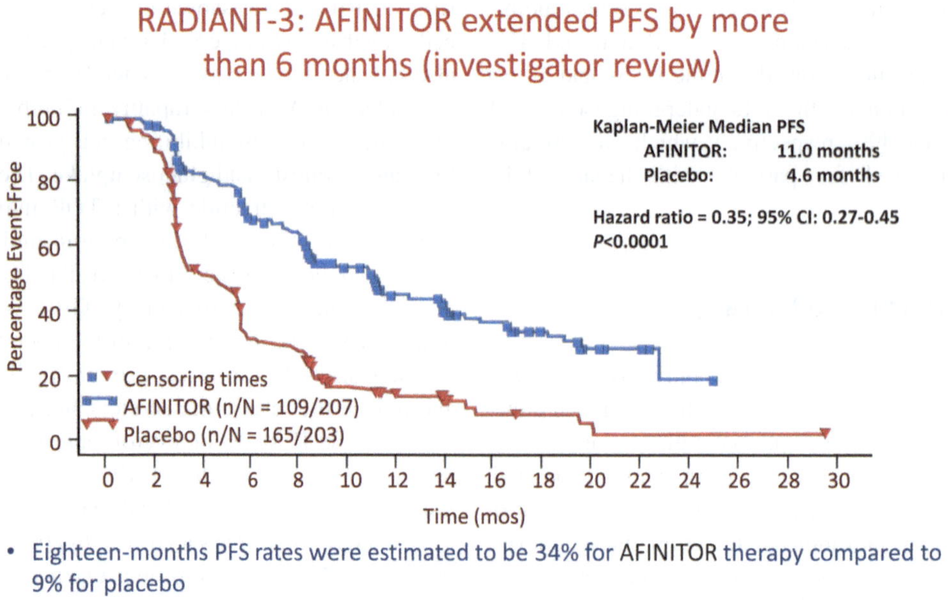

Fig. 12.11 Effects of everolimus (Affinitor) on progression-free survival in patients with metastatic NETs[197]

Fig. 12.12 Results of everolimus in five patients treated for over 24 months with everolimus 10 mg/day

	Pancreatic NET n = 5
Partial responses (PR)	2 (40)
Stable disease (SD)	5 (60)
Progressive disease (PD)	0 (0)
PFS (24 wk)	75%

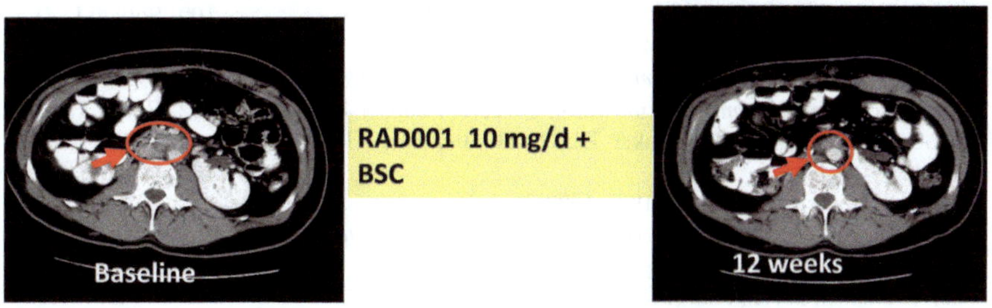

References

1. Boudreaux JP, Klimstra DS, Hassan MM, et al. *Pancreas*. 2010;39(6):753–66.
2. Boden G. Insulinoma and glucagonoma. *Semin Oncol*. 1987;14:253.
3. Vinik AI, Woltering EA, Warner RR, et al. Go VL; North American Neuroendocrine Tumor Society (NANETS). *Pancreas*. 2010;39(6):713–34.
4. Klimstra DS, Modlin IR, Coppola D, Lloyd RV, Suster S. *Pancreas*. 2010;39(6):707–12. Review.
5. Lew EA, Lewin KL, Zarchy T, Pisegna JR. *Am J Gastroenterol*. 1999 Jun;94(6):1692–4.
6. Saclarides TJ, Szekuga D, Staren ED. *Dis Col Rectum*. 1994;37:635–624.
7. Gaffey MJ, Mills SE, Lack EE. *Am J Surg Path*. 1990;14: 1010–1023.
8. Howard TJ, Stabile BE, Zinner MJ, et al. *Am J Surg*. 1990; 159(2):258–64.
9. Wang HS, Oh DS, Ohning GV, Pisegna JR. *J Mol Neurosci*. 2007;33(3):225–31.
10. Wawrukiewicz AS. *Cardiovasc Intervent Radiol*. 1982;5:318.
11. Breatnach RS. *J Comput Assist Tomogr*. 1985;9:25.
12. Wilkinson DS. *Trans St John's Hosp Dermatol Soc*. 1973;59:244.
13. Almdal TP. *Gut*. 1990;31:946.
14. Holst JJ. Glucagon-producing tumors. In: Cohen S, Soloway D, eds. *Hormone producing tumors of the gastrointestinal tract*. New York: Churchill Livingstone; 1978:57.
15. Marynick SP, Fagadau WR, Duncan LA. *Ann Intern Med*. 1980;93:453.
16. Abraira C. *Am J Clin Nutr*. 1984;39:351.
17. Shepherd ME. *J Am Acad Dermatol*. 1991;25:925.
18. Parr JH. *Postgrad Med J*. 1985;61:737.
19. Altimari AF. *Surgery*. 1986;100:989.
20. Rosenbaum A, Flourie B, Chagnon S, et al. *Digestion*. 1989;42(2):116–20.
21. Maton PN. *Digestive Dis Sci*. 1989;34:285.
22. Leichter SB. *Medicine*. 1980;59:100.
23. Stacpole PW. *Endocr Rev*. 1981;2:347.
24. Holst JJ, Helland S, Ingemansson S, et al. *Diabetologia*. 1979;17:151.
25. Stacpoole PW. *Endocr Rev*. 1981;2:347.
26. Jones B. *J Comput Assist Tomogr*. 1983;7:334.
27. Stevens FM. *Gut*. 1984;25:784.
28. Rowland KJ, Brubaker PL. *Am J Physiol Gastrointest Liver Physiol*. 2011;301(1):G1–8. Epub 2011 Apr 28. Review.
29. Doden G, Ryan IG, Eisenscmid BL, et al. *N Engl J Med*. 1986;314:1686.
30. Kasper CS. *Cutis*. 1992;49(2):120–2.
31. Rappaport KD, White JW. *J Mayo Clin Proc*. 1995;70(8):785–8.
32. Mozell E, Stenzel P, Woltering EA, et al. *Curr Probl Surg*. 1990;27(6):301–86.
33. Galbut DL, Markowitz AM. *Am J Surg*. 1980;139:682.
34. Gierchsky KE, Halse J, Mathisen W, et al. *Scand J Gastro*. 1980;15:129.
35. Glickman MH, Hart MJ, White TT. *Am J Surg*. 1980;140:119.
36. Le Quesne P, Nabarro JD, Kutz A, et al. *Br J Surg*. 1979;66:373.
37. Service FJ, dale AJ, Elveback LR, et al. *Mayo Clin Proc*. 1976;51:417.
38. Van Heerden JA, Edis AJ, Service FJ. *Ann Surg*. 1979;189:677.
39. Jaksic T, Yaman M, Thorner P, Wesson DK, Filler RM, Shandling B. *J Pediatr Surg*. 1992;27(10):1315–7.
40. Meleo K. *Probl Vet Med*. 1990;2(4):602–9.
41. Eckersley GN, Fockema A, Williams JH, et al. *J S Afr Vet Assoc*. 1987;58(4):187–92.
42. Sawicki PT, Baba T, Berger M, et al. *J Am Soc Nephrol*. 1992;3(4 Suppl):S64–8.
43. Svartberg J, Stridsberg M, Wilander E, et al. *J Intern Med*. 1996;239(2):181–5.
44. Garner PR, Tsang R. *Obstet Gynecol*. 1989;73(5 Pt 2):847–9.
45. Merimee TJ. *N Engl J Med*. 1974;291:1275.
46. Davidson MB. *Manual of Endocrinology and Metabolism*. 2nd ed. Boston: Little, Brown & Co; 1994:459.
47. Fajans SS, Vinik AI. *Endocrinol Metab Clin North Am*. 1989;18(1):45–74.
48. Merimee TJ. *Diabetes*. 1977;26:161.
49. Gutman RA. *N Engl J Med*. 1971;284:1003.
50. Sherman BM. *J Clin Endocrinol Metab*. 1972;35:271.

51. Cohen RM. *Metabolism*. 1986;35:1137.
52. Grunberger G, Weiner JL, Silverman R, et al. *Ann Int Med*. 1988;108:252.
53. Rendell M. *Acta Diabetol Lat*. 1983;20(2):105–113.
54. Bonser AM, Garcia-Webb P. *Ann Clin Biochem*. 1981;18(Pt 4): 200–206.
55. Grant CS. *Baillieres Clin Gastroenterol*. 1996;10(4):645–671.
56. Gray RK. *Radiology*. 1970;97:39.
57. Stark DA. *Radiology*. 1984;150:491.
58. Rossi P. *AJR*. 1985;144:57.
59. Vinayek R. *Gastroenterol Clin North Am*. 1990;19:197.
60. Berg CL. *Med Clin North Am*. 1991;75:903.
61. Day JP, Richter JE. *Gastroent Clin N Am*. 1990;19(3):587–607.
62. Hirschowitz BI. *Am J Gastroenterol*. 1997;92(4 Suppl):44S-48S.
63. Sugg SL, Norton JA, Fraker DL, et al. *Ann Surg*. 1993;218: 138–144.
64. van Heerden JA. *Surgery*. 1986;100:971.
65. Fishbeyn VA, Norton JA, Benya RV, et al. *Annals Intern Med*. 1993;119:199–206.
66. Thompson JC. *Ann Surg*. 1983;197:594.
67. Vinik AI. *Ann Intern Med*. 1986;105:956.
68. Kohan E, Oh D, Wang H, Hazany S, Ohning G, Pisegna JR. *Diagn Ther Endosc*. 2009;2009:298381.
69. Schjonsby H, Willassen Y. *Scand J Gastroenterol*. 1977;12: 205–207.
70. Pisegna JR, Lew E, Tarasova N, et al. *Gastroenterology*. 1998; 114(4):4797.
71. Pisegna JR, Lew EA, Martin P, et al. *Am J Gastroenterol*. 1999;94:2874–2880.
72. Pisegna JR, deWeerth A, Huppi K, et al. *Biochem Biophys Res Comm*. 1992;189:296–303.
73. Wank SA, Pisegna JR, de Weerth A. *Proc Natl Acad Sci USA*. 1992;89:8691–8695.
74. Wolfe MM, Jensen RT. *N Engl J Med*. 1987;317(19):1200–9.
75. Bloom SR, Long RG, Bryant MG, et al. *Gastroenterology*. 1980;78:1143.
76. Vezzadini C, Poggioli R, Casoni I, et al. *Panminerva Med*. 1996;38(4):255–8.
77. Arps H, Dietel M, Schulz A, et al. Virchows Arch. 1986: 408–497.
78. Oh DS, Wang HS, Ohning GV, Pisegna JR. *Clin Gastroenterol Hepatol*. 2006;4(12):1467–73. Epub 2006.
79. Fajans SS, Floyd JC. Fasting hypoglycemia in adults. *N Engl J Med*. 1976;294:766.
80. Domschke S, Domschke W, Bloom SR, et al. *Gut*. 1978; 29:1049.
81. Pisegna JR, Norton JA, Slimak GG, et al. *Gastroenterology*. 1992;102(3):767–78.
82. Richardson CT. *Gastroenterology*. 1985;89:357.
83. McArthur KE. *Gastroenterology*. 1985;88:939.
84. Stewart CA, Termanini B, Sutliff VE, et al. *Am J Obstet Gynecol*. 1997;176:224–33.
85. Maton PN. *Drugs*. 1996;52(1):33–44.
86. Frucht H. *Dig Dis Sci*. 1991;36:394.
87. Metz DC. *Gastroenterology*. 1992;103:1498.
88. Maton PN. *Aliment Pharmacol Ther*. 1991;5(Suppl 1):25.
89. Frucht H, Maton PN, Jensen RT. *Dig Dis Sci*. 1991;36:394–404.
90. Metz DC, Pisegna JR, Fishbeyn VA, et al. *Gastroenterology*. 1992;103:1498–1508.
91. Garnett WR. *Ann Pharmacother*. 1996;30(12):1425–36.
92. Metz DC, Pisegna JR, Ringham GL, et al. *Dig Dis Sci*. 1992;38:245–256.
93. Metz DC, Lew E, Forsmark CE, et al. *Gastroenterology*. 1998;114(4):G0926.
94. Pisegna JR, Huang M, Asvar C, et al. *Gastroenterology*. 1998; 114(4):G1065.
95. Lew EA, Pisegna JR, Starr JA, et al. *Gastroenterology*. 2000;118:696–704.
96. Nieto JM, Pisegna JR. *Expert Opin Pharmacother*. 2006;7(2): 169–75.
97. Helander HF, Rutgersson K, Helander KG, et al. *Gastroenterology*. 1992;27:875–883.
98. Waldum HL, Brenna E, Kleveland PM, et al. *Dig Dis*. 1995;13(1):25–38.
99. Cadiot G, Vissuzaine C, Potet F, et al. *Dig Dis Sci*. 1995;40(6): 1275–8.
100. Solvell L. *Digestion*. 1990;47(Suppl 1):59–63. discussion 76.
101. Solcia E, Capella C, Fiocca R, et al. *Am J Surg Pathol*. 1990;14(6):503–13.
102. Bordi C, D'Adda T, Azzoni C, et al. *Am J Surg Pathol*. 1995;19(Suppl 1):S8–19.
103. Delcore R, Friesen SR. *Surgery*. 1992;112(6):1016–22. discussion 1022–3.
104. O'Dorisio TM. *Endocrinol Metab Clin North Am*. 1989;18:545.
105. Zeng N, Kang T, Wong H, Walsh JH, Sachs GA, Pisegna JR. *J Clin Invest*. 1999;104:1383–1391.
106. Alberti KGMM, Oxbury J, Higgins G. *Br Med J*. 1972;1:87.
107. O'Dorisio TM, Mekhjian HS. VIPoma syndrome. In: Cohen S, Soloway RD, eds. *Hormone producing tumors of the pancreas*. New York: Churchil Livingstone; 1985:101.
108. Ronnov-Jenson D. *Eur J Clin Invest*. 1991;21:154.
109. Boden G, Shimoyama R. Somatostatinoma. In: Cohen S, Soloway RD, eds. *Hormone-producing tumors of the gastrointestinal tract*. New York: Churchill Livingstone; 1985:85.
110. Reber HA. In: Howard JM, ed. *Surgical Diseases of the Pancreas*. Lea & Febiger: Philadelphia; 1987:865.
111. Krejs GJ. *N Engl J Med*. 1971;301:285.
112. Lowry SF. *Surgery*. 1981;89:309.
113. Konomi K. *J Surg Oncol*. 1990;43:259.
114. Vinik AI, Strodel WE, Eckhauser FE, et al. *Endocrinol Clin N Am*. 1989;18:483–493.
115. Vinik AI, Strodel WE, Eckhauser FE, et al. *Semin Oncol*. 1987;14:263.
116. Galmiche JP, Chayvialle JA, Dubois PM, et al. Calcitonin-producing pancreatic somatostatinoma. *Gastroenterology*. 1980; 78:1577.
117. Konomi K, Chijiiwa K, Katsuta T, et al. *J Surg Oncol*. 1990; 43(4):259–65.
118. Walsh JH. Gastrointestinal hormones. In: Johnson LR, ed. *Physiology of the gastrointestinal tract*. New York: Raven; 1987.
119. Boden G, Sivitz MC, Owen OE. *Science*. 1975;190:163.
120. Koerker DJ, Ruth W, Chideckel E. *Science*. 1974;184:482.
121. Bloom SR, Mortimer CH, Thorner MO, et al. *Lancet*. 1974; 2:1106.
122. Schegel W, Rapits S, Harvey RF, et al. *Lancet*. 1977;2:166.
123. Ormsbee HS, Koehler SL, Telford GL. *Dig Dis*. 1978;23:781.
124. Reichlin S. Somatostatin. *N Engl J Med*. 1983;309:1495.
125. Samols E, Weir GC, Ramseur R, et al. *Metabolism*. 1978; 27:1219.
126. Boden G, Baile CA, McLauglin CL, et al. *Am J Physiol*. 1981; 241:E215.
127. Schusdziarra V. *Klin Wochenshr*. 1983;61:681.
128. Pipeleers D. *J Clin Endocrinol Metab*. 1979;49:572.
129. Axelrod L. *J Clin Endocrinol Metab*. 1981;52:886.
130. Wright J. *Clin Endocrinol*. 1980;12:603.
131. Swinburn BA. *Clin Endocrinol*. 1988;28:353.
132. Ohtsuki Y. *Acta Pathol Jpn*. 1989;39:141.
133. Soga J. *Eur J Cancer*. 1990;26:1107.
134. Hagen EC. *Pancreas*. 1992;7:98.
135. Maki M, Kaneko Y, Ohta Y, et al. *Intern Med*. 1995;34(7):661–5.
136. Kent RB, van Heerden JA, Weiland LH. *Ann Surg*. 1981;193:185.
137. Eckhauser FE, Cheung PS, Vinik A, et al. *Surgery*. 1986;100:978.

138. Erickson B, Oberg K, Skogseid B. *Acta Oncol*. 1989;28:373.
139. Grama D. *World J Surg*. 1992;16:632.
140. Rivier J, Spress J, Thorner M, Vale W. *Nature*. 1982;300:276.
141. Thorner MO, Perryman RL, Cronin MJ, et al. *J Clin Invest*. 1982;70:965.
142. Keogan MT, Baker ME. *Gastroint Endosc Clin N Am*. 1995; 5(1):31–59.
143. Pisegna JR, Doppman JL, Norton JA, et al. *Dig Dis Sci*. 1993;38:1318–1328.
144. Benya RV, Metz DA, Hijazi YM, et al. *Am J Gastroenterol*. 1993;88:258–265.
145. Termanini B, Gibril F, Doppman JL, et al. *Radiology*. 1997;202: 151–158.
146. Perry RR, Vinik AI. *Annu Rev Med*. 1996;47:57–68.
147. Modlin IM, Cornelius E, Lawton GP. *Arch Surg*. 1995;130(4):367–73. discussion 373–4.
148. Gorman B, Reading CC. *Semin Ultrasound CT MR*. 1995;16(4): 331–41.
149. Sugg SL, Norton JA, Fraker DL, et al. *Ann Surg*. 1993;218:138–144.
150. Meko JB, Norton JA. *Annu Rev Med*. 1995;46:395–411.
151. Cherner JA, Doppman JL, Norton JA, et al. *Ann Int Med*. 1986;105:841.
152. Maton PN, Miller DL, Doppman JL, et al. *Gastroenterology*. 1987;92:913.
153. Roche A, Raisonnier A, Gillon-Asavouret MC. *Radiology*. 1982;145:621.
154. Zeiger MA. *World J Surg*. 1993;17:448.
155. Rosch T. *N Engl J Med*. 1992;326:1721.
156. Rothmund M. *World J Surg*. 1990;14:393.
157. Passaro E Jr, Howard TJ, Sawicki MP, et al. *Arch Surg*. 1998;133(1):13–6.
158. Townsend CM Jr, Thompson JC. *Annu Rev Med*. 1985;36: 111–24.
159. Sheppard BC. *Surgery*. 1989;106:1108.
160. Thompson NW. *Henry Ford Hosp Med J*. 1992;40:195.
161. Frucht H. *Gastroenterology*. 1990;99:1622.
162. Mignon M. *World J Surg*. 1986;10:703.
163. Thompson NW. *World J Surg*. 1993;17:455.
164. Norton JA. *Ann Surg*. 1992;215:8.
165. Imamura M, Komoto I, Ota S, et al. *World J Gastroenterol*. 2011;17(10):1343–53.
166. Gedaly R, Daily MF, Davenport D, et al. *Arch Surg*. 2011;146(8):953–8.
167. Prinz RA. *Surgery*. 1981;90:713.
168. Marynick SP. *Ann Intern Med*. 1980;93:453.
169. Awrich AE. *J Surg Oncol*. 1981;17:321.
170. Strauss GM. *Ann Intern Med*. 1979;90:57.
171. Duncan LA. *Ann Intern Med*. 1982;97:930.
172. Altimari AF. *Surgery*. 1987;102:1009.
173. Moertel CG. *N Engl J Med*. 1980;303:1189.
174. Kvols LK. *Ann Intern Med*. 1987;107:162.
175. Wood SM. *Gut*. 1985;26:438.
176. Loubatieres A. *Ann NY Acad Sci*. 1968;150:226.
177. Porte D Jr. *J Clin Invest*. 1966;45:228.
178. Groen J. *Diabetes*. 1958;7:272.
179. Abramson EA. *Diabetes*. 1968;17:141.
180. Altszuler N. *Diabetes*. 1977;26:931.
181. Knopp RH. *Arch Intern Med*. 1972;130:904.
182. Brodows RG. *J Clin Endocrinol Metab*. 1974;38:159.
183. Hofeldt FD. *Diabetes*. 1974;23:192.
184. Federspil G. *Diabetologia*. 1974;10:189.
185. Ulbrecht JS. *Diabetes Care*. 1986;9:186.
186. Osei K. *Ann Intern Med*. 1985;103:223.
187. Broder LE. *Ann Intern Med*. 1973;79:108.
188. Fiebrich HB, Siemerink EJ, Brouwers AH, et al. *Oncologist*. 2011;16(6):783–7.
189. Thompson W. *World J Surg*. 1984;8:940.
190. Eckhauser FE. *Surgery*. 1986;100:978.
191. Geelhoed GW. *Surgery*. 1986;100:962.
192. Howard JM. *Gastroenterology*. 1983;84:1192.
193. Pisegna JR, Slimak GG, Metz DC, et al. *Gastroenterology*. 1993;105:1179–1183.
194. von Schrenck T. *Gastroenterology*. 1988;94:1326.
195. Chung MH, Pisegna J, et al. *Surgery*. 2001;130(6):954–62.
196. Wang HS, Oh DS, Ohning GV, Pisegna JR. *J Pharm Pharmacol*. 2006;58(12):1623–8.
197. Yao JC, Lombard-Bohas C, Baudin EJ. *Clin Oncol*. 2010;28(1): 69–76.
198. Yao JC, Shah MH, Ito T, et al. *N Engl J Med*. 2011;364:514–523.

Part IV

Metastatic Disease and Tumor Markers

Molecular Mechanisms of Tumor Metastasis

13

Andrew D. Rhim, Davendra Sohal, and Hiroshi Nakagawa

Introduction

The major cause of cancer-related death is metastatic disease. Defined quite simply, metastatic disease occurs when cancer cells from one organ translocate to another locale and establish new tumors. These lesions possess all of the hallmarks of cancer[1] and feature unchecked growth and invasive properties that frequently lead to incurable involvement of multiple organs. While recent research has led to significant advancements in the management of limited primary tumors, treatment of advanced metastatic disease continues to lag, and in the vast majority of cases, is nonexistent. However, with recent advances in molecular profiling of human specimens, modeling of human disease in genetically engineered mouse models of cancer, and more sensitive modes of radiographic and pathologic detection of tumors, our understanding of metastatic disease has increased dramatically and is poised to produce tangible gains for patients. Even as the study of metastasis has exploded over the past few years, many questions that have occupied researchers still remain: What is required for tumor cells to metastasize? What are the factors that specify tissue tropism within metastatic cells? When does metastasis occur? What is the latency between organ infiltration of individual disseminated cells and overt colonization? To which treatments are metastatic lesions susceptible? In this chapter, we will provide the groundwork for a general understanding of the biology of metastasis with special emphasis on cancers arising from the gastrointestinal tract. The understanding of these commonalities will provide for a foundation for the understanding of future discoveries that will address these questions, as well as evoke many others.

Tumor Microenvironment and Cell Heterogeneity in Metastasis

Metastasis encompasses wide arrays of biological processes including genetic and epigenetic changes within tumor cells, resulting in clonal evolution of metastatic cells or selection of unique cellular subpopulations with increased metastatic potential, cellular plasticity and motility. Metastasis begins by departure of cells from the primary tumor, involving collective as well as individual cancer cell invasion through the stroma, intravasation and extravasation from blood and lymphatic vessels, as well as settlement into metastatic sites such as lymph nodes and remote organs. These processes require a dynamic cross talk between tumor cells and the microenvironment sending mechanical and nonmechanical stimuli such as tissue stiffness, inflammation, growth factors, cytokines, hormones, low oxygen tension, limited nutrients, and energy sources. Tumor microenvironment comprises a variety of cellular components including immune cells, fibroblasts, and vascular endothelial cells. In addition, the tumor microenvironment undergoes dynamic changes along with tumor growth and even in response to therapeutic interventions, affecting tumor cell characteristics and functions through cell–cell and cell–extracellular matrix communications involving essential signaling pathways.

Stephen Paget (1855–1926), an English surgeon, first proposed the importance of tumor microenvironment as a common basis for cancer metastasis. In 1889, he reported that breast cancer metastasizes to specific organs such as the liver in a nonrandom fashion, proposing the "seed and soil" theory,[2] where cancer cells (seeds) require appropriate microenvironment (soil) in the destination organs to grow as a metastatic tumor. Consistent with Paget's theory, the incidence of remote metastasis depends upon the primary tumors.

A.D. Rhim, M.D. • H. Nakagawa, M.D., Ph.D. (✉)
Department of Medicine, Gastroenterology Division,
University of Pennsylvania School of Medicine, 421 Curie Blvd., Philadelphia, PA 19104, USA
e-mail: andrew.rhim@uphs.upenn.edu; nakagawh@mail.med.upenn.edu

D. Sohal, M.D., M.P.H.
Solid Tumor Oncology, Taussig Cancer Institute, Cleveland Clinic, 9500 Euclid Avenue, R35 Cleveland, OH 44195, USA
e-mail: sohald@ccf.org

A.R. Sepulveda and J.P. Lynch (eds.), *Molecular Pathology of Neoplastic Gastrointestinal Diseases*, Molecular Pathology Library 7,
DOI 10.1007/978-1-4614-6015-2_13,

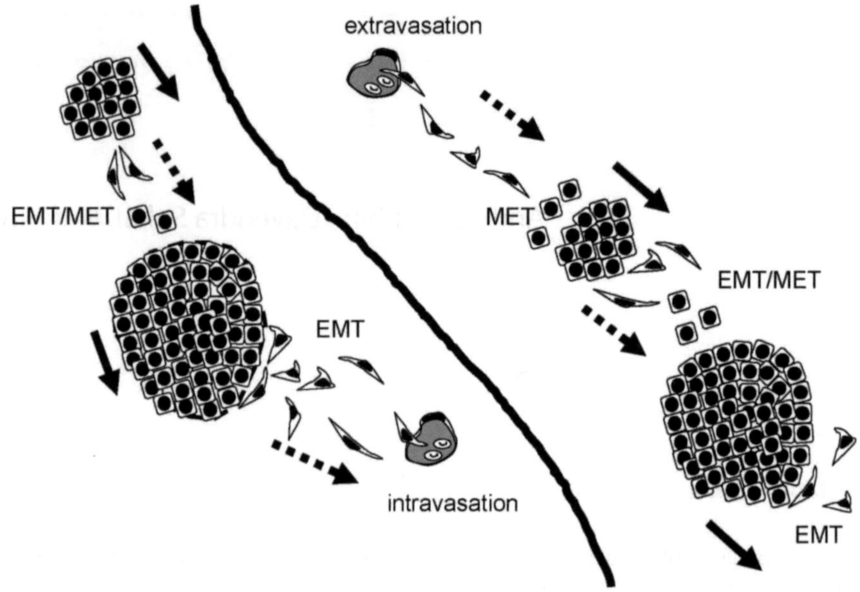

Fig. 13.1 Sequence of metastatic steps. Cancer metastasis involves local invasion, entry into the blood stream or lymph circulation (i.e., intravasation), persistence in the circulation, extravasation into distant organs, colonization, and metastatic growth of tumor cells. Invasion occurs either collectively (*arrows*) or individually (*broken arrows*). Cells may undergo epithelial-to-mesenchymal transition (EMT) and mesenchymal-to-epithelial transition (MET) during invasion through the tumor stroma where cancer cells are exposed to various factors from the microenvironment

For example, the ovary is a common metastasis site for GI cancers including colorectal and pancreatic carcinomas. In particular, ovarian metastasis of aggressive gastric carcinomas is known as Krukenberg tumors, featuring signet ring cells surrounded by an abundant dense fibrous tumor stroma.[3] James Ewing (1866–1943), an American pathologist, challenged Paget's hypothesis in 1929. He proposed that cancer metastasis depend upon the anatomical structure of the vascular system connecting primary tumors and destination organs. Ewing's view may hold for locally progressive diseases such as lymph node metastasis associated with lymphatic drainage from primary tumors as observed in many GI cancers. Nonetheless, the "Seed and Soil" hypothesis is applicable even for the early stages of tumor invasion as discussed in the following section, and is one of the key principles in cancer metastasis with respect to "tumor microenvironment," which is today a major focus of cancer research.

Histopathology of metastatic tumors often recapitulates that of primary tumors. While tumor grade is pathologically judged based on the extent of differentiation in the majority of tumor cells, an individual tumor exhibits substantive heterogeneity as noted in various GI cancers such as esophageal squamous cell carcinoma (ESCC)[4] and colorectal carcinomas (CRC).[5] At the invasive front, cancer cells tend to be dedifferentiated, losing cell–cell contact, and being disseminated into the adjacent stroma. Primary CRCs with liver metastasis contain more dedifferentiated cancer cells with indistinct polarity and an infiltrative growth pattern than those without metastasis.[6] Once metastasized to lymph nodes or remote organs, such cancer cells may form a tumor displaying morphological characteristics similar to primary tumors. Thus, tumor cells show a remarkable plasticity depending upon microenvironment as well as genetic changes as discussed below.

Genetic Changes Leading to Metastasis

Metastasis, in itself, refers to a phenomenon common to almost all cancers. Even though carcinomas may arise in different organs and driven by different genetic events, many share common sites of colonization. For example, the liver is a principal site of metastasis for colorectal, pancreatic, stomach, breast, and lung carcinomas.[7] However, some cancers show a certain degree of tissue tropism. This is exemplified by the fact that prostate cancer primarily metastasizes to bone in addition to local spread.[7] Indeed, it is very likely that the kinetics and driving genetic events for metastasis varies for each type of cancer. Nevertheless, it is helpful to deconstruct metastasis into a sequence of steps: local invasion, entry into the blood stream or lymph circulation, persistence in the circulation, extravasation into distant organs, colonization and metastatic growth (Fig. 13.1). Enough evidence now exists allowing us to begin to associate certain genes with the specific steps involved in metastasis (proposed by Nguyen and colleagues, Table 13.1[8]), similar to genetic progression models of tumorigenesis.[9]

Oncogenic transformation is required for a metastatic lesion to form. Thought to precede all other mutations, tumor initiating mutations confer many of the fundamental characteristics of cancer[1]: boundless proliferation, acquisition of progenitor-like characteristics, and tolerance of genomic instability.[8] Examples of such mutations include *KRAS*, *Erbb2*, *PTEN*, *APC*, *β-catenin*, *epidermal growth factor receptor* (*EGFR*), and *MYC*. Indeed it has been shown that tumors and metastatic lesions depend on these mutations to survive. Multiple studies in vitro and in vivo in gastrointestinal cancers exemplify this concept: *KRAS* in pancreatic cancers,[10] *KIT* in gastrointestinal stromal tumors (GIST[11]), *c-myc*

Table 13.1 Summary of metastasis-related genes (Adapted from[8])

Tumor initiation: Transformation, survival, anoikis resistance, growth, genomic instability
• Oncogenes (gain of function)
– *KRAS, β-catenin, EGFR, MYC, ERBB2*
• Tumor suppressors (loss of function)
– *APC, p53, PTEN, BRCA1, BRCA2*
Metastasis initiation: invasion, angiogenesis, endothelial penetration, circulation
• Gain of function
– *TWIST1, SNAIL1, SNAIL2, MET, ID1*
• Loss of function
– *mIR-126, mIR-335, KISS-1*
Metastasis progression: extravasation, survival, initiation of growth in distant organs
• *LOX, MMP1, ANGPTL4, PTGS2, COX2*
Metastasis virulence: organ specific effects
• *GM-CSF, PTHRP, IL6, IL11, TNFα*

in insulinomas,[12] and *β-catenin* in colon cancers.[13] However, while required, the presence of these tumor-initiating mutations is not sufficient for metastatic disease. This is best documented in many genetic mouse models of GI cancers, driven by tumor initiating mutations, in which almost all mice are born phenotypically normal and with no evidence of metastasis.

"Metastasis initiation genes" confer the ability for epithelial cells to become mobile in a process frequently referred to as epithelial-to-mesenchymal transition (EMT[8]) (Fig. 13.2). During an EMT, genes usually associated with stromal cells are activated, either by mutation or induction. Once activated, cancer cells gain the ability to invade through basement membranes, secrete enzymes to allow for penetration through the host organ and eventual entry into the blood circulation or lymphatic system. Examples of EMT mediators include the transcription factors TWIST1, SNAI1, SLUG, and ZEB1, as well as microRNAs such as miR-126 and miR-200a (suppression is seen in invading cells), and metastasis-associated in colon cancer (MACC1), a member of the hepatocyte growth factor signaling pathway. These genes are thought to mediate not only invasive properties that allow cells to enter the blood stream but also the ability to persist in the environments without cell attachment. For a more detailed discussion of EMT, please see the section entitled, "Importance of EMT."

Another set of genes is thought to mediate the ability for disseminated cancer cells to extravasate from the circulation, persist in distant organs, and establish thriving colonies. These genes have been termed as conferring "metastasis progression functions".[7] This set of genes has recently been established in models of metastatic breast cancer. Examples include matrix metalloproteinase 1 (MMP1), cyclooxygenase 2 (COX2), and lysyl oxidase (LOX). While these proteins have been shown to play prominent roles in inducing metastatic growth, many of these genes are also upregulated in the primary tumor. Thus, it has been suggested that these genes, while involved in a distal point of metastatic disease, may play a dual role early in tumorigenesis. For example, COX2 is known to be involved in cultivating the inflammatory microenvironment that supports cancer progression not only within the primary tumor but also in premalignant lesions in pancreatic and colorectal cancers.[14] LOX has also been shown to play an important role in cultivating the physical characteristics of the stromal environment surrounding epithelial structures, and it has been shown to directly affect the development of early invasive behaviors among transformed cells.[15] Further, in an experimental model of breast cancer, LOX secreted by the tumor has been shown to draw CD11b+ myeloid cells to sites of future metastasis.[16] These myeloid-derived cells are thought to "prime" the soil of the distant organ to allow for homing of disseminated cells to these immune-privileged sites. In addition to LOX, other genes have been implicated in targeting cancer cells to specific sites. Parathyroid-related protein (*PTHRP*) becomes significantly upregulated only in breast cancer cells that have colonized bone. This protein, along with interleukin-11 (IL-11), stimulates osteoclasts to create a local bone environment conducive for eventual metastatic growth.[17]

Thus, the past decade has ushered in a wave of insightful work that has shaped how we understand how cancer cells metastasize. We are now in a position to begin to translate findings in the mechanisms of metastasis to the clinical setting. Identification of mutations and upregulation of certain genes involved in dissemination and metastasis within primary tumors have already yielded valuable prognostic information for individual patients. Further, this work has initiated the development of compounds that specifically target metastasis-related genes for the purposes of treatment of late stage metastatic cancers as well as in the prophylaxis against metastatic seeding during treatment of a primary tumor. Despite these exciting advances, much work needs to be done, especially in gastrointestinal cancers where research has lagged behind breast and prostate cancers.

Importance of Epithelial to Mesenchymal Transition

Epithelial to mesenchymal transition (EMT) is a physiological process taking place in a reversible manner during embryonic development. EMT is marked by loss of epithelial characteristics and gain of mesenchymal characteristics (Fig. 13.2). Epithelial cells maintain apical–basolateral cell polarity, cell–cell contact through adherens junctions and desmosomes while mesenchymal traits include fibroblastic spindle-shaped morphology and an increased motility. During gastrulation and subsequent organogenesis, cells

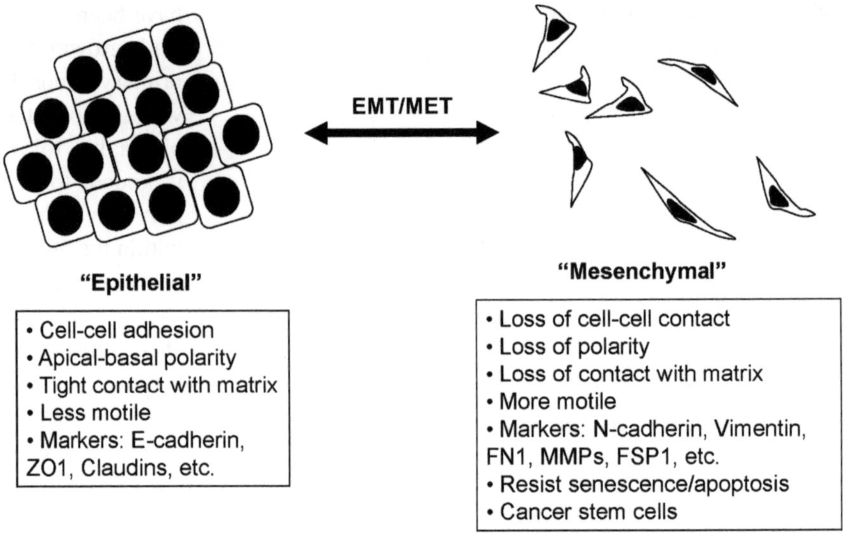

Fig. 13.2 EMT and MET Cancer cells exhibit plasticity during tumor invasion and metastasis by gaining epithelial and mesenchymal phenotypes in an interchangeable fashion

undergo EMT and mesenchymal to epithelial transition (MET) in a repetitive fashion to migrate to new tissue locations and differentiate into specific cell types in embryonic tissues. Gastrointestinal organs are derived from the foregut endoderm. EMT has been implied during the development of the liver[18] and the endocrine pancreas.[19] EMT also occurs during the wound healing process in response to injury, tissue regeneration, and pathological fibrosis.

EMT is critically involved in cancer invasion and metastasis through diverse mechanisms. First, EMT disrupts cell–cell adhesion allowing dissemination of tumor cells. Second, cancer cells undergoing EMT produce enzymes such as matrix metalloproteinases (MMPs), proteases degrading basement membrane and extracellular matrixes (ECM), and lysyl oxidases catalyzing collagen cross-linking. These molecules alter the tumor microenvironment and facilitate cancer cell invasion through tissues and intravasation into blood and lymph vessels. Third, EMT affects cell signaling activities through alterations of the cytoskeleton serving as platforms of diverse intracellular signaling pathways. For example, E-cadherin, the foremost epithelial markers and adhesion molecule downregulated during EMT, inhibits the activities of receptor tyrosine kinases (RTKs) such as epidermal growth factor receptor (EGFR), Insulin-like growth factor-1 receptor (IGF1R), and hepatocyte growth factor receptor cMET.[20] Amongst cell signaling pathways critically altered through EMT is integrin signaling that regulates cell motility, cytoskeleton, and cell survival through association with RTKs.[21] Fourth, tumor cells that have undergone EMT resist anoikis upon detachment from basement membrane. EMT also allows tumor cells to cope with other cellular stresses such as hypoxia and acidity in tissue microenvironment. In addition, EMT prevents tumor cells from undergoing apoptosis triggered by therapeutic agents. Finally, EMT is associated with putative cancer stem cells or tumor-initiating cells that may account for tumor cell heterogeneity in metastatic lesions.

EMT Markers and Regulatory Mechanisms

Despite an increasing body of in vitro evidence, the roles of EMT in cancer cell invasion and metastasis have been subjected to controversy[22] in part because of the issue of semantics and in part because EMT or EMT-like changes in vivo demands careful marker analysis and/or lineage tracing experiments due to its reversible, transient, and focal nature. In fact, it is often difficult to distinguish morphologically tumor cells that have undergone EMT from stromal fibroblasts within tumor tissues. However, imaging and cell fate mapping experiments have documented EMT in invasive tumor cells in vivo.[23] In human cancers, EMT is suggested by loss of E-cadherin and other epithelial markers (e.g., ZO1, Occludin, Claudins, cytokeratins) and concomitant upregulation of mesenchymal markers (e.g., N-cadherin, Vimentin, fibroblast specific protein-1, α-smooth muscle actin) (Fig. 13.2) as well as transcription factors (e.g., Twist, Snail, Slug, ZEB1, and ZEB2), repressing E-cadherin and transactivating various mesenchymal markers. Aberrant expression of these molecules has been documented in GI cancers including oral and esophageal squamous cell carcinoma, esophageal adenocarcinoma, gastric, pancreatic, hepatocellular, and colorectal carcinomas[24–43] and has been associated with invasion, metastasis, and usually poor prognosis. Most of these EMT markers have a plethora of biological functions that may influence EMT and its consequences directly or indirectly.

Cadherin Switching in EMT

E-cadherin is a calcium-dependent cell–cell adhesion molecule to maintain epithelial integrity. In human cancers, E-cadherin is inactivated partially or completely through loss of heterozygosity (LOH) and inactivating mutations, promoter hypermethylation, transcriptional repression, or endocytosis. LOH of human E-cadherin gene *CDH1* at chromosome 16q is common in breast, prostate, gastric, hepatocellular, and esophageal carcinomas.[44] Several somatic mutations in *CDH1* have been found in sporadic diffuse gastric carcinoma with epigenetic silencing as a more common mechanism than LOH for biallelic *CDH1* inactivation.[45,46] In addition, germ line mutations of *CDH1* have been identified in early-onset familial gastric carcinomas.[47,48] While mutations of *CDH1* are rare in other GI cancers,[44] hypermethylation on the *CDH1* promoter CpG island has been documented in hepatocellular and esophageal carcinomas.[49–51] Importantly, the methylation of CpG islands allows recruitment of histone deacetylases[52] and EMT-inducing transcriptional repressors such as Snail, ZEB1/δEF1, and ZEB2/SIP1 to silence E-cadherin gene expression.

As a transmembrane glycoprotein expressed at the cell junction, E-cadherin interacts physically with various catenins (e.g., β-catenin and p120ctn) and cytoskeleton, influencing directly or indirectly RTKs, Wnt, and other cell signaling pathways.[44] Loss of E-cadherin-mediated cell adhesion appears to be one rate-limiting step in the progression to invasive cancer in pancreatic β-cell carcinogenesis.[53] Combined loss of E-cadherin and p53 in mice accelerates development of invasive and metastatic mammary carcinomas although E-cadherin loss alone is not sufficient for full EMT.[54] In immortalized human breast epithelial cells, however, E-cadherin loss resulted in EMT, invasiveness, and metastasis with β-catenin nuclear translocation and twist induction.[55]

During EMT, loss of E-cadherin is accompanied by induction of nonepithelial cadherins such as N-cadherin and cadherin 11, and referred to as "cadherin switching."[56,57] N-cadherin contributes to squamous cell carcinoma cell invasion by suppression of E-cadherin-mediated cell adhesion and EMT.[58] N-cadherin augments fibroblast growth factor receptor (FGFR)-mediated extracellular signal-regulated kinase activation to stimulate MMP9 expression in breast cancer cells, thereby enhancing invasion and metastasis even in the presence of E-cadherin.[59–61] In transformed pancreatic ductal epithelial cells, oncogenic KRAS and mutant p53 regulate cell migration and invasion by modulating formation of a molecular complex consisting of N-cadherin, p120-catenin, and keratinocyte growth factor receptor, an isoform of FGFR.[62] N-cadherin also facilitates migration of melanoma cells upon loss of functional E-cadherin.[63]

Cell Signaling Pathways and Transcription Factors Regulating EMT

EMT is regulated by numerous growth factors, cytokines, and hormones present in the tumor microenvironment, cell signaling pathways, as well as transcription factors in cell-type and context-dependent manners.[64] Transforming growth factor (TGF)-β is one of the most potent EMT inducers[65] and TGF-β-mediated EMT occurs as a consequence of malignant transformation of epidermal keratinocytes and mammary epithelial cells.[66,67] However, many human cell lines fail to undergo EMT in response to TGF-β stimulation,[68] which may be accounted for by mutations in the TGF-β receptor and Smad4 in cancers. In fact, relatively favorable clinical outcomes in a subset of colorectal cancer patients associated with microsatellite instability may be accounted for by lack of EMT due to TGF-β receptor mutations.[69]

TGF-β signaling involves physical interactions between transcription factors ZEBs and receptor Smads (Smad2 and Smad3).[70,71] Other essential signaling pathways include Ras-MAPK, PI3, Wnt, and Notch.[64] They are likely responsible for EMT even in cells having impaired TGF-β signaling components. Zinc finger transcription factors Snail, Slug, ZEB1, and ZEB2 repress *CDH1* (E-cadherin) gene directly by binding the E-box *cis*-elements on its promoter region. Other transcription factors such as Twist, Goosecoid, FOXC2, and E47 regulate *CDH1* indirectly.[64] The expression and activities of individual transcription factors are variably regulated depending upon microenvironment. For example, Snail protein stability and nuclear localization are regulated by post-translational modifications. Wnt stabilizes Snail by inhibiting GSK3β-dependent phosphorylation, β-TrCP-directed ubiquitination, and proteasomal degradation, a mechanism similar to Wnt-mediated β-catenin stabilization and T-cell factor-dependent transcriptional activation.[72] NF-κB, an essential regulator in inflammatory response, also stabilizes Snail by preventing its GSK3β-dependent phosphorylation and degradation.[73] Hypoxia can activate Snail through HIF-1α-mediated induction of lysyl oxidases LOX and LOXL2 that catalyze oxidation of lysine residues, allowing stabilization of Snail protein.[74] HIF-1α also enhances Notch signaling,[75] whose intracellular domain transactivates the Snail promoter directly.[76] Interestingly, ZEB and the microRNA (miR)-205 and miR-200 family negatively regulate each other.[77–80] ZEB-mediated suppression of the miR-200 family leads to induction of the Notch ligand JAG1, another target for the miR-200 family members.[81,82] Thus, ZEBs may also induce Snail by activating Notch.

EMT, Senescence, and Cancer Stem Cell Theory

Invasive tumor cells may contain migratory cancer stem cells (CSCs), and aka tumor initiating cells that contribute to formation of metastatic tumors. EMT has been implicated in generation of CSCs.[83] To date, existence of CSCs or tumor initiating cells has been postulated for many tumor types including brain, pancreas, colon, prostate, and breast cancers.[84–89] Cell surface markers such as CD44 and CD24 have been used as CSC markers in addition to unique enzymatic activities (e.g., ABCG2 for side population and ALDH1).[90,91] Notch regulates EMT[92,93] as well as CSCs,[94] conferring resistance to chemotherapeutic agents and radiation,[94–96] Interestingly, EMT may also occur during the early stages of carcinogenesis to bypass oncogene-induced senescence.[97,98] Such a premise is in agreement with circulating tumor cells and early dissemination and metastasis as discussed in the following sections.

Circulating Tumor Cells

As mentioned previously, a consequence of EMT is thought to be the acquisition of invasive properties. In the context of cancer, EMT is theorized to lead to dissemination of cells throughout the systemic circulation and seeding of distant organs. Thus, cells that have entered into the circulation, circulating tumor cells (CTC), are purported to be the direct result of an EMT. A major paradox in the field revolves around the fact that CTC in human patients can be detected with the use of antibodies specific to epithelial epitopes such as EpCAM and cytokeratins.[99] Indeed, multiple reports have not only been able to show that epithelial marker-positive CTC can be detected in patients with carcinoma but also that CTC number roughly correlates to prognosis and response to treatment in multiple cancers, including breast, prostate, gastric, esophageal, and colon cancers.[100–104] At least three possibilities exist for these observations. First, EMT may not be required for hematogenous dissemination. Second, cells do not undergo a "complete" EMT; rather CTC can enter the circulation with a residual amount of epithelial epitopes that can be utilized for detection. Finally, once CTC enter the bloodstream, a phenotypic reversal begins—a mesenchymal to epithelial transition. Current technologies that utilize epithelial epitope detection to identify CTC are not able to discern which of these explanations may be correct; however, new technologies utilizing genetic mouse models of cancer progression may provide clarity on this muddled subject. It is interesting, however, that despite the fact that epithelial-based methods of CTC detection have been able to provide some clinical use, current technologies currently have not been able to be developed as a diagnostic modality; up to 40% of all biopsy-proven metastatic cancer patients will not have detectable CTC. This would suggest that a large number of CTC are devoid of epithelial epitopes or have so few epithelial epitopes that they escape the limit of detection of established modalities. The latter possibility is supported by the observation that newer, more sensitive microfluidic technologies that use epithelial antibodies can detect more CTC than older technologies.[105]

Timing of Dissemination and Metastasis

Cancer progression and metastasis has long been believed to progress in a step-wise manner.[106] This model, termed by many as the "linear progression model," holds that tumor cells accumulate mutations and genetic events within the primary tumor before they are able to disseminate and found a metastatic lesion.[107] Thus, it is within the primary cancer site that tumor cells are selected for a collection of genetic alterations that yield survival within a microenvironment that may be hypoxic and nutrient deprived. Indirectly, this model presupposes that tumor cells evolve to disseminate and colonize distant organs to survive and that metastases only occur late in the course of disease, once a large primary tumor (in which tumor hypoxia and nutrient deprivation are maximal) has been established. Evidence for this model first came from the general clinical observation that larger primary tumors of all types are associated with the greatest frequency of metastatic disease. On the molecular level, perhaps the strongest evidence for such a view was provided by Vogelstein and colleagues, where colonic adenomas were found to harbor unique mutations that were associated with worsening histologic grade.[9] This analysis has been replicated in other cancers, including breast cancer, with similar findings.[108]

On the other hand, two distinct clinical observations argue against the linear progression model. First, in many types of carcinomas, distant metastatic disease can be present even when the primary tumor is in the early stage or comparatively small. In breast cancer, approximately 5% of all patients with early stage tumors (T1M1 or T2M1) will have metastatic disease evident on cross-sectional imaging at the time of diagnosis.[109] In pancreatic cancer, even subcentimeter tumors have been known to be associated with high prevalence of metastatic disease.[110] Secondly, the linear progression model fails to explain the phenomenon of tumor of unknown primary. In this lethal disease, which accounts for 5–10% of all cancers diagnosed in the United States, patients present with multiple foci of tumors of similar size and of similar carcinoma-like histology without evidence of a primary tumor.[111] Thus, an alternative model of cancer progression has been proposed.

The "parallel progression model," reviewed by Klein,[112] posits that cancer cells disseminate to distant locales throughout tumorigenesis, likely beginning even before primary tumors can be detected. This model thus implies that the first cells that seed distant tissues may not have the exact collection of mutations that the resultant primary tumor may harbor, and that over time, metastatic lesions may evolve independently from sister cancer cells at the source organ. Additionally, this model also predicts that cancer cells may metastasize at multiple points during cancer progression, including late in tumorigenesis, when cells may be most proliferative. The main argument supporting this model involves considering the proliferative properties of both primary and metastatic lesions. Using colon cancer as an example, serial cross-sectional imaging have allowed for the estimation of the amount of time for a primary and metastatic lesion within the same individual to double in size. These studies estimated that the doubling time for both primary and metastatic tumors were surprisingly similar (130 vs. 109 days[113–115]). The results from studies of breast cancer were similar.[116–118] These studies also discovered that this relationship held despite the size of the primary tumor; in other words, no matter what the locale or size of the primary tumor, the rate of growth of the metastatic and primary lesions was always similar. These radiographic data have been confirmed in molecular analyses of cellular proliferation in pancreatic, breast, and prostate cancer.[119–122] Furthermore, in some cancers, such as pancreatic ductal adenocarcinoma (PDAC), the size of hepatic metastatic lesions are very similar to the primary tumor, when found at diagnosis.[123,124] Thus, based on a rather simple analysis, it would seem that a parallel progression model is most compatible with our current understanding of the kinetics of metastasis. Indeed, Christoph Klein, a major proponent of this view, calculated that to explain the kinetics of distant metastatic disease in resected T3 breast cancer (on average, women develop metastatic radiographically evident metastatic disease 20 months after surgery), the lesion doubling time had to be at least five times higher than the primary tumor if the metastases were seeded at the time of surgery[112]; data supporting such phenomenon have never been reported. Finally, in perhaps the best evidence to date supporting the parallel progression model, numerous reports have detailed the presence of disseminated prostate and mammary cells in the bone marrow of patients with carcinoma in situ and no primary tumor.[99,125–128]

Despite this burden of evidence, several things should be considered. First, all of the aforementioned data provide only indirect evidence for the parallel progression model (however, no direct data exist for the linear progression model either). While difficult to prove in humans, genetically engineered mouse models of spontaneous cancer progression may provide resolution to this controversy. Sophisticated tools that allow for the direct tracking of individual cancer cells as they disseminate are currently being developed. Second, as DNA sequencing technology has evolved dramatically, several studies have been published that would seem, on first blush, to refute the parallel progression hypothesis. Whole genome sequencing of tumors and metastases from patients have allowed for the mathematical modeling of cancer kinetics.[129] The most detailed examples come from pancreatic cancer.[120,130] Approximately 25–50% of all genetic alterations were shared amongst 24 matched primary tumor and metastatic lesion specimens. Based on this key finding and assumptions regarding the rate of genetic alteration and proliferation, the investigators estimated that the cell giving rise to a metastatic mass had to have been seeded within 3 years of diagnosis.[120] While these were landmark studies in their own right, numerous questions regarding the accuracy of their mathematical model, basic assumptions regarding proliferation of lesions, as well as the question of whether intra-tumor and intra-metastatic lesion heterogeneity was truly captured hinder the concreteness of their conclusions. Further, many of the genetic alterations that were captured in their analysis were involved in motility as well as play key roles in the dissemination of cancer cells to distant organs. Finally, some opponents of the parallel progression model maintain that genetic alterations are required in order for epithelial cells to disseminate and seed distant organs. This argument was recently debunked by a pivotal study by Varmus and colleagues.[131] In this elegant study, a phenotypically normal mammary cell line was genetically altered so that oncogenes could be activated upon treatment with doxycycline. These cells were then injected into the tail vein of immunocompromised mice. After a few days, half of the mice were given doxycycline to transform any cells that may have extravasated from the bloodstream and seeded any organ. In a brief period of time, only the doxycycline-treated mice developed multiple tumors in the liver and lungs. Thus, this constituted provide direct evidence of the inherent capacity for even "normal" epithelial cells to survive entry into the blood circulation and seed distant organs, providing proof-in-principle that cancer cells that may not have accumulated many mutations can indeed metastasize and survive in foreign environments.

Given the general mechanisms in cancer metastasis discussed above, we will focus in the following sections upon colorectal and pancreatic carcinomas, two specific cancers of digestive organs regarding their mechanisms, detection, models, and therapeutic targeting of invasion and metastasis.

Colorectal Cancer

Metastatic colorectal cancer is one of the most common problems encountered in oncology. The disease remains largely incurable; once metastases have set in, 5-year survival rates are only around 5%.[132] In comparison, for non-metastatic disease, 5-year survival is more than 70% with appropriate treatment.[132] Thus, understanding the mechanisms of metastases, early identification thereof, and appropriate therapeutic interventions can have a large impact on disease-specific morbidity and mortality.

Mechanisms of Invasion and Metastasis in Colorectal Cancer

Colorectal cancer has a well-defined path to metastatic disease: as the venous drainage of the colon (except the distal rectum) is directed towards the liver, colon cancer spreads to the adjacent lymph nodes and then the liver, from where it may spread to the lungs and beyond, via the inferior vena cava. Thus most metastatic colon cancer cases are detected with disease in the liver. Several mechanisms of this distant spread have been elucidated,[133,134] and will be discussed briefly here.

Tissue Destruction and Invasion Enzymes

The initial step in the egress of colorectal tumor cells from the primary organ is the invasion of adjacent tissues. Proteolytic enzymes, especially metalloproteinases, have been widely implicated in this process. MMP-7, also known as matrilysin, is the smallest metalloproteinase and participates in various steps of tumor spread.[135,136] Mouse models have demonstrated that MMP-7 induces loose cell aggregation when added to colon cancer cell lines; these convert to tight cell aggregates with the aid of E-cadherin, forming metastatic nodules in the liver.[137] In human tumor samples, the expression of MMP-7 is highly correlated with the presence of metastatic nodules, and transfection of MMP-7 into mice leads to remarkable metastatic disease without much alteration in the primary tumors.[138] In addition, in nude mice models, matrilysin-specific oligonucleotides have been shown to inhibit liver metastases from colon cancer.[139] Another important proteinase is the urokinase plasminogen activator (uPA). It is constitutively activated[140] and highly expressed in tumor cells[141] and has been shown to be correlated with poor survival in colon cancer.[142] GATA6 has been demonstrated to be an important regulator of uPA expression and promotes tumorigenesis and metastasis through this enzyme.[143] Mouse models have demonstrated that inhibition of urokinase by antisense mRNA can lead to suppression of colon cancer metastases.[144]

Lymphatic and Blood Vessel Neoproliferation

Angiogenesis is a critical step in cancer metastasis.[145] The molecular mechanism of angiogenesis has been widely studied; vascular endothelial growth factor (VEGF), with four isoforms, has been most strongly implicated as a mediator of lymphatic and blood vessel invasion and neoproliferation.[133,146] It is a direct mitogen of endothelial cells and acts via cell surface receptors—in human adults, VEGFR1 and VEGFR2 are mainly present on vascular endothelial cells, and VEGFR3 is mainly present on lymphatic endothelial cells.[147,148] Using experimental models, VEGF has been shown to play a role in various steps of angiogenesis—it participates in tumor invasion, endothelial cell proliferation and migration, and modulation of microvascular function.[149,150] Several other molecules also appear to play a role in this complex phenomenon; fibroblast growth factor, platelet-derived growth factor, transforming growth factors, and tumor necrosis factor being most prominent.[151]

More recently, the role of specific genes has been elucidated. KRAS, a downstream signaling molecule in the epidermal growth factor receptor (EGFR) pathway, may be a mediator in hypoxia-induced angiogenesis.[152] Similarly, bcl-2 and thymosin β4 have been shown to induce hypoxia inducible factor-1 (HIF-1) mediated overexpression of VEGF.[153,154] Interleukin-8 is another molecule implicated in tumor proliferation and angiogenesis.[155] Another gene expression analysis identified vimentin as a marker specific to tumor vasculature, with its inhibition antagonizing tumor microvasculature growth.[156] While these studies shed more light on angiogenesis, it remains to be seen if these genes will pan out as potential therapeutic targets.

Detection of Metastases in Colorectal Cancer

Early detection of malignancies is a key to good treatment outcomes. In colorectal cancer, early detection of metastases is also critical, since surgical resection of oligometastatic disease with/without other therapies can help achieve good long-term outcomes.[157,158] However, clinical symptoms and signs often appear when metastases are advanced, making imaging techniques important in detecting early lesions. Traditionally, helical computed tomography (CT) scans have been employed to detect metastatic disease in patients presenting with colorectal cancer; these achieve sensitivity of 75–85% and specificity of 95% for hepatic metastases.[159,160] In comparison, magnetic resonance imaging (MRI) performs slightly better, with sensitivity of over 85% and specificity of over 95%.[160,161] Positron emission tomography (PET) using 18-fluorodeoxyglucose (FDG) is becoming increasingly popular. This technique exploits the differential increase in glucose uptake by metabolically active cancerous cells

(Warburg effect), compared to the surrounding tissues.[162] Meta-analyses have shown that FDG-PET has sensitivity of 94% and specificity of over 95% for detecting liver metastases in colon cancer.[160,161] Thus, while specificities are comparable for all three modalities, MRI and PET appear to have higher sensitivities than CT. However, these estimates apply to liver metastases only; current guidelines and usual practice patterns favor the use of CT scans, as MRI is more cumbersome for the patient and MRI and PET are more operator dependent.[163]

Therapeutic Targeting of Invasion and Metastasis in Colorectal Cancer

First hypothesized as a therapeutic target in 1971,[164] angiogenesis is a prime candidate for effecting tumor control, given its prominent role in colon cancer metastasis. Bevacizumab is the first agent to specifically target this process. It is a VEGF inhibitor, although the exact molecular mechanism whereby it achieves clinical benefit remains uncertain.[165] It was shown to have clinical benefit in metastatic colorectal cancer in 2004.[166] However, it has not been beneficial in localized colon cancer treatment and, in metastatic disease also, overall survival benefit has not been seen.[167–169] This leads to important questions: Is targeting of other molecules in the VEGF pathway needed? Is angiogenesis control not enough to achieve durable clinical benefit? Does VEGF develop "escape" mechanisms that preclude sustained clinical responses? Further work in this field is ongoing, which may yield answers to some of these questions.

The other major pathway being targeted in metastatic colorectal cancer is the EGFR signaling cascade. The EGFR antibodies, cetuximab and panitumumab, improve progression-free survival and some data indicate an improvement in overall survival also.[170] However, not all patients benefit, and a basis for resistance to the antibodies has been elucidated—several studies have shown that EGFR antibodies are ineffective in cases where the *KRAS* gene is mutated.[171] Recent work has also implicated *NRAS* and *BRAF* mutations in nonefficacy of EGFR antibodies, making about 50% of cases ineligible for such therapy.[172] These mutations occur in one arm of the EGFR signaling cascade, which has two main downstream signal transduction pathways:

- MAPKinase (KRAS/NRAS–BRAF–MEK–ERK): affects cell cycle progression and cell proliferation.
- PI3Kinase (PI3K–PTEN–AKT–mTOR): affects anti-apoptotic and cell survival signals.

Mutations of genes in these pathways are commonly observed in colorectal cancer. Based on data in the literature, the proportions of cases harboring various mutations are as follows[173]:

MAPKinase Pathway

KRAS mutant	40–45%
NRAS mutant	2.5%
BRAF mutant	5–10%

PI3Kinase Pathway

PIK3CA mutant	15%
PTEN mutant	10–20%
AKT mutant	5%

Combined

KRAS/NRAS and PI3K mutant	10%

Preclinical data have shown that a *PIK3CA* or *PTEN* mutation (which leads to constitutive activation of the PI3K pathway) causes resistance of cancer cells to cetuximab.[174] Indirect evidence stems from preclinical work showing that *PIK3CA* mutation uncouples cell proliferation signaling from the KRAS pathway, leading to failure of inhibitors targeting the MAPK axis.[175] Initially, small studies showed conflicting roles of *PIK3CA* mutation in response to EGFR antibodies,[176,177] but a recent large study has demonstrated that *PIK3CA* mutation is associated with poor response to cetuximab.[172] Preclinical models indicate that in these tumors, inhibition of the PI3K axis may be required to achieve cancer control. Blocking the PI3K pathway in cancer cells with activating PI3K mutations has been shown to inhibit cell growth and induce apoptosis.[178,179] In addition, when mutations in both axes exist, dual inhibition—MEK and AKT/PI3K inhibitors—is required to control cell growth.[179,180] Thus work is ongoing on various inhibitors of these signal transduction molecules to see if collective inhibition of some or all constitutively activated genes will achieve clinical benefit.

Pancreatic Cancer

Pancreatic cancer remains a deadly disease: there are about 43,000 new cases each year in the US and 5-year overall survival remains less than 10%.[132] More importantly, these numbers have not changed in several decades and the mortality rate from pancreatic cancer appears to be rising.[132] The reason is that pancreatic cancer is often unresectable at diagnosis and nonsurgical systemic therapies have not achieved much clinical success. Conventional chemotherapeutic agents provide little benefit; therefore, understanding the molecular biology of this disease may allow the development of more effective targeted therapies.

Mechanisms of Invasion and Metastasis in Pancreatic Cancer

Pancreatic cancer appears to originate as an intraductal lesion, akin to breast cancer.[181,182] The acinar cells may also give rise to carcinoma via metaplasia to ductal cells. More than 80% of cases are diagnosed as advanced tumors, meaning that invasion or metastases have occurred. Molecular mechanisms for this aggressive behavior have been studied and the major candidates are discussed below.

KRAS

The EGF receptor impinges on the KRAS–BRAF–MEK–ERK signal transduction pathway. Mutations in *KRAS* can lead to constitutive activation of this pathway, causing uncontrolled cell cycle progression and cell growth. More than 95% of pancreatic adenocarcinoma specimens harbor *KRAS* mutations.[183,184] Mouse models have demonstrated that constitutive activation of KRAS can lead to development of neoplasia in the pancreas.[185,186] These lesions evolve from pancreatic intraductal neoplasms (PanIN) to invasive and metastatic carcinomas, akin to human tumors.[186,187] Other genes in the EGFR pathway are rarely mutated in pancreatic cancer—BRAF, PIK3CA, AKT, and PTEN alterations have been noted in the small number of cases where KRAS is wild type.[188,189] Thus the EGFR pathway seems to be almost universally aberrantly activated in pancreatic cancer, making it an attractive therapeutic target.

TP53

The tumor suppressor gene, p53, is frequently mutated in pancreatic cancer and an abnormal form is found in 50–75% of cases, usually a missense mutation.[190] This alteration is probably responsible for some of the genomic instability seen in pancreatic adenocarcinoma samples.[182] Recent work has better elucidated the role of p53 in pancreatic cancer.[191] Pancreatic cells with both *KRAS* mutations and *TP53* alterations progress rapidly to form invasive tumors. In the absence of *TP53* mutations, cells with *KRAS* mutations form premalignant lesions. Thus, *KRAS* and *TP53* mutations may form the "two-hit" genetic process leading to invasive pancreatic adenocarcinoma.[192]

CDKN2A/p16

Another gene that is frequently mutated is *CDKN2A*. As a tumor suppressor gene, it is silenced in many cases of familial pancreatic cancers which form a small proportion of all pancreatic cancers.[193] In conjunction with altered *KRAS*, silenced *CDKN2A* can lead to rapid progression of pancreatic neoplasms.[194]

Hedgehog Pathway

This embryonic signaling pathway is usually silent in adult life, but aberrant activation is seen in various disease states.[195] In mouse models of pancreatic cancer, hedgehog ligands are overexpressed, leading to development of PanIN lesions. These lesions also harbor *KRAS* mutations and blockade of hedgehog signaling appears to control pancreatic neoplasm growth.[196] In addition, hedgehog signaling has been implicated in the remarkable desmoplastic reaction seen in pancreatic tumors—the bulk of pancreatic adenocarcinoma mass is composed of fibrous tissue.[197] This increased hedgehog signaling is mediated via increased ligand expression in the stroma (paracrine stimulation) as well as increased Gli transcriptional activity in tumor epithelial cells.[185] The resultant fibrosis is thought to impair efficient drug delivery to the cancer cells in this disease and inhibition of hedgehog signaling leads to reduce desmoplasia and improved drug delivery in mouse models of pancreatic cancer.[198]

Mediators of Metastasis

The molecular mechanisms behind breakage of cells from the primary tumor and spread to distant sites remain nebulous. E-cadherin (an epithelial protein) switch to N-cadherin (a mesenchymal protein) may play a role in pancreatic cancer spread.[199] Like hedgehog signaling, β-catenin participates in the embryonic Wnt signaling pathway. It appears to be another mediator of pancreatic cancer metastasis and along with E-cadherin, it is frequently aberrantly expressed in tumor specimens.[200] Since it acts as a link between the actin cytoskeleton and surface E-cadherin, it may participate in cadherin switching and development of metastases.[182] Further, various genes involved in telomere dysfunction and cell-cycle control appear to be altered in this disease, with some present in primary tumors and others acquired during/after metastatic development.[201] Further focus on these candidate genes may shed more light on the molecular mechanisms behind pancreatic cancer spread.

Therapeutic Targeting of Invasion and Metastasis in Pancreatic Cancer

The prime target for molecular therapies for pancreatic cancer remains the *KRAS* gene. Since mutations thereof lead to constitutive activation of the EGFR pathway, inhibitors of EGFR have been tested in this disease. However, barring one study that showed minimal clinical benefit,[202] these agents have not been effective in this disease.[203,204] The obvious question is why, and what else should be tried. Exploratory analysis from the study that showed some benefit of erlotinib hints at *KRAS* mutations being predictive of nonresponse to EGFR inhibitors, but results remain inconclusive.[205] Preclinical models have, however, shown that in contrast to individual gene abnormalities, coordinated overexpression of the EGFR pathway genes is predictive of sensitivity to EGFR inhibitors.[206] In comparison, individual gene mutations in the RAS–RAF–MAPK arm of the EGFR signaling pathway render cells insensitive to growth inhibition by EGFR inhibitors; dual inhibition by EGFR inhibitors and MAPK inhibitors appears to be effective in such cases, in preclinical models.[207]

HER2, which belongs to the EGF family of receptors, has also been explored as a target in pancreatic cancer. Starting with breast cancer, HER2 inhibitors have gained clinical utility in gastric cancer also.[208] In preclinical models testing the hypothesis, trastuzumab, a monoclonal antibody against HER2, has shown growth inhibition of pancreatic cancer cells overexpressing HER2.[209] Some small clinical studies have hinted at some benefit; however, like EGFR inhibitors, this benefit is underwhelming.[210,211] Further studies are planned, but given the low rate of HER2 overexpression in pancreatic cancer, this therapeutic strategy may not yield the best results.[212]

Another important invasion and metastasis target is the vascular endothelial growth factor (VEGF) pathway. In pancreatic cancer, VEGF overexpression has been noted,[213] and preclinical models have shown a growth inhibitory effect of VEGF inhibitors on pancreatic cancer cell lines.[214] Monoclonal antibodies that target VEGF have shown clinical efficacy in a variety of human solid tumors. In pancreatic cancer, however, they have not shown much benefit. Several clinical trials have been conducted but VEGF inhibitors have failed to control metastatic disease.[215–217] The reasons remain unclear. A putative argument is that the abundant stroma in pancreatic cancer prevents efficient drug delivery to the tumor cells, preventing their control.[198] To address this issue, attention has been focused on hedgehog signaling. As described above, it is often aberrant in pancreatic cancer, and contributes to the strong desmoplastic reaction seen in this disease, making hedgehog signaling an attractive therapeutic target. Preclinical work has shown that hedgehog inhibition leads to marked reduction of in vitro invasiveness of pancreatic cancer cell lines, with a concomitant upregulation of E-cadherin, marking control of the epithelial-to-mesenchymal transition ("cadherin switch").[218] In addition, using mouse models, hedgehog inhibition has been shown to deplete the abundant stroma in pancreatic cancer, allowing better delivery of chemotherapy to the tumor cells.[198] Such agents are now being tested in early-phase clinical trials.

References

1. Hanahan D, Weinberg RA. Hallmarks of cancer: the next generation. *Cell*. 2011;144(5):646–74.
2. Paget S. Paget, Stephen paper reproduced from the Lancet, 1889. *Cancer Metastasis Rev*. 1989;8(2):98–101.
3. McCluggage WG, Wilkinson N. Metastatic neoplasms involving the ovary: a review with an emphasis on morphological and immunohistochemical features. *Histopathology*. 2005;47(3): 231–47.
4. Glickman JN. Section II: pathology and pathologic staging of esophageal cancer. *Semin Thorac Cardiovasc Surg*. 2003; 15(2):167–79.
5. Jass JR, Barker M, Fraser L, et al. APC mutation and tumour budding in colorectal cancer. *J Clin Pathol*. 2003;56(1):69–73.
6. Ono M, Sakamoto M, Ino Y, et al. Cancer cell morphology at the invasive front and expression of cell adhesion-related carbohydrate in the primary lesion of patients with colorectal carcinoma with liver metastasis. *Cancer*. 1996;78(6):1179–86.
7. Chiang AC, Massague J. Molecular basis of metastasis. *N Engl J Med*. 2008;359(26):2814–23.
8. Nguyen DX, Bos PD, Massague J. Metastasis: from dissemination to organ-specific colonization. *Nat Rev Cancer*. 2009;9(4): 274–84.
9. Fearon ER, Vogelstein B. A genetic model for colorectal tumorigenesis. *Cell*. 1990;61(5):759–67.
10. Singh A, Greninger P, Rhodes D, et al. A gene expression signature associated with "K-Ras addiction" reveals regulators of EMT and tumor cell survival. *Cancer Cell*. 2009;15(6):489–500.
11. Nakahara M, Isozaki K, Hirota S, et al. A novel gain-of-function mutation of c-kit gene in gastrointestinal stromal tumors. *Gastroenterology*. 1998;115(5):1090–5.
12. Pelengaris S, Khan M, Evan GI. Suppression of Myc-induced apoptosis in beta cells exposes multiple oncogenic properties of Myc and triggers carcinogenic progression. *Cell*. 2002;109(3): 321–34.
13. Peifer M. Beta-catenin as oncogene: the smoking gun. *Science*. 1997;275(5307):1752–3.
14. Wang S, Liu Z, Wang L, Zhang X. NF-kappaB signaling pathway, inflammation and colorectal cancer. *Cell Mol Immunol*. 2009;6(5):327–34.
15. Levental KR, Yu H, Kass L, et al. Matrix crosslinking forces tumor progression by enhancing integrin signaling. *Cell*. 2009; 139(5):891–906.
16. Erler JT, Bennewith KL, Cox TR, et al. Hypoxia-induced lysyl oxidase is a critical mediator of bone marrow cell recruitment to form the premetastatic niche. *Cancer Cell*. 2009;15(1):35–44.
17. Kang Y, Siegel PM, Shu W, et al. A multigenic program mediating breast cancer metastasis to bone. *Cancer Cell*. 2003;3(6): 537–49.
18. Su J, You P, Li WL, et al. The existence of multipotent stem cells with epithelial-mesenchymal transition features in the human liver bud. *Int J Biochem Cell Biol*. 2010;42(12):2047–55.
19. Rukstalis JM, Habener JF. Snail2, a mediator of epithelial-mesenchymal transitions, expressed in progenitor cells of the developing endocrine pancreas. *Gene Expr Patterns*. 2007;7(4):471–9.
20. Qian X, Karpova T, Sheppard AM, McNally J, Lowy DR. E-cadherin-mediated adhesion inhibits ligand-dependent activation of diverse receptor tyrosine kinases. *EMBO J*. 2004; 23(8):1739–48.
21. Guo W, Giancotti FG. Integrin signalling during tumour progression. *Nat Rev Mol Cell Biol*. 2004;5(10):816–26.
22. Tarin D, Thompson EW, Newgreen DF. The fallacy of epithelial mesenchymal transition in neoplasia. *Cancer Res*. 2005; 65(14):5996–6000.
23. Trimboli AJ, Fukino K, de Bruin A, et al. Direct evidence for epithelial-mesenchymal transitions in breast cancer. *Cancer Res*. 2008;68(3):937–45.
24. Bellovin DI, Bates RC, Muzikansky A, Rimm DL, Mercurio AM. Altered localization of p120 catenin during epithelial to mesenchymal transition of colon carcinoma is prognostic for aggressive disease. *Cancer Res*. 2005;65(23):10938–45.
25. Kim MA, Lee HS, Lee HE, Kim JH, Yang HK, Kim WH. Prognostic importance of epithelial-mesenchymal transition-related protein expression in gastric carcinoma. *Histopathology*. 2009;54(4):442–51.

26. Sun T, Zhao N, Zhao XL, et al. Expression and functional significance of Twist1 in hepatocellular carcinoma: its role in vasculogenic mimicry. *Hepatology*. 2010;51(2):545–56.
27. Yang MH, Chen CL, Chau GY, et al. Comprehensive analysis of the independent effect of twist and snail in promoting metastasis of hepatocellular carcinoma. *Hepatology*. 2009;50(5):1464–74.
28. Ohta H, Aoyagi K, Fukaya M, et al. Cross talk between hedgehog and epithelial-mesenchymal transition pathways in gastric pit cells and in diffuse-type gastric cancers. *Br J Cancer*. 2009;100(2):389–98.
29. Isohata N, Aoyagi K, Mabuchi T, et al. Hedgehog and epithelial-mesenchymal transition signaling in normal and malignant epithelial cells of the esophagus. *Int J Cancer*. 2009;125(5): 1212–21.
30. Bates RC, Bellovin DI, Brown C, et al. Transcriptional activation of integrin beta6 during the epithelial-mesenchymal transition defines a novel prognostic indicator of aggressive colon carcinoma. *J Clin Invest*. 2005;115(2):339–47.
31. Yu J, Ohuchida K, Mizumoto K, et al. MicroRNA, hsa-miR-200c, is an independent prognostic factor in pancreatic cancer and its upregulation inhibits pancreatic cancer invasion but increases cell proliferation. *Mol Cancer*. 2010;9:169.
32. Wellner U, Schubert J, Burk UC, et al. The EMT-activator ZEB1 promotes tumorigenicity by repressing stemness-inhibiting microRNAs. *Nat Cell Biol*. 2009;11(12):1487–95.
33. Schwock J, Bradley G, Ho JC, et al. SNAI1 expression and the mesenchymal phenotype: an immunohistochemical study performed on 46 cases of oral squamous cell carcinoma. *BMC Clin Pathol*. 2010;10:1.
34. Shioiri M, Shida T, Koda K, et al. Slug expression is an independent prognostic parameter for poor survival in colorectal carcinoma patients. *Br J Cancer*. 2006;94(12):1816–22.
35. Jethwa P, Naqvi M, Hardy RG, et al. Overexpression of Slug is associated with malignant progression of esophageal adenocarcinoma. *World J Gastroenterol*. 2008;14(7):1044–52.
36. Castro Alves C, Rosivatz E, Schott C, et al. Slug is overexpressed in gastric carcinomas and may act synergistically with SIP1 and Snail in the down-regulation of E-cadherin. *J Pathol*. 2007;211(5):507–15.
37. Natsugoe S, Uchikado Y, Okumura H, et al. Snail plays a key role in E-cadherin-preserved esophageal squamous cell carcinoma. *Oncol Rep*. 2007;17(3):517–23.
38. Usami Y, Satake S, Nakayama F, et al. Snail-associated epithelial-mesenchymal transition promotes oesophageal squamous cell carcinoma motility and progression. *J Pathol*. 2008;215(3):330–9.
39. Sasaki K, Natsugoe S, Ishigami S, et al. Significance of Twist expression and its association with E-cadherin in esophageal squamous cell carcinoma. *J Exp Clin Cancer Res*. 2009;28:158.
40. Ru GQ, Wang HJ, Xu WJ, Zhao ZS. Upregulation of twist in gastric carcinoma associated with tumor invasion and poor prognosis. *Pathol Oncol Res*. 2010;17:341–7.
41. Cates JM, Byrd RH, Fohn LE, Tatsas AD, Washington MK, Black CC. Epithelial-mesenchymal transition markers in pancreatic ductal adenocarcinoma. *Pancreas*. 2009;38(1):e1–6.
42. Jin H, Morohashi S, Sato F, et al. Vimentin expression of esophageal squamous cell carcinoma and its aggressive potential for lymph node metastasis. *Biomed Res*. 2010;31(2):105–12.
43. Javle MM, Gibbs JF, Iwata KK, et al. Epithelial-mesenchymal transition (EMT) and activated extracellular signal-regulated kinase (p-Erk) in surgically resected pancreatic cancer. *Ann Surg Oncol*. 2007;14(12):3527–33.
44. van Roy F, Berx G. The cell–cell adhesion molecule E-cadherin. *Cell Mol Life Sci*. 2008;65(23):3756–88.
45. Becker KF, Atkinson MJ, Reich U, et al. Exon skipping in the E-cadherin gene transcript in metastatic human gastric carcinomas. *Hum Mol Genet*. 1993;2(6):803–4.
46. Machado JC, Oliveira C, Carvalho R, et al. E-cadherin gene (CDH1) promoter methylation as the second hit in sporadic diffuse gastric carcinoma. *Oncogene*. 2001;20(12):1525–8.
47. Oliveira C, Seruca R, Carneiro F. Genetics, pathology, and clinics of familial gastric cancer. *Int J Surg Pathol*. 2006;14(1):21–33.
48. Guilford P, Hopkins J, Harraway J, et al. E-cadherin germline mutations in familial gastric cancer. *Nature*. 1998;392(6674): 402–5.
49. Nass SJ, Herman JG, Gabrielson E, et al. Aberrant methylation of the estrogen receptor and E-cadherin 5□ CpG islands increases with malignant progression in human breast cancer. *Cancer Res*. 2000;60(16):4346–8.
50. Kanai Y, Ushijima S, Tsuda H, Sakamoto M, Hirohashi S. Aberrant DNA methylation precedes loss of heterozygosity on chromosome 16 in chronic hepatitis and liver cirrhosis. *Cancer Lett*. 2000;148(1):73–80.
51. Takeno S, Noguchi T, Fumoto S, Kimura Y, Shibata T, Kawahara K. E-cadherin expression in patients with esophageal squamous cell carcinoma: promoter hypermethylation, Snail overexpression, and clinicopathologic implications. *Am J Clin Pathol*. 2004;122(1):78–84.
52. Koizume S, Tachibana K, Sekiya T, Hirohashi S, Shiraishi M. Heterogeneity in the modification and involvement of chromatin components of the CpG island of the silenced human CDH1 gene in cancer cells. *Nucleic Acids Res*. 2002;30(21):4770–80.
53. Perl AK, Wilgenbus P, Dahl U, Semb H, Christofori G. A causal role for E-cadherin in the transition from adenoma to carcinoma. *Nature*. 1998;392(6672):190–3.
54. Derksen PW, Liu X, Saridin F, et al. Somatic inactivation of E-cadherin and p53 in mice leads to metastatic lobular mammary carcinoma through induction of anoikis resistance and angiogenesis. *Cancer Cell*. 2006;10(5):437–49.
55. Onder TT, Gupta PB, Mani SA, Yang J, Lander ES, Weinberg RA. Loss of E-cadherin promotes metastasis via multiple downstream transcriptional pathways. *Cancer Res*. 2008;68(10):3645–54.
56. Hazan RB, Qiao R, Keren R, Badano I, Suyama K. Cadherin switch in tumor progression. *Ann N Y Acad Sci*. 2004;1014:155–63.
57. Wheelock MJ, Shintani Y, Maeda M, Fukumoto Y, Johnson KR. Cadherin switching. *J Cell Sci*. 2008;121(Pt 6):727–35.
58. Islam S, Carey TE, Wolf GT, Wheelock MJ, Johnson KR. Expression of N-cadherin by human squamous carcinoma cells induces a scattered fibroblastic phenotype with disrupted cell–cell adhesion. *J Cell Biol*. 1996;135(6 Pt 1):1643–54.
59. Nieman MT, Prudoff RS, Johnson KR, Wheelock MJ. N-cadherin promotes motility in human breast cancer cells regardless of their E-cadherin expression. *J Cell Biol*. 1999;147(3):631–44.
60. Hazan RB, Phillips GR, Qiao RF, Norton L, Aaronson SA. Exogenous expression of N-cadherin in breast cancer cells induces cell migration, invasion, and metastasis. *J Cell Biol*. 2000; 148(4):779–90.
61. Hulit J, Suyama K, Chung S, et al. N-cadherin signaling potentiates mammary tumor metastasis via enhanced extracellular signal-regulated kinase activation. *Cancer Res*. 2007;67(7):3106–16.
62. Deramaudt TB, Takaoka M, Upadhyay R, et al. N-cadherin and keratinocyte growth factor receptor mediate the functional interplay between Ki-RASG12V and p53V143A in promoting pancreatic cell migration, invasion, and tissue architecture disruption. *Mol Cell Biol*. 2006;26(11):4185–200.
63. Li G, Satyamoorthy K, Herlyn M. N-cadherin-mediated intercellular interactions promote survival and migration of melanoma cells. *Cancer Res*. 2001;61(9):3819–25.
64. Thiery JP, Acloque H, Huang RY, Nieto MA. Epithelial-mesenchymal transitions in development and disease. *Cell*. 2009;139(5):871–90.
65. Zavadil J, Bottinger EP. TGF-beta and epithelial-to-mesenchymal transitions. *Oncogene*. 2005;24(37):5764–74.

66. Cui W, Fowlis DJ, Bryson S, et al. TGFbeta1 inhibits the formation of benign skin tumors, but enhances progression to invasive spindle carcinomas in transgenic mice. *Cell*. 1996;86(4):531–42.
67. Miettinen PJ, Ebner R, Lopez AR, Derynck R. TGF-beta induced transdifferentiation of mammary epithelial cells to mesenchymal cells: involvement of type I receptors. *J Cell Biol*. 1994;127(6 Pt 2):2021–36.
68. Brown KA, Aakre ME, Gorska AE, et al. Induction by transforming growth factor-beta1 of epithelial to mesenchymal transition is a rare event in vitro. *Breast Cancer Res*. 2004;6(3):R215–31.
69. Pino MS, Kikuchi H, Zeng M, et al. Epithelial to mesenchymal transition is impaired in colon cancer cells with microsatellite instability. *Gastroenterology*. 2010;138(4):1406–17.
70. Postigo AA, Depp JL, Taylor JJ, Kroll KL. Regulation of Smad signaling through a differential recruitment of coactivators and corepressors by ZEB proteins. *EMBO J*. 2003;22(10):2453–62.
71. Postigo AA. Opposing functions of ZEB proteins in the regulation of the TGFbeta/BMP signaling pathway. *EMBO J*. 2003; 22(10):2443–52.
72. Yook JI, Li XY, Ota I, Fearon ER, Weiss SJ. Wnt-dependent regulation of the E-cadherin repressor snail. *J Biol Chem*. 2005; 280(12):11740–8.
73. Wu Y, Deng J, Rychahou PG, Qiu S, Evers BM, Zhou BP. Stabilization of snail by NF-kappaB is required for inflammation-induced cell migration and invasion. *Cancer Cell*. 2009;15(5):416–28.
74. Schietke R, Warnecke C, Wacker I, et al. The lysyl oxidases LOX and LOXL2 are necessary and sufficient to repress E-cadherin in hypoxia: insights into cellular transformation processes mediated by HIF-1. *J Biol Chem*. 2010;285(9):6658–69.
75. Gustafsson MV, Zheng X, Pereira T, et al. Hypoxia requires notch signaling to maintain the undifferentiated cell state. *Dev Cell*. 2005;9(5):617–28.
76. Sahlgren C, Gustafsson MV, Jin S, Poellinger L, Lendahl U. Notch signaling mediates hypoxia-induced tumor cell migration and invasion. *Proc Natl Acad Sci USA*. 2008;105(17):6392–7.
77. Burk U, Schubert J, Wellner U, et al. A reciprocal repression between ZEB1 and members of the miR-200 family promotes EMT and invasion in cancer cells. *EMBO Rep*. 2008;9(6):582–9.
78. Gregory PA, Bert AG, Paterson EL, et al. The miR-200 family and miR-205 regulate epithelial to mesenchymal transition by targeting ZEB1 and SIP1. *Nat Cell Biol*. 2008;10(5):593–601.
79. Korpal M, Lee ES, Hu G, Kang Y. The miR-200 family inhibits epithelial-mesenchymal transition and cancer cell migration by direct targeting of E-cadherin transcriptional repressors ZEB1 and ZEB2. *J Biol Chem*. 2008;283(22):14910–4.
80. Park SM, Gaur AB, Lengyel E, Peter ME. The miR-200 family determines the epithelial phenotype of cancer cells by targeting the E-cadherin repressors ZEB1 and ZEB2. *Genes Dev*. 2008;22(7):894–907.
81. Brabletz S, Bajdak K, Meidhof S, et al. The ZEB1/miR-200 feedback loop controls Notch signalling in cancer cells. *EMBO J*. 2011;30(4):770–82.
82. Vallejo DM, Caparros E, Dominguez M. Targeting Notch signalling by the conserved miR-8/200 microRNA family in development and cancer cells. *EMBO J*. 2011;30(4):756–69.
83. Mani SA, Guo W, Liao MJ, et al. The epithelial-mesenchymal transition generates cells with properties of stem cells. *Cell*. 2008;133(4):704–15.
84. Bonnet D, Dick JE. Human acute myeloid leukemia is organized as a hierarchy that originates from a primitive hematopoietic cell. *Nat Med*. 1997;3(7):730–7.
85. Singh SK, Hawkins C, Clarke ID, et al. Identification of human brain tumour initiating cells. *Nature*. 2004;432(7015):396–401.
86. Al-Hajj M, Wicha MS, Benito-Hernandez A, Morrison SJ, Clarke MF. Prospective identification of tumorigenic breast cancer cells. *Proc Natl Acad Sci USA*. 2003;100(7):3983–8.
87. Collins AT, Berry PA, Hyde C, Stower MJ, Maitland NJ. Prospective identification of tumorigenic prostate cancer stem cells. *Cancer Res*. 2005;65(23):10946–51.
88. Ricci-Vitiani L, Lombardi DG, Pilozzi E, et al. Identification and expansion of human colon-cancer-initiating cells. *Nature*. 2007;445(7123):111–5.
89. Simeone DM. Pancreatic cancer stem cells: implications for the treatment of pancreatic cancer. *Clin Cancer Res*. 2008;14(18): 5646–8.
90. Hirschmann-Jax C, Foster AE, Wulf GG, et al. A distinct "side population" of cells with high drug efflux capacity in human tumor cells. *Proc Natl Acad Sci USA*. 2004;101(39):14228–33.
91. Ginestier C, Hur MH, Charafe-Jauffret E, et al. ALDH1 is a marker of normal and malignant human mammary stem cells and a predictor of poor clinical outcome. *Cell Stem Cell*. 2007; 1(5):555–67.
92. Wang Z, Banerjee S, Li Y, Rahman KM, Zhang Y, Sarkar FH. Down-regulation of notch-1 inhibits invasion by inactivation of nuclear factor-kappaB, vascular endothelial growth factor, and matrix metalloproteinase-9 in pancreatic cancer cells. *Cancer Res*. 2006;66(5):2778–84.
93. Zhang P, Yang Y, Zweidler-McKay PA, Hughes DP. Critical role of notch signaling in osteosarcoma invasion and metastasis. *Clin Cancer Res*. 2008;14(10):2962–9.
94. Pannuti A, Foreman K, Rizzo P, et al. Targeting notch to target cancer stem cells. *Clin Cancer Res*. 2010;16(12):3141–52.
95. Wang Z, Li Y, Ahmad A, et al. Targeting notch signaling pathway to overcome drug resistance for cancer therapy. *Biochim Biophys Acta*. 2010;1806:258–67.
96. Wang Z, Li Y, Kong D, et al. Acquisition of epithelial-mesenchymal transition phenotype of gemcitabine-resistant pancreatic cancer cells is linked with activation of the notch signaling pathway. *Cancer Res*. 2009;69(6):2400–7.
97. Ansieau S, Bastid J, Doreau A, et al. Induction of EMT by twist proteins as a collateral effect of tumor-promoting inactivation of premature senescence. *Cancer Cell*. 2008;14(1):79–89.
98. Ansieau S, Hinkal G, Thomas C, Bastid J, Puisieux A. Early origin of cancer metastases: dissemination and evolution of premalignant cells. *Cell Cycle*. 2008;7(23):3659–63.
99. Pantel K, Brakenhoff RH, Brandt B. Detection, clinical relevance and specific biological properties of disseminating tumour cells. *Nat Rev Cancer*. 2008;8(5):329–40.
100. Cristofanilli M, Budd GT, Ellis MJ, et al. Circulating tumor cells, disease progression, and survival in metastatic breast cancer. *N Engl J Med*. 2004;351(8):781–91.
101. Sastre J, Maestro ML, Puente J, et al. Circulating tumor cells in colorectal cancer: correlation with clinical and pathological variables. *Ann Oncol*. 2008;19(5):935–8.
102. Stott SL, Hsu CH, Tsukrov DI, et al. Isolation of circulating tumor cells using a microvortex-generating herringbone-chip. *Proc Natl Acad Sci USA*. 2011;107(43):18392–7.
103. Nagrath S, Sequist LV, Maheswaran S, et al. Isolation of rare circulating tumour cells in cancer patients by microchip technology. *Nature*. 2007;450(7173):1235–9.
104. Hiraiwa K, Takeuchi H, Hasegawa H, et al. Clinical significance of circulating tumor cells in blood from patients with gastrointestinal cancers. *Ann Surg Oncol*. 2008;15(11):3092–100.
105. Maheswaran S, Haber DA. Circulating tumor cells: a window into cancer biology and metastasis. *Curr Opin Genet Dev*. 2010;20(1):96–9.
106. Cairns J. Mutation selection and the natural history of cancer. *Nature*. 1975;255(5505):197–200.
107. Klein G. Foulds' dangerous idea revisited: the multistep development of tumors 40 years later. *Adv Cancer Res*. 1998;72:1–23.
108. Olivier M, Langerod A, Carrieri P, et al. The clinical value of somatic TP53 gene mutations in 1,794 patients with breast cancer. *Clin Cancer Res*. 2006;12(4):1157–67.

109. Engel J, Eckel R, Kerr J, et al. The process of metastasisation for breast cancer. *Eur J Cancer*. 2003;39(12):1794–806.
110. Hidalgo M. Pancreatic cancer. *N Engl J Med*. 2010;362(17): 1605–17.
111. Abbruzzese JL, Abbruzzese MC, Hess KR, Raber MN, Lenzi R, Frost P. Unknown primary carcinoma: natural history and prognostic factors in 657 consecutive patients. *J Clin Oncol*. 1994; 12(6):1272–80.
112. Klein CA. Parallel progression of primary tumours and metastases. *Nat Rev Cancer*. 2009;9(4):302–12.
113. Bolin S, Nilsson E, Sjodahl R. Carcinoma of the colon and rectum–growth rate. *Ann Surg*. 1983;198(2):151–8.
114. Spratt JS, Meyer JS, Spratt JA. Rates of growth of human neoplasms: Part II. *J Surg Oncol*. 1996;61(1):68–83.
115. Finlay IG, Meek D, Brunton F, McArdle CS. Growth rate of hepatic metastases in colorectal carcinoma. *Br J Surg*. 1988;75(7):641–4.
116. Spratt JS Jr, Spratt TL. Rates of growth of pulmonary metastases and host survival. *Ann Surg*. 1964;159:161–71.
117. Peer PG, van Dijck JA, Hendriks JH, Holland R, Verbeek AL. Age-dependent growth rate of primary breast cancer. *Cancer*. 1993;71(11):3547–51.
118. Kusama S, Spratt JS Jr, Donegan WL, Watson FR, Cunningham C. The cross rates of growth of human mammary carcinoma. *Cancer*. 1972;30(2):594–9.
119. Okimura A, Hirano H, Nishigami T, et al. Immunohistochemical analyses of E-cadherin, beta-catenin, CD44s, and CD44v6 expressions, and Ki-67 labeling index in intraductal papillary mucinous neoplasms of the pancreas and associated invasive carcinomas. *Med Mol Morphol*. 2009;42(4):222–9.
120. Yachida S, Jones S, Bozic I, et al. Distant metastasis occurs late during the genetic evolution of pancreatic cancer. *Nature*. 2010;467(7319):1114–7.
121. Pence JC, Kizilbash AM, Kerns BJ, Marks JR, Iglehart JD. Proliferation index in various stages of breast cancer determined by Ki-67 immunostaining. *J Surg Oncol*. 1991;48(1):11–20.
122. Cheng L, Pisansky TM, Sebo TJ, et al. Cell proliferation in prostate cancer patients with lymph node metastasis: a marker for progression. *Clin Cancer Res*. 1999;5(10):2820–3.
123. Agarwal B, Correa AM, Ho L. Survival in pancreatic carcinoma based on tumor size. *Pancreas*. 2008;36(1):e15–20.
124. Frohlich A, Diederichs CG, Staib L, Vogel J, Beger HG, Reske SN. Detection of liver metastases from pancreatic cancer using FDG PET. *J Nucl Med*. 1999;40(2):250–5.
125. Sanger N, Effenberger KE, Riethdorf S, et al. Disseminated tumor cells in the bone marrow of patients with ductal carcinoma in situ. *Int J Cancer*. 2011;129:2522–6.
126. Husemann Y, Geigl JB, Schubert F, et al. Systemic spread is an early step in breast cancer. *Cancer Cell*. 2008;13(1):58–68.
127. Alix-Panabieres C, Riethdorf S, Pantel K. Circulating tumor cells and bone marrow micrometastasis. *Clin Cancer Res*. 2008; 14(16):5013–21.
128. Helo P, Cronin AM, Danila DC, et al. Circulating prostate tumor cells detected by reverse transcription-PCR in men with localized or castration-refractory prostate cancer: concordance with Cell Search assay and association with bone metastases and with survival. *Clin Chem*. 2009;55(4):765–73.
129. Parmigiani G, Boca S, Lin J, Kinzler KW, Velculescu V, Vogelstein B. Design and analysis issues in genome-wide somatic mutation studies of cancer. *Genomics*. 2009;93(1):17–21.
130. Campbell PJ, Yachida S, Mudie LJ, et al. The patterns and dynamics of genomic instability in metastatic pancreatic cancer. *Nature*. 2010;467(7319):1109–13.
131. Podsypanina K, Du YC, Jechlinger M, Beverly LJ, Hambardzumyan D, Varmus H. Seeding and propagation of untransformed mouse mammary cells in the lung. *Science*. 2008;321(5897):1841–4.
132. Edge S, Byrd DR, Compton CC, et al. *AJCC Cancer Staging Manual*. 7th ed. New York: Springer; 2010.
133. Royston D, Jackson DG. Mechanisms of lymphatic metastasis in human colorectal adenocarcinoma. *J Pathol*. 2009;217(5): 608–19.
134. Rudmik LR, Magliocco AM. Molecular mechanisms of hepatic metastasis in colorectal cancer. *J Surg Oncol*. 2005;92(4): 347–59.
135. Zucker S, Vacirca J. Role of matrix metalloproteinases (MMPs) in colorectal cancer. *Cancer Metastasis Rev*. 2004;23(1–2):101–17.
136. Wang WS, Chen PM, Su Y. Colorectal carcinoma: from tumorigenesis to treatment. *Cell Mol Life Sci*. 2006;63(6):663–71.
137. Kioi M, Yamamoto K, Higashi S, Koshikawa N, Fujita K, Miyazaki K. Matrilysin (MMP-7) induces homotypic adhesion of human colon cancer cells and enhances their metastatic potential in nude mouse model. *Oncogene*. 2003;22(54):8662–70.
138. Adachi Y, Yamamoto H, Itoh F, Hinoda Y, Okada Y, Imai K. Contribution of matrilysin (MMP-7) to the metastatic pathway of human colorectal cancers. *Gut*. 1999;45(2):252–8.
139. Hasegawa S, Koshikawa N, Momiyama N, et al. Matrilysin-specific antisense oligonucleotide inhibits liver metastasis of human colon cancer cells in a nude mouse model. *Int J Cancer*. 1998;76(6):812–6.
140. Lengyel E, Wang H, Gum R, Simon C, Wang Y, Boyd D. Elevated urokinase-type plasminogen activator receptor expression in a colon cancer cell line is due to a constitutively activated extracellular signal-regulated kinase-1–dependent signaling cascade. *Oncogene*. 1997;14(21):2563–73.
141. Harvey SR, Sait SN, Xu Y, Bailey JL, Penetrante RM, Markus G. Demonstration of urokinase expression in cancer cells of colon adenocarcinomas by immunohistochemistry and in situ hybridization. *Am J Pathol*. 1999;155(4):1115–20.
142. Ganesh S, Sier CF, Heerding MM, Griffioen G, Lamers CB, Verspaget HW. Urokinase receptor and colorectal cancer survival. *Lancet*. 1994;344(8919):401–2.
143. Belaguli NS, Aftab M, Rigi M, Zhang M, Albo D, Berger DH. GATA6 promotes colon cancer cell invasion by regulating urokinase plasminogen activator gene expression. *Neoplasia*. 2010;12(11):856–65.
144. Wang Y, Liang X, Wu S, Murrell GA, Doe WF. Inhibition of colon cancer metastasis by a 3′- end antisense urokinase receptor mRNA in a nude mouse model. *Int J Cancer*. 2001;92(2):257–62.
145. Folkman J. Angiogenesis in cancer, vascular, rheumatoid and other disease. *Nat Med*. 1995;1(1):27–31.
146. Leung DW, Cachianes G, Kuang WJ, Goeddel DV, Ferrara N. Vascular endothelial growth factor is a secreted angiogenic mitogen. *Science*. 1989;246(4935):1306–9.
147. Neufeld G, Cohen T, Gengrinovitch S, Poltorak Z. Vascular endothelial growth factor (VEGF) and its receptors. *FASEB J*. 1999;13(1):9–22.
148. Rmali KA, Puntis MC, Jiang WG. Tumour-associated angiogenesis in human colorectal cancer. *Colorectal Dis*. 2007;9(1):3–14.
149. Jain RK, Safabakhsh N, Sckell A, et al. Endothelial cell death, angiogenesis, and microvascular function after castration in an androgen-dependent tumor: role of vascular endothelial growth factor. *Proc Natl Acad Sci USA*. 1998;95(18):10820–5.
150. Warren RS, Yuan H, Matli MR, Gillett NA, Ferrara N. Regulation by vascular endothelial growth factor of human colon cancer tumorigenesis in a mouse model of experimental liver metastasis. *J Clin Invest*. 1995;95(4):1789–97.
151. Sund M, Zeisberg M, Kalluri R. Endogenous stimulators and inhibitors of angiogenesis in gastrointestinal cancers: basic science to clinical application. *Gastroenterology*. 2005;129(6):2076–91.
152. Zeng M, Kikuchi H, Pino MS, Chung DC. Hypoxia activates the K-ras proto-oncogene to stimulate angiogenesis and inhibit apoptosis in colon cancer cells. *PLoS One*. 2010;5(6):e10966.

153. Trisciuoglio D, Gabellini C, Desideri M, et al. Involvement of BH4 domain of bcl-2 in the regulation of HIF-1–mediated VEGF expression in hypoxic tumor cells. *Cell Death Differ.* 2011;18:1024–35.
154. Jo JO, Kim SR, Bae MK, et al. Thymosin beta4 induces the expression of vascular endothelial growth factor (VEGF) in a hypoxia-inducible factor (HIF)-1alpha-dependent manner. *Biochim Biophys Acta.* 1803;11:1244–51.
155. Ning Y, Manegold PC, Hong YK, et al. Interleukin-8 is associated with proliferation, migration, angiogenesis and chemosensitivity in vitro and in vivo in colon cancer cell line models. *Int J Cancer.* 2011;128:2038–49.
156. van Beijnum JR, Dings RP, van der Linden E, et al. Gene expression of tumor angiogenesis dissected: specific targeting of colon cancer angiogenic vasculature. *Blood.* 2006;108(7):2339–48.
157. Fernandez FG, Drebin JA, Linehan DC, Dehdashti F, Siegel BA, Strasberg SM. Five-year survival after resection of hepatic metastases from colorectal cancer in patients screened by positron emission tomography with F-18 fluorodeoxyglucose (FDG-PET). *Ann Surg.* 2004;240(3):438–47. discussion 447–50.
158. Abdalla EK, Vauthey JN, Ellis LM, et al. Recurrence and outcomes following hepatic resection, radiofrequency ablation, and combined resection/ablation for colorectal liver metastases. *Ann Surg.* 2004;239(6):818–25. discussion 825–7.
159. Valls C, Lopez E, Guma A, et al. Helical CT versus CT arterial portography in the detection of hepatic metastasis of colorectal carcinoma. *AJR Am J Roentgenol.* 1998;170(5):1341–7.
160. Niekel MC, Bipat S, Stoker J. Diagnostic imaging of colorectal liver metastases with CT, MR imaging, FDG PET, and/or FDG PET/CT: a meta-analysis of prospective studies including patients who have not previously undergone treatment. *Radiology.* 2010;257(3):674–84.
161. Floriani I, Torri V, Rulli E, et al. Performance of imaging modalities in diagnosis of liver metastases from colorectal cancer: a systematic review and meta-analysis. *J Magn Reson Imaging.* 2010;31(1):19–31.
162. Vander Heiden MG, Cantley LC, Thompson CB. Understanding the Warburg effect: the metabolic requirements of cell proliferation. *Science.* 2009;324(5930):1029–33.
163. Engstrom PF, Arnoletti JP, Benson AB 3rd, et al. NCCN Clinical Practice Guidelines in Oncology: colon cancer. *J Natl Compr Canc Netw.* 2009;7(8):778–831.
164. Folkman J. Tumor angiogenesis: therapeutic implications. *N Engl J Med.* 1971;285(21):1182–6.
165. O'Dwyer PJ. The present and future of angiogenesis-directed treatments of colorectal cancer. *Oncologist.* 2006;11(9):992–8.
166. Hurwitz H, Fehrenbacher L, Novotny W, et al. Bevacizumab plus irinotecan, fluorouracil, and leucovorin for metastatic colorectal cancer. *N Engl J Med.* 2004;350(23):2335–42.
167. Giantonio BJ, Catalano PJ, Meropol NJ, et al. Bevacizumab in combination with oxaliplatin, fluorouracil, and leucovorin (FOLFOX4) for previously treated metastatic colorectal cancer: results from the Eastern Cooperative Oncology Group Study E3200. *J Clin Oncol.* 2007;25(12):1539–44.
168. Wolmark N, Yothers G, O'Connell M, et al. A phase III trial comparing mFOLFOX6 to mFOLFOX6 plus bevacizumab in stage II or III carcinoma of the colon: Results of NSABP Protocol C-08. *J Clin Oncol.* 2009. p. abstr LBA4.
169. De Gramont A, Van Cutsem E, Tabernero J, et al. AVANT: Results from a randomized, three-arm multinational phase III study to investigate bevacizumab with either XELOX or FOLFOX4 versus FOLFOX4 alone as adjuvant treatment for colon cancer. *J Clin Oncol.* 2011;29:362.
170. Grothey A. EGFR antibodies in colorectal cancer: Where do they belong? *J Clin Oncol.* 2010;28:4668–70.
171. Karapetis CS, Khambata-Ford S, Jonker DJ, et al. K-ras mutations and benefit from cetuximab in advanced colorectal cancer. *N Engl J Med.* 2008;359(17):1757–65.
172. De Roock W, Claes B, Bernasconi D, et al. Effects of KRAS, BRAF, NRAS, and PIK3CA mutations on the efficacy of cetuximab plus chemotherapy in chemotherapy-refractory metastatic colorectal cancer: a retrospective consortium analysis. *Lancet Oncol.* 2010;11(8):753–62.
173. Bardelli A, Siena S. Molecular mechanisms of resistance to cetuximab and panitumumab in colorectal cancer. *J Clin Oncol.* 2010;28(7):1254–61.
174. Jhawer M, Goel S, Wilson AJ, et al. PIK3CA mutation/PTEN expression status predicts response of colon cancer cells to the epidermal growth factor receptor inhibitor cetuximab. *Cancer Res.* 2008;68(6):1953–61.
175. Halilovic E, She QB, Ye Q, et al. PIK3CA mutation uncouples tumor growth and cyclin D1 regulation from MEK/ERK and mutant KRAS signaling. *Cancer Res.* 2010;70(17):6804–14.
176. Prenen H, De Schutter J, Jacobs B, et al. PIK3CA mutations are not a major determinant of resistance to the epidermal growth factor receptor inhibitor cetuximab in metastatic colorectal cancer. *Clin Cancer Res.* 2009;15(9):3184–8.
177. Sartore-Bianchi A, Martini M, Molinari F, et al. PIK3CA mutations in colorectal cancer are associated with clinical resistance to EGFR-targeted monoclonal antibodies. *Cancer Res.* 2009;69(5):1851–7.
178. Brachmann SM, Hofmann I, Schnell C, et al. Specific apoptosis induction by the dual PI3K/mTor inhibitor NVP-BEZ235 in HER2 amplified and PIK3CA mutant breast cancer cells. *Proc Natl Acad Sci USA.* 2009;106(52):22299–304.
179. Serra V, Markman B, Scaltriti M, et al. NVP-BEZ235, a dual PI3K/mTOR inhibitor, prevents PI3K signaling and inhibits the growth of cancer cells with activating PI3K mutations. *Cancer Res.* 2008;68(19):8022–30.
180. She QB, Halilovic E, Ye Q, et al. 4E-BP1 is a key effector of the oncogenic activation of the AKT and ERK signaling pathways that integrates their function in tumors. *Cancer Cell.* 2010;18(1):39–51.
181. Hruban RH, Wilentz RE, Kern SE. Genetic progression in the pancreatic ducts. *Am J Pathol.* 2000;156(6):1821–5.
182. Mihaljevic AL, Michalski CW, Friess H, Kleeff J. Molecular mechanism of pancreatic cancer–understanding proliferation, invasion, and metastasis. *Langenbecks Arch Surg.* 2010;395(4):295–308.
183. Almoguera C, Shibata D, Forrester K, Martin J, Arnheim N, Perucho M. Most human carcinomas of the exocrine pancreas contain mutant c-K-ras genes. *Cell.* 1988;53(4):549–54.
184. Lohr M, Kloppel G, Maisonneuve P, Lowenfels AB, Luttges J. Frequency of K-ras mutations in pancreatic intraductal neoplasias associated with pancreatic ductal adenocarcinoma and chronic pancreatitis: a meta-analysis. *Neoplasia.* 2005;7(1):17–23.
185. Morris JP, Wang SC, Hebrok M. KRAS, Hedgehog, Wnt and the twisted developmental biology of pancreatic ductal adenocarcinoma. *Nat Rev Cancer.* 2011;10(10):683–95.
186. Hingorani SR, Petricoin EF, Maitra A, et al. Preinvasive and invasive ductal pancreatic cancer and its early detection in the mouse. *Cancer Cell.* 2003;4(6):437–50.
187. Habbe N, Shi G, Meguid RA, et al. Spontaneous induction of murine pancreatic intraepithelial neoplasia (mPanIN) by acinar cell targeting of oncogenic Kras in adult mice. *Proc Natl Acad Sci USA.* 2008;105(48):18913–8.
188. Calhoun ES, Jones JB, Ashfaq R, et al. BRAF and FBXW7 (CDC4, FBW7, AGO, SEL10) mutations in distinct subsets of pancreatic cancer: potential therapeutic targets. *Am J Pathol.* 2003;163(4):1255–60.
189. Asano T, Yao Y, Zhu J, Li D, Abbruzzese JL, Reddy SA. The PI 3-kinase/Akt signaling pathway is activated due to aberrant Pten

expression and targets transcription factors NF-kappaB and c-Myc in pancreatic cancer cells. *Oncogene*. 2004;23(53):8571–80.
190. Scarpa A, Capelli P, Mukai K, et al. Pancreatic adenocarcinomas frequently show p53 gene mutations. *Am J Pathol*. 1993;142(5): 1534–43.
191. Morton JP, Timpson P, Karim SA, et al. Mutant p53 drives metastasis and overcomes growth arrest/senescence in pancreatic cancer. *Proc Natl Acad Sci USA*. 2010;107(1):246–51.
192. Pellegata NS, Sessa F, Renault B, et al. K-ras and p53 gene mutations in pancreatic cancer: ductal and nonductal tumors progress through different genetic lesions. *Cancer Res*. 1994;54(6): 1556–60.
193. Caldas C, Hahn SA, da Costa LT, et al. Frequent somatic mutations and homozygous deletions of the p16 (MTS1) gene in pancreatic adenocarcinoma. *Nat Genet*. 1994;8(1):27–32.
194. Bardeesy N, Aguirre AJ, Chu GC, et al. Both p16(Ink4a) and the p19(Arf)-p53 pathway constrain progression of pancreatic adenocarcinoma in the mouse. *Proc Natl Acad Sci USA*. 2006;103(15): 5947–52.
195. Jiang J, Hui CC. Hedgehog signaling in development and cancer. *Dev Cell*. 2008;15(6):801–12.
196. Thayer SP, di Magliano MP, Heiser PW, et al. Hedgehog is an early and late mediator of pancreatic cancer tumorigenesis. *Nature*. 2003;425(6960):851–6.
197. Bailey JM, Swanson BJ, Hamada T, et al. Sonic hedgehog promotes desmoplasia in pancreatic cancer. *Clin Cancer Res*. 2008; 14(19):5995–6004.
198. Olive KP, Jacobetz MA, Davidson CJ, et al. Inhibition of Hedgehog signaling enhances delivery of chemotherapy in a mouse model of pancreatic cancer. *Science*. 2009;324(5933):1457–61.
199. Nakajima S, Doi R, Toyoda E, et al. N-cadherin expression and epithelial-mesenchymal transition in pancreatic carcinoma. *Clin Cancer Res*. 2004;10(12 Pt 1):4125–33.
200. Al-Aynati MM, Radulovich N, Riddell RH, Tsao MS. Epithelial-cadherin and beta-catenin expression changes in pancreatic intraepithelial neoplasia. *Clin Cancer Res*. 2004;10(4):1235–40.
201. Campbell PJ, Yachida S, Mudie LJ, et al. The patterns and dynamics of genomic instability in metastatic pancreatic cancer. *Nature*. 2010;467(7319):1109–13.
202. Moore MJ, Goldstein D, Hamm J, et al. Erlotinib plus gemcitabine compared with gemcitabine alone in patients with advanced pancreatic cancer: a phase III trial of the National Cancer Institute of Canada Clinical Trials Group. *J Clin Oncol*. 2007;25(15): 1960–6.
203. Philip PA, Benedetti J, Corless CL, et al. Phase III study comparing gemcitabine plus cetuximab versus gemcitabine in patients with advanced pancreatic adenocarcinoma: Southwest Oncology Group-directed intergroup trial S0205. *J Clin Oncol*. 2010; 28(22):3605–10.
204. Cascinu S, Berardi R, Labianca R, et al. Cetuximab plus gemcitabine and cisplatin compared with gemcitabine and cisplatin alone in patients with advanced pancreatic cancer: a randomised, multicentre, phase II trial. *Lancet Oncol*. 2008;9(1):39–44.
205. da Cunha Santos G, Dhani N, Tu D, et al. Molecular predictors of outcome in a phase 3 study of gemcitabine and erlotinib therapy in patients with advanced pancreatic cancer: National Cancer Institute of Canada Clinical Trials Group Study PA.3. *Cancer*. 2010;116(24):5599–607.
206. Jimeno A, Tan AC, Coffa J, et al. Coordinated epidermal growth factor receptor pathway gene overexpression predicts epidermal growth factor receptor inhibitor sensitivity in pancreatic cancer. *Cancer Res*. 2008;68(8):2841–9.
207. Jimeno A, Rubio-Viqueira B, Amador ML, et al. Dual mitogen-activated protein kinase and epidermal growth factor receptor inhibition in biliary and pancreatic cancer. *Mol Cancer Ther*. 2007;6(3):1079–88.
208. Bang YJ, Van Cutsem E, Feyereislova A, et al. Trastuzumab in combination with chemotherapy versus chemotherapy alone for treatment of HER2–positive advanced gastric or gastro-oesophageal junction cancer (ToGA): a phase 3, open-label, randomised controlled trial. *Lancet*. 2010;376(9742):687–97.
209. Kimura K, Sawada T, Komatsu M, et al. Antitumor effect of trastuzumab for pancreatic cancer with high HER-2 expression and enhancement of effect by combined therapy with gemcitabine. *Clin Cancer Res*. 2006;12(16):4925–32.
210. Buchler P, Reber HA, Eibl G, et al. Combination therapy for advanced pancreatic cancer using Herceptin plus chemotherapy. *Int J Oncol*. 2005;27(4):1125–30.
211. Safran H, Iannitti D, Ramanathan R, et al. Herceptin and gemcitabine for metastatic pancreatic cancers that overexpress HER-2/neu. *Cancer Invest*. 2004;22(5):706–12.
212. Mihaljevic A, Buchler P, Harder J, et al. A prospective, non-randomized phase II trial of Trastuzumab and Capecitabine in patients with HER2 expressing metastasized pancreatic cancer. *BMC Surg*. 2009;9:1.
213. Itakura J, Ishiwata T, Friess H, et al. Enhanced expression of vascular endothelial growth factor in human pancreatic cancer correlates with local disease progression. *Clin Cancer Res*. 1997;3(8): 1309–16.
214. Baker CH, Solorzano CC, Fidler IJ. Blockade of vascular endothelial growth factor receptor and epidermal growth factor receptor signaling for therapy of metastatic human pancreatic cancer. *Cancer Res*. 2002;62(7):1996–2003.
215. Kindler HL, Ioka T, Richel DJ, et al. Axitinib plus gemcitabine versus placebo plus gemcitabine in patients with advanced pancreatic adenocarcinoma: a double-blind randomised phase 3 study. *Lancet Oncol*. 2011;12:256–62.
216. Kindler HL, Niedzwiecki D, Hollis D, et al. Gemcitabine plus bevacizumab compared with gemcitabine plus placebo in patients with advanced pancreatic cancer: phase III trial of the Cancer and Leukemia Group B (CALGB 80303). *J Clin Oncol*. 2010; 28(22):3617–22.
217. Van Cutsem E, Vervenne WL, Bennouna J, et al. Phase III trial of bevacizumab in combination with gemcitabine and erlotinib in patients with metastatic pancreatic cancer. *J Clin Oncol*. 2009; 27(13):2231–7.
218. Feldmann G, Dhara S, Fendrich V, et al. Blockade of hedgehog signaling inhibits pancreatic cancer invasion and metastases: a new paradigm for combination therapy in solid cancers. *Cancer Res*. 2007;67(5):2187–96.

Circulating Tumor Cells and Nucleic Acids for Tumor Diagnosis

14

Loren Joseph

Introduction

"There are no free lunches" is an assertion popularized by the economist Milton Friedman. A blood based biomarker for solid tumors that can access the entire tumor genome/transcriptome could potentially guide treatment selection, sharpen prognosis, monitor treatment response, detect minimal residual disease (MRD), and possibly enable population screening. This seems to offer a "free lunch" for molecular pathology. The analysis of circulating tumor cells (CTC) and circulating tumor nucleic acids (CNA) each hold the promise of meeting these objectives.[1] These are not the first promising cancer biomarkers but unlike biochemical and immunological biomarkers, CTC and CNA methods do not target a single moiety and provide a wide range of pan-tumor and patient-specific markers.[2-5]

The first observation of CTC was reported in 1869,[6] and the first observation of circulating tumor nucleic acids was reported in 1972.[7] Advances in immunohistochemistry, image cytometry, and molecular biology have converged to the point where circulating tumor cells can be analyzed by methods ranging from morphology[8] through 10-color immunohistochemistry[9] and FISH[10,11] to whole genome analysis of single cells.[12] Cell-free circulating tumor nucleic acids (genomic DNA, mRNA, miRNA) can be quantified and analyzed for changes like mutation and methylation using common methods.

A better understanding of CTCs *might* also offer insights into the biology of tumor progression and metastasis.[13-15] The majority of CTC do NOT form metastases, dormant or active. The problem of determining when CTC should be worrisome will be familiar to pathologists: a similar question is raised by detection of isolated tumor cells in tissues. Complicating interpretation is that before resection, CTC arise in metastases and reseed the primary.[16-18] CTC can persist following resection of a primary tumor in the absence of detectable metastases; this could present a window into tumor "dormancy".

Most work on circulating tumor cells has been directed at breast and prostate cancer. Colon cancer, in contrast, uncommonly presents with metastasis; nonetheless, disseminated tumor cells are present in the bone marrow of many or most patients with colon cancer. CTC and tumor CNA are present in a substantial proportion of patients at all stages of primary gastrointestinal malignancies and in the majority with stage IV.[19-24]

Most studies have been small scale with casual rigor in design. A few have studied CTC for chemosensitivity.[25,26] A specific assay format for CTC has received FDA approval following large prospective trials: the change in CTC number following therapy *may* be used as one of the several criteria for changing therapy for metastatic colon, breast and prostate cancer.[27] Three exciting studies have shown the successful application of CTC/CNA analysis to monitor minimal residual disease (MRD) by targeting tumor-specific mutations and gene rearrangements.[3,4,28] The rationale is attractively simple. Profiles of circulating microRNA show promise for robust detection of primary epithelial tumors. The NIH directory of clinical trials lists 80 approved or active trials which include analysis of CTC/CNA, in sixteen CTC/CNA is the main focus (http://www.cancer.gov/search—accessed 01-06-11). Whether or not CTC and CNA assays will add a "free lunch" to the lab test menu awaits the outcome of large prospective clinical trials.

Terminology. "Circulating tumor cells" (*CTC*) can originate in EITHER primary OR metastatic tumors.[16,17] "Disseminated tumor cells" (*DTC*) are individual tumor-derived cells found in any site other than the circulation, such as lymph nodes or bone marrow. "Isolated tumor cell" (*ITC*) is defined in the TNM classification so as to include "micrometastasis": "single

L. Joseph, M.D. (✉)
Department of Pathology, The University of Chicago, 5841 S. Maryland Avenue, Chicago, IL 60637, USA
e-mail: ljlj@midway.uchicago.edu

A.R. Sepulveda and J.P. Lynch (eds.), *Molecular Pathology of Neoplastic Gastrointestinal Diseases*, Molecular Pathology Library 7,
DOI 10.1007/978-1-4614-6015-2_14, © Springer Science+Business Media New York 2013

malignant cells or a few tumor cells in microclusters", not more than 0.2 mm in diameter, present within a lymph node.[29] "Circulating nucleic acids" (*CNA*) refer to nucleic acids found in serum or plasma free of cells, the prefix "cf" will be used to denote "cell free" for clarity as needed (e.g., cf-mRNA). Context should make clear if CNA refers to baseline levels or tumor-derived CNA.

Circulating Tumor Cells

Historical Background

The origin of the term "metastasis" traces to an 1829 publication by Jean Claude Recamier.[30] It was natural to speculate on the existence of circulating tumor cells but it was not until 1869 that circulating tumor cells were described, albeit in an autopsy.[6]

Biology

A Circulating Epithelial Cell Is Presumed to Be Neoplastic. Many studies are designed to determine the effect of CTC number on prognosis and so do not include a "healthy subject" arm. Early studies took pains to demonstrate that circulating epithelial cells, putative CTC, had karyotype abnormalities consistent with those of the primary.[31] CTC occur at low levels if at all in "healthy" subjects, or those with adenomas or inflammatory disease.[24,32,33] The presence of genomic alterations in the CTC in an apparently healthy subject would raise concern, but would not be proof of malignancy rather than dysplasia.

The Earliest Tumor Stage Can Generate CTC. There is a modest correlation of stage with increasing incidence of CTC and number of CTC. A low level has been reported in association with colonic adenomas.[32,34]

Not All Tumors Generate CTC. CTC have been identified up to 80% of many tumors types including gastrointestinal malignancies. The level of CTC varies widely, possibly all tumors shed CTC but some below the level of detection. The determinants are unclear. Anatomic position and size of tumor are NOT determinants in any obvious way. Variation in neoangiogenesis, altered motility, altered adhesion, and predisposition to apoptosis are all considerations.[35] Although gene signatures of primary tumors have been proposed to correlate with propensity for metastasis they have not been assessed with respect to presence or levels of CTC.[36-38]

The Mechanisms by Which Tumor Cells Intravasate to Become CTC Are Uncertain. Bockhorn et al, in a paper entertainingly subtitled "Do cancer cells crawl into vessels, or are they pushed?", presented evidence that most CTC are apoptotic.[39] This might explain, in part, how so many CTC give rise to so few DTC even though other work shows that most CTC do enter the tissues. Although several xenograft studies show high levels of apoptosis, however, most studies of CTC in humans do not *report* on apoptotic cells.[40-43] This might reflect a difference from the animal models, but *might* also reflect a bias against apoptotic cells during enrichment or in analysis.[41,44] An antibody against a neo-epitope of cytokeratin 18, which is generated in apoptosis, can be shown to mark apoptotic epithelial cells, benign and malignant. It can be used for example with the CellSearch system but is NOT part of the FDA-approved system.[41,44]

Investigation of the mechanism of CTC generation requires animal studies of human tumor xenografts (or murine tumor transplants). The study of CTC from spontaneous tumors even in animals genetically predisposed to tumors would face challenges presented by the uncertain time course and the small blood volume available to sample. Studies using intravital microscopy have helped unravel how tumor cells intravasate (and extravasate).[45-48] Chang and Tomaso implicated the development of mosaic blood vessels within tumors as providing an egress. Access to the vasculature would seem to be a requirement[49-53] but connections from the lymphatics are much less studied and their use as an alternative exit cannot be dismissed.[54-56] Whether CTC come from the periphery, the central region of a primary, or both is unknown. There is evidence that they show an altered response to hypoxia.[57]

CTC Are Rare. The concentration of CTC varies widely as a function of the patient tested and the analytical method. Typical measurement ranges from extremely rare (1 per billion nucleated blood cells) to merely very rare (1 per 10,000,000). Assay sensitivity and specificity is often determined by assaying patient samples "spiked" with cells from a tumor cell line. While a useful indicator, this probably overestimates performance in practice. There is no gold standard, so it is hard to assess the rate of false negatives with clinical specimens. Given the low concentration, the total number of CTC generated daily might seem surprisingly high after factoring in the half-life and blood volume. One of the few studies to address this experimentally in mice calculated $3–4 \times 10^6$ cells shed/g tumor/24 h.[58]The commonly cited estimate of 10^9 tumor cells/g (1 cm diameter) has been criticized as too large, but even so millions of CTC traverse the vasculature every day in many patients.[59]

CTC Half-Life Is on the Order of Hours. Measurement of CTC before and after resection of a tumor gave an estimate of 1–2 h in circulation in one study and a more global estimate of 24 h to reach an undetectable level (at most ten half-lives).[60,61] An animal study in which labeled tumor cells were injected intravenously (not exactly mimicking the clinical scenario) showed 80% removed within 2–4 h. Many "settle out" in the vasculature. Many extravasate but most do NOT become a long-lived DTC). Many are actively removed in the liver or possibly lung.

No single operational definition of circulating epithelial tumor cells identifies all ctc, not all circulating malignant epithelial tumor cells appear epithelial. Because of their rarity, CTC have to be enriched from samples. Immunoselection is the most common method; the EpCam antigen and cytokeratins (after the cells have been permeabilized) are the most common target antigens. Neither marker is ideal.[62-65] In epithelial–mesenchymal transformation (*EMT*) epithelial cells take on a mesenchymal phenotype. If one believes EMT is a real process[66] one must consider the possibility it is reflected in CTC.[67,68] Immunoselection or immunodetection for epithelial markers could miss CTC altered by EMT. Size can be used to separate blood cells (small) from CTC (large), some implementations are rapid and simple; however, epithelial tumor cells can be smaller than the typical cut-off.[69] In contrast negative selection, in which only hematopoietic cells are removed, captures both EMT-modified and aberrant epithelial cells providing considerable enrichment for analysis.[70]

CTC often do not travel alone. Early reports described "tumor emboli" consisting of epithelial tumor cells, platelets, and neutrophils.[71-73] The evidence suggested that tumor emboli formed metastases more efficiently than did isolated CTC. Konstantopoulos reviewed recent literature on the role of platelets and of fibrinogen in metastasis.[74] Most CTC-centric studies take little note of platelet or neutrophil fellow-travelers. This might reflect that most methods to isolate CTC do not show emboli. Filter-based size selection methods like ISET can show mixed CTC clusters. It is not clear if other methods disrupt clusters, preferentially select single cells or discount clusters in image analysis.

CTC show genomic heterogeneity. A macroscopic tumor can be composed of a single dominant clone or of several divergent clones with both common and distinct genomic changes.[75,76] Navin et al reported a detailed study of heterogeneity in breast cancers and a discussion of the conceptual issues in analysis.[77] The size of the genomically homogenous region will vary inversely with the resolution of the method for genetic analysis. This picture is complicated by the recent finding that CTC *from* metastases can home to the primary.[16,17] It follows that CTC at any given time *could* vary widely with respect to genomic sequence. A small number of studies using FISH analysis has shown significant variation among CTC (and a low but still surprising level of abnormalities in the few CTC from "normals".[10,78] DTC, which arise at different times over the lifetime of the primary tumor also show prominent genetic divergence from each other and from the primary.[12,79]

DTC must originate as CTC, most CTC do not become DTC (sleeper cells, sleepwalking cells, and zombie cells). "Tumor dormancy" refers to an inferred state of disseminated tumor cells to account for the late appearance of metastatic disease years after resection of the primary.[60,80-82] Since CTC can be observed long after resection of a primary tumor, they must originate from a population of proliferating disseminated tumor cells in an equilibrium state, perhaps held in check by the microenvironment and/or the immune system. There is minimal evidence for a separate long-lived CTC compartment.

Dormant tumor cells can be likened to secret agents, planted years ahead of time ("sleeper cells"). The activating influences are unknown. Whether every DTC could potentially be activated is unknown. Presumably all DTC originate as CTC but the sheer number of CTC compared to DTC implies that most CTC do not become DTC even if the CTC extravasate. Whether or not most CTC *could* give rise to DTC if only they were to lodge in a receptive location is unknown: these CTC could be likened to "sleepwalking" cells. Many CTC are apoptotic ("zombie cells"?). The inefficient nature of this process is illustrated by an arresting *clinical* study.[83] In the study by Tarin 29 subjects with both malignant ascites AND peritoneovenous shunts were monitored, some for months. 15 subjects underwent autopsy. Some subjects were free of remote metastases even at autopsy, and most metastases identified were small.

Most DTC Are Probably not CTC in Transit. Techniques like Ki67 staining show that most DTC are not proliferating ("dormant"). This does NOT exclude the possibility that the DTC found in any given biopsy is actually a nonproliferating CTC caught in transit as by freeze-frame. In one animal model study, cells of a breast cancer line were loaded with fluorescent nanospheres and injected i.v. into mice.[84] Most cells settled into the liver. DTC with high levels of fluor could be identified for months, showing that the cells were not proliferating; however quiescent is not the same as "immobile".[84,85] CTC were not assayed.

CTC: Methods

The methods can be categorized with respect to the three phases of the process—collection, enrichment, and detection/analysis.

Collection

There have been few explicit studies of preanalytical variables such as the time to processing.[86,87] The only parameter uniformly reported is the collection volume, with typical values ranging from 5 to 20 ml. The most published work is for the CellSearch method which uses collection tubes containing a proprietary fixative as well as an anticoagulant.[24,86,88,89] Fixation provides flexibility in work flow; this is important for multi-institutional trials with a common laboratory and for reference labs.

Enrichment

Red Cell Lysis

Most protocols require removal of RBC prior to analysis. Typically this is achieved either by osmotic RBC lysis or density gradient centrifugation, followed by multiple washes. Each step carries the risk of CTC loss. The CTC-chip *flows* 5 ml whole blood past thousands of microscale "pillars" decorated with antibody, avoiding lysis and centrifugation.[2] The lack of RBC lysis *might* explain in part the high levels of CTC found with this system relative to other systems.

The 2009 N.I.H. conference "Circulating Tumor Cells: Emerging Technologies for Diagnosis, Prognosis, and Treatment" highlighted a wide variety common as well as uncommon methods such as dielectric cell separation[90] and photoacoustic flowmetry.[91] This does not exhaust the variety described in the literature.[46,92-96] An intriguing functional selection method plates peripheral cells on chorioamniotic membrane coated tissue culture plates.[97,98] The DEPArray system employs dielectrophoretic separation using tens of thousands of programmable "cages" which can separate individual cells followed by imaging and permits individual cell recovery, all on a silicon chip integrated with a microfluidic cartridge.[99]

The most common approaches fall into three categories:

- Flow cytometry/sorting
- Selection by size (filtration)
- Immunomagnetic selection (positive or negative)

Flow Cytometric/Cytometric Methods

Current flow sorters can process 50,000 cells/s so it is feasible albeit nontrivial to look for CTC as is shown in the studies by Low et al.[46] Low et al also describe a novel marker for CTC: a fluorescently labeled folate analog which binds tightly to the high-affinity folate receptor commonly expressed on epithelial tumors.[100] Sorting permits post-detection analysis by methods like FISH.[101,102]

Size Selection

Circulating epithelial tumor cells are *generally* larger than hematopoietic cells.[69] Filter-based size selection using an 8 μm opening is typical. Microfluidic size selection methods have also been described.[93] The large cells which are retained can be transferred on the filter to a slide for IHC or FISH studies or pooled and studied by PCR. Commercial systems are available: ISET (Isolation by Size of Epithelial Tumor cells).[69] The system could underestimate CTC by missing small tumor cells, especially those undergoing EMT. Occasional large nonepithelial cells which are captured should be flagged by the subsequent detection method. ISET is the *only* method so far shown to consistently capture clusters of CTC, keeping them intact. The limited evidence indicates that the process does NOT *produce* CTC clusters.

Positive Immunoselection

Immunoselection can be performed manually using magnetic beads or with automated instruments. A tissue-agnostic approach is to perform immunocapture with an antibody directed at a pan-epithelial target. EpCAM and cytokeratins (typically 7, 18, 19 and 20) are the most common targets for positive selection. EpCAM (CD326) is implicated in adhesion, it is NOT universally expressed on CTC.[62,103] There are differences in performance among the several EpCAM specific monoclonals. Antolovic et al investigated the effects of different EpCAM specific antibodies in CTC enrichment.[104] mAb BerEP4 and mAb KS1/4 recognize different epitopes. Detection was performed using anti-CK20 IHC. Of 39 patients 11 were positive with BerEP4 enrichment, 5 positive with KS1/4, none with both antibodies. Compounding problems, EpCAm expression can be lost in EMT. The cytokeratins (CK) are intracellular antigens so a permeabilization step is necessary prior to selection or detection. CK can be upregulated on granulocytes in inflammation, so immunoselection for CK will be problematic as will detection if selection does not exclude granulocytes.[105,106]

Antibodies specific for a particular tissue, such as CEA, have also been used. In most such studies the selected cells were pooled and analysis was limited to PCR (mRNA for expression or DNA for mutations) rather than cell-by-cell analysis as with IHC. The commercial AdnaTest uses a mixture of anti-EpCAM and anti-MUC1 antibodies; however, this selects any cell positive for EpCAM OR MUC1 (or both). Peripheral blood cells recovered by nonspecific interactions should be invisible if the gene target is tissue-specific (for mRNA) and/or mutations are only present in CTC (for DNA) both of which are plausible assumptions. This also presupposes that normal epithelial cells do NOT circulate or at least not at the level of CTC.

Negative Immunoselection

Antibodies such as anti-CD45 can be used to enrich by negative selection.[70,107] CD45 is expressed on most peripheral blood cells but NOT on epithelial cells, malignant or benign. Lara et al typically reduce the number of blood cells from 4×10^9 to 8×10^3 cells per mL, at which point analysis by IHC/FISH is feasible. Using this approach CTCs were detected in 20 of 32 head and neck cancer patients.[107] The average number of CTCs detected was 22 per mL of blood with the number ranging from 1 to 282 CTC/ml. This method should also capture and possibly detect EMT altered CTCs.

CTC Methods of Analysis

Morphology. Surprisingly few studies have reported morphologic assessments.[8,108] One study asserts that CTC reflect the morphology of the primary tumor in the sense that inspection of the CTC permitted differentiation among breast/colon/prostate/lung in many cases. The cytologic appearance of EMT has not been described.

Ploidy. DAPI staining is widely used primarily to ensure only intact cells are studied. Although there is a long tradition of studying DNA ploidy in tumors by image cytometry, this has received little attention with respect to CTC.

IHC. This is the most common technique for selection and enumeration of CTC. A CTC is typically defined as an EpCAM positive (or cytokeratin positive), CD45-negative cell with an intact DAPI-stained nucleus. Image analysis with carefully matched highly multiplexed fluorescent antibodies is feasible. Uhr et al described a 10-plex system.[9] Negative immunoselection requires scanning more cells than does positive immunoselection. Although Balasubramanian et al[70] describe using confocal microscopy there are higher throughput systems such as the imaging cytometer which permits morphologic imaging of cells and can incorporate both IHC and cytogenetic FISH images (cells are labeled before flow). Samples would have to be enriched.[109] In the FAST system the entire specimen is spread on a large slide. The cells are fixed and then stained. The entire slide is scanned by a laser cytometer.[110,111]

Cytogenetics. Karyotyping was important in early studies to confirm the relationship of CTC to the corresponding primary tumors. More recently FISH has been applied both to trace clonal evolution and to look at pharmacogenetic predictors like HER2 amplification in breast cancer. Patient/tumor-specific translocations could be suitable for FISH as well as RT-PCR analysis of CTC to detect MRD.[28]

Gene Expression. Numerous tumor specific targets (e.g., CEA, guanyl cyclase) as well as epithelial markers (EpCAM, keratins) have been tested by RT-PCR in CTC. Most reports have relied on qualitative detection (present, absent) even when using real-time PCR. Quantitative PCR could provide greater reliability as would validation of cut-offs.

Mutation Detection. Detection of specific mutations, such as Kras2 in a metastasis generally but not invariably reflects the status of the primary tumor.[112] A similar disagreement can be seen when CTC are analyzed but is much less studied.[10] As with gene expression, validation of sensitivity and specificity is often limited.

Whole Genome/Transcriptome Amplification. CTC and CNA yield little nucleic acid for analysis. Whole genome or whole transcriptome amplification can be applied, enabling use of microarrays or NextGen sequencing.[113-116] Whole-transcriptome amplification of CTC by Smirnov et al generated a five-gene profile which could distinguish among CTC of colon, prostate and breast cancer as well as from normal profiles with 94% accuracy.[113]

In Vivo Detection (Animal Models). Tumor xenografts either expressing GFP or preloaded with a fluor-like FITC-dextran are injected into an immunodeficient mouse, then monitored by fluorescent microscopy through temporary skin flaps or permanent "surgical windows". This approach can offer insight into the generation of CTC within the tumor as well as on circulation kinetics.[117]

CNA

History of CNA Analysis

The earliest demonstration of cell-free DNA in blood was in 1948.[118] The first report of CNA in association with solid tumors was, arguably, in 1972 or 1977.[7,119] An increased level of *total* DNA in the serum of patients with malignancy was seen relative to serum of healthy patients. Elevated levels of CNA in autoimmune disorders, especially lupus, had already been reported. It was much more recently shown that mRNA, microRNA, and methylated DNA can be routinely measured in cell-free serum and plasma.

The advent of PCR enabled demonstrations that the same mutation in a primary tumor could often be found in the corresponding CNA. Kras-2 was by far the most commonly studied gene. In a prospective study Kras2 mutations were identified in the CNA of 3.8% (of 1,098 subjects) and TP53 mutations in 5.5% (of 550 subjects) of patients with bladder cancer, but Kras and TP53 mutations were ALSO found in CNA from 1% and 3% respectively of healthy controls.[120] Mutations were found in smokers without known tumors.

Detection of mutations in cfDNA occasionally presaged the clinical detection of cancer.

Fleischacker et al provides an exhaustive summary of the literature on CNA through 2006.[121] The survey covers literature on point mutations, microsatellite variation, loss of heterozygosity, methylation, and RNA expression. As a result of the limited experimental design, the early studies mainly serve as proof of principle—that alterations can be identified in the CNA of many cancer patients.

"Personalized medicine" is a current touchstone of optimal medical care. Genomic/transcriptomic analysis of a tumor can identify point mutations, insertions–deletions, and fusion transcripts which are present in the tumor (or at least the dominant clone) and then used for literally "personalized" monitoring of minimal residual disease by analysis of CTC, CNA, or both.[2-4,28]

Much current work is directed at the measurement of circulating methylated promoter sequences, microRNA profiles, and tumor-specific mutations. MicroRNA expression signatures show robust performance in classifying epithelial cancers including "tumors of unknown origin".[122,123] Profiling of circulating miRNA appears very promising for detection of solid tumors.[124-128] Whole genome amplification of tumor CNA has been successful for moderate scale SNP/LOH analysis.[129] The few published NextGen Sequencing studies of CNA for copy number are technically unsatisfactory.[130,131] Next Generation Sequencing of fetal DNA in the maternal circulation (an example, after all, of circulating neoplastic DNA) *has been* analyzed successfully by Next Generation Sequencing for copy number variation.[132]

CNA: Biology

Source of CNA Circulating DNA, mRNA, and miRNA are present at low levels in all people. The basal level of CNA reflects normal cell turnover primarily from hematopoietic cells. A study of a sex-mismatched bone marrow transplant recipient showed that most cfDNA came from the donor.[133] It is a leap to generalize from a result in a bone marrow transplantation patient, but this conclusion supports expectations. Elevated levels of cfDNA have been reported in conditions such as stroke and lupus and after radiation therapy.[134-138] In many but not all cancer patients, the level of total circulating DNA is elevated.[139-143] The proportion of CNA derived from CTC (as distinct from primary tumor) has not been determined. In some cases a rise in total cfDNA has preceded clinical detection of cancer.[140,141]

That some cancer patients had elevated cell-free DNA did NOT prove that the cell-free DNA came from the tumor rather than immune or stromal cells. The demonstration that the primary tumor and CNA often contained the same mutation or loss of heterozygosity supported the conclusion that some increased DNA came from the tumor cells.[144,145] Xenograft studies of human tumors in immunosuppressed mice showed the cfDNA is overwhelmingly of human origin. The reported fraction of tumor DNA ranges from 3 to 93%, a summary statistic cited in the review by Ziegler et al.[146] Jahr undertook a novel approach, measuring levels of rearranged T-cell receptor gene sequences and of methylated selectin promoter in cfDNA, reasoning that these would reflect the inflammatory and endothelial (stromal) components.[147] Failing to see signals for the study concluded that most cfDNA in cancer patients is tumoral in origin.

Whether cfDNA originating from tumor cells is generated by apoptosis or necrosis has been decided both ways. DNA from necrotic cells is suggested to be high MW (>10,000 kb) whereas DNA from apoptotic cells is shorter, typically showing a ladder pattern with "rungs" 180 bp apart, reflecting nucleosomal packaging.[148,149] Jahr et al looked at CNA in subjects with a variety of tumors and found both short and long DNA fragments.

DNA. Circulating DNA is thought to be carried in nucleoprotein complexes. Circulating nucleoproteins, including the specifically methylated histones have been implicated, but it has not been shown that the bulk of cfDNA is present in such complexes.[149-152] The fate of various CNA is uncertain. cfDNA disappears rapidly, with a half-life of 4–30 min, as judged by study of circulating fetal DNA.[153]

Methylated DNA. Methylation of DNA in promoter sequences can turn gene expression down or off. Methylation of the promoter for MLH1 in many sporadic microsatellite unstable colon cancers is a classic example. Methylated DNA promoter sequences, including MLH1, can be detected in CNA.[154,155] Conditions, such as aging and inflammation are associated with increased methylation of varying combinations of promoters; whereas some drugs can decrease methylation.

mRNA. Measureable cell-free mRNA is present in the circulation despite the reputation of RNA for "fragility". Serum has potent RNAse activity: exogenous RNA added to serum shows a half-life on the order of seconds.[156] The leading explanation is that the cf-mRNA is present in either a proteolipid complex or an intact microvesicle.[157,158]

miRNA. Mature miRNAs are 20–25 nucleotide long RNA molecules. Each miRNA includes a "seed sequence" which matches, imperfectly, corresponding sequences in tens or hundreds of mRNA. Mature miRNAs regulate these mRNA either by inhibiting translation or promoting degradation. The stability of miRNA in blood, serum, and plasma is striking. After incubation of aliquots of whole blood at 4°, 25°, or for up to 4 days "housekeeping" microRNAs were readily demonstrated with modest change (unpublished). As for circulating mRNA, experimental evidence shows that circulating miRNA is present in micro-vesicles, proteolipid complexes (perhaps from microvesicles), and in exosomes.[159,160] Analysis of circulating miRNA in cancer was reported in 2008.[124] Kosaka has already reviewed 20 studies which primarily correlate cf-miRNA expression profiles with the presence of specific solid tumors.[126]

CNA Methods

Collection of Sample. The level in serum is invariably higher than in plasma, the difference attributable to the progressive release of nucleic acids from hematopoietic cells lysed in the evolving clot. The difference increases with the delay in separation. Many current studies still underestimate the effect of preanalytic variation in boosting apparent cfDNA (probably all CNA) levels.[161-164] Platelets, which do not contain genomic DNA, do contain both mRNA and miRNA.

Purification of CAN. Standard methods for purification of nucleic acids from blood cells can be used provided they do not loose low-molecular weight CNA. Commercial kits specific for cfDNA are available. Molecular diagnostic laboratories routinely isolate viral RNA and DNA from plasma.

Size of CNA. Notwithstanding the debate over apoptotic versus necrotic origins, much cfDNA is less than 500 bp.[165] As noted, mature miRNAs are already small. Accurate sizing and concentration measurement in this range can be obtained using microfluidic instruments such as the BioAgilent 2000.

Nucleic Acid Quantitation. UV spectrophotometric absorption is insufficiently sensitive. Fluorescent dye-binding methods, using agents like PicoGreen™ (DNA) and Ribogreen™ (RNA) are satisfactory.[166] The typical diploid human cell contains 6.6 pg of total DNA. 1,000 cells would correspond to 6.6 ng, this is near the lower limit reported for cfDNA/ml blood. Contrast this with intact CTC: 1,000 CTC/ml is a high level.

Jung compared 7 reports and found means ranging from 6 to 650 ng/ml of plasma.[167] The largest study, including 776 controls, showed a median plasma cfDNA of 26 ng/ml, a mean of 67 ng/ml but a standard deviation of 405 ng/ml. Fleischhacker gives an exhaustive listing in various cancers and controls.[121]

Mutation Detection/DNA Copy Number/Gene Expression/miRNA Expression. As for any DNA or RNA source, if the region of interest can be amplified, it can then be studied by various methods including real-time PCR and sequencing. The often small amount of CNA limits direct use of high-throughput methods like microarray and Next Generation Sequencing but as noted above whole genome/transcriptome/miRNome amplification can overcome this, albeit at risk of distorting relative levels. Digital PCR methods like BEAMING, can provide quantitative analysis of mutations, copy number, or expression level with greater sensitivity and accuracy than does typical real-time PCR or microarrays but with limited multiplexing.[168,169]

Methylation Detection of methylated CpG sites is challenging. Numerous methods are in use.[170,171] A common feature is bisulfite treatment of the DNA sample prior to PCR amplification. Traditional protocols destroy up to 90% of the input DNA which makes working with small amounts of cfDNA especially challenging. Auwera et al showed correlated levels of methylated cfDNA and CTC numbers.[172] This leaves open the question of whether the methylated sequences derive from CTC or from the primary tumor. Auwera did NOT test for methylated sequences *in* the CTC. The highly parallel BEAMING method noted above has been modified and shown to work with circulating methylated DNA sequences.[169] The authors describe a bisulfite treatment protocol which leaves 99.4% of the DNA intact.

CTC and CNA in Specific Gastrointestinal Malignancies

The following sections summarize recent findings, organized by anatomic site, for CTC, circulating methylated DNA (promoters), mRNA, and microRNA.

Esophageal Cancer and CTC

A tour-de-force study by Stocklein et al examined the question of how closely DTC reflect the primary tumor and each other at the genomic level. The data impacts the uncertainty over whether DTC arise "early" or "late" in the evolution of the primary tumor. A parallel study of CTC could help dissect the relationship of CTC and DTC. This study looked at paired primary tumors and bone marrows from 104 consecutive patients with esophageal cancer (adeno and squamous) and disaggregated lymph node preparations from 18 of these patients. DTC were identified by staining for cytokeratins or EpCAM. 38 bone marrows and 9 lymph node preps demonstrated 1 or more DTC. Sixty DTC were individually selected by micromanipulation. The DNA from each cell underwent whole genome amplification and was then assayed by comparative genomic hybridization (CGH) (not by array). Twenty-two DTC showed amplification of the region 17q12–21, which encompasses HER2. Quantitative PCR confirmed amplification of the HER2 locus in 11 of the 22 cells. Focal amplifications including HER2 but less than 5 Mb in extent would have been missed by CGH. Amplification of 17q12–21 could also encompass a region short of HER2 but still contain other significant genes. In cases where more than one DTC came from the same case, the two or three cells showed similar CGH profiles including HER2 status. In the several cases with one DTC from LN and one from bone marrow, the profiles shared the 17q12–21 amplification but were otherwise distinct. Perplexingly (or intriguingly) amplification was seen in only about 15% of the primaries without close correlation with the finding in DTC.

Fourteen studies since 2000 have examined CTC in patients with esophageal cancer, none examined CTC morphologically or immunohistochemically.[22,173-186] Eleven used RT-PCR to detect RNA transcripts of epithelial-specific genes in mRNA prepared from the mononuclear population of peripheral blood after density gradient centrifugation. In total these studies encompassed 883 patients, most were squamous carcinoma. The most frequently target was CEA. Other genes used to infer the presence of esophageal CTC were survivin, deltaNp63, SCC antigen 1, SCCA2, Eya4 (eyes absent 4) hTERT, and cytokeratin 20. One study looked p16 deletion and cyclin D1 amplification at the DNA level in CTC (and plasma).

CEA expression has been observed in activated lymphocytes.[187] Although some studies[178] report a narrow window between patients and healthy controls, most find minimal CEA mRNA in the healthy controls. The likeliest explanation (other than PCR contamination) is that the stringency of the cut-off varies among studies. Ito et al find CK20 transcripts present in the PBMC of most healthy controls, with considerable overlap with the level in patients with esophageal cancer.[178] Contamination with activated lymphocytes has been described several times.[106] Six reports do not report quantitative results even when they use real-time PCR.

Survivin is of uncertain function beyond ability to inhibit apoptosis in selected settings. Survivin mRNA is present in the basal layer of the epidermis (and in other epithelia) but not in the intermediate or superficial layers. SCCA1 (Squamous Cell Carcinoma Antigen 1) is a member of the ovalbumin family of serine protease inhibitors. SCCA2 is a homologue found in tandem with SCCA1. SCCA1 mRNA is present at the mRNA level in lymphocytes at a very low level compared to that in epithelial cells but this could be significant relative to the level in CTC.[179] "deltaNp63" is an isoform of p63, a homologue of p53, implicated as a marker of epithelial stem cells.[188] In normal subjects expression of deltaNp63 is confined to the basal layer of stratified epithelium. In normal cells p53 targets deltaNp63 for degradation. Eya4 ("eyes absent 4") not surprisingly was first identified in drosophila. The protein has tyrosine and ser/thr phosphatase activity, beyond that little is known of its function.

The highest rate of positivity for CTC was found with survivin, with the proportion of positive cases ranging from 51 to 88%.[22,174] Grimminger did a short-term study looking only at the response to neoadjuvant therapy.[175] In that study expression of survivin in CTC was associated with a higher likelihood of a minor response but no incidence of a major response. In other studies elevated survivin levels were loosely correlated with worse outcome.

Li et al show increasing rates of positivity in correlation with worsening esophageal histology (normal, hyperplasia, dysplasia, cancer) for hTERT—24%, 30%, 52% and 80% respectively. Eya4 showed inferior discrimination at each stage.

Kaganoi et al looked at SCCA mRNA in CTC preoperatively and intraoperatively in 70 patients. 23/70 patients were positive for CTC preoperatively and 24/70 were positive for CTC collected intraoperatively but only 13 of these had also been positive in the pre-op sample. Of the patient's positive for CTC at admission, 17/23 recurred; of those negative 11/47 recurred. For those positive intraoperatively 16/24 recurred, and of those negative intraoperatively, 12/46 recurred. Of those negative in both assays, only 4/36 recurred.

These studies differ not only in the targets chosen but also in the clinical parameters: volume of blood sample, time of sampling (pre-op, intra-op, post-op), and treatment prior to surgery (for example in the Kaganoi study some subjects had chemo which might affect CTC levels), distribution of stages and length of follow-up.

Esophageal Cancer and CNA

Esophageal cfDNA. Takeshita et al measured CCND amplification (11q13) in plasma DNA in 96 patients using the level of the dopamine receptor locus as a control (11q22–23).[189] Although there was a trend toward increased recurrence in patients with a high ratio, it did not reach statistical significance but in multivariate regression analysis it did reach statistical significance.

Esophageal Cancer and Methylated CNA

Four other reports have examined CNA in esophageal cancer. All four looked at methylation markers.[177,190-192] Kawakami measured methylated APC promoter sequences in peripheral blood.[190] 13 of 52 patients with methylated APC in their primary tumor had methylated sequences detected in the plasma. Of the 13, 11 were adenocarcinomas. None of the controls (20 healthy subjects, 23 with gastritis, 11 with Barrett's metaplasia) showed circulating methylated APC promoter. The authors calculate a "hypermethylation" index, the ratio of methylated to nonmethylated sequences and determined a cut-off. Six of 52 plasma samples were considered "hypermethylated," all six had survival of less than 6 months, the non-"hypermethylated" subjects had a 50% survival rate of approximately 2 years.

Hoffmann et al looked at methylation of the APC and DAPK (Death associated protein kinase) promoters.[191,193,194] Of 59 patients, 61% were positive for one or both markers. Use of both makers led to significant discrimination with respect to survival (<2.5 years) with a p-value of 0.03.

Presurgical neoadjuvant chemoradiation was seen to significantly decrease levels of methylated promoter detected in plasma (an encouraging sign of treatment effect but an obstacle to developing a useful biomarker). Pretreatment DAPK promoter methylation had by far the strongest independent effect on survival but might be functioning as a surrogate marker for adenocarcinoma).

The study by Ikoma et al is the only study so far to look at CTC and plasma.[177] 44 patients were studied by RT-PCR for CEA and for specific methylated sites in p16, E-cadherin and RAR-beta. Mononuclear cells were isolated by density gradient from 5 ml of whole blood to measure CEA by RT-PCR. Another 5 ml aliquot was centrifuged sequentially three times to obtain cell-free plasma for detection of methylated DNA by qualitative PCR. CEA was detected in 12 patients (27%). Fourteen patients (32%) showed methylation in one or more promoters. Twenty-three patients had an abnormality in one of the assays. Methylation status of the primary tumors was not provided; no information was given regarding clinical parameters such as outcome.

Esophageal Cancer: Circulating miRNA

Xie tabulates the results of four miRNA profiling studies of esophageal cancers including adenocarcinomas and squamous cell carcinomas.[122] At the time of this writing there are no published studies of circulating miRNA in patients with esophageal cancer.

Gastric Cancer: CTC

Literature review identified 20 studies in the period 2000–2010.[195-215] These encompass 1,546 subjects (excluding controls), 13 had fewer than 100 subjects. Mimori et al looked at 810 patients (and 29 controls), extracting total RNA from whole blood (the discussion implies this was interpreted as reflecting CTC) and performing real-time PCR for CEA, CK-7, CK-19, and VEGFR-1.[203] 30% of all subjects were positive for one or more markers in peripheral blood (48% in bone marrow). Kolodziejczyk screened 268 consecutive patients with gastric cancer under consideration for chemotherapy followed by gastrectomy.[200] Samples were drawn before starting chemotherapy and just before surgery. Flow sorted CD45(−) cells screened for CTC by IHC for cytokeratins. Only 32 subjects showed CTC or DTC (bone marrow) (12%). The level of DTC but NOT CTC showed a response to chemotherapy, but the DTC "responders" showed a lower 3 year survival. Fourteen studies report correlation of one or more clinical parameters with the level of CTC.

Three studies looked at CTC directly; the others applied RT-PCR to detect gene expression or miRNA expression. Matsusaka et al used the CellSearch System to follow 52 patients with metastatic gastric cancer, each of whom had demonstrable CTC, to determine if the CTC level could stratify patient responses to therapy.[202] Patients were tested at baseline, then 2 weeks and 4 weeks after initiation of chemotherapy. The analysis concluded that a CTC level >= 4 CTC (per 7.5 ml) at either 2 weeks or 4 weeks correlated with worse outcomes (OS of 3.5 and 4.0 months respectively) than for subjects who had <4 CTC at those time points (OS 11.7 and 11.4 months). The differences in outcome, stratified by CTC, were held to be significant with $p<0.001$ independent of other parameters by univariate and multivariate analysis.

Some of the gene expression studies of CTC which do not use IHC or other imaging modality give ambiguous descriptions of the source of RNA. "RNA from the blood" could mean cells, plasma, or whole blood. If just red cells are lysed and the resulting supernatant processed for RNA it is possible that CNA will be processed and mistaken for RNA from CTC. The targets of gene expression studies included cytokeratins, survivin, MUC1, c-MET, MAGE-1 and -2, uPAR, VEGF, VEGFR-1, CEA, MT1-MMP, and CD44v6. Several studies compared CTC and DTC. Kita et al analyzed the presence of uPAR, CEA, CK-7, and CK-19 mRNA in DTC (bone marrow) and CTC (blood) in 846 patients with gastric cancer, by far the largest study of DTC/CTC in gastric cancer.[199] uPAR was the most discriminating marker. Using a stringent cut-off uPAR positive DTC were present in 51% and positive CTC in 48% of all patients. uPAR expression in both DTC and CTC showed statistically significant correlation with depth of invasion, stage, and distant metastases. Only CTC uPAR was an independent prognostic factor for distant metastasis by multivariate analysis. What appears to be the same large patient group was also studied for the utility of MT1-MMP and VEGFR-1 as biomarkers. Each gene reflects a potentially distinct role and each was found in DTC and CTC of patients with gastric cancer, but the proportion of positive patients was much smaller than for uPAR.

Chen et al provide one of the few comparative evaluations measuring CTC by both IHC and by RT-PCR.[196] Cells isolated on a ficoll gradient were subsequently either immunoselected with magnetic beads coated with antibody to CK20. IHC was performed for CEA, hTERT, CD34, and CD45. The methods section does not explicitly state the source of RNA, exegesis of the discussion suggests that it was from "whole blood" with the assumption that free circulating mRNA is negligible. Real-time PCR was performed for CK20 and beta-actin. IHC detected CTC in 25/60 (42%) of cases, none in gastritis controls ($n=20$). QPCR detected transcripts for CK20 in 32 of the 60 subjects (53%) and none in the gastritis controls. All 25 cases identified by IHC were also positive by QPCR. No clinical associations such as outcome were presented.

Gastric Cancer and CNA

Methylation. Despite several surveys of methylation in gastric cancer so far only one study of methylated sequences in plasma was identified for gastric cancer.[216,217] Bernal *et al* evaluated methylation of 24 genes in primary gastric carcinoma tissues from 32 cases. 11 genes were hypermethylated in at least 50% of cases. Of these seven genes were in a statistically significant association with the signet cell variant which could be validated in a second set. Of these only APC and Reprimo promoters showed significant methylation in plasmas paired with the tumors, and only Reprimo methylation was seen in plasma from asymptomatic cases. Reprimo participates in the p53 mediated cell cycle arrest at G2.[218] Methylation of Reprimo has been demonstrated in gastric cancer in an independent study by Luo et al as well as in other malignancies, both in the primary tumors and in the plasma (pancreas, prostate, bladder, lung)[218-221]

Gastric Cancer: miRNA. Xie et al reviewed miRNA profiling studies for all gastrointestinal malignancies, including nine studies of gastric cancers.[122] They list all discriminating miRNA from the individual studies.

Zhou et al analyzed miRNA expression in circulating *tumor cells* of patients with gastric carcinoma.[215] Zou et al looked at 90 patients—41 had pre-op samples, 49 had post-op samples drawn within 3 weeks of surgery, and 29 controls. The pre-op and post-op samples are from DIFFERENT sets of patients! miR-17 and miR-106a levels were each increased (normalized to the small RNA RNU6) in the patients with tumors relative to the controls but with moderate overlap. Both miRNA levels were decreased after surgery but remained higher than controls.

Tsujiura et al looked at several miRNA (miR-21, 17-5-p, -106a, -106b, and let-7a) in the *plasma* of 69 patients with gastric cancer, sampling both pre and post-op, and 30 healthy controls.[222] miRNA was also extracted from matching primary tumors where possible. Each of the five miRNA distinguished patients from controls ($p=0.006$) with let-7a decreased and the others increased in concentration. The miRNA(s) used for normalization is not given. Of various formulae tested by the authors, the miR-106a/let-7 ratio gave the highest AUC, 0.8979. No mention is made of confirming this conclusion with an independent validation set.

Colon Cancer and CTC

Sergeant et al reviewed all studies of CRC in which CTC were measured by *quantitative* RT-PCR.[223] Only 12 studies in the period 1999–2007 met their criteria for adequate study design. The sample size ranged from 27 to 168. The studies varied widely with respect to the cell selection method, gene(s) analyzed, and the time points sampled (preoperative, intraoperative, postoperative). Three studies did NOT indicate the collection time. Given the range of study designs any conclusions must be limited. Sergeant et al concluded that in the four studies with adequate published information, there IS evidence of an association of increased numbers of CTC (inferred from RT-PCR) with stage but NO evidence for an effect on disease-free or overall survival.

A comprehensive review, by Rahbari et al, employed a complex meta-analysis of the entire literature through June 2009.[224] The review included studies of peripheral blood CTC and bone marrow DTC. Studies were required to have more than 20 subjects and to provide sufficient information that a hazard ratio could be calculated for relapse-free survival and/or overall survival. The initial scan retrieved 1,864 studies. Of these 1,825 did NOT meet the criteria. The remaining 36 studies, including only five of the reports accepted by Sergeant, were analyzed in detail. The 36 studies encompass 3,094 subjects with sample sizes ranging from 20 to 438 patients (median of 67). Twenty-nine studies used only RT-PCR for detection of CTC. Target genes included cytokeratin 20 ($n=15$ studies), CK19 ($n=4$), CK18 ($n=2$), Kras2 ($n=4$), CEA ($n=14$), survivin, EphB4, Laminin, MAT, GalNAc, MAGE-A3, c-Met, EGFR, IL10, p63, and hTERT. The review assessed six categories of bias, the only category in which a significant number of reports failed (16/36) was lack of control for confounding. Undeterred, the reviewers performed subgroup and factor interaction analysis, finally drawing two conclusions:

- If CTC were present the recurrence free survival (RFS) as well as overall survival (OS) were each significantly decreased (hazard ratios 3.24 [95% CI: 2.06–5.10]) and 2.28[1.55–3.38]). DTC positivity was of marginal significance.
- The perioperative time point was the most significant for both RFS and OS.

To identify relevant publications available after the period covered by Rahbari et al, PubMed was searched for the single Mesh term "neoplastic cells, circulating". Eight substantive studies were identified.[20,25,104,108,225-228]

Miller et al reviewed three *prospective* large multicenter studies CTC in metastatic disease using the CellSearch system, one each for metastatic breast, prostate, and colon cancer, which form the core for the FDA approval of CTC measurement using a specific reagent kit and a specific instrument. This system uses magnetic nanoparticles coated with anti-EpCAM antibodies for selection. The fixed cells are permeabilized and labeled with DAPI (to stain nuclei), anti-CK-Phycoerythrin, directed at the *intra*cellular cytokeratins 8, 18, and 19 (characteristic of epithelial cells), anti-CD45-Allophycocyanin to highlight retained leukocytes. The cells are scanned and the images analyzed semiautomatically with operator interaction. This system require that the CTC express BOTH EpCAM and cytokeratins. FISH analysis is possible but NOT part of the FDA-approved application.

FDA approval is for measurement of change in CTC number as an acceptable guide to changing therapy in patients with metastatic CRC..[19,24,229] Patients were serially monitored. For CRC the cut-off for "positivity" was >3 CTC/7.5 ml of whole blood. Of 295 normals, 3% had 1 or more putative CTC and none had greater than 5 CTC. Of 255 subjects with various benign diseases (all sites) 7% had one or more CTC, 0.5% had more than 10 CTC. Of 413 patients with metastatic CRC, 47% had one or more CTC, 18.2% had 5 or more CTC, 11.6% had 10 or more, 2% had 50 or more (the table does NOT list 3 CTC as a stratification cut-off). Patients with greater than 3 CTC showed an overall survival of 8.5 months, patients with less than 3 CTC showed an OS of 19.1 months. The discussion notes that results are significantly operator dependent despite the partially automated image analysis. Normal subjects showed a mean of 53 unclassified cells, patients with metastatic CRC showed a mean of 223 unclassified cells. These are large numbers in an assay where a change of one CTC/sample can have major impact on clinical action. Patients who converted from positive to negative even weeks after treatment had significantly improved outcomes. The authors recommended confirmation of a trend prior to clinical action. CTC measurement outperformed CEA measurement.

Operative manipulation can transiently increase the number of CTC.[230,231] A seemingly natural concern is that a large efflux of CTC might increase risk of metastases. Given the large number of CTC circulating daily in some subjects this would not seem a compelling concern unless there is a qualitative difference in the CTC released or if surgical stress changed the systemic or microenvironmental response to the CTC. The limited evidence is inconclusive.

Peach et al reviewed nine studies colon cancer in which sampling of peripheral CTC took place 24 h or more after surgery, when most CTC released by trauma, should be absent.[232] Six of nine studies showed the CTC count was an independent adverse prognostic factor.

Wong et al studied 462 patients using a manual bead-based immunoselection for EpCAM followed by manual IHC for CK20.[34] 62% of 132 patients with CRC were positive, 6% of 50 patients with adenomas were positive, and none of 160 patients with benign or no disease. The authors note that chromosome 17 aneusomy was seen in 90% of the CK20 positive cases. Hardingham et al using immunoselection and RT-PCR found CTC in 3/30 patients with adenomas and in 4/34 patients with ulcerative colitis.[32]

Colon Cancer: CNA

Methylated CNA. Numerous methylated promoter sequences have been identified in colon cancer.[233] Methylated hMLH1 promoter sequences have been detected in serum of patients with microsatellite unstable colon cancer.[154] In nine cases with hMLH1 promoter hypermethylation, three cases showed promoter methylation in the serum. Methylated hMLH1 promoter sequences were NOT identified in the serum of patients in whom the primary did not show hypermethylation. p16 promoter hypermethylation occurs in colorectal (as well as esophageal and gastric cancers) with the incidence often increasing with stage. Two studies reported detection of p16 methylation in serum of colorectal cancer patients. Zou et al looked at matching tissue and serum samples from 52 patients with cancer, 34 with adenomatous polyps, and 10 healthy individuals.[234] p16 hypermethylation was present in 20/52 (38%) of the cancer tissues. Of those 20 cases, 14 matching sera showed p16 hypermethylation (70%). No methylated p16 promoter sequences were detected in the sera of the other cancer cases, patients with adenomas, or healthy controls. Nakayama et al looked at matched tumor, remote normal mucosa, and serum samples in 168 cases of colorectal cancer. The text appears to assert that in all 99 positive tumors, the matching serum also showed at least weak p16 promoter hypermethylation whereas controls showed no methylation in serum, but a figure in the text suggests only 30–40% of sera from patients showed substantial methylation.[235,236]

Among the interesting recently identified genes methylated in colorectal cancer is HPP1 (Hyperplastic Polyposis Gene 1, aka TMEFF2, ["transmembrane containing epidermal growth factor and follistatin domains"]).[237] HPP1 is expressed in epithelium along the GI tract and in pericryptal myofibroblasts. The function is unclear. Sabbioni and Wallner have each shown that methylated HPP1 promoter sequences can be detected in serum of patients with colon cancer. Sabbioni found hypermethylation in 83% of tumors and none in control tissues.[238] Methylated HPP1 promoter sequences were identified in serum. Wallner et al identified HPP1 promoter methylation in the sera of 13% of 24 patients with local CRC, 36% of 14 with metastatic disease, and none in 20 healthy controls.[239]

Model et al used methylation-specific microarrays to assay colorectal samples: 115 metastatic cancers, 89 adenocarcinomas, 55 polyps, 31 inflammatory bowel mucosa, and 67 healthy mucosae.[240] Promising candidates included TMEFF2 (HPP1), ZDHHC22, SLITRK1, SLC32A1, DLX5, GSK3B, NGFR, and PCDH17 all of which distinguished colon neoplasia not just from normal colon but also from other tissues, especially blood (important for application to CNA). Ten markers were confirmed by real-time PCR on an independent set of 149 adenocarcinomas. Methylation of an additional marker, ALX4, showed high specificity for colon tissue BUT in both normal and malignant colon.

A second large survey used "methylation microarrays" followed by quantitative PCR confirmation.[241] This time candidates were chosen not just for minimal expression in normal tissue but also for minimal expression in blood cells. The three top candidates still included NGFR and TMEFF2 but now also SEPT9. A member of the septin protein family,

SEPT9 was discovered as a fusion partner in leukemia. The function of this class of proteins is uncertain but involves, in part, binding to the metaphase plate during mitosis. Loss of SEPT9 leads to loss of chromosome segregation. SEPT9 was present not only in the plasma of 69% of CRC patients but also in 14% of controls.

Subsequent work extended analysis of the performance of SEPT9 in plasma, looking at 379 CRC patients and 179 controls split over several test and validation groups, with comparable performance to the initial report.[242] This study included ALX4, identified earlier as a potential biomarker. ALX4, also known as Aristaless 4, is a homeobox gene with a known target sequence. ALX4 was also flagged by Zou et al in a survey of primary tumors.[243] He et al described a triplex Methylight assay for TMEFF2, SEPT9, and ALX4 in analysis of peripheral blood.[244] The combined assay showed 84% sensitivity and 87% specificity for primary tumors and 81% sensitivity and 90% specificity for cell-free methylated DNA in peripheral blood.

Zou et al identified methylation of several genes in addition to ALX4 in a high proportion of primary tumors: BMP3, EYA2, and vimentin, each methylated in approximately 70% of cases.[243] Detection in adenomas ranged from 48% for EYA2 and 72% for vimentin to 89% for ALX4. Frequency in normal epithelial ranged from 5% to 10%. This group also extensively studied fecal DNA markers and shown that methylation of the first (untranslated) exon of vimentin is an analytically robust marker. A methyl-binding protein domain immobilized on a column was used to enhance detection in the discovery phase. Without the enrichment column methylated vimentin sequence was only detected in a single cancer

Li et al used MethylBEAMING in an elegant high tech study of methylated vimentin promoter sequence in circulating DNA and in fecal DNA from patients with colorectal cancer: plasmas from 110 normal controls and from 81 patients with colorectal cancer, evenly distributed over all four Duke's stages.[168,169] Methylation of the vimentin promoter had been already demonstrated in primary tumors and fecal samples in colorectal cancer.[245,246] Fecal samples were from 38 normal controls, 20 patients with adenomas, and 22 from patents with colorectal cancer (against multiple stages). In 2 ml of peripheral blood from normal subjects a mean of 3,170 DNA vimentin exon 1 fragments were detected. Of these, on average, 0.6 vimentin exon 1 fragments were methylated per sample (only eight samples had >1 methylated molecule). The CRC patients showed a mean of 8,240 total vimentin exon 1 fragments and a mean of 335 methylated fragments. In fecal DNA, normal subjects showed a mean of 47,3000 total vimentin exon 1 fragments with 1% methylated, subjects with an adenoma showed 69,600 total fragments with 3.8% methylated, and cancer patients (all stages) showed 236,000 fragments with 7.3% methylated. Viewed differently the authors give the sensitivity for plasma as 59% overall and specificity as 93%. For Dukes A and B, curable stages, sensitivity was 52%. For the fecal study, using the optimal cut-off, 45% of patients with adenomas and 41% of patients with colorectal cancer were positive, only 5% of healthy subjects were positive.

The sensitivity and specificity of several of the tests for circulating methylated sequences might not seem high enough to be clinically useful for screening populations but they appear significantly better than the statistics for fecal occult blood testing.

Colon Cancer and Circulating miRNA

There are numerous miRNA profiles of primary colon cancer tumors, but none of CTC or plasma.

Conclusion

The role of circulating tumor cells (CTC) in the cancer ecosystem (the primary, the stroma, the metastases, the disseminated tumor cells, and immune cells) could remain elusive even as a clinical role is defined. It is tempting to dismiss circulating tumor nucleic acids as debris; however, uptake of tumor miRNA has been shown for normal cells and free DNA can activate elements of the immune system. Several findings merit emphasis:

- Circulating tumor cells can number in the millions per day but very few become disseminated tumor cells, even fewer give rise to metastases.
- Circulating tumor cells can originate in the primary or in a metastasis but can also persist after complete resection even in the absence of known metastases.
- Determinants of the level of circulating tumor cells and/or nucleic acids are unknown.
- The half-life of CTC, based on limited data, is on the order of several hours. Many are apoptotic.
- Direct detection of CTC is complicated by epithelial–mesenchymal transformation as well as the lack of uniform marker expression even in the absence of EMT.
- Limited data shows genomic heterogeneity among CTC and with respect to the primary.

With respect to future clinical applications one can, with some confidence or foolhardiness, commit to print a few predictions:

Expanded Applications for Monitoring the Effectiveness of Therapy

This is the one area for which the FDA has already approved a test. Because of genomic heterogeneity it is not clear that genomic analysis of CTC/CNA alone will dictate therapy.

Monitoring Minimal Residual Disease

As whole genome/transcriptome analysis of primary tumors becomes commonplace, data on translocations and deletions will enable sensitive detection of persisting or recurrent disease by analysis of CTC or CNA. Because of genomic heterogeneity and continued "evolution" more than one abnormality will have to be assayed. Development and validation of such personalized diagnostics will be costly at first. Proving clinical benefit will require long-term clinical studies.

Screening Populations at Risk

Analysis of CTC and CNA, especially microRNA and methylated DNA, will each be evaluated as screening tests for populations at risk. None of these tests will be perfect biomarkers but should offer significant improvements on current biomarkers like fecal occult blood (or "none" in the case of esophageal cancer).

References

1. Maheswaran S, Haber DA. Circulating tumor cells: a window into cancer biology and metastasis. *Curr Opin Genet Dev*. 2010;20(1):96–99.
2. Nagrath S, Sequist LV, Maheswaran S, et al. Isolation of rare circulating tumour cells in cancer patients by microchip technology. *Nature*. 2007;450(7173):1235–1239.
3. Maheswaran S, Sequist LV, Nagrath S, et al. Detection of mutations in EGFR in circulating lung-cancer cells. *N Engl J Med*. 2008;359(4):366–377.
4. Leary RJ, Kinde I, Diehl F, et al. Development of personalized tumor biomarkers using massively parallel sequencing. *Sci Transl Med*. 2010;2(20):20.
5. Müller V, Alix-Panabières C, Pantel K. Insights into minimal residual disease in cancer patients: Implications for anti-cancer therapies. *Eur J Cancer*. 2010;46(7):1189–1197.
6. Ashworth TR. A case of cancer in which cells similar to those in the tumours were seen in the blood after death. *Med J Aust*. 1869;14:146–147.
7. Perlin E, Moquin RB. Serum DNA levels in patients with malignant disease. *Am J Clin Pathol*. 1972;58(5):601–602.
8. Marrinucci D, Bethel K, Bruce RH, et al. Case study of the morphologic variation of circulating tumor cells. *Hum Pathol*. 2007;38(3):514–519.
9. Horton AP, Kumar K, Liu H, et al. Quantitative immunophenotyping of circulating tumor cells in blood using microfluidic screening chip integrated with hyperspectral microscope. 2009.
10. Swennenhuis JF, Tibbe AGJ, Levink R, Sipkema RCJ, Terstappen LWMM. Characterization of circulating tumor cells by fluorescence in situ hybridization. *Cytometry A*. 2009;75(6):520–527.
11. Ntouroupi TG, Ashraf SQ, McGregor SB, et al. Detection of circulating tumour cells in peripheral blood with an automated scanning fluorescence microscope. *Br J Cancer*. 2008;99(5):789–795.
12. Stoecklein NH, Hosch SB, Bezler M, et al. Direct genetic analysis of single disseminated cancer cells for prediction of outcome and therapy selection in esophageal cancer. *Cancer Cell*. 2008;13(5):441–453.
13. Pantel K, Alix-Panabières C, Riethdorf S. Cancer micrometastases. *Nat Rev Clin Oncol*. 2009;6(6):339–351.
14. Yachida S, Jones S, Bozic I, et al. Distant metastasis occurs late during the genetic evolution of pancreatic cancer. *Nature*. 2010;467(7319):1114–1117.
15. Nguyen DX, Massague J. Genetic determinants of cancer metastasis. *Nat Rev Genet*. 2007;8(5):341–352.
16. Aguirre-Ghiso JA. On the theory of tumor self-seeding: implications for metastasis progression in humans. *Breast Cancer Res*. 2010;12(2):304.
17. Kim MY, Oskarsson T, Acharyya S, et al. Tumor self-seeding by circulating cancer cells. *Cell*. 2009;139(7):1315–1326.
18. Hölzel D, Eckel R, Emeny RT, Engel J. Distant metastases do not metastasize. *Cancer Metastasis Rev*. 2010;29(4):737–750.
19. Cohen SJ, Punt CJ, Iannotti N, et al. Relationship of circulating tumor cells to tumor response, progression-free survival, and overall survival in patients with metastatic colorectal cancer. *J Clin Oncol*. 2008;26(19):3213–3221.
20. Cohen SJ, Punt CJ, Iannotti N, et al. Prognostic significance of circulating tumor cells in patients with metastatic colorectal cancer. *Ann Oncol*. 2009;20(7):1223–1229.
21. Lalmahomed ZS, Kraan J, Gratama JW, Mostert B, Sleijfer S, Verhoef C. Circulating tumor cells and sample size: the more, the better. *J Clin Oncol*. 2010;3:1–2.
22. Hoffmann AC, Warnecke-Eberz U, Luebke T, et al. Survivin mRNA in peripheral blood is frequently detected and significantly decreased following resection of gastrointestinal cancers. *J Surg Oncol*. 2007;95(1):51–54.
23. Hiraiwa K, Takeuchi H, Hasegawa H, et al. Clinical significance of circulating tumor cells in blood from patients with gastrointestinal cancers. *Ann Surg Oncol*. 2008;15(11):3092–3100.
24. Allard WJ, Matera J, Miller MC, et al. Tumor cells circulate in the peripheral blood of all major carcinomas but not in healthy subjects or patients with nonmalignant diseases. *Clin Cancer Res*. 2004;10(20):6897–6904.
25. Yen LC, Yeh YS, Chen CW, et al. Detection of KRAS oncogene in peripheral blood as a predictor of the response to cetuximab plus chemotherapy in patients with metastatic colorectal cancer. *Clin Cancer Res*. 2009;15(13):4508–4513.
26. Gazzaniga P, Naso G, Gradilone A, et al. Chemosensitivity profile assay of circulating cancer cells: prognostic and predictive value in epithelial tumors. *Int J Cancer*. 2010;126(10):2437–2447.
27. Miller MC, Doyle GV, Terstappen LW. Significance of circulating tumor cells detected by the Cell Search System in patients with metastatic breast colorectal and prostate cancer. *J Oncol*. 2010;2010:617421.
28. Stott SL, Lee RJ, Nagrath S, et al. Isolation and characterization of circulating tumor cells from patients with localized and metastatic prostate cancer. *Sci Transl Med*. 2010;2(25):25ra23.
29. de Mascarel I, MacGrogan G, Debled M, Brouste V, Mauriac L. Distinction between isolated tumor cells and micrometastases in breast cancer: is it reliable and useful? *Cancer*. 2008;112(8):1672–1678.
30. Talmadge JE, Fidler IJ. AACR centennial series: the biology of cancer metastasis: historical perspective. *Cancer Res*. 2010;70(14):5649–5669.
31. Fehm T, Sagalowsky A, Clifford E, et al. Cytogenetic evidence that circulating epithelial cells in patients with carcinoma are malignant. *Clin Cancer Res*. 2002;8(7):2073–2084.
32. Hardingham JE, Hewett PJ, Sage RE, et al. Molecular detection of blood-borne epithelial cells in colorectal cancer patients and in patients with benign bowel disease. *Int J Cancer*. 2000;89(1):8–13.
33. Wong CS, Cheung MT, Ma BB, et al. Isolated tumor cells and circulating CK20 mRNA in pN0 colorectal cancer patients. *Int J Surg Pathol*. 2008;16(2):119–126.
34. Wong SC, Chan CM, Ma BB, et al. Clinical significance of cytokeratin 20-positive circulating tumor cells detected by a refined

immunomagnetic enrichment assay in colorectal cancer patients. *Clin Cancer Res*. 2009;15(3):1005–1012.
35. Kim S-J, Fidler IJ. The pathogenesis of cancer metastasis: relevance to therapy. *Principles of Cancer Biotherapy*. 2009:1–24.
36. Bockhorn M, Roberge S, Sousa C, Jain RK, Munn LL. Differential gene expression in metastasizing cells shed from kidney tumors. *Cancer Res*. 2004;64(7):2469–2473.
37. Ramaswamy S, Ross KN, Lander ES, Golub TR. A molecular signature of metastasis in primary solid tumors. *Nat Genet*. 2003;33(1):49–54.
38. Fidler IJ, Kripke ML. Genomic analysis of primary tumors does not address the prevalence of metastatic cells in the population. *Nat Genet*. 2003;34(1):23.
39. Bockhorn M, Jain RK, Munn LL. Active versus passive mechanisms in metastasis: do cancer cells crawl into vessels, or are they pushed? *Lancet Oncol*. 2007;8(5):444–448.
40. Holmgren L, O'Reilly MS, Folkman J. Dormancy of micrometastases: balanced proliferation and apoptosis in the presence of angiogenesis suppression. *Nat Med*. 1995;1(2):149–153.
41. Larson CJ, Moreno JG, Pienta KJ, et al. Apoptosis of circulating tumor cells in prostate cancer patients. *Cytometry A*. 2004;62(1): 46–53.
42. Linder S, Havelka AM, Ueno T, Shoshan MC. Determining tumor apoptosis and necrosis in patient serum using cytokeratin 18 as a biomarker. *Cancer Lett*. 2004;214(1):1–9.
43. Mehes G, Witt A, Kubista E, Ambros PF. Circulating breast cancer cells are frequently apoptotic. *Am J Pathol*. 2001;159(1):17–20.
44. Rossi E, Basso U, Celadin R, et al. M30 Neoepitope expression in epithelial cancer: quantification of apoptosis in circulating tumor cells by Cell Search analysis. *Clin Cancer Res*. 2010; 16(21):5233.
45. Lohela M, Werb Z. Intravital imaging of stromal cell dynamics in tumors. *Curr Opin Genet Dev*. 2010;20(1):72–78.
46. He W, Wang H, Hartmann LC, Cheng J-X, Low PS. In vivo quantitation of rare circulating tumor cells by multiphoton intravital flow cytometry. *Proc Natl Acad Sci USA*. 2007;104(28): 11760–11765.
47. Condeelis J, Segall JE. Intravital imaging of cell movement in tumours. *Nat Rev Cancer*. 2003;3(12):921–930.
48. Friedl P, Gilmour D. Collective cell migration in morphogenesis, regeneration and cancer. *Nat Rev Mol Cell Biol*. 2009;10(7): 445–457.
49. Liotta LA, Kleinerman J, Saidel GM. Quantitative relationships of intravascular tumor cells, tumor vessels, and pulmonary metastases following tumor implantation. *Cancer Res*. 1974;34(5): 997–1004.
50. Chang YS, di Tomaso E, McDonald DM, Jones R, Jain RK, Munn LL. Mosaic blood vessels in tumors: frequency of cancer cells in contact with flowing blood. *Proc Natl Acad Sci USA*. 2000;97(26): 14608–14613.
51. Folkman J. Can mosaic tumor vessels facilitate molecular diagnosis of cancer? *Proc Natl Acad Sci USA*. 2001;98(2):398–400.
52. Wyckoff JB, Jones JG, Condeelis JS, Segall JE. A critical step in metastasis: in vivo analysis of intravasation at the primary tumor. *Cancer Res*. 2000;60(9):2504–2511.
53. Hashizume H, Baluk P, Morikawa S, et al. Openings between defective endothelial cells explain tumor vessel leakiness. *Am J Pathol*. 2000;156(4):1363–1380.
54. Ji R-C. Lymphatic endothelial cells, tumor lymphangiogenesis and metastasis: New insights into intratumoral and peritumoral lymphatics. *Cancer Metastasis Rev*. 2006;25(4):677–694.
55. Sleeman J, Schmid A, Thiele W. Tumor lymphatics. *Semin Cancer Biol*. 2009;19(5):285–297.
56. Pries AR, Hopfner M, le Noble F, Dewhirst MW, Secomb TW. The shunt problem: control of functional shunting in normal and tumour vasculature. *Nat Rev Cancer*. 2010;10(8):587–593.
57. Ameri K, Luong R, Zhang H, et al. Circulating tumour cells demonstrate an altered response to hypoxia and an aggressive phenotype. *Br J Cancer*. 2010;102(3):561–569.
58. Butler TP, Gullino PM. Quantitation of cell shedding into efferent blood of mammary adenocarcinoma. *Cancer Res*. 1975;35(3): 512–516.
59. Del Monte U. Does the cell number 10(9) still really fit one gram of tumor tissue? *Cell Cycle*. 2009;8(3):505–506.
60. Meng S, Tripathy D, Frenkel EP, et al. Circulating tumor cells in patients with breast cancer dormancy. *Clin Cancer Res*. 2004;10(24):8152–8162.
61. Patel H, Le Marer N, Wharton RQ, et al. Clearance of circulating tumor cells after excision of primary colorectal cancer. *Ann Surg*. 2002;235(2):226.
62. Sieuwerts AM, Kraan J, Bolt J, et al. Anti-epithelial cell adhesion molecule antibodies and the detection of circulating normal-like breast tumor cells. *J Natl Cancer Inst*. 2009;101(1):61–66.
63. Dimmler A, Gerhards R, Betz C, et al. Transcription of cytokeratins 8, 18, and 19 in bone marrow and limited expression of cytokeratins 7 and 20 by carcinoma cells: inherent limitations for RT-PCR in the detection of isolated tumor cells. *Lab Invest*. 2001;81(10):1351–1361.
64. Vlems F, Soong R, Diepstra H, et al. Effect of blood sample handling and reverse transcriptase-polymerase chain reaction assay sensitivity on detection of CK20 expression in healthy donor blood. *Diagn Mol Pathol*. 2002;11(2):90–97.
65. Vlems FA, Ladanyi A, Gertler R, et al. Reliability of quantitative reverse-transcriptase-PCR-based detection of tumour cells in the blood between different laboratories using a standardised protocol. *Eur J Cancer*. 2003;39(3):388–396.
66. Tarin D, Thompson EW, Newgreen DF. The fallacy of epithelial mesenchymal transition in neoplasia. *Cancer Res*. 2005;65(14):5996–6000. discussion 6000–5991.
67. Bonnomet A, Brysse A, Tachsidis A, et al. Epithelial-to-mesenchymal transitions and circulating tumor cells. *J Mammary Gland Biol Neoplasia*. 2010;7:1–13.
68. Aktas B, Tewes M, Fehm T, Hauch S, Kimmig R, Kasimir-Bauer S. Stem cell and epithelial-mesenchymal transition markers are frequently overexpressed in circulating tumor cells of metastatic breast cancer patients. *Breast Cancer Res*. 2009;11(4):R46.
69. Vona G, Sabile A, Louha M, et al. Isolation by size of epithelial tumor cells: a new method for the immunomorphological and molecular characterization of circulating tumor cells. *Am J Pathol*. 2000;156(1):57–63.
70. Balasubramanian P, Yang L, Lang JC, et al. Confocal images of circulating tumor cells obtained using a methodology and technology that removes normal cells. *Mol Pharm*. 2009;6(5):1402–1408.
71. Fidler IJ. Metastasis: guantitative analysis of distribution and fate of tumor embolilabeled with 125 I-5-iodo-2′-deoxyuridine. *J Natl Cancer Inst*. 1970;45(4):773–782.
72. Fidler IJ. The relationship of embolic homogeneity, number, size and viability to the incidence of experimental metastasis. *Eur J Cancer*. 1973;9(3):223–227.
73. Liotta LA, Saidel MG, Kleinerman J. The significance of hematogenous tumor cell clumps in the metastatic process. *Cancer Res*. 1976;36(3):889–894.
74. Konstantopoulos K, Thomas SN. Cancer cells in transit: the vascular interactions of tumor cells. *Annu Rev Biomed Eng*. 2009;11(1):177–202.
75. Losi L, Baisse B, Bouzourene H, Benhattar J. Evolution of intratumoral genetic heterogeneity during colorectal cancer progression. *Carcinogenesis*. 2005;26(5):916–922.
76. Torres L, Ribeiro FR, Pandis N, Andersen JA, Heim S, Teixeira MR. Intratumor genomic heterogeneity in breast cancer with clonal divergence between primary carcinomas and lymph node metastases. *Breast Cancer Res Treat*. 2007;102(2):143–155.

77. Navin N, Krasnitz A, Rodgers L, et al. Inferring tumor progression from genomic heterogeneity. *Genome Res*. 2010;20(1):68–80.
78. Katz RL, He W, Khanna A, et al. Genetically abnormal circulating cells in lung cancer patients: an antigen-independent fluorescence in situ hybridization-based case–control study. *Clin Cancer Res*. 2010;16(15):3976–3987.
79. Klein CA. Parallel progression of primary tumours and metastases. *Nat Rev Cancer*. 2009;9(4):302–312.
80. Alix-Panabières C, Riethdorf S, Pantel K. Circulating tumor cells and bone marrow micrometastasis. *Clin Cancer Res*. 2008;14(16):5013–5021.
81. Röcken M. Early tumor dissemination, but late metastasis: insights into tumor dormancy. *J Clin Invest*. 2010;120(6):1800–1803.
82. Eyles J, Puaux A-L, Wang X, et al. Tumor cells disseminate early, but immunosurveillance limits metastatic outgrowth, in a mouse model of melanoma. *J Clin Invest*. 2010;120(6):2030–2039.
83. Tarin D, Price JE, Kettlewell MG, Souter RG, Vass AC, Crossley B. Mechanisms of human tumor metastasis studied in patients with peritoneovenous shunts. *Cancer Res*. 1984;44(8):3584–3592.
84. Naumov GN, MacDonald IC, Chambers AF, Groom AC. Solitary cancer cells as a possible source of tumour dormancy? *Semin Cancer Biol*. 2001;11(4):271–276.
85. Goodison S, Kawai K, Hihara J, et al. Prolonged dormancy and site-specific growth potential of cancer cells spontaneously disseminated from nonmetastatic breast tumors as revealed by labeling with green fluorescent protein. *Clin Cancer Res*. 2003;9(10 Pt 1):3808–3814.
86. Lam NYL, Rainer TH, Chiu RWK, Lo YMD. EDTA is a better anticoagulant than heparin or citrate for delayed blood processing for plasma DNA analysis. *Clin Chem*. 2004;50(1):256–257.
87. Benoy IH, Elst H, Van Dam P, et al. Detection of circulating tumour cells in blood by quantitative real-time RT-PCR: effect of pre-analytical time. *Clin Chem Lab Med*. 2006;44(9):1082–1087.
88. Kagan M, Howard D, Bendele T, et al. A sample preparation and analysis system for identification of circulating tumor cells. *J Clin Ligand Assay*. 2002;25(1):104–110.
89. Allard WJ, Hayes DF, Repollet MI, et al. A cellular preservative improves the specificity and yield of circulating tumor cells in carcinoma patients 2003.
90. Gascoyne PRC, Noshari J, Anderson TJ, Becker FF. Isolation of rare cells from cell mixtures by dielectrophoresis. *Electrophoresis*. 2009;30(8):1388–1398.
91. Viator JA, Gupta S, Goldschmidt BS, et al. Gold nanoparticle mediated detection of prostate cancer cells using photoacoustic flowmetry with optical reflectance. *J Biomed Nanotechnol*. 2010;6(2):187–191.
92. Tkaczyk ER, Zhong CF, Ye JY, et al. In vivo monitoring of multiple circulating cell populations using two-photon flow cytometry. *Opt Commun*. 2008;281(4):888–894.
93. Zheng S, Lin H, Liu J-Q, et al. Membrane microfilter device for selective capture, electrolysis and genomic analysis of human circulating tumor cells. *J Chromatogr A*. 2007;1162(2):154–161.
94. Lee H, Sun E, Ham D, Weissleder R. Chip-NMR biosensor for detection and molecular analysis of cells. *Nat Med*. 2008;14(8):869–874.
95. Galanzha EI, Shashkov EV, Tuchin VV, Zharov VP. In vivo multispectral, multiparameter, photoacoustic lymph flow cytometry with natural cell focusing, label-free detection and multicolor nanoparticle probes. *Cytometry*. 2008;73A(10):884–894.
96. Neugebauer U, Clement JH, Bocklitz T, Krafft C, Popp J. Identification and differentiation of single cells from peripheral blood by Raman spectroscopic imaging. *J Biophoton*. 2010;3:579–87.
97. Paris PL, Kobayashi Y, Zhao Q, et al. Functional phenotyping and genotyping of circulating tumor cells from patients with castration resistant prostate cancer. *Cancer Lett*. 2009;277(2):164–173.
98. Lu J, Fan T, Zhao Q, et al. Isolation of circulating epithelial and tumor progenitor cells with an invasive phenotype from breast cancer patients. *Int J Cancer*. 2010;126(3):669–683.
99. Fuchs AB, Romani A, Freida D, et al. Electronic sorting and recovery of single live cells from microlitre sized samples. *Lab Chip*. 2006;6(1):121.
100. Sega EI, Low PS. Tumor detection using folate receptor-targeted imaging agents. *Cancer Metastasis Rev*. 2008;27(4):655–664.
101. Georgakoudi I, Solban N, Novak J, et al. In vivo flow cytometry: a new method for enumerating circulating cancer cells. *Cancer Res*. 2004;64(15):5044–5047.
102. Hu Y, Fan L, Zheng J, et al. Detection of circulating tumor cells in breast cancer patients utilizing multiparameter flow cytometry and assessment of the prognosis of patients in different CTCs levels. *Cytometry A*. 2010;77(3):213–219.
103. Deng G, Herrler M, Burgess D, Manna E, Krag D, Burke JF. Enrichment with anti-cytokeratin alone or combined with anti-EpCAM antibodies significantly increases the sensitivity for circulating tumor cell detection in metastatic breast cancer patients. *Breast Cancer Res*. 2008;10(4):R69.
104. Antolovic D, Galindo L, Carstens A, et al. Heterogeneous detection of circulating tumor cells in patients with colorectal cancer by immunomagnetic enrichment using different EpCAM-specific antibodies. *BMC Biotechnol*. 2010;10:35.
105. Krüger WH, Jung R, Detlefsen B, et al. Interference of cytokeratin-20 and mammaglobin-reverse-transcriptase polymerase chain assays designed for the detection of disseminated cancer cells. *Med Oncol*. 2001;18(1):33–38.
106. Jung R, Petersen K, Krüger W, et al. Detection of micrometastasis by cytokeratin 20 RT-PCR is limited due to stable background transcription in granulocytes. *Br J Cancer*. 1999;81(5):870–873.
107. Lara O, Tong X, Zborowski M, et al. Enrichment of rare cancer cells through depletion of normal cells using density and flow-through, immunomagnetic cell separation. *Exp Hematol*. 2004;32(10):891–904.
108. Marrinucci D, Bethel K, Lazar D, et al. Cytomorphology of circulating colorectal tumor cells:a small case series. *J Oncol*. 2010;2010:861341. doi:10.1155/2010/861341.
109. Basiji DA, Ortyn WE, Liang L, Venkatachalam V, Morrissey P. Cellular image analysis and imaging by flow cytometry. *Clin Lab Med*. 2007;27(3):653–670.
110. Hsieh HB, Marrinucci D, Bethel K, et al. High speed detection of circulating tumor cells. *Biosens Bioelectron*. 2006;21(10):1893–1899.
111. Gerstner AOH, Laffers W, Tárnok A. Clinical applications of slide-based cytometry - an update. *J Biophoton*. 2009;2(8–9):463–469.
112. Baldus SE, Schaefer K-L, Engers R, Hartleb D, Stoecklein NH, Gabbert HE. Prevalence and heterogeneity of KRAS, BRAF, and PIK3CA mutations in primary colorectal adenocarcinomas and their corresponding metastases. *Clin Cancer Res*. 2010;16(3):790–799.
113. Smirnov DA, Zweitzig DR, Foulk BW, et al. Global gene expression profiling of circulating tumor cells. *Cancer Res*. 2005;65(12):4993–4997.
114. Ozsolak F, Ting DT, Wittner BS, et al. Amplification-free digital gene expression profiling from minute cell quantities. *Nature Methods*. 2010;2165:1–4.
115. Paliwal A, Vaissière T, Herceg Z. Quantitative detection of DNA methylation states in minute amounts of DNA from body fluids. *METHODS*. 2010;16:1–6.
116. Polzer B, Hartmann CH, Klein CA. *Genome and transcriptome analysis of single tumor cells*. Weinheim: Wiley-VCH Verlag GmbH & Co KGaA; 2009.
117. Alexander S, Koehl GE, Hirschberg M, Geissler EK, Friedl P. Dynamic imaging of cancer growth and invasion: a modified

skin-fold chamber model. *Histochem Cell Biol.* 2008;130(6): 1147–1154.
118. Mandel P, Metais P. Les acides nucleiques du plasma sanguin chez l'hommes. *C R Acad Sci (Paris).* 1948;142:241–243.
119. Leon SA, Shapiro B, Sklaroff DM, Yaros MJ. Free DNA in the serum of cancer patients and the effect of therapy. *Cancer Res.* 1977;37:646–650.
120. Gormally E, Vineis P, Matullo G, et al. TP53 and KRAS2 mutations in plasma DNA of healthy subjects and subsequent cancer occurrence: a prospective study. *Cancer Res.* 2006;66(13): 6871–6876.
121. Fleischhacker M, Schmidt B. Circulating nucleic acids (CNAs) and cancer–a survey. *Biochim Biophys Acta.* 2007;1775(1): 181–232.
122. Xie L, Qian X, Liu B. MicroRNAs: novel biomarkers for gastrointestinal carcinomas. *Mol Cell Biochem.* 2010;27:1–9.
123. Rosenwald S, Gilad S, Benjamin S, et al. Validation of a microRNA-based qRT-PCR test for accurate identification of tumor tissue origin. *Mod Pathol.* 2010;23(6):814–823.
124. Mitchell PS, Parkin RK, Kroh EM, et al. Circulating microRNAs as stable blood-based markers for cancer detection. *Proc Natl Acad Sci USA.* 2008;105(30):10513–10518.
125. Lodes MJ, Caraballo M, Suciu D, Munro S, Kumar A, Anderson B. Detection of cancer with serum miRNAs on an oligonucleotide microarray. *PLoS One.* 2009;4(7):e6229.
126. Kosaka N, Iguchi H, Ochiya T. Circulating microRNA in body fluid: A new potential biomarker for cancer diagnosis and prognosis. *Cancer Sci.* 2010;101:2087–2092.
127. Shen J, Todd NW, Zhang H, et al. Plasma microRNAs as potential biomarkers for non-small-cell lung cancer. *Lab Invest.* 2011;91:579–87.
128. Bishop JA, Benjamin H, Cholakh H, Chajut A, Clark DP, Westra WH. Accurate classification of non-small cell lung carcinoma using a novel microRNA-based approach. *Clin Cancer Res.* 2010;16(2):610–619.
129. Li J, Harris L, Mamon H, et al. Whole genome amplification of plasma-circulating DNA enables expanded screening for allelic imbalance in plasma. *J Mol Diagn.* 2006;8(1):22–30.
130. Van der Vaart M, Semenov DV, Kuligina EV, Richter VA, Pretorius PJ. Characterisation of circulating DNA by parallel tagged sequencing on the 454 platform. *Clinica Chimica Acta.* 2009;409(1–2):21–27.
131. Beck J, Urnovitz HB, Mitchell WM, Schutz E. Next generation sequencing of serum circulating nucleic acids from patients with invasive ductal breast cancer reveals differences to healthy and nonmalignant controls. *Mol Cancer Res.* 2010;8(3):335–342.
132. Fan HC, Blumenfeld YJ, Chitkara U, Hudgins L, Quake SR. Noninvasive diagnosis of fetal aneuploidy by shotgun sequencing DNA from maternal blood. *Proc Natl Acad Sci USA.* 2008;105(42):16266–16271.
133. Lui YY, Chik KW, Chiu RW, Ho CY, Lam CW, Lo YM. Predominant hematopoietic origin of cell-free DNA in plasma and serum after sex-mismatched bone marrow transplantation. *Clin Chem.* 2002;48(3):421–427.
134. Rainer TH, Wong LK, Lam W, et al. Prognostic use of circulating plasma nucleic acid concentrations in patients with acute stroke. *Clin Chem.* 2003;49(4):562–569.
135. Raptis L, Menard HA. Quantitation and characterization of plasma DNA in normals and patients with systemic lupus erythematosus. *J Clin Invest.* 1980;66(6):1391–1399.
136. Gornik I, Wagner J, Gašparović V, Lauc G, Gornik O. Free serum DNA is an early predictor of severity in acute pancreatitis. *Clin Biochem.* 2008;42(1–2):38–43.
137. Stroun M, Anker P. Prehistory of the notion of circulating nucleic acids in plasma/serum (CNAPS): birth of a hypothesis. *Ann N Y Acad Sci.* 2006;1075:10–20.
138. Cheng C, Omura-Minamisawa M, Kang Y, Hara T, Koike I, Inoue T. Quantification of circulating cell-free DNA in the plasma of cancer patients during radiation therapy. *Cancer Sci.* 2009;100(2):303–309.
139. Shapiro B, Chakrabarty M, Cohn EM, Leon SA. Determination of circulating DNA levels in patients with benign or malignant gastrointestinal disease. *Cancer.* 1983;51(11):2116–2120.
140. Gormally E, Hainaut P, Caboux E, et al. Amount of DNA in plasma and cancer risk: a prospective study. *Int J Cancer.* 2004;111(5):746–749.
141. Gormally E, Caboux E, Vineis P, Hainaut P. Circulating free DNA in plasma or serum as biomarker of carcinogenesis: practical aspects and biological significance. *Mutat Res.* 2007;635(2–3): 105–117.
142. Beck J, Urnovitz HB, Riggert J, Clerici M, Schutz E. Profile of the circulating DNA in apparently healthy individuals. *Clin Chem.* 2009;55(4):730–738.
143. Yoon K-A, Park S, Lee SH, Kim JH, Lee JS. Comparison of circulating plasma DNA levels between lung cancer patients and healthy controls. *J Mol Diagn.* 2009;11(3):182–185.
144. Chen XQ, Stroun M, Magnenat JL, et al. Microsatellite alterations in plasma DNA of small cell lung cancer patients. *Nat Med.* 1996;2(9):1033–1035.
145. Mulcahy HE, Lyautey J, Lederrey C, et al. Plasma DNA K-ras mutations in patients with gastrointestinal malignancies. *Ann N Y Acad Sci.* 2000;906:25–28.
146. Ziegler A, Zangemeister-Wittke U, Stahel RA. Circulating DNA: a new diagnostic gold mine? *Cancer Treat Rev.* 2002;28(5): 255–271.
147. Jahr S, Hentze H, Englisch S, et al. DNA fragments in the blood plasma of cancer patients: quantitations and evidence for their origin from apoptotic and necrotic cells. *Cancer Res.* 2001;61(4): 1659–1665.
148. Stroun M, Maurice P, Vasioukhin V, et al. The origin and mechanism of circulating DNA. *Ann N Y Acad Sci.* 2000;906: 161–168.
149. Thierry AR, Mouliere F, Gongora C, et al. Origin and quantification of circulating DNA in mice with human colorectal cancer xenografts. *Nucl Acids Res.* 2010;21:1–17.
150. Kawamura MT, Paschoal ME, da Costa Carvalho MD. In vitro interaction of serum protein with circulating DNA of lung cancer patient. *Int J Mol Med.* 1999;4(2):187–190.
151. Fournie GJ, Courtin JP, Laval F, et al. Plasma DNA as a marker of cancerous cell death. Investigations in patients suffering from lung cancer and in nude mice bearing human tumours. *Cancer Lett.* 1995;91(2):221–227.
152. Deligezer U, Akisik EE, Erten N, Dalay N. Sequence-specific histone methylation is detectable on circulating nucleosomes in plasma. *Clin Chem.* 2008;54(7):1125–1131.
153. Lo YM, Zhang J, Leung TN, Lau TK, Chang AM, Hjelm NM. Rapid clearance of fetal DNA from maternal plasma. *Am J Hum Genet.* 1999;64(1):218–224.
154. Grady WM, Rajput A, Lutterbaugh JD, Markowitz SD. Detection of aberrantly methylated hMLH1 promoter DNA in the serum of patients with microsatellite unstable colon cancer. *Cancer Res.* 2001;61(3):900–902.
155. Leung WK, To K-F, Man EPS, et al. Quantitative detection of promoter hypermethylation in multiple genes in the serum of patients with colorectal cancer. *Am J Gastroenterol.* 2005;100(10): 2274–2279.
156. Tsui NBY, Ng EKO, Lo YMD. Stability of endogenous and added RNA in blood specimens, serum, and plasma. *Clin Chem.* 2002;48(10):1647–1653.
157. El-Hefnawy T, Raja S, Kelly L, et al. Characterization of amplifiable, circulating RNA in plasma and its potential as a tool for cancer diagnostics. *Clin Chem.* 2004;50(3):564–573.

158. Garcia JM, Garcia V, Pena C, et al. Extracellular plasma RNA from colon cancer patients is confined in a vesicle-like structure and is mRNA-enriched. *RNA*. 2008;14(7):1424–1432.
159. Hunter MP, Ismail N, Zhang X, et al. Detection of microRNA expression in human peripheral blood microvesicles. *PLoS One*. 2008;3(11):e3694.
160. Rosell R, Wei J, Taron M. Circulating MicroRNA signatures of tumor-derived exosomes for early diagnosis of non-small-cell lung cancer. *Clin Lung Cancer*. 2009;10(1):8–9.
161. Jen J, Wu L, Sidransky D. An overview on the isolation and analysis of circulating tumor DNA in plasma and serum. *Ann N Y Acad Sci*. 2000;906:8–12.
162. Sozzi G, Roz L, Conte D, et al. Effects of prolonged storage of whole plasma or isolated plasma DNA on the results of circulating DNA quantification assays. *J Natl Cancer Inst*. 2005;97(24): 1848–1850.
163. Page K, Powles T, Slade MJ, et al. The importance of careful blood processing in isolation of cell-free DNA. *Ann N Y Acad Sci*. 2006;1075:313–317.
164. Xue X, Teare MD, Holen I, Zhu YM, Woll PJ. Optimizing the yield and utility of circulating cell-free DNA from plasma and serum. *Clin Chim Acta*. 2009;404(2):100–104.
165. Schmidt B, Weickmann S, Witt C, Fleischhacker M. Integrity of cell-free plasma DNA in patients with lung cancer and nonmalignant lung disease. *Ann N Y Acad Sci*. 2008;1137:207–213.
166. Wu T-L, Zhang D, Chia J-H, K-h T, Sun C-F, Wu JT. Cell-free DNA: measurement in various carcinomas and establishment of normal reference range. *Clin Chim Acta*. 2002;321(1–2):77–87.
167. Jung K, Fleischhacker M, Rabien A. Cell-free DNA in the blood as a solid tumor biomarker—A critical appraisal of the literature. *Clin Chim Acta*. 2010;411(21–22):1611–1624.
168. Li M, Diehl F, Dressman D, Vogelstein B, Kinzler KW. BEAMing up for detection and quantification of rare sequence variants. *Nat Methods*. 2006;3(2):95–97.
169. Li M, Chen WD, Papadopoulos N, et al. Sensitive digital quantification of DNA methylation in clinical samples. *Nat Biotechnol*. 2009;27(9):858–863.
170. Sepulveda AR, Jones D, Ogino S, et al. CpG methylation analysis–current status of clinical assays and potential applications in molecular diagnostics: a report of the Association for Molecular Pathology. *J Mol Diagn*. 2009;11(4):266–278.
171. Tierling S, Schuster M, Tetzner R, Walter J. A combined HM-PCR/SNuPE method for high sensitive detection of rare DNA methylation. *Epigenetics Chromatin*. 2010;3(1):12.
172. Van der Auwera I, Elst HJ, Laere SJV, et al. *The presence of circulating total DNA and methylated genes is associated with circulating tumour cells in blood from breast cancer patients*. 2009;100(8):1277–1286.
173. Brabender J, Vallbohmer D, Grimminger P, et al. ERCC1 RNA expression in peripheral blood predicts minor histopathological response to neoadjuvant radio-chemotherapy in patients with locally advanced cancer of the esophagus. *J Gastrointest Surg*. 2008;12(11):1815–1821.
174. Cao M, Yie SM, Wu SM, et al. Detection of survivin-expressing circulating cancer cells in the peripheral blood of patients with esophageal squamous cell carcinoma and its clinical significance. *Clin Exp Metastasis*. 2009;26(7):751–758.
175. Grimminger P, Vallbohmer D, Hoffmann A, et al. Quantitative analysis of survivin RNA expression in blood as a non-invasive predictor of response to neoadjuvant radiochemotherapy in esophageal cancer. *J Surg Oncol*. 2009;100(6):447–451.
176. Hashimoto T, Kajiyama Y, Tsutsumi-Ishii Y, Nagaoka I, Tsurumaru M. Circulating micrometastases of esophageal cancer detected by carcinoembryonic antigen mRNA reverse transcriptase-polymerase chain reaction: clinical implications. *Dis Esophagus*. 2008;21(8):690–696.
177. Ikoma D, Ichikawa D, Ueda Y, et al. Circulating tumor cells and aberrant methylation as tumor markers in patients with esophageal cancer. *Anticancer Res*. 2007;27(1B):535–539.
178. Ito H, Kanda T, Nishimaki T, Sato H, Nakagawa S, Hatakeyama K. Detection and quantification of circulating tumor cells in patients with esophageal cancer by real-time polymerase chain reaction. *J Exp Clin Cancer Res*. 2004;23:455–464.
179. Kaganoi J, Shimada Y, Kano M, Okumura T, Watanabe G, Imamura M. Detection of circulating oesophageal squamous cancer cells in peripheral blood and its impact on prognosis. *Br J Surg*. 2004;91(8):1055–1060.
180. Koike M, Hibi K, Kasai Y, Ito K, Akiyama S, Nakao A. Molecular detection of circulating esophageal squamous cell cancer cells in the peripheral blood. *Clin Cancer Res*. 2002;8(9):2879.
181. Liu Z, Jiang M, Zhao J, Ju H. Circulating tumor cells in perioperative esophageal cancer patients: quantitative assay system and potential clinical utility. *Clin Cancer Res*. 2007;13(10):2992–2997.
182. Nakamura T, Yasumura T, Hayashi K, et al. Immunocytochemical detection of circulating esophageal carcinoma cells by immunomagnetic separation. *Anticancer Res*. 2000;20(6C):4739–4744.
183. Nakashima S, Natsugoe S, Matsumoto M, et al. Clinical significance of circulating tumor cells in blood by molecular detection and tumor markers in esophageal cancer. *Surgery*. 2003;133(2):162–169.
184. Setoyama T, Natsugoe S, Okumura H, et al. Carcinoembryonic antigen messenger RNA expression in blood predicts recurrence in esophageal cancer. *Clin Cancer Res*. 2006;12(20):5972.
185. Tanaka K, Yano M, Motoori M, et al. CEA-antigen and SCC-Antigen mRNA expression in peripheral blood predict hematogenous recurrence after resection in patients with esophageal cancer. *Ann Surg Oncol*. 2010;22:1–8.
186. Xi L, Nicastri DG, El-Hefnawy T, Hughes SJ, Luketich JD, Godfrey TE. Optimal markers for real-time quantitative reverse transcription PCR detection of circulating tumor cells from melanoma, breast, colon, esophageal, head and neck, and lung cancers. *Clin Chem*. 2007;53(7):1206–1215.
187. Jung R, Kruger W, Hosch S, et al. Specificity of reverse transcriptase polymerase chain reaction assays designed for the detection of circulating cancer cells is influenced by cytokines in vivo and in vitro. *Br J Cancer*. 1998;78(9):1194–1198.
188. Ratovitski EA, Patturajan M, Hibi K, Trink B, Yamaguchi K, Sidransky D. p53 associates with and targets Delta Np63 into a protein degradation pathway. *Proc Natl Acad Sci USA*. 2001;98(4):1817–1822.
189. Takeshita H, Ichikawa D, Komatsu S, et al. Prediction of CCND1 amplification using plasma DNA as a prognostic marker in oesophageal squamous cell carcinoma. *Br J Cancer*. 2011;102(9): 1378–1383.
190. Kawakami K, Brabender J, Lord RV, et al. Hypermethylated APC DNA in plasma and prognosis of patients with esophageal adenocarcinoma. *J Natl Cancer Inst*. 2000;92(22):1805–1811.
191. Hoffmann AC, Vallbohmer D, Prenzel K, et al. Methylated DAPK and APC promoter DNA detection in peripheral blood is significantly associated with apparent residual tumor and outcome. *J Cancer Res Clin Oncol*. 2009;135(9):1231–1237.
192. Hibi K, Taguchi M, Nakayama H, et al. Molecular detection of p16 promoter methylation in the serum of patients with esophageal squamous cell carcinoma. *Clin Cancer Res*. 2001;7(10): 3135–3138.
193. Kuester D, Dar AA, Moskaluk CC, et al. Early involvement of death-associated protein kinase promoter hypermethylation in the carcinogenesis of Barrett's esophageal adenocarcinoma and its association with clinical progression. *Neoplasia*. 2007;9(3):236–245.
194. Schildhaus HU, Krockel I, Lippert H, Malfertheiner P, Roessner A, Schneider-Stock R. Promoter hypermethylation of p16INK4a, E-cadherin, O6-MGMT, DAPK and FHIT in adenocarcinomas of

the esophagus, esophagogastric junction and proximal stomach. *Int J Oncol*. 2005;26(6):1493–1500.
195. Bertazza L, Mocellin S, Marchet A, et al. Survivin gene levels in the peripheral blood of patients with gastric cancer independently predict survival. *J Transl Med*. 2009;7:111.
196. Chen X-M, Chen G-Y, Wang Z-R, Zhu F-S, Wang X-L, Zhang X. Detection of micrometastasis of gastric carcinoma in peripheral blood circulation. *World J Gastroenterol*. 2004;10(6):804–808.
197. Czopek J, Bialas M, Rudzki Z, et al. The relationship between gastric cancer cells circulating in the blood and microsatellite instability positive gastric carcinomas. *Aliment Pharmacol Ther*. 2002;16(Suppl 2):128–136.
198. Illert B, Fein M, Otto C, et al. Disseminated tumor cells in the blood of patients with gastric cancer are an independent predictive marker of poor prognosis. *Scand J Gastroenterol*. 2005;40(7): 843–849.
199. Kita Y, Fukagawa T, Mimori K, et al. Expression of uPAR mRNA in peripheral blood is a favourite marker for metastasis in gastric cancer cases. *Br J Cancer*. 2009;100(1):153–159.
200. Kolodziejczyk P, Pituch-Noworolska A, Drabik G, et al. The effects of preoperative chemotherapy on isolated tumour cells in the blood and bone marrow of gastric cancer patients. *Br J Cancer*. 2007;97(5):589–592.
201. Majima T, Ichikura T, Takayama E, Chochi K, Mochizuki H. Detecting circulating cancer cells using reverse transcriptase-polymerase chain reaction for cytokeratin mRNA in peripheral blood from patients with gastric cancer. *Jpn J Clin Oncol*. 2000;30(11):499.
202. Matsusaka S, Chin K, Ogura M, et al. Circulating tumor cells as a surrogate marker for determining response to chemotherapy in patients with advanced gastric cancer. *Cancer Sci*. 2010;101: 1067–71.
203. Mimori K, Fukagawa T, Kosaka Y, et al. A large-scale study of MT1-MMP as a marker for isolated tumor cells in peripheral blood and bone marrow in gastric cancer cases. *Ann Surg Oncol*. 2008;15(10):2934–2942.
204. Mimori K, Fukagawa T, Kosaka Y, et al. Hematogenous metastasis in gastric cancer requires isolated tumor cells and expression of vascular endothelial growth factor receptor-1. *Clin Cancer Res*. 2008;14(9):2609–2616.
205. Noh YH, Im G, Ku JH, Lee YS, Ahn MJ. Detection of tumor cell contamination in peripheral blood by RT-PCR in gastrointestinal cancer patients. *J Korean Med Sci*. 1999;14(6):623–628.
206. Park SC, Park JG, Yang HK. Detection of cancer cells in peripheral blood of stomach cancer patients using RT-PCR amplification of tumour-specific mRNAs. *Aliment Pharmacol Ther*. 2002; 16(2):137–144.
207. Pituch-Noworolska A, Drabik G, Szatanek R, et al. Immunophenotype of isolated tumour cells in the blood, bone marrow and lymph nodes of patients with gastric cancer. *Pol J Pathol*. 2007;58(2):93–97.
208. Shin JH, Chung J, Kim HO, et al. Detection of cancer cells in peripheral blood of stomach cancer patients using RT-PCR amplification of tumour-specific mRNAs. *Aliment Pharmacol Ther*. 2002;16(Suppl 2):137–144.
209. Sumikura S, Ishigami S, Natsugoe S, et al. Disseminated cancer cells in the blood and expression of sialylated antigen in gastric cancer. *Cancer Lett*. 2003;200(1):77–83.
210. Szatanek R, Drabik G, Baran J, et al. Detection of isolated tumour cells in the blood and bone marrow of patients with gastric cancer by combined sorting, isolation and determination of MAGE-1, -2 mRNA expression. *Oncol Rep*. 2008;19(4):1055–1060.
211. Wang D-R, Chen G-Y, Liu X-L, et al. CD44v6 in peripheral blood and bone marrow of patients with gastric cancer as micro-metastasis. *World J Gastroenterol*. 2006;12(1):36–42.
212. Wu C-H, Lin S-R, Yu F-J, et al. Development of a high-throughput membrane-array method for molecular diagnosis of circulating tumor cells in patients with gastric cancers. *Int J Cancer*. 2006;119(2):373–379.
213. Wu CH, Lin SR, Hsieh JS, et al. Molecular detection of disseminated tumor cells in the peripheral blood of patients with gastric cancer: evaluation of their prognostic significance. *Dis Markers*. 2006;22(3):103–109.
214. Yie SM, Lou B, Ye SR, et al. Detection of survivin-expressing circulating cancer cells (CCCs) in peripheral blood of patients with gastric and colorectal cancer reveals high risks of relapse. *Ann Surg Oncol*. 2008;15(11):3073–3082.
215. Zhou H, Guo JM, Lou YR, et al. Detection of circulating tumor cells in peripheral blood from patients with gastric cancer using microRNA as a marker. *J Mol Med*. 2010;88(7):709–717.
216. Kang GH, Lee S, Cho NY, et al. DNA methylation profiles of gastric carcinoma characterized by quantitative DNA methylation analysis. *Lab Invest*. 2008;88(2):161–170.
217. Bernal C, Aguayo F, Villarroel C, et al. Reprimo as a potential biomarker for early detection in gastric cancer. *Clin Cancer Res*. 2008;14(19):6264–6269.
218. Ohki R, Nemoto J, Murasawa H, et al. Reprimo, a new candidate mediator of the p53-mediated cell cycle arrest at the G2 phase. *J Biol Chem*. 2000;275(30):22627–22630.
219. Luo J, Zhu Y, Yang G, Gong L, Wang B, Liu H. Loss of Reprimo and S100A2 expression in human gastric adenocarcinoma. *Diagn Cytopathol*. 2011;39:752–7.
220. Hamilton JP, Sato F, Greenwald BD, et al. Promoter methylation and response to chemotherapy and radiation in esophageal cancer. *Clin Gastroenterol Hepatol*. 2006;4(6):701–708.
221. Hamilton JP, Sato F, Jin Z, et al. Reprimo methylation is a potential biomarker of Barrett's-Associated esophageal neoplastic progression. *Clin Cancer Res*. 2006;12(22):6637–6642.
222. Tsujiura M, Ichikawa D, Komatsu S, et al. Circulating microRNAs in plasma of patients with gastric cancers. *Br J Cancer*. 2010;102(7):1174–1179.
223. Sergeant G, Penninckx F, Topal B. Quantitative RT-PCR detection of colorectal tumor cells in peripheral blood–a systematic review. *J Surg Res*. 2008;150(1):144–152.
224. Rahbari NN, Aigner M, Thorlund K, et al. Meta-analysis shows that detection of circulating tumor cells indicates poor prognosis in patients with colorectal cancer. *Gastroenterology*. 2010;138(5): 1714–1726.
225. Lagoudianakis EE, Kataki A, Manouras A, et al. Detection of epithelial cells by RT-PCR targeting CEA, CK20, and TEM-8 in colorectal carcinoma patients using OncoQuick density gradient centrifugation system. *J Surg Res*. 2009;155(2):183–190.
226. Garrigos N, Gallego J, Guillen-Ponce C, et al. Circulating tumour cell analysis as an early marker for relapse in stage II and III colorectal cancer patients: a pilot study. *Clin Transl Oncol*. 2010; 12(2):142–147.
227. Konigsberg R, Gneist M, Jahn-Kuch D, et al. Circulating tumor cells in metastatic colorectal cancer: efficacy and feasibility of different enrichment methods. *Cancer Lett*. 2010;293(1):117–123.
228. Yang MJ, Chiu HH, Wang HM, et al. Enhancing detection of circulating tumor cells with activating KRAS oncogene in patients with colorectal cancer by weighted chemiluminescent membrane array method. *Ann Surg Oncol*. 2010;17(2):624–633.
229. Miller MC, Doyle GV, Terstappen LWMM. Significance of circulating tumor cells detected by the cell search system in patients with metastatic breast colorectal and prostate cancer. *J Oncol*. 2010;2010:1–9.
230. Harless WW. Revisiting perioperative chemotherapy: the critical importance of targeting residual cancer prior to wound healing. *BMC Cancer*. 2009;9:118.

230. Wind J, Tuynman JB, Tibbe AGJ, et al. Circulating tumour cells during laparoscopic and open surgery for primary colonic cancer in portal and peripheral blood. *Eur J Surg Oncol*. 2009;35(9): 942–950.
232. Peach G, Kim C, Zacharakis E, Purkayastha S, Ziprin P. Prognostic significance of circulating tumour cells following surgical resection of colorectal cancers: a systematic review. *Br J Cancer*. 2010;102(9):1327–1334.
233. Kim MS, Lee J, Sidransky D. DNA methylation markers in colorectal cancer. *Cancer Metastasis Rev*. 2010;29(1):181–206.
234. Zou H-Z, Yu B-M, Wang Z-W, et al. Detection of aberrant p16 methylation in the serum of colorectal cancer patients. *Clin Cancer Res*. 2002;8(1):188–191.
235. Nakayama H, Hibi K, Taguchi M, et al. Molecular detection of p16 promoter methylation in the serum of colorectal cancer patients. *Cancer Lett*. 2002;188(1–2):115–119.
236. Nakayama G, Hibi K, Kodera Y, Koike M, Fujiwara M, Nakao A. P16 methylation in serum as a potential marker for the malignancy of colorectal carcinoma. *Anticancer Res*. 2007;27(5A):3367–3370.
237. Ebert MPA, Mooney SH, Tonnes-Priddy L, et al. Hypermethylation of the TPEF/HPP1 gene in primary and metastatic colorectal cancers. *Neoplasia*. 2005;7(8):771–778.
238. Sabbioni S, Miotto E, Veronese A, et al. Multigene methylation analysis of gastrointestinal tumors: TPEF emerges as a frequent tumor-specific aberrantly methylated marker that can be detected in peripheral blood. *Mol Diagn*. 2003;7(3–4):201–207.
239. Wallner M, Herbst A, Behrens A, et al. Methylation of serum DNA is an independent prognostic marker in colorectal cancer. *Clin Cancer Res*. 2006;12(24):7347–7352.
240. Model F, Osborn N, Ahlquist D, et al. Identification and validation of colorectal neoplasia-specific methylation markers for accurate classification of disease. *Mol Cancer Res*. 2007;5(2): 153–163.
241. Lofton-Day C, Model F, Devos T, et al. DNA methylation biomarkers for blood-based colorectal cancer screening. *Clin Chem*. 2008;54(2):414–423.
242. Tänzer M, Balluff B, Distler J, et al. Performance of epigenetic markers SEPT9 and ALX4 in plasma for detection of colorectal precancerous lesions. *PLoS ONE*. 2010;5(2):e9061.
243. Zou H, Harrington JJ, Shire AM, et al. Highly methylated genes in colorectal neoplasia: implications for screening. *Cancer Epidemiol Biomarkers Prev*. 2007;16(12):2686–2696.
244. He Q, Chen H-Y, Bai E-Q, et al. Development of a multiplex MethyLight assay for the detection of multigene methylation in human colorectal cancer. *Cancer Genet Cytogenet*. 2010;202(1): 1–10.
245. Chen W-D, Han ZJ, Skoletsky J, et al. Detection in fecal DNA of colon cancer-specific methylation of the nonexpressed vimentin gene. *JNCI J Natl Cancer Inst*. 2005;97(15):1124–1132.
246. Shirahata A, Sakata M, Sakuraba K, et al. Vimentin methylation as a marker for advanced colorectal carcinoma. *Anticancer Res*. 2009;29(1):279–281.

15 Serological Markers of Digestive Tract Cancers

Jorge L. Sepulveda

Introduction

In this chapter we will consider circulating protein markers for esophageal (EC), gastric (GC), and colorectal (CRC) cancers. Specific nucleic acids and circulating tumor cells have shown considerable potential as markers for gastrointestinal (GI) tumors and are covered in other chapters. We will focus first into the well-established, commonly available markers, namely the glycoprotein carcinoembryonic antigen (CEA) and the sialylated glycoprotein CA 19-9, and then we will review emerging markers for each GI tumor, discussing potential practical approaches for developing clinically useful applications.

In current clinical practice, serum markers are used mainly for staging and post-therapy surveillance of gastrointestinal tumors. The only recommendation for clinical use of these markers, in guidelines published by several expert group organizations, is that CEA measurements should be used for staging, therapy monitoring, and recurrence prediction in patients with colorectal cancer (see Table 15.1). No specific markers are currently recommended for routine use in gastric or esophageal cancer. Despite this paucity of widely accepted biochemical markers for GI tumors, there is a great need for reliable, sensitive, and specific markers for the following clinical applications:

1. *Screening* for early stage cancers in the general population: the main obstacle to generalized screening tests is that all of the commercially available markers and many of the markers in development tend to be negative in the great majority of early stage, localized cancers, and attain acceptable sensitivity only in advanced, widespread tumors. Additionally, specificity needs to be very high to screen a general population; otherwise, given the low prevalence of tumors in the population, most positive results will be false positive. Given their low sensibility at early stages and less than desirable specificity, none of these markers is recommended for screening in populations with low pretest probabilities of the cancer.
2. *Diagnosis* of cancer when symptoms or other signs increase the pretest probability of cancer and in patients at high risk for cancer development: given the same lack of sensitivity at early stages mentioned above, these markers should not be used to rule out tumors; however, in conjunction with other diagnostic modalities, certain positive tumor marker measurements may help to point the diagnostician in the right direction.
3. *Tumor sizing and staging*: for many of the tumor markers, there is a good correlation with tumor size, especially for those markers that are released from the tumor (in contrast with "host response" markers), and this is one reason why these markers attain higher levels in more advanced stages. However, currently, there is no generally accepted staging protocol involving GI tumor markers.
4. *Prognosis evaluation*: while there is a good correlation with survival for some of the markers, there is no widely accepted prognostic evaluation algorithm incorporating any of the GI tumor markers because of poor accuracy of the prediction or lack of sufficient data.
5. *Predict response to therapy*: as rational therapies targeting pathogenic mechanism are developed, markers will be needed to predict response to these often highly expensive treatments. An example is the measurement of her2/neu amplification for predicting response to *Herceptin* in breast cancer. The plasma protein markers currently available cannot be used effectively to predict response to therapy in GI tumors.
6. *Monitor effectiveness of therapy*: This is an accepted use of GI tumor markers such as CEA and CA19-9, as patients with elevations of these markers produced by the tumor will show a significant decrease in levels (typically greater than 50%) with effective therapy. Complete remission

J.L. Sepulveda, M.D., Ph.D. (✉)
Department of Pathology & Cell Biology, Columbia University, New York, NY, USA
e-mail: jls2282@columbia.edu

A.R. Sepulveda and J.P. Lynch (eds.), *Molecular Pathology of Neoplastic Gastrointestinal Diseases*, Molecular Pathology Library 7,
DOI 10.1007/978-1-4614-6015-2_15, © Springer Science+Business Media New York 2013

Table 15.1 Recommendations by various expert groups for clinical use of CEA in colorectal cancer

Application	ASCO[126,161–164]	EGTM[165–167]	ESMO[168–172]	NCCN[86]	NACB[67,173]	LOE	SOR
Screening	No	No	None published	None published	No	IV/V	A
Preoperative staging, prognosis	Yes, if it could assist in staging or surgical treatment planning	Yes, in combination with standard factors	Yes	Yes, as part of a complete staging workup	Yes, combined with other factors, if it would aid planning surgical treatment	III	C
Postoperative surveillance (Stage II–III)	Yes, if a patient is candidate for surgery or systemic therapy	Yes, candidates for aggressive surgical resection or chemotherapy if recurrence is detected	Yes	Yes, candidates for aggressive surgical resection if recurrence is detected	Yes, if patient is candidate for liver resection or systemic chemotherapy	I	A
Frequency after surgery	q3 Mo × 3y	q2-3 Mo × 3y		q3–6 Mo × 2 y → q6 Mo × 3 y	q3 Mo × 3y		
Monitoring advanced disease (Stage IV)	Yes	Yes, ideally in combination with radiology	Yes, if initially elevated, after 2-3Mo of therapy	Yes, for T2 or greater lesions	Yes, especially for disease that cannot be evaluated by other modalities	III	B
Frequency for advanced disease	q1–3 Mo during active treatment	q2–3 Mo during therapy	q2–3 Mo during therapy	q3 Mo × 2 y → q6 Mo × 3–5 y			

Modified from[67]

ASCO American Society for Clinical Oncology, *EGTM* European Group on Tumor Markers, *ESMO* European Society for Medical Oncology, *NCCN* National Comprehensive Cancer Network, *NACB* National Academy of Clinical Biochemistry. *Mo* months, *y* years, *LOE* Level of evidence: I, evidence from prospective, controlled, high-powered studies specifically designed to test the marker, or from a meta-analysis, pooled analysis or overview of level II or III studies; II, marker data obtained from a prospective therapeutic trial; III: large prospective studies; IV, small retrospective studies; V, small pilot studies., *SOR* Strength of Recommendation from the NACB: A—(A) high (further research is very unlikely to change the panel's confidence in the estimate of effect); (B) moderate (further research is likely to have an important impact on the panel's confidence in the estimate of effect and is likely to change the estimate); (C) low (further research is very likely to have an important effect on the panel's confidence in the estimate of effect and is likely to change the estimate

Table 15.2 CEACAM genes expressed in humans

Gene	Synonyms	Expression	PM
CEACAM1	Biliary glycoprotein, BGP1, CD66a	Ubiquitous, especially GI epithelia	TM
CEACAM3	CGM1, W264; W282; CD66d;	Granulocytes	TM
CEACAM4	NCA; CGM7	Granulocytes	TM
CEACAM5	CEA, CD66e, DKFZp781M2392	Epithelia	GPI
CEACAM6	NCA; CEAL; CD66c; CEACAM6	Epithelia, lung, spleen, granulocytes	GPI
CEACAM7	CGM2	Epithelia	GPI
CEACAM8	CD67; CGM6; CD66b; NCA-95	Granulocytes	GPI
CEACAM16	CEAL2	Cerebellum (mouse)	Sec
CEACAM18		Widespread	Sec
CEACAM19	CEAL1; MGC105097	Squamous epithelia (mouse)	TM
CEACAM20	UNQ9366	Intestine, thymus (mouse)	TM
CEACAM21	FLJ13540; R29124_1; MGC119874	Hypothalamus	TM

PM plasma membrane insertion mode, *TM* transmembrane, *GPI* glycophosphatidylinositol linked, *Sec* secreted

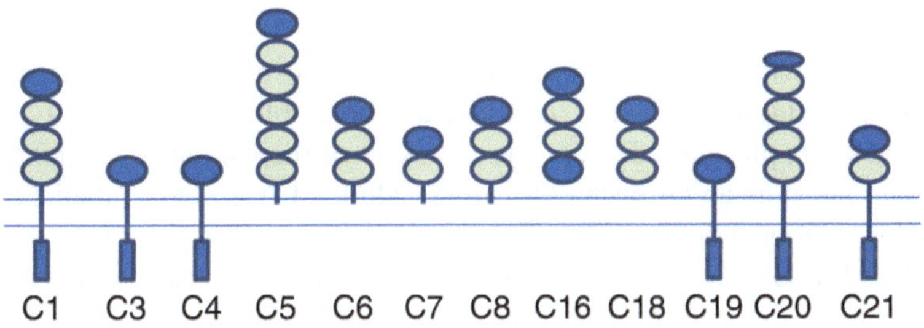

Fig. 15.1 Structure of CEACAM proteins expressed in humans. Each ellipse represents a Ig-like extracellular domain, dark IgV-like, light IgC-like (adapted from ref.240)

cannot be established by tumor marker measurements, but persistent elevation should be considered as evidence of tumor persistence, provided that alternative explanations for the marker elevation can be excluded.

7. *Screen for cancer recurrence*: This is also a widely accepted use of current GI tumor markers, as tumors that expressed the biomarkers before therapy most often re-express them upon relapse. The Working Group on Tumor Marker Criteria suggests that an increase of at least 25% or a linear increase in a marker's level in three consecutive samples is consistent with progressive disease and tumor recurrence.[1] However, due to significant false-positive and false-negative tumor marker results, complementary recurrence screening methods, including various imaging modalities, should be used.

Carcinoembryonic Antigen (CEA)

The carcinoembryonic antigen was first described by Gold and Freedman after immunizing rabbits with an extract from a colon cancer patient.[2] Since then, it has become the most widely used marker for CRC, and the only serum protein marker incorporated in current recommendations for diagnosis, treatment and follow-up of GI cancers.

Biochemistry

The carcinoembryonic antigen, also named CEACAM5, gp180 or CD66e is a member of the CEA family of genes. The CEA family is part of the immunoglobulin superfamily, and consists of the CEA subgroup and the pregnancy-specific glycoprotein (PSG) subgroup. The CEA family in humans comprises 23 genes located within a 1.2 Mb cluster on the long arm of chromosome 19, of which 18 are expressed and 11 are pseudogenes.[3,4] The CEA subgroup in humans (Table 15.2 and Fig. 15.1) comprises 6 transmembrane proteins, 4 membrane glycosylphosphatidyl inositol (GPI) -anchored glycoproteins (CEACAM5-CEACAM8), and 2 secreted proteins (CEACAM16 and 18), while the PSG group consists of 10 soluble members (PSG1–PSG10), secreted from trophoblast cells. GPI-anchoring results from a hydrophobic signal peptide coding for attachment of the phosphatidyl-glycol moiety that allows insertion of the protein into the membrane and more fluid movement to areas of interest, as demonstrated by the apical location of CEA. GPI moieties are typically linked to sugar moieties on the protein, most commonly through an alpha-6 linkage between the inositol of GPI and a glucosamine residue. The GPI tail can be cleaved with GPI phospholipase D expressed in colon cancer cells, resulting in solubilization of CEA.[5] There is some experimental evidence that CEA released from tumor cells may have a role in metastatic spreading to the liver.[6] Interestingly, the GPI-anchored CEACAM proteins tend to be upregulated in tumors, while the transmembrane CEACAMs are typically downregulated.

The CEA protein consists of 641 aminoacid residues and 45–55% carbohydrate, resulting in heterogeneous molecules with molecular masses ranging from 150 to 300 kDa, and is encoded by mRNAs 2.6 kb transcribed from five to six exons with alternative splicing and polyadenylation sites. Meconium CEA (NCA-2) differs from colon CEA in reactivity with various monoclonal antibodies, probably reflecting different post-translational modifications.[7]

Expression and Regulation

CEA is widely expressed in fetal GI tract and other tissues, including meninges, cartilage and bone, blood vessel walls, placenta, dermis, muscle layers of the stomach and intestine and bronchioles.[8] In the adult, CEA is shutdown in most cells, although expression is maintained at low levels in some adult tissues such as colon mucosa,[9] squamous esophageal mucosa,[10] squamous uterine cervical mucosa,[11] rare thymic epithelial cells in Hassall's corpuscles,[12] tracheal, bronchial, and bronchiolar epithelium and alveolar type I pneumocytes,[13] and sweat and sebaceous glands.[14]

High-level reexpression of CEA in epithelial carcinomas provides a mechanism for selective identification and targeting of these cancer cells. This tight regulation can be reproduced with a fragment containing the CEA basic promoter (–266 to +102 bp around the transcription start site), and robust expression with preserved tissue specificity can be achieved by adding the CEA enhancer located –6.1 to –4.0 kb upstream of the start site.[15] Specific targeting of a suicide gene to xenographed colon cancer was achieved using calcium phosphate nanoparticle mediated delivery of fusion construct containing the CEA promoter and the cytosine deaminase enzyme cDNA, therefore rendering the cells more susceptible to 5-fluorocytosine.[16] The promoter apparently works even in tumors without detectable CEA.[17]

CEA expression is stimulated by transforming growth factor beta (TGFβ), possibly as a regulator of cell adhesion and differentiation during embryonic development, and its expression in embryonic development mimics that of TGFβ.[8,15] The effects of TGFβ signaling on CEA expression appear to be mediated by *Smad* transcription factors, as suggested by low CEA expression in TGFβ-unresponsive gastric cancer cells and in *Smad3* knockout mice.[18]

Functional Aspects of CEA

Adhesion

Extracellular domains are involved in homotypic and heterotypic interactions between CEACAM family members, and in general these interactions play an important role in binding targets, including adhesion to other mammalian cells and bacteria. For example, CEA cooperates with CD44 variants to bind to E- and L-selectin ligands on endothelial cells and resisthigh shear stress, which may be important for the metastatic ability of colon cancer cells.[19] Binding of bacteria to the apical surface of enterocytes expressing CEACAM molecules, followed by shedding of microvesicles or cleavage of GPI linkages provides a mechanism for regulating the amount of bacteria attached to the mucosa.[20]

Cell Differentiation

Expression of CEA (and the related CEACAM6 GPI-linked molecule) generally inhibits differentiation in a variety of cell types, including myoblasts[21] and pre-adipocytes,[22] and overexpression of CEACAM5 or CEACAM6 in colonic epithelial cells results in loss of cell polarity and tissue architecture in culture and in a nude mouse model of colonic differentiation.[23] These anti-differentiation effects appear to have been selected most likely for embryologic purposes during evolution of the ancestral transmembrane-anchored CEACAM1, which does not have these effects, to the GPI-linked CEACAM5 and CEACAM6.[22]

Immunomodulation

CEA is expressed at low levels in the apical surface of adult colonic enterocytes and goblet cells,[4,24] where it may bind bacteria, regulating bacterial colonization and promoting the immune response.[20,25] Expression at the basolateral surface is found mostly in embryonic and tumor cells and may impart an immunosuppressive function by binding CD8, in conjunction with CD1d, and activating suppressor T-cells.[26] Since tumor cells frequently have loss of polarity and express CEA in the entire cell surface,[24] CEA may play a similar immunosuppressive function in colon cancer cells. Additionally, CEA was shown to decrease killing of colon cancer cells by natural killer (NK)[27] and lymphocyte-activated killer (LAK) cells.[28] It has been speculated that immunoinhibitory CEACAM molecules appeared during mammalian evolution to play a role in fetal tolerance in species with invasive trophoblastic growth.[29]

Metastasis and Tumor Survival

Injection of nude mice with CEA enhances growth of colon CA tumors.[30,31] Expression of the human chromosomal region containing CEA and CEACAM6 in transgenic mice induced enlarged colons with severe hyperplasia, dysplasia, and serrated adenomas.[32] Overexpression of CEA and

CEACAM6 in colonic cells lines disrupted their ability to form glandular structures and increased their tumorigenicity in nude mice.[23] Interestingly, in contrast with the GPI-anchored CEA and CEACAM6 molecules, CEACAM1 appears to have antitumor[33] and pro-apoptotic[34] effects and shows decreased expression in about a quarter of human colon cancers.[35]

In addition to the above-mentioned role of CEACAM molecules in adhesion and immune modulation, mechanisms of enhanced tumorigenesis potentially include:

1. Induction of interleukin-10 and resulting inhibition of the up-regulation of the inducible nitrogen oxide synthase (iNOS) in Kupfer cells.[36] Up-regulation of iNOS results in ischemic injury to the circulating tumor cells as they enter the liver microvasculature and CEA may prevent this effect.
2. Interaction of CEA with Kupfer cells also leads to release of cytokines such as IL-1β, IL-6, and TNFα, which increase expression of adhesion molecules (primarily ICAM-1) by sinusoidal endothelial cells, resulting in increased attachment of tumor cells.[37,38]
3. Inhibition of colon CA anoikis, a form of apoptosis induced by cellular detachment from the extracellular matrix, by binding to and blocking the pro-apoptotic effect of TRAIL-R2 (DR5) receptor.[39] The importance of this mechanism is highlighted by the failure of a CEA construct lacking the TRAIL-R2 binding domain to enhance experimental liver metastasis of colon cancer cells.
4. CEA and CEACAM6 modulate clustering of integrin alpha-5/beta-1 resulting in increased binding to fibronectin, enhanced cellular adhesion to the extracellular matrix with a fibronectin "cocoon" around the cells, and resistance to anoikis. Interaction of CEA with the integrins initiated signal transduction through integrin linked kinase, protein kinase B (PKB/Akt), and the mitogen-activated protein kinase cascade and appears to lead to inactivation of the intrinsic apoptosis pathway.[40-42]
5. Colon cancer apoptosis under different conditions (confluence, treatment with 5-fluorouracil, UV light or IFNγ, and in vivo) was significantly increased by selective inactivation of CEA expression with a ribozyme.[43,44]

CEA as Target

Imaging

Given its association with CRC, in particular more advanced and metastatic tumors, it makes sense to use CEA as targeting marker for localizing tumors by imaging. For example, positron emission tomography (PET) and single-photon emission computed tomography (SPECT) with pre-targeted anti-CEA antibodies identified human colon tumors in mice lungs, while ^{18}F-fludeoxyglucose labeling failed.[45] Pre-targeting with antibody, followed by addition of the radioisotope improves imaging in humans.[46] Imaging with fluorescent-labeled antibodies against CEA was used to visualize CEA-expressing xenographed tumors in mice[47] and may soon be used to help surgeons distinguish residual tumor tissue during colon cancer resections. CEA-Scan (a ^{99m}Tc-labeled anti-CEA $F_{ab'}$ fragment) has been approved by the United States Food and Drug Administration (FDA) for cancer imaging and should facilitate further studies of CEA as an imaging tumor marker.[48]

Circulating Tumor Cell Capture

Beads coupled to anti-CEA antibodies can be used to capture circulating tumor cells (CTC) expressing CEA, allowing quantification of CTC levels as well as subsequent molecular analysis on the purified cells.[49,50] Currently, most capture methods, including the FDA-approved CellSearch® test from Veridex, LLC (Raritan, NJ), use pan-epithelial-specific markers, such as cytokeratins and Er-B4, but CEA and other tumor markers have the potential to increase the specificity of the assay.

CEA as Target for Therapy

Given its role in tumor progression and survival, it is encouraging that ribozyme mediated inactivation of endogenous CEA expression in HT29 human CRC cells was followed by apoptosis and inhibition of metastatic growth in nude mice.[43,44] In addition to its specific inhibition to counter tumor promoting activities, CEA has been used as a homing target for more aggressive, nonspecific experimental therapies. Promising results have been seen with CEA-targeted radiation therapy in mice[51,52] and in humans,[53] immunotherapy with CEA-DNA vaccines,[54] CEA-stimulated dendritic cells[55] or T-cells,[56,57] and gene therapy using viral vectors expressing CEA binding domains.[58] However, these therapies need to carefully modulate the balance between anti-cancer effectiveness and toxicity due to CEA expression in normal tissues.[59]

Further refinements of ribozyme technology allow a combination of both approaches by simultaneous inactivation of CEA and expression by trans-splicing of the "suicidal gene" thymidine kinase, thereby conferring increased susceptibility of CEA-expressing cells to gancyclovir treatment.[60] Another ingenious approach uses an anti-CEA single chain antibody fused to cytosine deaminase to target colon cancer cells for 5-fluorocytosine therapy.[61] An important consideration for the use of CEA as target for therapy is that CEA expression in tumors does not necessarily correlate with CEA serum levels,[62] and therefore serum levels should not be used to select patients for CEA-directed therapy.

Assays

CEA was first detected in serum with a radioimmunoassay in 1969, which demonstrated levels above 20 ng/mL in 15 of 15 recurrent or metastatic colon CA patients, levels above the 2.5 ng/mL detection limit in 19 of 20 with preoperative or residual cancer, and undetectable levels in patients with no residual colon cancer, non-GI cancers, non-cancer GI diseases, and normal subjects including pregnant women.[63] Although these results were overly optimistic compared to subsequent studies, they launched the foundation for the use of CEA to detect cancer colon recurrence.

Most commonly used current CEA assays are performed on high throughput, automated, random-access analyzers using electrochemiluminescence detection, which have replaced manual, labor-intensive, and expensive radioimmunoassays. In general, a capture antibody is immobilized in a solid phase, such as magnetic beads, and CEA is purified from the sample after binding to the capture antibody and washing of unbound materials. Detection uses another anti-CEA antibody, which is coupled to an enzyme such as alkaline phosphatase. For chemiluminescence detection, a substrate such as Lumi Phos 530 is added and upon reaction with the enzyme generates light that can be measured with high sensitivity and low background by luminometers. Alternatively, the detection antibody may be coupled to a chemiluminescent chemical such as an acridinium ester. Other antibody-coupled enzymes may generate a colored product that can be measured with a spectrophotometer, but these are subject to higher background and more interference and are not commonly used in routine assays for clinical purposes. More experimental detection methods are pushing further the limits of detection of CEA. For example, a microchip assay using beads coated with a CEA capture antibody and a second anti-CEA antibody coupled to gold beads and thermal lens microscopy for detection achieved analytical sensitivities several times lower than conventional enzyme-linked immunoassays.[64] It is important to note that CEA is a complex molecule, with multiple glycosylation sites and alternative epitopes, and results from one method cannot be directly compared to another method, especially if different antibodies and calibrator materials are used.

Typically, the capture and/or the detection antibodies are mouse monoclonal antibodies, therefore, these assays may be subject to interference by human anti-mouse antibodies (HAMA). Excess turbidity in the sample, such as highly lipemic serum, can also interfere with assays using colorimetric or chemiluminescent detection. Another source of potential confounding results is the hook effect, which results from excessive amounts of antigen interfering with the formation of detectable antigen–antibody complexes and therefore resulting in falsely low measurements. In all these cases, dilution of the sample often removes some or all of the interfering substances. If the CEA levels after adjustment for the dilution factor are higher than the undiluted levels, an interference is possibly present. Other strategies involve removal of interfering immunoglobulins, e.g., with blocking reagents, polyethylene glycol precipitation, or anti-immunoglobulin columns.

Use of CEA in Colon Cancer

The major clinical use of CEA measurements is as an adjunct to assessing and monitoring the extent of colon cancer disease. While initially hoped to be tumor specific, it soon became evident that individuals with several non-neoplastic conditions, including chronic smokers, had elevations in CEA levels. Therefore, this marker has limited utility for general screening, but as a quantitative test, it has been shown to correlate with the extent of colon cancer growth, with higher levels being seen in more advanced cancers with worse prognosis. The serum levels of CEA depend on the amount synthesized by the tumor, the number of CEA-expressing cells in the tumor and their degree of differentiation, CEA release from tumors by secretion, GPI-cleavage, and cell death, the vascularization of the tumor, amount of necrosis, catabolism of CEA by the liver, and renal elimination. As a general rule, benign conditions express lower level of CEA (typically < 10 ng/mL) and tend to remain stable over time, whereas CEA levels often increase with tumor progression. Recommendations for the use of CEA and other tumor markers in clinical care of patients with colon cancer are summarized in Fig. 15.2.

Screening

In a review of colon cancer markers, Hundt et al[65] summarized performance characteristics of CEA from 19 studies published before July 2006. Overall sensitivity varied from 43 to 69% but was highly dependent on Dukes stage, ranging from 8 to 52% for Dukes A, 22 to 59% for Dukes B, 38 to 72% for Dukes C, and 69 to 96% for Dukes D. CEA was more often than not below cutoff in non-metastatic colon cancers (stages A–C). Specificity was dependent on the CEA analytical cutoff and on the selected population of controls, and ranged from 55 to 100%. Lower specificity was observed with cutoffs below 4 ng/ml and in benign GI disorders. In general, the *use of CEA for screening and detection of early colon cancer in healthy individuals is not recommended because of poor sensitivity and optimal specificity.*[66,67] Even though it is not recommended for screening healthy, asymptomatic individuals, a study in Singapore found that up to 7.4% of asymptomatic patients whose only indication for endoscopy was an elevated CEA had a malignancy, including colon, stomach, lung and ovarian cancer.[68] Once an elevated CEA is found, it is probably best to investigate the patient for possible malignancy.

- **CEA cannot be used in screening of healthy subjects for early CRC [LOE, IV/V; SOR, A]**
- **Preoperative CEA concentrations might be used in combination with other factors in planning surgical treatment.**
- **Patients with increased concentrations of CEA (e.g., >5 μg/L) should be evaluated for the presence of distant metastases [LOE, III; SOR, C].**
- **Preoperative CEA concentrations should not be used at present to select patients for adjuvant chemotherapy [LOE, III; SOR, C].**
- **CEA should be measured every 3 months in patients with stage II or III CRC for at least 3 years after diagnosis if the patient is a candidate for surgery or systemic therapy of metastatic disease [LOE, I; SOR, A].**
- **In patients with advanced CRC undergoing systemic therapy, regular CEA determinations should be carried out.**
- **A confirmed CEA increase (e.g., >30%) suggests progressive disease provided the possibility of false-positive elevations can be excluded [LOE, III; SOR, B].**
- **Routine measurement of CA19.9, CA 242, or TIMP-1 is not recommended [LOE, III/IV; SOR, B/C].**

Fig. 15.2 National Academy of Clinical Biochemistry Laboratory Medicine Practice Guidelines for use of tumor markers in colorectal cancer (created from data in [67]). LOE and SOE as in Table 15.1

Planning Therapy, Staging, and Evaluating Prognosis

CEA can be used conjunctly with other diagnostic modalities to evaluate extension of disease and plan surgical treatment. However, CEA should not be used to select patients for adjuvant therapy.[67] While there is no formal prognostic evaluation algorithm incorporating CEA, the College of American Pathologists[69] and The American Joint Committee on Cancer[70] have determined that CEA is a category I prognostic factor for CRC and should be incorporated in staging protocols, together with tumor TNM stage and residual tumor following surgery. Category I includes "factors definitively proven to be of prognostic import based on evidence from multiple statistically robust published trials and generally used in patient management".[69] For example, pre-op CEA>5 ng/ml was significantly associated with worst prognosis in colon cancer (5-year disease free survival 71% vs 82%), particularly in stage II tumors,[71] and CEA may be useful to select patients with stage II tumors that may be benefited from adjuvant chemotherapy.[72] *All patients with CEA elevations (*e.g., *>5 ng/mL) should be evaluated for the presence of distant metastases.*

Postoperative Surveillance

A major role of CEA measurement is in the evaluation of the CRC patient postsurgery, with the goals of monitoring effectiveness of therapy, providing reassurance to patients and health providers, and detecting recurrence or metastases. After curative resection, the overall 5-year recurrence rate of CRC is about 40%, including 12% local recurrence, nearly 20% liver metastasis, 8% pulmonary metastasis, and 30% other recurrences.[73] After curative surgical resection of CRC, CEA levels tend to revert to normal, while persistently elevated CEA is associated with residual tumor. Quantitative meta-analysis of 20 studies examining the performance of CEA in 4,285 patients following resection of colon CA arrived at an overall sensitivity of 64% for detection of cancer recurrence with 90% specificity. Using weighted

Table 15.3 Diagnostic accuracy of CEA for detection of recurrences of CRC following curative surgery, based on data from[73]

Outcome	Sensitivity	Specificity	PPV	Number of Patients
Local recurrence	60	86	2.8	1,305
Liver metastasis	73	91	8.3	1,293
Lung metastasis	56	83	3.4	525
Other recurrence	70	73	2.6	380

PPV Positive predictive value. Numbers are in percentages

meta-regression, the optimal cutoff to achieve optimal diagnostic yield was 2.2 mg/dL, corresponding to derived specificity and sensitivity of 84%, still insufficient for use in isolation.[74] Another meta-analysis determined the diagnostic accuracy of CEA for detection of local recurrence and liver, pulmonary, and other recurrences[73] (Table 15.3). It is important to note that while the specificities range from 73 to 91%, the positive predictive values are very low, around 3% for detection of local recurrences and 8% for detection of liver metastasis (Table 15.3).

Other meta-analysis studies have also concluded that intensive follow-up including CEA testing resulted in a small but statistically significant improvement in survival. In two of these studies, intensive surveillance was associated with improved outcome only if CEA was included.[75,76] In general, early surgical intervention in patients with recurrent disease detected by increases in CEA levels may improve survival in up to 35% of patients.[77] A nomogram incorporating patient age, tumor location, preoperative CEA, T stage, numbers of positive and negative lymph nodes, lymphovascular invasion, perineural invasion, and use of postoperative chemotherapy was developed to help predict post-operative cancer recurrence and showed a concordance index of 0.77, better than the categorical staging system of the American Joint Committee on Cancer.[78] Another nomogram incorporating CEA was developed to predict survival after hepatic resection for metastatic colon CA.[79] Note that there is no correlation of serum CEA with tumor CEA or histopathologic features, even though high serum CEA predicts worse outcome,[80] and therefore both CEA and morphological findings should be used for outcome prediction.

While the period between CEA elevation and detection of recurrence (lead time) may reflect the speed of tumor growth, there was no statistically significant correlation between lead time and re-resection rate or survival in a study of 4,841 resected colon cancer patients, probably because the average CEA lead time (about 5 months) is too short to have a significant impact.[81] Markers that can detect recurrence with improved lead time relative to CEA, allowing more timely intervention before relapsing tumor or metastases become extensive, may offer better opportunity for improvements in outcomes.

These studies lead to the recommendation that CEA be measured every 2–3 months in stage II-III patients for at least 3 years, if the patients are candidates for surgery or systemic treatment in the event of cancer recurrence or metastatic disease (Table 15.1). Monitoring after 5 years is not advised, as over 80% of the recurrences occur during the first 3 years, and therefore the positive predictive value of CEA elevations will considerably decrease.[82] Monitoring of early stage CRC with CEA or imaging does not appear cost effective, as less than 1% of the patients would benefit from such approach.[73,83] In stage II, CEA levels >5 ng/mL together with stage T4 and lymphovascular or perineural invasion identified patients with lower 5-year survival that should potentially be considered for adjuvant chemotherapy.[84] Stage IV (Dukes D) patients are also poor candidates for follow-up, as surgery is rarely effective.[73]

Monitoring should include at a minimum imaging and CEA measurements for optimal sensitivity in detecting CRC recurrences. In one study, the combination of CEA and CT imaging detected over 90% of the asymptomatic recurrences post-resection of CRC.[85] If CEA is used alone, a lower cutoff (e.g., 2.2 ng/mL or a 30% increase) should be used for increased sensitivity, followed by imaging and endoscopy for confirmation. The NCCN Colon Cancer Panel recommends that *patients with confirmed elevations of CEA post-surgical resection,* e.g., *a 30% increase confirmed a month later, should undergo physical examination, colonoscopy, and chest, abdominal, and pelvic CT scans.*[86] PET-CT should be considered but it is extremely rare to detect CRC recurrence if CT scans are negative. Imaging studies, if initially negative, should be repeated every 3 months until recurrence is identified or CEA stabilizes or decreases. With negative imaging studies, "blind" laparotomy or laparoscopy is not indicated solely based on the CEA elevation, as most elevations will be false positives.[73]

Similarly, patients that fail to decrease CEA within 3–4 weeks postsurgery may be at high risk for early recurrence and should undergo aggressive follow-up. A study of 600 patients with CRC and elevated preoperative CEA levels found that persistently elevated postoperative CEA levels were a strong predictor of recurrence, particularly as liver metastases.[87] In another study of CRC patients with preoperative CEA levels >5 ng/mL showed that a drop ≥60% in CEA levels was associated with better 5-year survival rates.[88]

Compliance with these recommendations appears poor. For example, a recent study of nearly 10,000 patients with curative resection for colon cancer found that only 17% had appropriate follow-up at the recommended frequency, while 60% were tested less frequently and 23% above guideline recommendations.[89] Under testing was more frequent in older individuals and minorities.

Monitoring Response to Chemotherapy

In patients with advanced or metastatic disease, CEA levels are often elevated, and a sustained decrease in CEA levels correlates with good response to treatment. For example, a CEA doubling time of >13.8 days had a sensitivity of 86% with 85% specificity to detect disease progression, while patients that responded to therapy had CEA half-life of <3.4 days.[90] The doubling time or half-life is calculated from an exponential-regressive curve connecting a minimum of three consecutive, semilogarithmic-transformed CEA values, which can be implemented in widely available worksheet programs.

CEA is the marker of choice for monitoring the response of metastatic disease to chemotherapy and should be used in conjunction with imaging and other clinical assessment modalities. Testing should be done for the duration of chemotherapy with a testing interval of 2–3 months. An increase of at least 30%, when confirmed by a repeat measurement within 1 month, is considered evidence of cancer recurrence or metastatic disease, after ruling out early effects of chemotherapy or another cause for CEA elevation.

Caution: certain treatments (such as 5-FU, levamisole, irinotecan, and oxaliplatin) can cause temporary elevations of CEA, probably as a consequence of release by dying tumor cells, which may be associated with better outcomes.[91-93] For example, a CEA flare, defined as a ≥15% increase of ≥4 μg/L followed by a decrease of ≥15%, had an objective response rate of 73%, compared to 11% for patients with CEA increasing ≥15% in two consecutive measurements.[94] Other studies have supported these findings.[91,95] *Early CEA elevations should not be interpreted as failure to respond, and changes in therapy should not be based on CEA alone in the first 4–6 months of chemotherapy.*

Monitoring Colon Cancer with Negative CEA

CEA is elevated only in about 50% of patients with colon cancer, ranging from 0 to 15% in stage A to 65 to 80% in stage D. Therefore, other markers are necessary to monitor patients with CEA levels below cutoff. In addition to the use of CA19-9, other promising markers are discussed below.

Use of CEA in Gastric Cancer

CEA is actually expressed in the vast majority of gastric cancers (over 90%), particularly of the intestinal type, but expression in the tumor tissue by immunohistochemistry has little correlation with serum levels.[96] The National Academy of Clinical Biochemistry states that "although carcinoembryonic antigen and CA 19-9 have been proposed for use in gastric cancer,... none of these markers can currently be recommended for routine clinical use".[97]

Screening

CEA is insensitive for early detection of GC, with positivity rates below 20%. In advanced GC, the positivity rates are higher but usually below 50%. Highly elevated CEA in nonmetastatic GC appears to be associated with signet ring morphology and poorly differentiated tumors with massive local infiltration.[98] Another study showed good correlation between CEA elevation and serosal invasion.[99]

Monitoring

A study of 258 patients post-gastrectomy for GC showed low sensitivity and specificity of both CEA and CA19-9 for prediction of recurrence of gastric cancer.[100] These authors observed a false-positive rate of 15% in GC patients post-gastrectomy, especially in patients with conditions that tend to elevate CEA, such as smoking, and liver, renal, or pulmonary diseases. Positive predictive values were particularly low after gastrectomy for early stage GC, with recurrence rates below 3%, while the sensitivity for recurrence even in advanced stage GC was not very high (37% in GC, compared to 80% for colon cancer). A different study confirmed a low positivity rate of CEA for GC (around 20%) but showed higher sensitivity (79%) for detection of recurrences in CEA-positive tumors with a specificity of 94% with the same cutoff of >5 ng/ml.[101] As in CRC, about 20% of patients undergoing chemotherapy for GC demonstrate early surges in CEA levels, occurring in the first few months of treatment, which should not be interpreted as indicators of progressive disease.[102]

Prognostication

The value of CEA levels in predicting gastric cancer prognosis is a topic of controversy. An older multicentric study of 2,768 GC patients showed that pre-gastrectomy CEA levels strongly correlated with stage, lymph node metastases, and histopathology and had independent prognostic value.[103] A study of 810 patients in Korea[96] showed significantly worse prognosis in 9% of patients with serum CEA >7 ng/mL (5-year survival of 80.7% vs 48%). In a study of 549 Japanese patients with GC undergoing gastrectomy, CEA levels above 5 ng/mL were found in 19.5% of the patients, and the levels significantly correlated with depth of invasion, hepatic metastases, and rates of curative resection.[104] In multivariate analysis, CEA>10 ng/mL, nodal involvement, and depth of invasion were significant predictors of prognosis.[104] In another study, CEA>10 ng/mL correlated with worse survival, lymph node metastases, and depth of tumor invasion, although the difference between CEA-positive and CEA-negative tumors was not large enough to be useful as a single prognostic factor in an individual patient.[105] In a separate study, patients with ascites fluid CEA (aCEA) levels >5 ng/ml had an average survival of 2.3 months compared to 7.4 months with aCEA below the cutoff; no such correlation was found with serum CEA in these patients.[106] Peritoneal lavage CEA >0.4 ng/mL also correlated with worse survival in a study of 229 Japanese patients.[107] CEA and CA19-9 levels were of no independent prognostic value in predicting survival of GC patients,[108] although combination with pro-inflammatory proteins IL6 and CRP increased their predictive value.[109] Combination of CEA with CA19-9 and CA125 showed increased sensitivity and specificity for predicting worse prognosis.[99] A comparison of CEA, CA 19-9, CA 72-4, and AFP showed correlation of individual markers with metastasis locations, but only CA72-4 showed specific independent prognostic value, with a 3.8-fold higher risk of death.[110] *In summary, while more research is needed to determine the appropriate combination of markers for GC prognostic evaluation and none of the markers are currently recommended for follow-up of GC, it seems reasonable to provide more intensive follow-up for GC patients determined to have elevated levels of CEA, CA19-9, CA72-4, or CA125.*

CEA in Esophageal Cancer

CEA is expressed in about 60% of squamous cell tumors and most adenocarcinomas of the esophagus, and although elevations in the serum are found in only a minority of those patients, it can be used as a marker to monitor effectiveness of therapy.[111] For example, while CEA >5 ng/mL was present in only 19% of the patients with EC before resection, elevations above the threshold occurred in 55% of the patients with recurring disease, with 90% specificity.[112] Squamous cell carcinomas (ESCC) are better followed with squamous cell markers, such as squamous cell cancer antigen (SCC), but CEA elevations are seen in a few cases and may be useful to monitor response to therapy. For example, while only 4.2% of the patients with ESCC and CEA elevations above 3.3 ng/ml responded to chemotherapy, the complete response rate for those patients with low CEA was 48% in one study.[113] Interestingly, measurement of CEA mRNA in the serum of patients with ESCC had higher sensitivity and specificity than serum CEA or SCC protein levels for detection of postoperative recurrences.[114]

CEA in Non-GI Tumors

CEA is nonspecific for the gastrointestinal tract, and many other tumors can result in increased levels of CEA in the serum:

- Non-small cell Lung carcinomas (65%)
- Small cell Lung carcinomas (30%)
- Pancreatic carcinomas (25–55%)
- Biliary carcinomas (50%)
- Breast carcinomas (40%)
- Squamous uterine cervical carcinomas (40%)
- Ovarian tumors (25%)
- Thymomas[12]
- Medullary thyroid carcinomas[115,116]
- Salivary gland tumors[117]

False-Positive CEA Results

In a study in a central laboratory in Sweden, the overall incidence of false-positive and false-negative CEA results in the general population was 4%. However, in patients with GI tumors, elevations in CEA unrelated to tumor progression are more frequent. For example, CEA (and CA19-9) remained elevated in 14% of 151 patients that had curative gastrectomy.[118] Some of the patients had benign conditions associated with elevated CEA (see below), while in other patients the levels of CEA and CA19-9 spontaneously decreased 1–2 months after the operation. These false-positive elevations are less common with curative CRC resections, enhancing their value for monitoring of recurrence in these tumors, compared to GC.[100]

It is important to distinguish biological false positives, which represent true elevations of CEA not resulting from a neoplastic condition, from analytical false-positive results, which are caused by instrument malfunction or interferences with the assay and were discussed above. CEA elevations in benign diseases rarely exceed 10 ng/mL. In the following list of CEA biologic false-positives, numbers indicate approximate frequency of CEA elevations:

- Benign GI diseases
  - Rectal polyps (5%)
  - Inflammatory bowel diseases (15–90% depending on activity)
  - Diverticulitis (20%)
  - Gastric ulcer (15%)
  - Atrophic gastritis (25%)
  - Pancreatitis (20–50%)
- Various renal and hepatic diseases may affect CEA levels, as these organs are involved in its metabolism and elimination
  - Acute hepatitis (50–85%)
  - Chronic Hepatitis (20–30%)
  - Cirrhosis (15–80%)
  - Alcoholic liver disease (50–90%)
  - Biliary obstruction (50%)
  - Chronic renal failure (40%)
- Benign lung diseases
  - Pulmonary emphysema (15–30%)
  - Chronic bronchitis (15–70% depending on activity)
  - Cystic fibrosis (50%)
  - Pneumonia (45%)
  - Tuberculosis (35%)
  - Sarcoidosis[119]
  - Eosinophilic bronchiolitis[120]

- Benign fibrocystic breast disease (15%)
- Hypothyroidism following chemoradiation therapy involving the thyroid—CEA decreased after thyroxine supplementation[121]
- Circulating immune complexes with CEA can falsely elevate the CEA levels because of the reduction in clearance
- Anecdotally, high levels of CEA can persist post-curative resection of colon cancer for several years without any evidence of tumor development or any of the causes above[122]

Importantly, mild elevations of CEA can be seen in healthy individuals, correlating with smoking and advanced age. In a study of 276 healthy volunteers, smokers had higher mean levels of CEA (2.7 vs 1.9 ng/mL) and nearly 5% of the smokers had levels >5 ng/mL, although the CEA levels declined to nonsmoker range within 3 months of smoking cessation.[123] In both groups, CEA levels increased with age.

False-Negative CEA Results

About 50% of the patients with CRC have normal levels of CEA, particularly patients with localized disease and poorly differentiated tumors. Among patients with truly elevated CEA, there are some conditions that may result in falsely decreased CEA levels, including hemodilution, such as parenteral nutrition and blood transfusion, and the presence of CEA containing immune complexes in the plasma.[124] Analytic interferences by anti-mouse antibodies can cause either false increases or decreases in CEA levels.

Other Glycoprotein Markers

The CA series of antigens are carbohydrate moieties of glycoproteins with complex patterns of glycosylation, recognized by specific antibodies (Table 15.4). The most commonly used marker for monitoring of GI tumors is CA19-9, although CA 72-4 has shown some promising characteristics. In general, sensitivities above 50% were observed only for advanced and metastatic GI cancers.

CA 19-9

This antigen is related to the Lewis^a red blood cell antigen, structurally a sialylated Lewis^a lacto-fucopenteose II ganglioside, and was discovered in 1981 by Koprowski et al., in patients with gastric, colon, and pancreatic cancer.[125] Since it requires the Lewis gene product, 1,4-fucosyl-transferase, it is absent in Le^{a-b-} individuals, which comprise approximately 5% of the general population, and therefore cannot be used as a tumor marker in this population. The main application of CA19-9 measurement is for detection of recurrences of pancreatic cancer, since it is elevated in about 80% of patients with pancreatic adenocarcinoma. Patients with locally advanced or metastatic pancreatic cancer receiving active therapy should be monitored every 1–3 months as recommended by ASCO.[126] CA19-9 is also elevated in a variety of other tumors, including hepatobiliary, gastric, colorectal, breast, endometrial, and salivary carcinomas, and in a variety of benign conditions that include lung, renal, and liver disease, and up to 20% of patients with pancreatitis. In one report, persistent elevation of CA19-9 ranging from 112 to 1,338 IU/ml was observed in patients followed for up to 7 years without biliary or pancreatic tumors but with pulmonary fibrosis, diabetes, non-ulcer dyspepsia, obesity, acute diarrhea, colon diverticula, or gastric ulcer.[127]

Colorectal Cancer

While only present in a minority of patients with resectable CRC (around 20%), CA19-9 elevation is an independent predictor of adverse prognosis in CRC and may complement CEA for that purpose.[128,129] A study in Japan concluded that computed tomography (CT), CA19-9, and CEA were the first abnormal test in 73, 25, and 22% of recurrences of resected CRC, respectively.[130] While imaging was superior to the serum markers, CA19-9 was able to detect recurrence earlier than CT in 27% of the patients. In patients with liver metastases of CRC, elevated CA19-9 (but not CEA) is a good predictor of extrahepatic metastases.[131]

Gastric Cancer

Similarly to CRC, the positivity rate for CA19-9 is low in GC (around 18%), but the sensitivity for detection of recurrences in CA19-9-positive tumors is 60%, with a specificity of 93% at a cutoff of 100 U/ml.[101] A multicenter, prospective study in Japan of 321 patients with resected GC showed that the combination of CEA and CA19-9 had a sensitivity of 85% for detection of tumor recurrence, compared to 66% for CEA alone.[132] Even in patients with preoperative-elevated CEA and/or CA19-9 (45%), the levels increased again at recurrence. CA19-9 correlated well with lymph node metastasis, clinical stage, vascular invasion, and tumor size but not with survival in a study of 75 resectable, non-metastatic GC patients, suggesting that recurrence after surgical removal of non-metastatic GC is not predictable from preoperative CA19-9 levels.[108] Another study in 166 patients showed that preoperative CA19-9 correlated with clinical stage and was an independent prognostic factor in resected GC.[99] CA19-9 has moderate sensitivity (38%) to detect peritoneal metastasis of GC,[133] and appears more sensitive than CEA for that purpose, while CEA is more sensitive to detect liver metastasis.[134] In another study, elevated CA19-9 had an odds ratio of 4.4–4.5 to predict liver and lymph node metastasis in GC.[135]

Table 15.4 Glycoprotein tumor markers

	Chemical structure	Breast	Ovary	Lung	Prostate	Hepato-biliary	Pancreas	Colon	Stomach	Esophagus	Other cancers
CA 15–3	MUC-1 (Epsialin)	6–83[a]	64	71		28	80	63			
CA 27.29	MUC-1 (Epsialin)	6–86[a]									
CA 549	MUC-1 (Epsialin)	11–83[a]	50	33	40						
CA 125	Mucin MUC16	30[a]	80–90	5–25			50–60	35	40[a]		Endometrial/ cervix
MCA (B12)	Mucin-like	25–90	Few		Few						Endometrial/ cervix
DU-PAN-2	Positive in Le^{a-b-}		Few	Few		44	48–72		Few		
CA 195	Sialylated $Le^{a}+Le^{a}$		Few				76–82	71	Few		
CA 19-9	Sialylated Le^{xa}	15				30–67	70–100	18–65	13–47	30	Endometrial
CA 242	Sialylated Le^{a}-like			30–65			57–82	33–85	44		
CA 50	Sialylated Le^{a}+afucosyl sialylated Le^{a}	Few	Few	Few	Few	14–78/58–70	80–97	24–67	41–78	41–71	Renal, bladder
CA 72-4	Sialylated Tn	Few	24	36			70	25–43	40–84	50	

Numbers indicate percentage of tumors with elevation in the specific marker. Adapted from[174]
[a]in metastatic disease

As with CEA, early surges in the levels of CA19-9 in GC patients treated with chemotherapy should not be interpreted as treatment failures.[102]

CA 72-4

The CA72-4 glycoprotein is a mucin-like molecule with a molecular mass of over 1,000 kDa carrying the sialylated Tn blood group antigen.[136] It appears more specific and less sensitive than CEA for GI malignancies, with sensitivities of 56%, 32%, and 18% for CRC, GC, and EC, respectively, in one study[137] and specificities of more than 95%.[138] Addition of CA72-4 to CEA significantly increased the detection of CRC[139] but not of CRC recurrences.[140] A recent study using a time-resolved immunofluorometric assay showed a sensitivity of 84% with a specificity of 99% of CA72-4 for newly diagnosed GC.[141] Another study showed sensitivity of 48% for GC, which increased to 61% when combined with CEA and CA19-9.[142] While preoperative CA72-4 was elevated in only 20% of GC, post-gastrectomy recurrences showed elevations in 51% of the cases with a specificity of 97%.[143] CA72-4 is elevated in about 1–7% of benign GI conditions. While the low sensitivity of CA72-4 precludes its use as the sole marker for detection of GI cancers, its high specificity allows its addition in combination with other markers and may provide an useful target for molecular imaging and directed chemotherapy.[144]

CA 125

The CA125 antigen is present in mucin 16 (MUC16), a cell-surface associated single-pass type I membrane protein that can be cleaved and secreted into the extracellular space following phosphorylation of its intracellular domain. The main use of CA125 is to monitor epithelial ovarian cancer, but there are a few studies showing limited utility in GI cancers. For example, elevations of CA125 have a sensitivity of 39% and specificity of 98% to detect peritoneal metastasis of GC.[133] In another study, all GC patients with CA125 >35 U/ml had peritoneal metastasis compared to only 23% of patients with CA125 <35 U/ml.[145] The main problem with this assay is its lack of specificity, as up to 64% of patients with liver cirrhosis, and 20–40% of patients with other GI and liver diseases have elevated CA125.

CA 242

This antigen is similar to CA19-9 but consists of a different sialylated Le^a epitope. Following radical gastrectomy for GC, CA242 may be more sensitive to detect lung metastases, while CA19-9 is a better predictor of peritoneal metastasis, and CEA appears more sensitive for liver metastases.[134] It has a slightly better AUC than CA19-9 as an adverse prognosis factor in CRC, with a 5 year recurrence rate of 77% for CA 242-positive cases vs. 44% for CA 242-negative.[129] Use of CA 242 in combination with CEA increased the overall sensitivity for metastases, e.g., from 84% with CEA alone to 88% with the combination of CEA and CA 242.[146] CA 242 is elevated in 5–33% of benign GI conditions.

CA50

This antigen is also recognized by the CA19-9 antibody and is composed of sialylated Le^a and the afucosyl form of sialylated Le^a. It can be elevated in a variety of tumors, including pancreas, CRC and GC, but it is also elevated in 12–46% of benign diseases involving pancreas, liver, or biliary tract, limiting its usefulness as a tumor marker.

Promising Markers for Colon Cancer

A meta-analysis of CRC biomarkers published in 2007 reported 52 serum protein markers with overall sensitivity ranging from 18% to 65%,[65] many listed in Table 15.5 together with other potential biomarkers for which sensitivity and specificity data were available. No single marker is clearly superior for detection of CRC, and further study of new markers and possible marker combinations are necessary to achieve sensitive biochemical detection of CRC. For example, combining CEA measurement with detection of six autoantibodies achieved 92% sensitivity and 96% specificity for CRC detection.[147]

As an illustration of the slow progress in CRC biomarker development, the DR-70® (FDP) test (AMDL Diagnostics, Tustin, CA) is the first assay cleared by the FDA for monitoring CRC since the approval of CEA in 1982. Sensitivity and specificity are comparable to CEA, but this can be a useful assay in patients with CRC and low levels of CEA.[148]

Promising Markers in Gastric and Esophageal Cancer

Gastric and esophageal carcinomas have also been the subject of several studies examining potential biomarkers, a few examples of which are listed in Table 15.6. The standard biomarker for monitoring esophageal squamous cell carcinomas is the squamous cell antigen (SCA), which is elevated in a variety of squamous cell carcinomas, including those affecting the esophageal mucosa. It can be elevated in about 40–50% of the patients with squamous cell carcinoma of the

Table 15.5 Promising biomarkers associated with colorectal cancer

Marker	Sensitivity	Specificity	Pubmed 2009–2011	Reference
CA 19-9	18–65	80–100	68	65a
VEGF	36–91	61–100	66	65a 175
Antitumor antigen panel	61	90	23	158,176
TIMP-1	55	95	10	177,178
u-PA	76	80–96	8	179
sCD26	80–100	72–90	7	180,181
α-Defensins 1-3	69	100	7	182,183
M2-PK	56–85	76–90	6	184,185
OPN	30–65	56–85	5	186
CA 72-4	25–43	95–98	4	65a
CA 242	33–55	89–96	4	65a
TPA-M	70	96	4	187
SLEX	25	96	3	188
TATI	74	34	3	189
Laminin	89	88	3	190
Nicotinamide *N*-Methyltransferase	51	95	3	191
Anti-CEA	79	90	3	192
GM-CSF	80	70	3	193
Fibrin degradation DR-7	65–80	67–93	3	148,194
CCSA-2	78	97	3	195
sP-selectin	21	94–99	2	196
Prolactin	77	98	2	197
α-Defensin 6 (DEFA6)	69	83	2	198
Cystatin SN	28	95	2	199
Migration inhibitory factor	47	91	2	200
SIMA	36	90–95	1	201
SIMA-I	27	89	1	202
SIMA-II	19	89	1	202
Anti-p53	15–28	100	1	65a
IL-3	55	80	1	203
Progesterone	57–64	37–40	1	204
Dermokine βγ	29–36	92	1	205
Seprase	42	95	1	151
Desmin	55	80	1	156
Anti-DDX-48	10	100	0	206
Anti-Fas	33	100	0	207
Anti-NCC-ST 439	27	94	0	208
BSP	88–96	100	0	186
CA 195	71	71–100	0	209
CA 50	24–67	51–99	0	65a
CA M26	22	99	0	210
CA M29	12	99	0	210
CA M43	42–74	92–99	0	211,212
Cancer Procoagulant	86	82	0	213
CO 29.11	41	95–97	0	214
Free PSA (women)	35	93	0	215
GST enzymes	89	77–85	0	216
NCA50-90	35	95	0	217
PA 8-15	45	87–95	0	218
SCF	89	17	0	203
Tenascin	25	95	0	219

(continued)

Table 15.5 (continued)

Marker	Sensitivity	Specificity	Pubmed 2009–2011	Reference
Villin	51	87–97	0	220
α-L-fucosidase	69	85	0	221

"Pubmed" refers to the number of articles published between 2009 and 2011 referring the specific marker
[a]Data from Hundt et al.[65]

Table 15.6 Examples of promising biomarkers for detection of gastric (GC) and esophageal (EC) carcinomas

Marker	Outcome	Sensitivity	Specificity	References
CA72-4+M2-PK	EC Detection	74	95	222
MMP-9	EC Detection	70	60	223
sVEGF-C	EC Detection	60	78	224
anti-CDC25B	EC Detection	57	91	225
MMP-9 (serum)	GC Detection	83	66	226
TIMP-1	GC Detection	17–89	97	227,228
MG7	GC Detection	84	87	229
MIF	GC Detection	84	92	230
M2-pyruvate kinase	GC Detection	62	89	231
IL18	GC Detection	52	83	232
MUC1/5 AC alternative glycosylation	GC Detection	25–42	90	233
IPO-38	GC Detection	57	90	234
Pepsinogen I/II+hsCRP	GC Detection—Early	74	70	235
ITIH3	GC Detection—Early	96	66	236
IL6	GC Detection—Advanced	82	67	237
IL6	GC Lymph node metastasis	87	58	237
Reg4+Olfactomedin 4	GC Detection (Stage 1–4)	52–88	95	238
Soluble E-cadherin	GC Detection -Recurrence	47–59	75–81	239

esophagus and is associated with worse prognosis.[149,150] It is also elevated in a variety of benign diseases of the skin (such as psoriasis, pemphigus, and eczema), lungs (tuberculosis, sarcoidosis, and pleural effusions), and other tissues with squamous epithelia, limiting its use for diagnostic purposes.

Proteomic Approaches to GI Tumor Markers

It is evident that single markers are of insufficient diagnostic accuracy to screen for GI tumors, especially at early stages. Combinatorial approaches using several protein markers, which can be labeled as low-multiplex proteomics, have been shown to improve sensitivity and specificity for tumor detection.[151] For example, a protein chip using 12 markers (CEA, alpha-fetoprotein, CA 19-9, CA 242, CA 15-3, CA 125, prostate specific antigen, free-PSA, neuron-specific enolase, human chorionic gonadotropin-beta, human growth hormone, and ferritin) detected GC with sensitivities varying from 37% in stage I to 50% in stage IV tumors.[152] More comprehensive, unbiased proteomic approaches aim at identifying additional biomarkers differentially expressed by tumors. However, the approach using comprehensive proteomics has been somewhat disappointing. Most of the studies with serum proteomics identified peptides derived from secondary alterations in abundant serum proteins induced by tumor-associated proteases. These approaches are unlikely to result in useful markers because of the lack of specificity. For example, surface-enhanced laser desorption/ionization (SELDI) based proteomics identified peptides derived from complement C3a des-Arg, alpha1-antitrypsin, and transferrin, all nonspecific to colon cancer, as having diagnostic potential.[153] Another SELDI study in gastric cancer identified five peaks that predicted survival with 84% sensitivity and 85% specificity, but the nature of the peptides was not further specified.[154] A separate study using four unidentified peaks revealed a sensitivity of 93% and specificity of 90% for detection of GC.[155] Despite these promising results, good reproducibility of these findings has not yet been achieved.

In contrast to serum proteomics, differential proteomic analysis of tumor vs. non-tumor tissue samples can reveal tumor-associated proteins of potential diagnostic use. An example is the identification of desmin and ZF protein 829 by 2D gel comparison of normal tissue and CRC.[156]

Unfortunately, the delivery of tumor proteins to the plasma is affected by many factors, including tumor vascularization, degree of inflammation, necrosis, and fibrotic response. The study of tumor-associated membrane-expressed proteins may obviate some of these limitations and identify biomarkers more likely to be released in circulation. For example, differential labeling of membranes from CRC versus normal mucosa, using the iTraq procedure, identified CEA, CEACAM6, claudin-1, HLA class I histocompatibility antigen A-1, tapasin, and mitochondrial solute carrier family 25A4 as differentially expressed in CRC.[157]

An alternative approach to identify diagnostically useful markers is the detection of autoantibodies against tumor-enriched/modified proteins. For example, Liu et al. used enzyme-linked immunosorbent assay (ELISA) to identify antibodies against Imp1, p62, Koc, p53, and c-myc full-length recombinant proteins in CRC, achieving a combined sensitivity of 61% and a specificity of 90%.[158] Adding CEA to the panel increased the sensitivity to 83%. A proteomic approach using 2D-gel electrophoresis followed by immunoblotting with sera from GC patients resulted in the identification of GRP78 as a target for autoantibodies in 28% of GC patients versus 0/20 controls.[159] A recent study used a high density protein array containing 37,830 clones expressing recombinant proteins to identify patterns of autoantibodies that distinguished symptomatic from asymptomatic CRC patients.[160]

Conclusions

Serum protein biomarkers offer the potential to diagnose and monitor GI tumors with simple, quantitative, easily automated, and inexpensive assays. Unfortunately, the diagnostic accuracy of current and most prospective markers is insufficient to recommend their use in isolation for tumor detection, especially in the general population. In contrast, the role of serum protein markers in monitoring the response to treatment is well accepted, particularly for CEA and CRC. The list of newer, potential markers is large and likely to expand at an increasing rate, especially in consequence of large-scale "omic" approaches. While comprehensive proteomic approaches are unlikely to be used in the near future, combinatorial panels of selected markers offering increased sensitivity and specificity are expected to replace single biomarkers in the evaluation of patients with GI tumors.

References

1. Bonfrer JM. Working Group on Tumor Marker Criteria (WGTMC). *Tumour Biol.* 1990;11(5):287–288.
2. Gold P, Freedman SO. Demonstration of tumor-specific antigens in human colonic carcinomata by immunological tolerance and absorption techniques. *J Exp Med.* 1965;121:439–462.
3. Zebhauser R, Kammerer R, Eisenried A, McLellan A, Moore T, Zimmermann W. Identification of a novel group of evolutionarily conserved members within the rapidly diverging murine Cea family. *Genomics.* 2005;86(5):566–580.
4. Hammarstrom S. The carcinoembryonic antigen (CEA) family: structures, suggested functions and expression in normal and malignant tissues. *Semin Cancer Biol.* 1999;9(2):67–81.
5. Naghibalhossaini F, Ebadi P. Evidence for CEA release from human colon cancer cells by an endogenous GPI-PLD enzyme. *Cancer Lett.* 2006;234(2):158–167.
6. Pakdel A, Naghibalhossaini F, Mokarram P, Jaberipour M, Hosseini A. Regulation of carcinoembryonic antigen release from colorectal cancer cells. *Mol Biol Rep.* 2012;39:3695–3704.
7. Bjerner J, Lebedin Y, Bellanger L, et al. Protein epitopes in carcinoembryonic antigen. Report of the ISOBM TD8 workshop. *Tumour Biol.* 2002;23(4):249–262.
8. Huang JQ, Turbide C, Daniels E, Jothy S, Beauchemin N. Spatiotemporal expression of murine carcinoembryonic antigen (CEA) gene family members during mouse embryogenesis. *Development.* 1990;110(2):573–588.
9. Zimmermann W, Ortlieb B, Friedrich R, von Kleist S. Isolation and characterization of cDNA clones encoding the human carcinoembryonic antigen reveal a highly conserved repeating structure. *Proc Natl Acad Sci USA.* 1987;84(9):2960–2964.
10. Sanders DS, Wilson CA, Bryant FJ, et al. Classification and localisation of carcinoembryonic antigen (CEA) related antigen expression in normal oesophageal squamous mucosa and squamous carcinoma. *Gut.* 1994;35(8):1022–1025.
11. Sanders DS, Stocks SC, Milne DM, Milne GA, Hopwood D, Kerr MA. Membranous expression of carcinoembryonic antigen (CEA) in the normal cervical squamous mucosa. *J Pathol.* 1992;167(1):77–82.
12. Savino W, Durand D, Dardenne M. Immunohistochemical evidence for the expression of the carcinoembryonic antigen by human thymic epithelial cells in vitro and in neoplastic conditions. *Am J Pathol.* 1985;121(3):418–425.
13. Nouwen EJ, Pollet DE, Eerdekens MW, Hendrix PG, Briers TW, De Broe ME. Immunohistochemical localization of placental alkaline phosphatase, carcinoembryonic antigen, and cancer antigen 125 in normal and neoplastic human lung. *Cancer Res.* 1986;46(2):866–876.
14. Metze D, Luger TA. Ultrastructural localization of carcinoembryonic antigen (CEA) glycoproteins and epithelial membrane antigen (EMA) in normal and neoplastic sweat glands. *J Cutan Pathol.* 1996;23(6):518–529.
15. Nyati MK, Sreekumar A, Li S, et al. High and selective expression of yeast cytosine deaminase under a carcinoembryonic antigen promoter-enhancer. *Cancer Res.* 2002;62(8):2337–2342.
16. Zhang G, Liu T, Chen YH, et al. Tissue specific cytotoxicity of colon cancer cells mediated by nanoparticle-delivered suicide gene in vitro and in vivo. *Clin Cancer Res.* 2009;15(1):201–207.
17. Dabrowska A, Szary J, Kowalczuk M, Szala S, Ugorski M. CEA-negative glioblastoma and melanoma cells are sensitive to cytosine deaminase/5-fluorocytosine therapy directed by the carcinoembryonic antigen promoter. *Acta Biochim Pol.* 2004; 51(3):723–732.
18. Han SU, Kwak TH, Her KH, et al. CEACAM5 and CEACAM6 are major target genes for Smad3-mediated TGF-beta signaling. *Oncogene.* 2008;27(5):675–683.
19. Thomas SN, Zhu F, Schnaar RL, Alves CS, Konstantopoulos K. Carcinoembryonic antigen and CD44 variant isoforms cooperate to mediate colon carcinoma cell adhesion to E- and L-selectin in shear flow. *J Biol Chem.* 2008;283(23):15647–15655.
20. Baranov V, Hammarstrom S. Carcinoembryonic antigen (CEA) and CEA-related cell adhesion molecule 1 (CEACAM1), apically expressed on human colonic M cells, are potential receptors for microbial adhesion. *Histochem Cell Biol.* 2004;121(2):83–89.

21. Screaton RA, Penn LZ, Stanners CP. Carcinoembryonic antigen, a human tumor marker, cooperates with Myc and Bcl-2 in cellular transformation. *J Cell Biol.* 1997;137(4):939–952.
22. Naghibalhossaini F, Yoder AD, Tobi M, Stanners CP. Evolution of a tumorigenic property conferred by glycophosphatidyl-inositol membrane anchors of carcinoembryonic antigen gene family members during the primate radiation. *Mol Biol Cell.* 2007; 18(4):1366–1374.
23. Ilantzis C, DeMarte L, Screaton RA, Stanners CP. Deregulated expression of the human tumor marker CEA and CEA family member CEACAM6 disrupts tissue architecture and blocks colonocyte differentiation. *Neoplasia.* 2002;4(2):151–163.
24. Baranov V, Yeung MM, Hammarstrom S. Expression of carcinoembryonic antigen and nonspecific cross-reacting 50-kDa antigen in human normal and cancerous colon mucosa: comparative ultrastructural study with monoclonal antibodies. *Cancer Res.* 1994;54(12):3305–3314.
25. Leusch HG, Drzeniek Z, Markos-Pusztai Z, Wagener C. Binding of Escherichia coli and Salmonella strains to members of the carcinoembryonic antigen family: differential binding inhibition by aromatic alpha-glycosides of mannose. *Infect Immun.* 1991;59(6):2051–2057.
26. Allez M, Brimnes J, Shao L, Dotan I, Nakazawa A, Mayer L. Activation of a unique population of CD8(+) T cells by intestinal epithelial cells. *Ann N Y Acad Sci.* 2004;1029:22–35.
27. Prado IB, Laudanna AA, Carneiro CR. Susceptibility of colorectal-carcinoma cells to natural-killer-mediated lysis: relationship to CEA expression and degree of differentiation. *Int J Cancer.* 1995;61(6):854–860.
28. Kammerer R, von Kleist S. CEA expression of colorectal adenocarcinomas is correlated with their resistance against LAK-cell lysis. *Int J Cancer.* 1994;57(3):341–347.
29. Kammerer R, Zimmermann W. Coevolution of activating and inhibitory receptors within mammalian carcinoembryonic antigen families. *BMC Biol.* 2010;8:12.
30. Hostetter RB, Augustus LB, Mankarious R, et al. Carcinoembryonic antigen as a selective enhancer of colorectal cancer metastasis. *J Natl Cancer Inst.* 1990;82(5):380–385.
31. Jessup JM, Thomas P. Carcinoembryonic antigen: function in metastasis by human colorectal carcinoma. *Cancer Metastasis Rev.* 1989;8(3):263–280.
32. Chan CH, Camacho-Leal P, Stanners CP. Colorectal hyperplasia and dysplasia due to human carcinoembryonic antigen (CEA) family member expression in transgenic mice. *PLoS One.* 2007;2(12):e1353.
33. Leung N, Turbide C, Olson M, Marcus V, Jothy S, Beauchemin N. Deletion of the carcinoembryonic antigen-related cell adhesion molecule 1 (Ceacam1) gene contributes to colon tumor progression in a murine model of carcinogenesis. *Oncogene.* 2006;25(40):5527–5536.
34. Leung N, Turbide C, Balachandra B, Marcus V, Beauchemin N. Intestinal tumor progression is promoted by decreased apoptosis and dysregulated Wnt signaling in Ceacam1−/− mice. *Oncogene.* 2008;27(36):4943–4953.
35. Song JH, Cao Z, Yoon JH, et al. Genetic alterations and expression pattern of CEACAM1 in colorectal adenomas and cancers. *Pathol Oncol Res.* 2011;17:67–74.
36. Jessup JM, Samara R, Battle P, Laguinge LM. Carcinoembryonic antigen promotes tumor cell survival in liver through an IL-10-dependent pathway. *Clin Exp Metastasis.* 2004;21(8):709–717.
37. Minami S, Furui J, Kanematsu T. Role of carcinoembryonic antigen in the progression of colon cancer cells that express carbohydrate antigen. *Cancer Res.* 2001;61(6):2732–2735.
38. Gangopadhyay A, Lazure DA, Thomas P. Adhesion of colorectal carcinoma cells to the endothelium is mediated by cytokines from CEA stimulated Kupffer cells. *Clin Exp Metastasis.* 1998; 16(8):703–712.
39. Samara RN, Laguinge LM, Jessup JM. Carcinoembryonic antigen inhibits Anoikis in colorectal carcinoma cells by interfering with trail-R2 (DR5) signaling. *Cancer Res.* 2007;67(10):4774–4782.
40. Camacho-Leal P, Zhai AB, Stanners CP. A co-clustering model involving alpha5beta1 integrin for the biological effects of GPI-anchored human carcinoembryonic antigen (CEA). *J Cell Physiol.* 2007;211(3):791–802.
41. Ordonez C, Zhai AB, Camacho-Leal P, Demarte L, Fan MM, Stanners CP. GPI-anchored CEA family glycoproteins CEA and CEACAM6 mediate their biological effects through enhanced integrin alpha5beta1-fibronectin interaction. *J Cell Physiol.* 2007;210(3):757–765.
42. Camacho-Leal P, Stanners CP. The human carcinoembryonic antigen (CEA) GPI anchor mediates anoikis inhibition by inactivation of the intrinsic death pathway. *Oncogene.* 2008;27(11):1545–1553.
43. Wirth T, Soeth E, Czubayko F, Juhl H. Inhibition of endogenous carcinoembryonic antigen (CEA) increases the apoptotic rate of colon cancer cells and inhibits metastatic tumor growth. *Clin Exp Metastasis.* 2002;19(2):155–160.
44. Soeth E, Wirth T, List HJ, et al. Controlled ribozyme targeting demonstrates an antiapoptotic effect of carcinoembryonic antigen in HT29 colon cancer cells. *Clin Cancer Res.* 2001;7(7):2022–2030.
45. Sharkey RM, Karacay H, Vallabhajosula S, et al. Metastatic human colonic carcinoma: molecular imaging with pretargeted SPECT and PET in a mouse model. *Radiology.* 2008;246(2):497–507.
46. Aarts F, Boerman OC, Sharkey RM, et al. Pretargeted radioimmunoscintigraphy in patients with primary colorectal cancer using a bispecific anticarcinoembryonic antigen CEA X anti-di-diethylenetriaminepentaacetic acid F(ab')2 antibody. *Cancer.* 2010;116(4 Suppl):1111–1117.
47. Kaushal S, McElroy MK, Luiken GA, et al. Fluorophore-conjugated anti-CEA antibody for the intraoperative imaging of pancreatic and colorectal cancer. *J Gastrointest Surg.* 2008; 12(11):1938–1950.
48. Hong H, Sun J, Cai W. Radionuclide-based cancer imaging targeting the carcinoembryonic antigen. *Biomark Insights.* 2008;3:435–451.
49. Park S, Lee B, Kim I, et al. Immunobead RT-PCR versus regular RT-PCR amplification of CEA mRNA in peripheral blood. *J Cancer Res Clin Oncol.* 2001;127(8):489–494.
50. Douard R, Moutereau S, Serru V, et al. Immunobead multiplex RT-PCR detection of carcinoembryonic genes expressing cells in the blood of colorectal cancer patients. *Clin Chem Lab Med.* 2005;43(2):127–132.
51. Liu Z, Jin C, Yu Z, et al. Radioimmunotherapy of human colon cancer xenografts with 131I-labeled anti-CEA monoclonal antibody. *Bioconjug Chem.* 2010;21(2):314–318.
52. Liu Z, Jin C, Yu Z, et al. Radioimmunotherapy of human colon cancer xenografts with 131I-labeled anti-CEA monoclonal antibody. *Bioconjug Chem.* 2010;21(2):314–318.
53. Buchegger F, Roth A, Allal A, et al. Radioimmunotherapy of colorectal cancer liver metastases: combination with radiotherapy. *Ann N Y Acad Sci.* 2000;910:263–269. discussion 9–70.
54. Mori F, Giannetti P, Peruzzi D, et al. A therapeutic cancer vaccine targeting carcinoembryonic antigen in intestinal carcinomas. *Hum Gene Ther.* 2009;20(2):125–136.
55. Ojima T, Iwahashi M, Nakamura M, et al. Successful cancer vaccine therapy for carcinoembryonic antigen (CEA)-expressing colon cancer using genetically modified dendritic cells that express CEA and T helper-type 1 cytokines in CEA transgenic mice. *Int J Cancer.* 2007;120(3):585–593.
56. Shibaguchi H, Luo NX, Kuroki M, et al. A fully human chimeric immune receptor for retargeting T-cells to CEA-expressing tumor cells. *Anticancer Res.* 2006;26(6A):4067–4072.
57. Hou Y, Kavanagh B, Fong L. Distinct CD8+ T cell repertoires primed with agonist and native peptides derived from a tumor-associated antigen. *J Immunol.* 2008;180(3):1526–1534.

58. Li HJ, Everts M, Pereboeva L, et al. Adenovirus tumor targeting and hepatic untargeting by a coxsackie/adenovirus receptor ectodomain anti-carcinoembryonic antigen bispecific adapter. *Cancer Res*. 2007;67(11):5354–5361.
59. Bos R, van Duikeren S, Morreau H, et al. Balancing between antitumor efficacy and autoimmune pathology in T-cell-mediated targeting of carcinoembryonic antigen. *Cancer Res*. 2008;68(20):8446–8455.
60. Jung HS, Lee SW. Ribozyme-mediated selective killing of cancer cells expressing carcinoembryonic antigen RNA by targeted trans-splicing. *Biochem Biophys Res Commun*. 2006;349(2):556–563.
61. Zamboni S, Mallano A, Flego M, et al. Genetic construction, expression, and characterization of a single chain anti-CEA antibody fused to cytosine deaminase from yeast. *Int J Oncol*. 2008;32(6):1245–1251.
62. Guadagni F, Roselli M, Cosimelli M, et al. Quantitative analysis of CEA expression in colorectal adenocarcinoma and serum: lack of correlation. *Int J Cancer*. 1997;72(6):949–954.
63. Thomson DMP, Krupey J, Freedman SO, Gold P. The radioimmunoassay of Circulating carcinoembryonic antigen of the human digestive system. *Proc Natl Acad Sci USA*. 1969;64(1):161–167.
64. Sato K, Tokeshi M, Kimura H, Kitamori T. Determination of carcinoembryonic antigen in human sera by integrated bead-bed immunoassay in a microchip for cancer diagnosis. *Anal Chem*. 2001;73(6):1213–1218.
65. Hundt S, Haug U, Brenner H. Blood markers for early detection of colorectal cancer: a systematic review. *Cancer Epidemiol Biomarkers Prev*. 2007;16(10):1935–1953.
66. Duffy MJ. Carcinoembryonic antigen as a marker for colorectal cancer: is it clinically useful? *Clin Chem*. 2001;47(4):624–630.
67. Sturgeon CM, Duffy MJ, Stenman UH, et al. National Academy of Clinical Biochemistry laboratory medicine practice guidelines for use of tumor markers in testicular, prostate, colorectal, breast, and ovarian cancers. *Clin Chem*. 2008;54(12):e11-e79.
68. Lim YK, Kam MH, Eu KW. Carcinoembryonic antigen screening: how far should we go? *Singapore Med J*. 2009;50(9):862–865.
69. Compton CC, Fielding LP, Burgart LJ, et al. Prognostic factors in colorectal cancer. College of American Pathologists Consensus Statement 1999. *Arch Pathol Lab Med*. 2000;124(7):979–994.
70. Compton C, Fenoglio-Preiser CM, Pettigrew N, Fielding LP. American Joint Committee on Cancer Prognostic Factors Consensus Conference: Colorectal Working Group. *Cancer*. 2000;88(7):1739–1757.
71. Huh JW, Oh BR, Kim HR, Kim YJ. Preoperative carcinoembryonic antigen level as an independent prognostic factor in potentially curative colon cancer. *J Surg Oncol*. 2010;101(5):396–400.
72. Ogata Y, Murakami H, Sasatomi T, et al. Elevated preoperative serum carcinoembrionic antigen level may be an effective indicator for needing adjuvant chemotherapy after potentially curative resection of stage II colon cancer. *J Surg Oncol*. 2009;99(1):65–70.
73. Kievit J. Follow-up of patients with colorectal cancer: numbers needed to test and treat. *Eur J Cancer*. 2002;38(7):986–999.
74. Tan E, Gouvas N, Nicholls RJ, Ziprin P, Xynos E, Tekkis PP. Diagnostic precision of carcinoembryonic antigen in the detection of recurrence of colorectal cancer. *Surg Oncol*. 2009;18(1):15–24.
75. Bruinvels DJ, Stiggelbout AM, Kievit J, van Houwelingen HC, Habbema JD, van de Velde CJ. Follow-up of patients with colorectal cancer. A meta-analysis. *Ann Surg*. 1994;219(2):174–182.
76. Figueredo A, Rumble RB, Maroun J, et al. Follow-up of patients with curatively resected colorectal cancer: a practice guideline. *BMC Cancer*. 2003;3:26.
77. Hida J, Yasutomi M, Shindoh K, et al. Second-look operation for recurrent colorectal cancer based on carcinoembryonic antigen and imaging techniques. *Dis Colon Rectum*. 1996;39(1):74–79.
78. Weiser MR, Landmann RG, Kattan MW, et al. Individualized prediction of colon cancer recurrence using a nomogram. *J Clin Oncol*. 2008;26(3):380–385.
79. Kattan MW, Gonen M, Jarnagin WR, et al. A nomogram for predicting disease-specific survival after hepatic resection for metastatic colorectal cancer. *Ann Surg*. 2008;247(2):282–287.
80. Li M, Li JY, Zhao AL, Gu J. Colorectal cancer or colon and rectal cancer? Clinicopathological comparison between colonic and rectal carcinomas. *Oncology*. 2007;73(1–2):52–57.
81. Chen CH, Hsieh MC, Lai CC, et al. Lead time of carcinoembryonic antigen elevation in the postoperative follow-up of colorectal cancer did not affect the survival rate after recurrence. *Int J Colorectal Dis*. 2010;25(5):567–571.
82. Sargent D, Sobrero A, Grothey A, et al. Evidence for cure by adjuvant therapy in colon cancer: observations based on individual patient data from 20,898 patients on 18 randomized trials. *J Clin Oncol*. 2009;27(6):872–877.
83. Chao M, Gibbs P. Caution is required before recommending routine carcinoembryonic antigen and imaging follow-up for patients with early-stage colon cancer. *J Clin Oncol*. 2009;27(36):e279-e280. author reply e81.
84. Quah HM, Chou JF, Gonen M, et al. Identification of patients with high-risk stage II colon cancer for adjuvant therapy. *Dis Colon Rectum*. 2008;51(5):503–507.
85. Chau I, Allen MJ, Cunningham D, et al. The value of routine serum carcino-embryonic antigen measurement and computed tomography in the surveillance of patients after adjuvant chemotherapy for colorectal cancer. *J Clin Oncol*. 2004;22(8):1420–1429.
86. NCCN Colon Cancer Panel. Colon Cancer. 2010 [updated 9/10/2010; cited 2010 9/30/2010]; Available from: http://www.nccn.org/professionals/physician_gls/PDF/colon.pdf.
87. Lin JK, Lin CC, Yang SH, et al. Early postoperative CEA level is a better prognostic indicator than is preoperative CEA level in predicting prognosis of patients with curable colorectal cancer. *Int J Colorectal Dis*. 2011;26:1135–1141.
88. Lee WS, Baek JH, Kim KK, Park YH. The prognostic significant of percentage drop in serum CEA post curative resection for colon cancer. *Surg Oncol*. 2012;21:45–51.
89. Cooper GS, Kou TD, Reynolds HL Jr. Receipt of guideline-recommended follow-up in older colorectal cancer survivors: a population-based analysis. *Cancer*. 2008;113(8):2029–2037.
90. Iwanicki-Caron I, Di Fiore F, Roque I, et al. Usefulness of the serum carcinoembryonic antigen kinetic for chemotherapy monitoring in patients with unresectable metastasis of colorectal cancer. *J Clin Oncol*. 2008;26(22):3681–3686.
91. Ailawadhi S, Sunga A, Rajput A, Yang GY, Smith J, Fakih M. Chemotherapy-induced carcinoembryonic antigen surge in patients with metastatic colorectal cancer. *Oncology*. 2006;70(1):49–53.
92. An X, Ding PR, Xiang XJ, et al. Carcinoembryonic antigen surge in metastatic colorectal cancer patients responding to irinotecan combination chemotherapy. *Biomarkers*. 2010;15(3):243–248.
93. Sorbye H, Dahl O. Carcinoembryonic antigen surge in metastatic colorectal cancer patients responding to oxaliplatin combination chemotherapy: implications for tumor marker monitoring and guidelines. *J Clin Oncol*. 2003;21(23):4466–4467.
94. Strimpakos AS, Cunningham D, Mikropoulos C, Petkar I, Barbachano Y, Chau I. The impact of carcinoembryonic antigen flare in patients with advanced colorectal cancer receiving first-line chemotherapy. *Ann Oncol*. 2010;21(5):1013–1019.
95. Wang WS, Lin JK, Lin TC, et al. Carcinoembryonic antigen in monitoring of response to systemic chemotherapy in patients with metastatic colorectal cancer. *Int J Colorectal Dis*. 2001;16(2):96–101.
96. Park SH, Ku KB, Chung HY, Yu W. Prognostic significance of serum and tissue carcinoembryonic antigen in patients with gastric adenocarcinomas. *Cancer Res Treat*. 2008;40(1):16–21.
97. Sturgeon CM, Duffy MJ, Hofmann BR, et al. National Academy of Clinical Biochemistry Laboratory Medicine Practice Guidelines for use of tumor markers in liver, bladder, cervical, and gastric cancers. *Clin Chem*. 2010;56(6):e1-e48.

98. Horie Y, Miura K, Matsui K, et al. Marked elevation of plasma carcinoembryonic antigen and stomach carcinoma. *Cancer.* 1996;77(10):1991–1997.
99. Zhang YH, Li Y, Chen C, Peng CW. Carcinoembryonic antigen level is related to tumor invasion into the serosa of the stomach: study on 166 cases and suggestion for new therapy. *Hepatogastroenterology.* 2009;56(96):1750–1754.
100. Ohtsuka T, Nakafusa Y, Sato S, Kitajima Y, Tanaka M, Miyazaki K. Different roles of tumor marker monitoring after curative resections of gastric and colorectal cancers. *Dig Dis Sci.* 2008; 53(6):1537–1543.
101. Qiu MZ, Lin JZ, Wang ZQ, et al. Cutoff value of carcinoembryonic antigen and carbohydrate antigen 19–9 elevation levels for monitoring recurrence in patients with resectable gastric adenocarcinoma. *Int J Biol Markers.* 2009;24(4):258–264.
102. Kim HJ, Lee KW, Kim YJ, et al. Chemotherapy-induced transient CEA and CA19–9 surges in patients with metastatic or recurrent gastric cancer. *Acta Oncol.* 2009;48(3):385–390.
103. Sakamoto J, Nakazato H, Teramukai S, et al. Association between preoperative plasma CEA levels and the prognosis of gastric cancer following curative resection. Tumor Marker Committee, Japanese Foundation for Multidisciplinary Treatment of Cancer, Tokyo, Japan. *Surg Oncol.* 1996;5(3):133–139.
104. Ishigami S, Natsugoe S, Hokita S, et al. Clinical importance of preoperative carcinoembryonic antigen and carbohydrate antigen 19–9 levels in gastric cancer. *J Clin Gastroenterol.* 2001;32(1):41–44.
105. Kim DY, Kim HR, Shim JH, Park CS, Kim SK, Kim YJ. Significance of serum and tissue carcinoembryonic antigen for the prognosis of gastric carcinoma patients. *J Surg Oncol.* 2000; 74(3):185–192.
106. Jung M, Jeung HC, Lee SS, et al. The clinical significance of ascitic fluid CEA in advanced gastric cancer with ascites. *J Cancer Res Clin Oncol.* 2010;136(4):517–526.
107. Yamamoto M, Baba H, Toh Y, Okamura T, Maehara Y. Peritoneal lavage CEA/CA125 is a prognostic factor for gastric cancer patients. *J Cancer Res Clin Oncol.* 2007;133(7):471–476.
108. Dilege E, Mihmanli M, Demir U, et al. Prognostic value of preoperative CEA and CA 19–9 levels in resectable gastric cancer. *Hepatogastroenterology.* 2010;57(99–100):674–677.
109. Lukaszewicz-Zajac M, Mroczko B, Gryko M, Kedra B, Szmitkowski M. Comparison between clinical significance of serum proinflammatory proteins (IL-6 and CRP) and classic tumor markers (CEA and CA 19–9) in gastric cancer. *Clin Exp Med.* 2011;11:89–96.
110. Ucar E, Semerci E, Ustun H, Yetim T, Huzmeli C, Gullu M. Prognostic value of preoperative CEA, CA 19–9, CA 72–4, and AFP levels in gastric cancer. *Adv Ther.* 2008;25(10):1075–1084.
111. Bhatnagar J, Heroman W, Murphy M, Austin GE. Immunohistochemical detection of carcinoembryonic antigen in esophageal carcinomas: a comparison with other gastrointestinal neoplasms. *Anticancer Res.* 2002;22(3):1849–1857.
112. Clark GW, Ireland AP, Hagen JA, Collard JM, Peters JH, DeMeester TR. Carcinoembryonic antigen measurements in the management of esophageal cancer: an indicator of subclinical recurrence. *Am J Surg.* 1995;170(6):597–600. discussion –1.
113. Yi Y, Li B, Sun H, et al. Predictors of sensitivity to chemoradiotherapy of esophageal squamous cell carcinoma. *Tumour Biol.* 2010;31(4):333–340.
114. Setoyama T, Natsugoe S, Okumura H, et al. Carcinoembryonic antigen messenger RNA expression in blood predicts recurrence in esophageal cancer. *Clin Cancer Res.* 2006;12(20 Pt 1): 5972–5977.
115. Cvejic D, Savin S, Golubovic S, Paunovic I, Tatic S, Havelka M. Galectin-3 and carcinoembryonic antigen expression in medullary thyroid carcinoma: possible relation to tumour progression. *Histopathology.* 2000;37(6):530–535.
116. Gill S, Cosolo W, Herbertson RA, Berlangieri SU, Scott AM. Medullary carcinoma of the thyroid in a patient with colon cancer and a rising carcinoembryonic antigen level. *Intern Med J.* 2009;39(4):264–265.
117. Angelov A, Klissarova A, Dikranian K. Radioimmunological and immunohistochemical study of carcinoembryonic antigen in pleomorphic adenoma and mucoepidermoid carcinoma of the salivary glands. *Gen Diagn Pathol.* 1996;141(3–4):229–234.
118. Ohtsuka T, Sato S, Kitajima Y, Tanaka M, Nakafusa Y, Miyazaki K. False-positive findings for tumor markers after curative gastrectomy for gastric cancer. *Dig Dis Sci.* 2008;53(1):73–79.
119. Gallagher DJ, Libby DM, Kemeny N. Elevated carcinoembryonic antigen and sarcoidosis masquerading as metastatic colon cancer. *Clin Colorectal Cancer.* 2009;8(3):172–174.
120. Yanagitani N, Shimizu Y, Kazama T, Dobashi K, Ishizuka T, Mori M. Eosinophilic bronchiolitis indicating eosinophilic airway disease with overexpression of carcinoembryonic antigen in sinus and bronchiole: case report. *J Biol Regul Homeost Agents.* 2010;24(1):99–102.
121. Kawaguchi G, Abe E, Sasamoto R, Sasai K. Elevation of serum carcinoembryonic antigen level in a patient with hypothyroidism after radiation therapy for cervical esophageal cancer. *Int J Clin Oncol.* 2010;15(1):104–108.
122. Hsu TC. Unusual elevation of CEA in a patient with history of colon cancer. *Jpn J Clin Oncol.* 2006;36(12):811–813.
123. Alexander JC, Silverman NA, Chretien PB. Effect of age and cigarette smoking on carcinoembryonic antigen levels. *JAMA.* 1976;235(18):1975–1979.
124. Fuchs C, Krapf F, Kern P, Hoferichter S, Jager W, Kalden JR. CEA-containing immune complexes in sera of patients with colorectal and breast cancer–analysis of complexed immunoglobulin classes. *Cancer Immunol Immunother.* 1988;26(2):180–184.
125. Koprowski H, Herlyn M, Steplewski Z, Sears HF. Specific antigen in serum of patients with colon carcinoma. *Science.* 1981; 212(4490):53–55.
126. Locker GY, Hamilton S, Harris J, et al. ASCO 2006 update of recommendations for the use of tumor markers in gastrointestinal cancer. *J Clin Oncol.* 2006;24(33):5313–5327.
127. Ventrucci M, Pozzato P, Cipolla A, Uomo G. Persistent elevation of serum CA 19–9 with no evidence of malignant disease. *Dig Liver Dis.* 2009;41(5):357–363.
128. Basbug M, Arikanoglu Z, Bulbuller N, et al. Prognostic value of preoperative CEA and CA 19–9 levels in patients with colorectal cancer. *Hepatogastroenterology.* 2011;58(106):400–405.
129. Yang XQ, Chen C, Peng CW, Liu SP, Li Y. Carbohydrate antigen 242 highly consists with carbohydrate antigen 19–9 in diagnosis and prognosis of colorectal cancer: study on 185 cases. *Med Oncol.* 2012;29:1030–1036.
130. Kawamura YJ, Tokumitsu A, Mizokami K, Sasaki J, Tsujinaka S, Konishi F. First alert for recurrence during follow-up after potentially curative resection for colorectal carcinoma: CA 19–9 should be included in surveillance programs. *Clin Colorectal Cancer.* 2010;9(1):48–51.
131. Sasaki A, Kawano K, Inomata M, Shibata K, Matsumoto T, Kitano S. Value of serum carbohydrate antigen 19–9 for predicting extrahepatic metastasis in patients with liver metastasis from colorectal carcinoma. *Hepatogastroenterology.* 2005;52(66): 1814–1819.
132. Takahashi Y, Takeuchi T, Sakamoto J, et al. The usefulness of CEA and/or CA19–9 in monitoring for recurrence in gastric cancer patients: a prospective clinical study. *Gastric Cancer.* 2003;6(3):142–145.
133. Hwang GI, Yoo CH, Sohn BH, et al. Predictive value of preoperative serum CEA, CA19–9 and CA125 levels for peritoneal metastasis in patients with gastric carcinoma. *Cancer Res Treat.* 2004;36(3):178–181.

134. Choi SR, Jang JS, Lee JH, et al. Role of serum tumor markers in monitoring for recurrence of gastric cancer following radical gastrectomy. *Dig Dis Sci*. 2006;51(11):2081–2086.
135. Nakagoe T, Sawai T, Tsuji T, et al. Predictive factors for preoperative serum levels of sialy Lewis(x), sialyl Lewis(a) and sialyl Tn antigens in gastric cancer patients. *Anticancer Res*. 2002;22(1A):451–458.
136. Sheer DG, Schlom J, Cooper HL. Purification and composition of the human tumor-associated glycoprotein (TAG-72) defined by monoclonal antibodies CC49 and B72.3. *Cancer Res*. 1988;48(23):6811–6818.
137. Lopez JB, Royan GP, Lakhwani MN, Mahadaven M, Timor J. CA 72–4 compared with CEA and CA 19–9 as a marker of some gastrointestinal malignancies. *Int J Biol Markers*. 1999;14(3):172–177.
138. Guadagni F, Roselli M, Cosimelli M, et al. CA 72–4 serum marker–a new tool in the management of carcinoma patients. *Cancer Invest*. 1995;13(2):227–238.
139. Carpelan-Holmstrom M, Louhimo J, Stenman UH, Alfthan H, Jarvinen H, Haglund C. Estimating the probability of cancer with several tumor markers in patients with colorectal disease. *Oncology*. 2004;66(4):296–302.
140. Carpelan-Holmstrom M, Louhimo J, Stenman UH, Alfthan H, Jarvinen H, Haglund C. CEA, CA 242, CA 19–9, CA 72–4 and hCGbeta in the diagnosis of recurrent colorectal cancer. *Tumour Biol*. 2004;25(5–6):228–234.
141. Sheng SL, Wang Q, Huang G. Development of time-resolved immunofluorometric assays for CA 72–4 and application in sera of patients with gastric tumors. *Clin Chim Acta*. 2007;380(1–2): 106–111.
142. Mattar R. Alves de Andrade CR, DiFavero GM, Gama-Rodrigues JJ, Laudanna AA. Preoperative serum levels of CA 72–4, CEA, CA 19–9, and alpha-fetoprotein in patients with gastric cancer. *Rev Hosp Clin Fac Med Sao Paulo*. 2002;57(3):89–92.
143. Marrelli D, Pinto E, De Stefano A, Farnetani M, Garosi L, Roviello F. Clinical utility of CEA, CA 19–9, and CA 72–4 in the follow-up of patients with resectable gastric cancer. *Am J Surg*. 2001;181(1):16–19.
144. Zou P, Povoski SP, Hall NC, et al. 124I-HuCC49deltaCH2 for TAG-72 antigen-directed positron emission tomography (PET) imaging of LS174T colon adenocarcinoma tumor implants in xenograft mice: preliminary results. *World J Surg Oncol*. 2010;8:65.
145. Fujimura T, Kinami S, Ninomiya I, et al. Diagnostic laparoscopy, serum CA125, and peritoneal metastasis in gastric cancer. *Endoscopy*. 2002;34(7):569–574.
146. Hall NR, Finan PJ, Stephenson BM, Purves DA, Cooper EH. The role of CA-242 and CEA in surveillance following curative resection for colorectal cancer. *Br J Cancer*. 1994;70(3):549–553.
147. Ran Y, Hu H, Zhou Z, et al. Profiling tumor-associated autoantibodies for the detection of colon cancer. *Clin Cancer Res*. 2008;14(9):2696–2700.
148. Small-Howard AL, Harris H. Advantages of the AMDL-ELISA DR-70 (FDP) assay over carcinoembryonic antigen (CEA) for monitoring colorectal cancer patients. *J Immunoassay Immunochem*. 2010;31(2):131–147.
149. Shimada H, Nabeya Y, Okazumi S, et al. Prediction of survival with squamous cell carcinoma antigen in patients with resectable esophageal squamous cell carcinoma. *Surgery*. 2003;133(5): 486–494.
150. Ikeda K, Terashima M, Ishida K, et al. Clinical significance of serum levels of SCC antigen in patients with esophageal squamous cell carcinoma. *Gan To Kagaku Ryoho*. 1988;15(4 Pt 1):677–682.
151. Wild N, Andres H, Rollinger W, et al. A combination of serum markers for the early detection of colorectal cancer. *Clin Cancer Res*. 2010;16(24):6111–6121.
152. Chen C, Chen LQ, Chen LD, Yang GL, Li Y. Evaluation of tumor markers biochip C12 system in the diagnosis of gastric cancer and the strategies for improvement: analysis of 100 cases. *Hepatogastroenterology*. 2008;55(84):991–997.
153. Ward DG, Suggett N, Cheng Y, et al. Identification of serum biomarkers for colon cancer by proteomic analysis. *Br J Cancer*. 2006;94(12):1898–1905.
154. Qiu FM, Yu JK, Chen YD, Jin QF, Sui MH, Huang J. Mining novel biomarkers for prognosis of gastric cancer with serum proteomics. *J Exp Clin Cancer Res*. 2009;28:126.
155. Lim JY, Cho JY, Paik YH, Chang YS, Kim HG. Diagnostic application of serum proteomic patterns in gastric cancer patients by ProteinChip surface-enhanced laser desorption/ionization time-of-flight mass spectrometry. *Int J Biol Markers*. 2007;22(4):281–286.
156. Ma Y, Peng J, Liu W, et al. Proteomics identification of desmin as a potential oncofetal diagnostic and prognostic biomarker in colorectal cancer. *Mol Cell Proteomics*. 2009;8(8):1878–1890.
157. Chen JS, Chen KT, Fan CW, et al. Comparison of membrane fraction proteomic profiles of normal and cancerous human colorectal tissues with gel-assisted digestion and iTRAQ labeling mass spectrometry. *FEBS J*. 2010;277(14):3028–3038.
158. Liu W, Wang P, Li Z, et al. Evaluation of tumour-associated antigen (TAA) miniarray in immunodiagnosis of colon cancer. *Scand J Immunol*. 2009;69(1):57–63.
159. Tsunemi S, Nakanishi T, Fujita Y, et al. Proteomics-based identification of a tumor-associated antigen and its corresponding autoantibody in gastric cancer. *Oncol Rep*. 2010;23(4):949–956.
160. Kijanka G, Hector S, Kay EW, et al. Human IgG antibody profiles differentiate between symptomatic patients with and without colorectal cancer. *Gut*. 2010;59(1):69–78.
161. American Society of Clinical Oncology. Clinical practice guidelines for the use of tumor markers in breast and colorectal cancer. Adopted on May 17, 1996 by the American Society of Clinical Oncology. *J Clin Oncol*. 1996;14(10):2843–2877.
162. Bast RC Jr, Ravdin P, Hayes DF, et al. 2000 update of recommendations for the use of tumor markers in breast and colorectal cancer: clinical practice guidelines of the American Society of Clinical Oncology. *J Clin Oncol*. 2001;19(6):1865–1878.
163. Desch CE, Benson AB 3rd, Somerfield MR, et al. Colorectal cancer surveillance: 2005 update of an American Society of Clinical Oncology practice guideline. *J Clin Oncol*. 2005;23(33): 8512–8519.
164. Guillem JG, Wood WC, Moley JF, et al. ASCO/SSO review of current role of risk-reducing surgery in common hereditary cancer syndromes. *J Clin Oncol*. 2006;24(28):4642–4660.
165. Klapdor R, Aronsson A, Duffy M, Hansson L, Khalifa R, Lamerz R. Tumour markers in gastrointestinal cancers–EGTM recommendations. European Group on Tumour Markers. *Anticancer Res*. 1999;19(4A):2811–2815.
166. Duffy MJ, van Dalen A, Haglund C, et al. Clinical utility of biochemical markers in colorectal cancer: European Group on Tumour Markers (EGTM) guidelines. *Eur J Cancer*. 2003;39(6):718–727.
167. Duffy MJ, van Dalen A, Haglund C, et al. Tumour markers in colorectal cancer: European Group on Tumour Markers (EGTM) guidelines for clinical use. *Eur J Cancer*. 2007;43(9):1348–1360.
168. Van Cutsem EJ. Advanced colorectal cancer: ESMO clinical recommendations for diagnosis, treatment and follow-up. *Ann Oncol*. 2007;18(Suppl 2):ii25-ii26.
169. Van Cutsem E, Oliveira J. Advanced colorectal cancer: ESMO clinical recommendations for diagnosis, treatment and follow-up. *Ann Oncol*. 2009;20(Suppl 4):61–63.
170. Van Cutsem E, Nordlinger B, Cervantes A. Advanced colorectal cancer: ESMO Clinical Practice Guidelines for treatment. *Ann Oncol*. 2010;21(Suppl 5):v93-v97.
171. Balmana J, Castells A, Cervantes A. Familial colorectal cancer risk: ESMO Clinical Practice Guidelines. *Ann Oncol*. 2010; 21(Suppl 5):v78-v81.

172. Van Cutsem E, Dicato M, Arber N, et al. Molecular markers and biological targeted therapies in metastatic colorectal cancer: expert opinion and recommendations derived from the 11th ESMO/ World Congress on Gastrointestinal Cancer, Barcelona, 2009. *Ann Oncol*. 2010;21(Suppl 6):vi1-vi10.
173. Fleisher M, Dnistrian A, Sturgeon C, Lamerz R, Witliff J. *Practice guidelines and recommendations for use of tumor markers in the clinic. Tumor Markers: physiology, pathobiology, technology and clinical applications*. Washington, DC: AACC Press; 2002:33–63.
174. Chan DW, Booth RA, Diamandis E. Tumor markers. In: Burtis C, Ashwood E, Bruns D, eds. *Tietz textbook of clinical chemistry and molecular diagnostics*. St. Louis, MI: Elsevier; 2006.
175. Tsai WS, Changchien CR, Yeh CY, et al. Preoperative plasma vascular endothelial growth factor but not nitrite is a useful complementary tumor marker in patients with colorectal cancer. *Dis Colon Rectum*. 2006;49(6):883–894.
176. Babel I, Barderas R, Diaz-Uriarte R, Martinez-Torrecuadrada JL, Sanchez-Carbayo M, Casal JI. Identification of tumor-associated autoantigens for the diagnosis of colorectal cancer in serum using high density protein microarrays. *Mol Cell Proteomics*. 2009;8(10):2382–2395.
177. Holten-Andersen MN, Christensen IJ, Nielsen HJ, et al. Total levels of tissue inhibitor of metalloproteinases 1 in plasma yield high diagnostic sensitivity and specificity in patients with colon cancer. *Clin Cancer Res*. 2002;8(1):156–164.
178. Nielsen HJ, Brunner N, Jorgensen LN, et al. Plasma TIMP-1 and CEA in detection of primary colorectal cancer: a prospective, population based study of 4509 high-risk individuals. *Scand J Gastroenterol*. 2011;46:60–90.
179. Huber K, Kirchheimer JC, Sedlmayer A, Bell C, Ermler D, Binder BR. Clinical value of determination of urokinase-type plasminogen activator antigen in plasma for detection of colorectal cancer: comparison with circulating tumor-associated antigens CA 19–9 and carcinoembryonic antigen. *Cancer Res*. 1993;53(8):1788–1793.
180. Cordero OJ, Ayude D, Nogueira M, Rodriguez-Berrocal FJ, de la Cadena MP. Preoperative serum CD26 levels: diagnostic efficiency and predictive value for colorectal cancer. *Br J Cancer*. 2000;83(9):1139–1146.
181. Cordero OJ, Imbernon M, Chiara LD, et al. Potential of soluble CD26 as a serum marker for colorectal cancer detection. *World J Clin Oncol*. 2011;2(6):245–261.
182. Melle C, Ernst G, Schimmel B, et al. Discovery and identification of alpha-defensins as low abundant, tumor-derived serum markers in colorectal cancer. *Gastroenterology*. 2005;129(1):66–73.
183. van den Broek I, Sparidans RW, Engwegen JY, et al. Evaluation of human neutrophil peptide-1, -2 and –3 as serum markers for colorectal cancer. *Cancer Biomark*. 2010;7(2):109–115.
184. Haug U, Rothenbacher D, Wente MN, Seiler CM, Stegmaier C, Brenner H. Tumour M2-PK as a stool marker for colorectal cancer: comparative analysis in a large sample of unselected older adults vs colorectal cancer patients. *Br J Cancer*. 2007;96(9): 1329–1334.
185. Hathurusinghe HR, Goonetilleke KS, Siriwardena AK. Current status of tumor M2 pyruvate kinase (tumor M2-PK) as a biomarker of gastrointestinal malignancy. *Ann Surg Oncol*. 2007;14(10):2714–2720.
186. Fedarko NS, Jain A, Karadag A, Van Eman MR, Fisher LW. Elevated serum bone sialoprotein and osteopontin in colon, breast, prostate, and lung cancer. *Clin Cancer Res*. 2001;7(12):4060–4066.
187. Fernandes LC, Kim SB, Matos D. Cytokeratins and carcinoembryonic antigen in diagnosis, staging and prognosis of colorectal adenocarcinoma. *World J Gastroenterol*. 2005;11(5):645–648.
188. Kawahara M, Chia D, Terasaki PI, et al. Detection of sialylated LewisX antigen in cancer sera using a sandwich radioimmunoassay. *Int J Cancer*. 1985;36(4):421–425.
189. Pasanen P, Eskelinen M, Kulju A, Penttila I, Janatuinen E, Alhava E. Tumour-associated trypsin inhibitor (TATI) in patients with colorectal cancer: a comparison with CEA, CA 50 and CA 242. *Scand J Clin Lab Invest*. 1995;55(2):119–124.
190. Saito N, Kameoka S. Serum laminin is an independent prognostic factor in colorectal cancer. *Int J Colorectal Dis*. 2005;20(3): 238–244.
191. Roessler M, Rollinger W, Palme S, et al. Identification of nicotinamide N-methyltransferase as a novel serum tumor marker for colorectal cancer. *Clin Cancer Res*. 2005;11(18):6550–6557.
192. Albanopoulos K, Armakolas A, Konstadoulakis MM, et al. Prognostic significance of circulating antibodies against carcinoembryonic antigen (anti-CEA) in patients with colon cancer. *Am J Gastroenterol*. 2000;95(4):1056–1061.
193. Mroczko B, Szmitkowski M, Okulczyk B, Piotrowski Z. Granulocyte-macrophage-colony stimulating factor in patients with colorectal cancer. *Folia Histochem Cytobiol*. 2001;39(Suppl 2):110–111.
194. Kerber A, Trojan J, Herrlinger K, Zgouras D, Caspary WF, Braden B. The new DR-70 immunoassay detects cancer of the gastrointestinal tract: a validation study. *Aliment Pharmacol Ther*. 2004;20(9):983–987.
195. Leman ES, Schoen RE, Magheli A, Sokoll LJ, Chan DW, Getzenberg RH. Evaluation of colon cancer-specific antigen 2 as a potential serum marker for colorectal cancer. *Clin Cancer Res*. 2008;14(5):1349–1354.
196. Ferroni P, Roselli M, Martini F, et al. Prognostic value of soluble P-selectin levels in colorectal cancer. *Int J Cancer*. 2004;111(3):404–408.
197. Soroush AR, Zadeh HM, Moemeni M, Shakiba B, Elmi S. Plasma prolactin in patients with colorectal cancer. *BMC Cancer*. 2004; 4:97.
198. Nam MJ, Kee MK, Kuick R, Hanash SM. Identification of defensin alpha6 as a potential biomarker in colon adenocarcinoma. *J Biol Chem*. 2005;280(9):8260–8265.
199. Yoneda K, Iida H, Endo H, et al. Identification of Cystatin SN as a novel tumor marker for colorectal cancer. *Int J Oncol*. 2009;35(1):33–40.
200. Lee H, Rhee H, Kang HJ, et al. Macrophage migration inhibitory factor may be used as an early diagnostic marker in colorectal carcinomas. *Am J Clin Pathol*. 2008;129(5):772–779.
201. Pinczower GD, Gianello RD, Williams RP, Preston BN, Preston H, Linnane AW. Monoclonal antibody 4D3 detects small intestinal mucin antigen (SIMA)–glycoprotein in the serum of patients with colorectal cancer. *Int J Cancer*. 1993;54(3): 391–396.
202. Eskelinen M, Pasanen P, Janatuinen E, Pettersson N, Linnane A, Alhava E. Small intestinal mucin antigen (SIMA); a novel tumour marker in colorectal cancer? *Anticancer Res*. 1995;15(5B): 2351–2356.
203. Mroczko B, Szmitkowski M, Wereszczynska-Siemiatkowska U, Okulczyk B. Stem cell factor (SCF) and interleukin 3 (IL-3) in the sera of patients with colorectal cancer. *Dig Dis Sci*. 2005;50(6):1019–1024.
204. Kuru B, Ozaslan C, Yalman K, Camlybel M. Serum progesterone levels in patients with gastric and colorectal cancers. *Acta Chir Belg*. 2002;102(2):122–125.
205. Tagi T, Matsui T, Kikuchi S, et al. Dermokine as a novel biomarker for early-stage colorectal cancer. *J Gastroenterol*. 2010;45:1201–1211.
206. Xia Q, Kong XT, Zhang GA, Hou XJ, Qiang H, Zhong RQ. Proteomics-based identification of DEAD-box protein 48 as a novel autoantigen, a prospective serum marker for pancreatic cancer. *Biochem Biophys Res Commun*. 2005;330(2):526–532.
207. Reipert BM, Tanneberger S, Pannetta A, et al. Increase in autoantibodies against Fas (CD95) during carcinogenesis in the human

colon: a hope for the immunoprevention of cancer? *Cancer Immunol Immunother*. 2005;54(10):1038–1042.
208. Yamaguchi A, Kurosaka Y, Ishida T, et al. Clinical significance of tumor marker NCC-ST 439 in large bowel cancers. *Dis Colon Rectum*. 1991;34(10):921–924.
209. Kornek G, Depisch D, Temsch EM, Scheithauer W. Comparative analysis of cancer-associated antigen CA-195, CA 19–9 and carcinoembryonic antigen in diagnosis, follow-up and monitoring of response to chemotherapy in patients with gastrointestinal cancer. *J Cancer Res Clin Oncol*. 1991;117(5):493–496.
210. Yedema KA, Kenemans P, Wobbes T, et al. Carcinoma-associated mucin serum markers CA M26 and CA M29: efficacy in detecting and monitoring patients with cancer of the breast, colon, ovary, endometrium and cervix. *Int J Cancer*. 1991;47(2):170–179.
211. Goodgame R, Kiefe C, Rose E, Sutton F, Brown J, Alpert E. Clinical evaluation of M43: a novel cancer-associated mucin epitope. *Cancer Res*. 1993;53(12):2803–2809.
212. van Kamp GJ, von Mensdorff-Pouilly S, Kenemans P, et al. Evaluation of colorectal cancer-associated mucin CA M43 assay in serum. *Clin Chem*. 1993;39(6):1029–1032.
213. Kozwich DL, Kramer LC, Mielicki WP, Fotopoulos SS, Gordon SG. Application of cancer procoagulant as an early detection tumor marker. *Cancer*. 1994;74(4):1367–1376.
214. Herlyn M, Blaszczyk M, Bennicelli J, et al. Selection of monoclonal antibodies detecting serodiagnostic human tumor markers. *J Immunol Methods*. 1985;80(1):107–116.
215. Duraker N, Can D, Parilti M. Measurement of serum total and free prostate-specific antigen in women with colorectal carcinoma. *Br J Cancer*. 2002;86(2):203–206.
216. Severini G. Glutathione S-transferase activity in patients with cancer of the digestive tract. *J Cancer Res Clin Oncol*. 1993;120 (1–2):112–114.
217. Kuroki M, Matsushita H, Matsumoto H, Hirose Y, Senba T, Yamamoto T. Nonspecific cross-reacting antigen-50/90 (NCA-50/90) as a new tumor marker. *Anticancer Res*. 1999;19(6C): 5599–5606.
218. Arai M, Sakamoto K, Otsuka H, Yokoyama Y, Akagi M. Detection of tumor associated antigen, PA8–15, in sera from pancreatic and gastrointestinal carcinoma patients. *Jpn J Clin Oncol*. 1990;20(2):145–153.
219. Riedl S, Bodenmuller H, Hinz U, et al. Significance of tenascin serum level as tumor marker in primary colorectal carcinoma. *Int J Cancer*. 1995;64(1):65–69.
220. Dudouet B, Jacob L, Beuzeboc P, et al. Presence of villin, a tissue-specific cytoskeletal protein, in sera of patients and an initial clinical evaluation of its value for the diagnosis and follow-up of colorectal cancers. *Cancer Res*. 1990;50(2):438–443.
221. Ayude D, Fernandez-Rodriguez J, Rodriguez-Berrocal FJ, et al. Value of the serum alpha-L-fucosidase activity in the diagnosis of colorectal cancer. *Oncology*. 2000;59(4):310–316.
222. Schneider J, Bitterlich N, Schulze G. Improved sensitivity in the diagnosis of gastro-intestinal tumors by fuzzy logic-based tumor marker profiles including the tumor M2-PK. *Anticancer Res*. 2005;25(3A):1507–1515.
223. Mroczko B, Kozlowski M, Groblewska M, et al. The diagnostic value of the measurement of matrix metalloproteinase 9 (MMP-9), squamous cell cancer antigen (SCC) and carcinoembryonic antigen (CEA) in the sera of esophageal cancer patients. *Clin Chim Acta*. 2008;389(1–2):61–66.
224. Kozlowski M, Kowalczuk O, Milewski R, Chyczewski L, Niklinski J, Laudanski J. Serum vascular endothelial growth factors C and D in patients with oesophageal cancer. *Eur J Cardiothorac Surg*. 2010;38(3):260–267.
225. Dong J, Zeng BH, Xu LH, et al. Anti-CDC25B autoantibody predicts poor prognosis in patients with advanced esophageal squamous cell carcinoma. *J Transl Med*. 2010;8:81.
226. Wu CY, Wu MS, Chiang EP, et al. Plasma matrix metalloproteinase-9 level is better than serum matrix metalloproteinase-9 level to predict gastric cancer evolution. *Clin Cancer Res*. 2007;13(7):2054–2060.
227. Mroczko B, Groblewska M, Lukaszewicz-Zajac M, Bandurski R, Kedra B, Szmitkowski M. Pre-treatment serum and plasma levels of matrix metalloproteinase 9 (MMP-9) and tissue inhibitor of matrix metalloproteinases 1 (TIMP-1) in gastric cancer patients. *Clin Chem Lab Med*. 2009;47(9):1133–1139.
228. Wang CS, Wu TL, Tsao KC, Sun CF. Serum TIMP-1 in gastric cancer patients: a potential prognostic biomarker. *Ann Clin Lab Sci*. 2006;36(1):23–30.
229. Jin B, Wang X, Jin Y, et al. Detection of serum gastric cancer-associated MG7-Ag from gastric cancer patients using a sensitive and convenient ELISA method. *Cancer Invest*. 2009;27(2): 227–233.
230. Xia HH, Yang Y, Chu KM, et al. Serum macrophage migration-inhibitory factor as a diagnostic and prognostic biomarker for gastric cancer. *Cancer*. 2009;115(23):5441–5449.
231. Kumar Y, Tapuria N, Kirmani N, Davidson BR. Tumour M2-pyruvate kinase: a gastrointestinal cancer marker. *Eur J Gastroenterol Hepatol*. 2007;19(3):265–276.
232. Thong-Ngam D, Tangkijvanich P, Lerknimitr R, Mahachai V, Theamboonlers A, Poovorawan Y. Diagnostic role of serum interleukin-18 in gastric cancer patients. *World J Gastroenterol*. 2006;12(28):4473–4477.
233. Xu Y, Zhang L, Hu G. Potential application of alternatively glycosylated serum MUC1 and MUC5AC in gastric cancer diagnosis. *Biologicals*. 2009;37(1):18–25.
234. Hao Y, Yu Y, Wang L, et al. IPO-38 is identified as a novel serum biomarker of gastric cancer based on clinical proteomics technology. *J Proteome Res*. 2008;7(9):3668–3677.
235. Chung HW, Kim JW, Lee JH, et al. Comparison of the validity of three biomarkers for gastric cancer screening: carcinoembryonic antigen, pepsinogens, and high sensitive C-reactive protein. *J Clin Gastroenterol*. 2009;43(1):19–26.
236. Chong PK, Lee H, Zhou J, et al. ITIH3 is a potential biomarker for early detection of gastric cancer. *J Proteome Res*. 2010;9(7): 3671–3679.
237. Ashizawa T, Okada R, Suzuki Y, et al. Clinical significance of interleukin-6 (IL-6) in the spread of gastric cancer: role of IL-6 as a prognostic factor. *Gastric Cancer*. 2005;8(2):124–131.
238. Oue N, Sentani K, Noguchi T, et al. Serum olfactomedin 4 (GW112, hGC-1) in combination with Reg IV is a highly sensitive biomarker for gastric cancer patients. *Int J Cancer*. 2009;125(10):2383–2392.
239. Chan AO, Chu KM, Lam SK, et al. Early prediction of tumor recurrence after curative resection of gastric carcinoma by measuring soluble E-cadherin. *Cancer*. 2005;104(4):740–746.
240. Kammerer R, Zimmermann W. Coevolution of activating and inhibitory receptors within mammalian carcinoembryonic antigen families. *BMC Biol*. 2012;8:12.

Index

A.R. Sepulveda and J.P. Lynch (eds.), *Molecular Pathology of Neoplastic Gastrointestinal Diseases*, Molecular Pathology Library 7,
DOI 10.1007/978-1-4614-6015-2, © Springer Science+Business Media New York 2013

MIX
Papier aus verantwortungsvollen Quellen
Paper from responsible sources
FSC® C105338

If you have any concerns about our products,
you can contact us on
ProductSafety@springernature.com

In case Publisher is established outside the EU,
the EU authorized representative is:
Springer Nature Customer Service Center GmbH
Europaplatz 3, 69115 Heidelberg, Germany

Printed by Libri Plureos GmbH
in Hamburg, Germany